T0293829

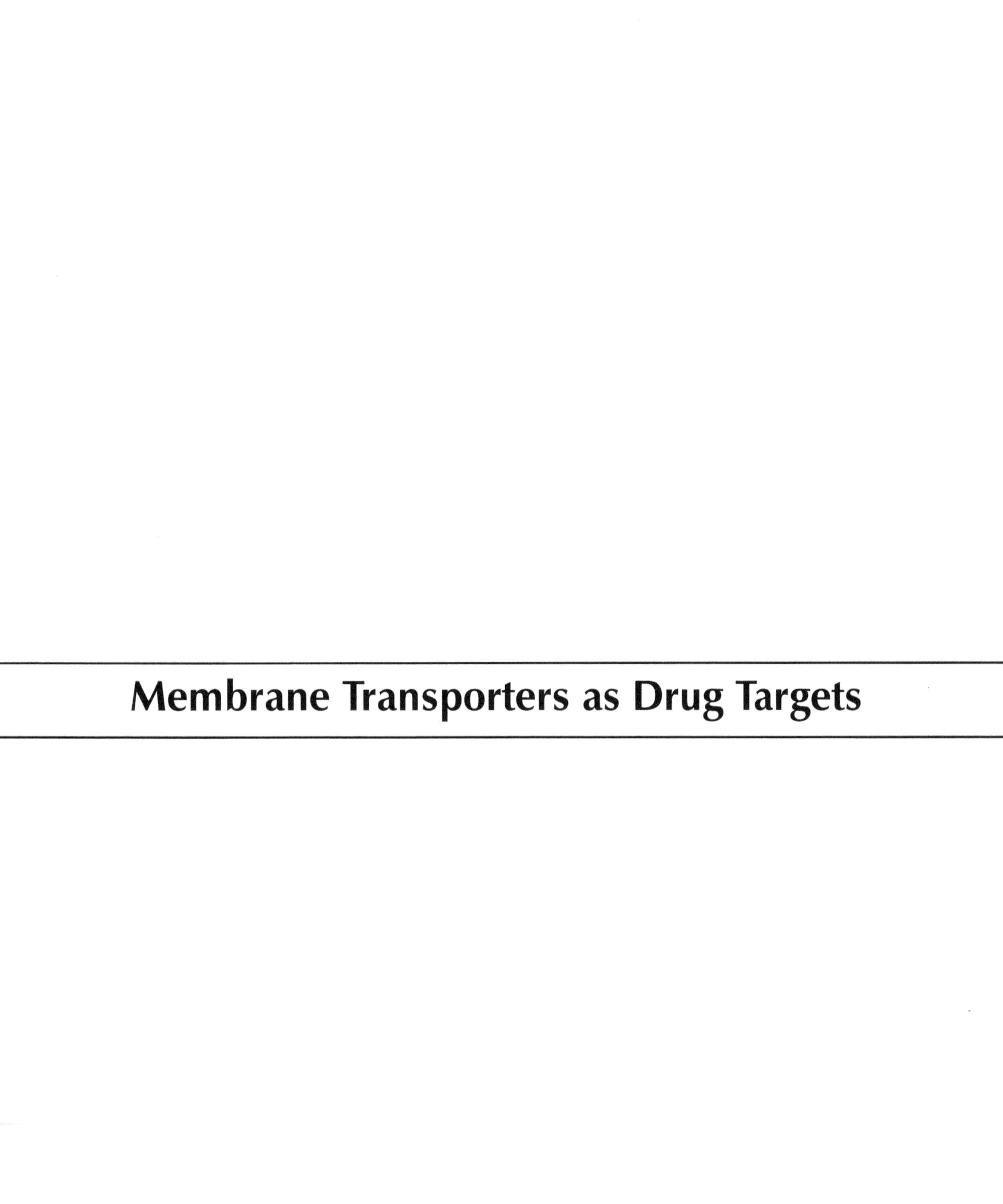

Membrane Transporters as Drug Targets

Membrane Transporters as Drug Targets

Editor: Henry Williams

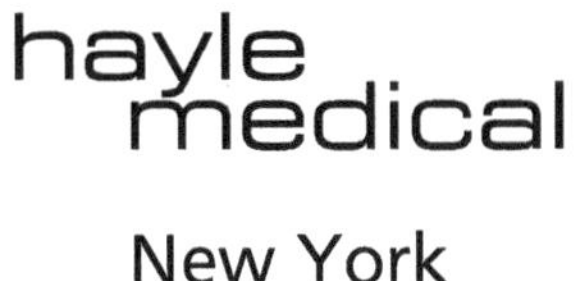

New York

Hayle Medical,
750 Third Avenue, 9th Floor,
New York, NY 10017, USA

Visit us on the World Wide Web at:
www.haylemedical.com

ISBN 978-1-64647-599-5 (Hardback)

Cataloging-in-Publication Data

Membrane transporters as drug targets / edited by Henry Williams.
p. cm.
Includes bibliographical references and index.
ISBN 978-1-64647-599-5
1. Drug targeting. 2. Drugs--Physiological transport. 3. Drug carriers (Pharmacy).
4. Carrier proteins. 5. Drug receptors. I. Williams, Henry.
RM301.63 M46 2023
615.7--dc23

Contents

Preface ... VII

Chapter 1 **P2RX7 Purinoceptor as a Therapeutic Target—The Second Coming?** ... 1
Chris N. J. Young and Dariusz C. Górecki

Chapter 2 **Drug Interactions with the Ca^{2+}-ATPase from Sarco(Endo)Plasmic Reticulum (SERCA)** ... 15
Francesco Tadini-Buoninsegni, Serena Smeazzetto, Roberta Gualdani and Maria Rosa Moncelli

Chapter 3 **Ligand Screening Systems for Human Glucose Transporters as Tools in Drug Discovery** ... 23
Sina Schmidl, Cristina V. Iancu, Jun-yong Choe and Mislav Oreb

Chapter 4 **Moving the Cellular Peptidome by Transporters** ... 30
Rupert Abele and Robert Tampé

Chapter 5 **Targeting Channels and Transporters in Protozoan Parasite Infections** ... 43
Anna Meier, Holger Erler and Eric Beitz

Chapter 6 **The Emerging Role of microRNAs in Aquaporin Regulation** ... 66
André Gomes, Inês V. da Silva, Cecília M. P. Rodrigues, Rui E. Castro and Graça Soveral

Chapter 7 **Pancreatic Aquaporin-7: A Novel Target for Anti-Diabetic Drugs?** ... 74
Leire Méndez-Giménez, Silvia Ezquerro, Inês V. da Silva, Graça Soveral, Gema Frühbeck and Amaia Rodríguez

Chapter 8 **Nutritional Stress Induced by Amino Acid Starvation Results in Changes for Slc38 Transporters in Immortalized Hypothalamic Neuronal Cells and Primary Cortex Cells** ... 84
Sofie V. Hellsten, Rekha Tripathi, Mikaela M. Ceder and Robert Fredriksson

Chapter 9 **The Physiopathological Role of the Exchangers Belonging to the SLC37 Family** ... 96
Anna Rita Cappello, Rosita Curcio, Rosamaria Lappano, Marcello Maggiolini and Vincenza Dolce

Chapter 10 **The Sodium Sialic Acid Symporter from *Staphylococcus aureus* has Altered Substrate Specificity** ... 113
Rachel A. North, Weixiao Y. Wahlgren, Daniela M. Remus, Mariafrancesca Scalise, Sarah A. Kessans, Elin Dunevall, Elin Claesson, Tatiana P. Soares da Costa, Matthew A. Perugini, S. Ramaswamy, Jane R. Allison, Cesare Indiveri, Rosmarie Friemann and Renwick C. J. Dobson

Chapter 11 **Interaction of the New Monofunctional Anticancer Agent Phenanthriplatin with Transporters for Organic Cations** 124
Anna Hucke, Ga Young Park, Oliver B. Bauer, Georg Beyer, Christina Köppen, Dorothea Zeeh, Christoph A. Wehe, Michael Sperling, Rita Schröter, Marta Kantauskaitė, Yohannes Hagos, Uwe Karst, Stephen J. Lippard and Giuliano Ciarimboli

Chapter 12 **Targeting Endoplasmic Reticulum and/or Mitochondrial Ca^{2+} Fluxes as Therapeutic Strategy for HCV Infection** 133
Rosella Scrima, Claudia Piccoli, Darius Moradpour and Nazzareno Capitanio

Chapter 13 **Aquaporins as Targets of Dietary Bioactive Phytocompounds** 145
Angela Tesse, Elena Grossini, Grazia Tamma, Catherine Brenner, Piero Portincasa, Raul A. Marinelli and Giuseppe Calamita

Chapter 14 **VDAC1 as Pharmacological Target in Cancer and Neurodegeneration: Focus on its Role in Apoptosis** 158
Andrea Magrì, Simona Reina and Vito De Pinto

Chapter 15 **Mechanisms of Aquaporin-Facilitated Cancer Invasion and Metastasis** 175
Michael L. De Ieso and Andrea J. Yool

Chapter 16 **The Expression of AQP1 is Modified in Lung of Patients with Idiopathic Pulmonary Fibrosis: Addressing a Possible New Target** 195
Ana Galán-Cobo, Elena Arellano-Orden, Rocío Sánchez Silva, José Luis López-Campos, César Gutiérrez Rivera, Lourdes Gómez Izquierdo, Nela Suárez-Luna, María Molina-Molina, José A. Rodríguez Portal and Miriam Echevarría

Chapter 17 **Identification of Loop D Domain Amino Acids in the Human Aquaporin-1 Channel Involved in Activation of the Ionic Conductance and Inhibition by AqB011** 204
Mohamad Kourghi, Michael L. De Ieso, Saeed Nourmohammadi, Jinxin V. Pei and Andrea J. Yool

Chapter 18 **The Human SLC7A5 (LAT1): The Intriguing Histidine/Large Neutral Amino Acid Transporter and its Relevance to Human Health** 216
Mariafrancesca Scalise, Michele Galluccio, Lara Console, Lorena Pochini and Cesare Indiveri

Permissions

List of Contributors

Index

Preface

Membranes bind all cells together, and the lipid bilayer of cell membranes is extremely impervious for most water-soluble compounds. Membrane transport processes that have been identified in many biological events occur during the formation of electrochemical potentials, uptake of nutrients, removal of wastes, endocytotic internalization of macromolecules, and oxygen transport in respiration. Specific transport proteins catalyze the flow of ions, nutrients, and metabolites across cellular membranes. These transport proteins are studied within pharmaceutical science in order to understand their impact on drug absorption, distribution, metabolism, and elimination (ADME), as well as drug safety. Several neurological diseases have been linked to altered CNS transporter expression. As a result, many transport proteins have emerged as pharmacological targets. In this book, various advancements related to the use of membrane transporters as drug targets have been discussed in detail. It aims to equip students and experts with the advanced topics and upcoming concepts in this area of study.

This book is a result of research of several months to collate the most relevant data in the field.

When I was approached with the idea of this book and the proposal to edit it, I was overwhelmed. It gave me an opportunity to reach out to all those who share a common interest with me in this field. I had 3 main parameters for editing this text:

1. Accuracy - The data and information provided in this book should be up-to-date and valuable to the readers.

2. Structure - The data must be presented in a structured format for easy understanding and better grasping of the readers.

3. Universal Approach - This book not only targets students but also experts and innovators in the field, thus my aim was to present topics which are of use to all.

Thus, it took me a couple of months to finish the editing of this book.

I would like to make a special mention of my publisher who considered me worthy of this opportunity and also supported me throughout the editing process. I would also like to thank the editing team at the back-end who extended their help whenever required.

Editor

1

P2RX7 Purinoceptor as a Therapeutic Target—The Second Coming?

Chris N. J. Young[1,2] *and Dariusz C. Górecki*[1,3*]

[1] *Molecular Medicine Laboratory, Institute of Biomedical and Biomolecular Sciences, School of Pharmacy and Biomedical Sciences, University of Portsmouth, Portsmouth, United Kingdom,* [2] *Faculty of Health and Life Sciences, The School of Allied Health Sciences, De Montfort University, Leicester, United Kingdom,* [3] *The General Karol Kaczkowski Military Institute of Hygiene and Epidemiology, Warsaw, Poland*

Correspondence:
Dariusz C. Górecki
darek.gorecki@port.ac.uk

The P2RX7 receptor is a unique member of a family of extracellular ATP (eATP)-gated ion channels expressed in immune cells, where its activation triggers the inflammatory cascade. Therefore, P2RX7 has been long investigated as a target in the treatment of infectious and inflammatory diseases. Subsequently, P2RX7 signaling has been documented in other physiological and pathological processes including pain, CNS and psychiatric disorders and cancer. As a result, a range of P2RX7 antagonists have been developed and trialed. Interestingly, the recent crystallization of mammalian and chicken receptors revealed that most widely-used antagonists may bind a unique allosteric site. The availability of crystal structures allows rational design of improved antagonists and modeling of binding sites of the known or presumed inhibitors. However, several unanswered questions limit the cogent development of P2RX7 therapies. Firstly, this receptor functions as an ion channel, but its chronic stimulation by high eATP causes opening of the non-selective large pore (LP), which can trigger cell death. Not only the molecular mechanism of LP opening is still not fully understood but its function(s) are also unclear. Furthermore, how can tumor cells take advantage of P2RX7 for growth and spread and yet survive overexpression of potentially cytotoxic LP in the eATP-rich environment? The recent discovery of the feedback loop, wherein the LP-evoked release of active MMP-2 triggers the receptor cleavage, provided one explanation. Another mechanism might be that of cancer cells expressing a structurally altered P2RX7 receptor, devoid of the LP function. Exploiting such mechanisms should lead to the development of new, less toxic anticancer treatments. Notably, targeted inhibition of P2RX7 is crucial as its global blockade reduces the immune and inflammatory responses, which have important anti-tumor effects in some types of malignancies. Therefore, another novel approach is the synthesis of tissue/cell specific P2RX7 antagonists. Progress has been aided by the development of *p2rx7* knockout mice and new conditional knock-in and knock-out models are being created. In this review, we seek to summarize the recent advances in our understanding of molecular mechanisms of receptor activation and inhibition, which cause its re-emergence as an important therapeutic target. We also highlight the key difficulties affecting this development.

Keywords: ATP, cancer, DMD, inflammation, large pore, P2X7, P2RX7 KO mouse

INTRODUCTION

P2RX7 is a 595aa protein belonging to the ionotropic purinergic P2X subfamily which consists of seven members, P2X1-7 (Burnstock and Knight, 2004). P2Xs represent an ancient form of purine chemical messenger reception, with relatives now cloned from species as diverse as *Homo sapiens* and *Dictyostelium* (Burnstock and Verkhratsky, 2012). All family members are trimeric ligand-gated ion channels displaying a preference for cations. Their subunits comprise intracellular N and C termini, two transmembrane domains and a large intervening extracellular region containing the ATP binding site (Surprenant et al., 1996). P2RX7, originally characterized by Cockcroft and Gomperts as the ATP^{4-} receptor in rat mast cells (Cockcroft and Gomperts, 1980) was previously also known by the name of P2Z receptor, responsible for the eATP-dependent lysis of macrophages (Surprenant et al., 1996). This confusion arose in part due to its many characteristics, which make this receptor entirely distinct from other P2Xs. These include uniquely lower affinity for eATP: $EC_{50} > 1$ mM at physiological ion concentrations (Yan et al., 2010) and the ability to induce membrane blebbing and cell death. As such, P2RX7 is perhaps best known for its role in regulating innate and adaptive immune responses and is expressed on virtually all cell types of the immune system (Burnstock and Knight, 2017). Macrophages and microglia express high levels of P2RX7 (He et al., 2017; Young et al., 2017) and are perhaps the best studied cells in relation to receptor function both *in vitro* and *in/ex vivo* (Csóka et al., 2015). However, P2RX7 has a huge functional repertoire being involved in phenomena as diverse as inflammation (Rissiek et al., 2015), proliferation (Monif et al., 2010), migration and invasion (Qiu et al., 2014), metabolism (Amoroso et al., 2012), autophagy (Young et al., 2015), cell death (Massicot et al., 2013), and neurotransmission (Sperlágh et al., 2002). P2RX7 over-expression and over-activation have been implicated in numerous physiological/pathophysiological processes where, intriguingly, P2RX7 activation can result in both positive and negative outcomes depending on a host of factors such as intensity and duration of the agonist stimulus (Hanley et al., 2012), severity of pathogen virulence/infection (Figliuolo et al., 2017), the cell type (Cortés-Garcia et al., 2016; Young et al., 2017), extracellular ion concentration (Virginio et al., 1997), phospholipid membrane composition (Karasawa et al., 2017), co-factor activity (Migita et al., 2016), enzymatic processing (Young et al., 2017), polymorphic variations (Fuller et al., 2009; Ursu et al., 2014), and non-ATP agonist activation (Hong et al., 2009). The latter occurs during innate immune responses through the release of damage-associated molecular patterns (DAMPs; e.g., DNA, RNA, HMGB1, etc.) or pathogen-associated molecular patterns (PAMPs, e.g., LPS) either directly or via Toll-like receptors (TLRs). Specifically, TLR2 and TLR4 have been found to directly interact with P2RX7 via biglycan (Babelova et al., 2009). Classically, once eATP activates P2RX7, TLR4-mediated pro-IL-1β processing is followed by potassium efflux, NLRP3/ASC inflammasome assembly and caspase-1-dependent IL-1β maturation and release (Perregaux and Gabel, 1994; Pelegrin et al., 2008; Dubyak, 2012). Other P2RX7-dependent inflammatory activators include IL-6, ROS (Munoz et al., 2017), other caspases and MMPs (Gu and Wiley, 2006; Young et al., 2017). P2RX7 role in the adaptive immune response is to directly activate T cell populations, being a pre-requisite for IL-2 release, to orchestrate the balance between Treg and T helper cell populations, with receptor activation favoring the formation of T helpers and its blockade having the opposite effect (Schenk et al., 2011; Cekic and Linden, 2016). However, while its role in macrophages, microglia, and T cells has been researched extensively, our understanding of the role of P2RX7 in other immune cell types is still evolving. Neutrophils, for example, first thought devoid of P2RX7 expression in humans (Martel-Gallegos et al., 2010), have risen to the fore with the recent demonstration of neutrophil-mediated orchestration of the IL-1β/NLRP3 response in BMDNs (Karmakar et al., 2016). Exploration of tumor-associated immune cell populations has also led to the discovery that macrophages and microglia are not the only cells to express high levels of P2RX7. Tumors also display upregulated P2RX7 expression, reaching levels far exceeding that of macrophages (Young et al., 2017). In fact, all tumor types listed in The Cancer Genome Atlas were found to have upregulated levels of *P2RX7* expression, with sub-type-specific mutation patterns highlighting the significant potential for novel therapeutic approaches in this area (Young et al., 2017).

Compared to other P2X receptors, P2RX7 possesses an extra-long intracellular C-terminus with additional 200 amino acids. Mutations at various locations in this region have been associated with loss of diverse physiological functions such as LPS binding (Denlinger et al., 2001), post-translational modifications (Gonnord et al., 2009), membrane targeting (Smart et al., 2003) and large pore formation (Feng et al., 2006). P2RX7 stimulation at lower-end eATP doses opens a cation-selective plasma membrane channel permeable to Ca^{2+}, Na^{+}, and K^{+}. Chronic/sustained eATP dosing reveals the second facet to P2RX7 signaling; the formation of a non-selective large pore (LP), permeable to molecules of up to 900 Da, such as dyes (EtBr, 314 Da; YO-PRO-1, 376 Da and Lucifer Yellow, 457 Da Adinolfi et al., 2005). Thus, P2RX7 can display the properties of a prototypic cytotoxic receptor. The inherent insensitivity to eATP coupled with dire consequences of receptor over-stimulation prompted the belief that this low agonist affinity might be a safe-guard against potentially damaging receptor-mediated inflammatory cascade activation through the release of IL-1β, additional eATP or other DAMPs. Indeed, although healthy interstitial eATP levels are maintained at nanomolar levels or below, it has been shown that the eATP concentration around sites of inflammation can increase several fold (Morciano et al., 2017). For example, eATP around damaged cells or dystrophic muscle fibers can reach 5–10 mM (Di Virgilio, 2000; Hetherington et al., 2001) and in the tumor microenvironment, levels of $>700\,\mu$M have been recorded (Pellegatti et al., 2008). The tonic, low-level vs. chronic high-level receptor

Abbreviations: eATP, extracellular Adenosine Triphosphate; BMDNs, Bone Marrow Derived Neutrophils; DAMPs, Danger Associated Molecular Patterns; PAMPs, Pathogen Associated Molecular Patterns; TLR, Toll-like receptor; NLRP3, NOD-like receptor protein 3; MMP, Matrix metalloproteinase; IL, Interleukin.

stimulation have very different outcomes, indeed. Moreover, the balance and fine tuning of the molecular controls that govern these responses may underlie some of the most exciting new possibilities for therapeutic manipulation. Efforts in this area have been hampered by the lack of a P2RX7 crystal structure. However, recent successful crystallizations and 3-D reconstructions include both the 356 aa (without the C-terminal tail) Panda (*Ailuropoda melanoleuca)* pdP2RX7 (Karasawa and Kawate, 2016) as well as the truncated variant (lacking 27 N- and 214 C-terminal aa residues) of the chicken ckP2RX7 (Kasuya et al., 2017). These developments permit rational mechanistic studies (Karasawa and Kawate, 2016) with exciting novel insights into the specific mechanisms of both permeability and drug interactions. Appreciating the number of recent reviews on P2RX7 as a therapeutic target (Burnstock and Knight, 2017; Di Virgilio et al., 2018a; Savio et al., 2018) in this paper we discuss recent developments in P2RX7 drug design and repurposing, highlighting the potential new therapeutic applications of these drugs in human disorders.

RECENT DEVELOPMENTS IN P2RX7 CRYSTALLOGRAPHY

Crystal structures for zebrafish P2RX4 (Kawate et al., 2009), then human P2RX3 (Mansoor et al., 2016) gave the first insights into conserved mechanisms of action: the ATP binding pocket, subunit interactions and conformation changes upon agonist binding (i.e., predictions of gating and opening) (Hattori and Gouaux, 2012). Individual subunits of these crystallized receptors (zebrafish and human alike) adopt "dolphin-shaped" conformations (see Kawate et al., 2009; Karasawa and Kawate, 2016). The aforementioned recent crystallizations of both ckP2RX7 (Kasuya et al., 2017) and pdP2RX7 (Karasawa and Kawate, 2016) confirmed this structure. 3-D reconstructions of trimeric subunit interactions also confirm three equivalent ATP binding site locations at subunit interfaces. More excitingly, the pdP2RX7 structure has revealed a completely novel allosteric site situated in the groove formed between two adjacent subunits, which is completely distinct from the ATP binding site (Karasawa and Kawate, 2016). ckP2RX7 and pdP2RX7 share ~62 and 85% homology with human P2RX7A (Karasawa and Kawate, 2016), respectively. Unfortunately, both crystal structures lack the C-terminal, intracellular tail region, so important for the receptor function (see below). Achieving the complete P2RX7 3-D structural resolution remains an unclaimed trophy. However, even the partial pdP2RX7 structure has revealed some unexpected features. When expressed in liposomes, the pdP2RX7 triggered LP formation despite lacking the C-terminus. The proposed mechanism was the regulatory dependence of the P2RX7 large pore on the membrane lipid composition, where the cholesterol level played a significant role: increases in membrane cholesterol correlated with reductions in membrane fluidity and LP formation in this liposome-based system (Karasawa et al., 2017). The singularly unique aspect of the pdP2RX7 3-D modeling however, was the discovery of a new allosteric binding site, distinct from the ATP-binding pocket, at each subunit interface. The structurally unrelated antagonists A740003, A804598, AZ10606120, GW791343, and JNJ47965567 all were shown to bind this allosteric "groove" between subunit faces (Karasawa and Kawate, 2016). Kawate et al., used functional fluorescence anisotropy-based assays to show that these compounds effectively act as "door-stops" or "wedges," preventing the narrowing of this groove during the turret-like conformational rotation during channel dilation upon agonist binding. Mutational replacement of residues with "bulkier" cysteines resulted in effective narrowing of the inter-subunit groove and reduced channel opening kinetics. Thus, we now know that it is the spatial filling of this new inter-subunit non-competitive hydrophobic pocket, which is the determining factor in antagonist selectivity and potency. The pocket itself is composed of β-strand residues (β4, β13, and β14) with hydrophobic interactions at positions deep inside the pocket (F95, F103, M105, F293, and V312) (Karasawa and Kawate, 2016). See **Figure 1** for structural representations of the eATP binding pocket and the allosteric antagonist binding groove.

The remaining limitation is the structural resolution (~3.2~3.6 Å), which does not currently facilitate definitive predictions of bond angles or side chain-drug interactions. However, the main dimensions of the pocket are clearly defined and this finding have opened the door for significant strategic antagonist developments through targeted screening and rational design approaches. Moreover, with the apparent absence of this allosteric site in the known P2RX3 and P2RX4 crystal structures, there is a potential for the development of highly P2RX7-selective drugs. However, since ATP binding was also found to narrow the groove (Karasawa and Kawate, 2016), further functional studies are required to determine the accessibility of this allosteric site under conditions of high eATP concentration. Hence, the groove might theoretically be less accessible due to continued receptor activation, which could have implications for therapeutic applications. Moreover, positive allosteric agonists such as polymyxin B (Ferrari et al., 2004) may share this novel allosteric site or indeed may occupy other distinct sites. Such intricacies remain unresolved but the crystal structure makes further studies possible.

P2RX7 KINETICS: CHANNEL BECOMES PORE?

It was the 3-D structure predictions of P2RX4, which first suggested ion flux upon agonist binding to be initiated through the rotation of six helical transmembrane domains of the trimeric receptor (Hattori and Gouaux, 2012). Once TM2 Val335-Leu346 moves, the channel gate is opened and current may flow as directed by the membrane potential (Li et al., 2008). However, P2RX7 ion flux studies at the upper-end eATP concentrations (typical for damaged tissues) are hampered by what appears to be the biphasic nature of the channel, leading to a second mode of opening. Given that pathological P2RX7 responses have been linked to the activation of this large pore, this has been a singularly enigmatic and controversial issue in the P2RX7 field. Chronic receptor activation under the appropriate conditions

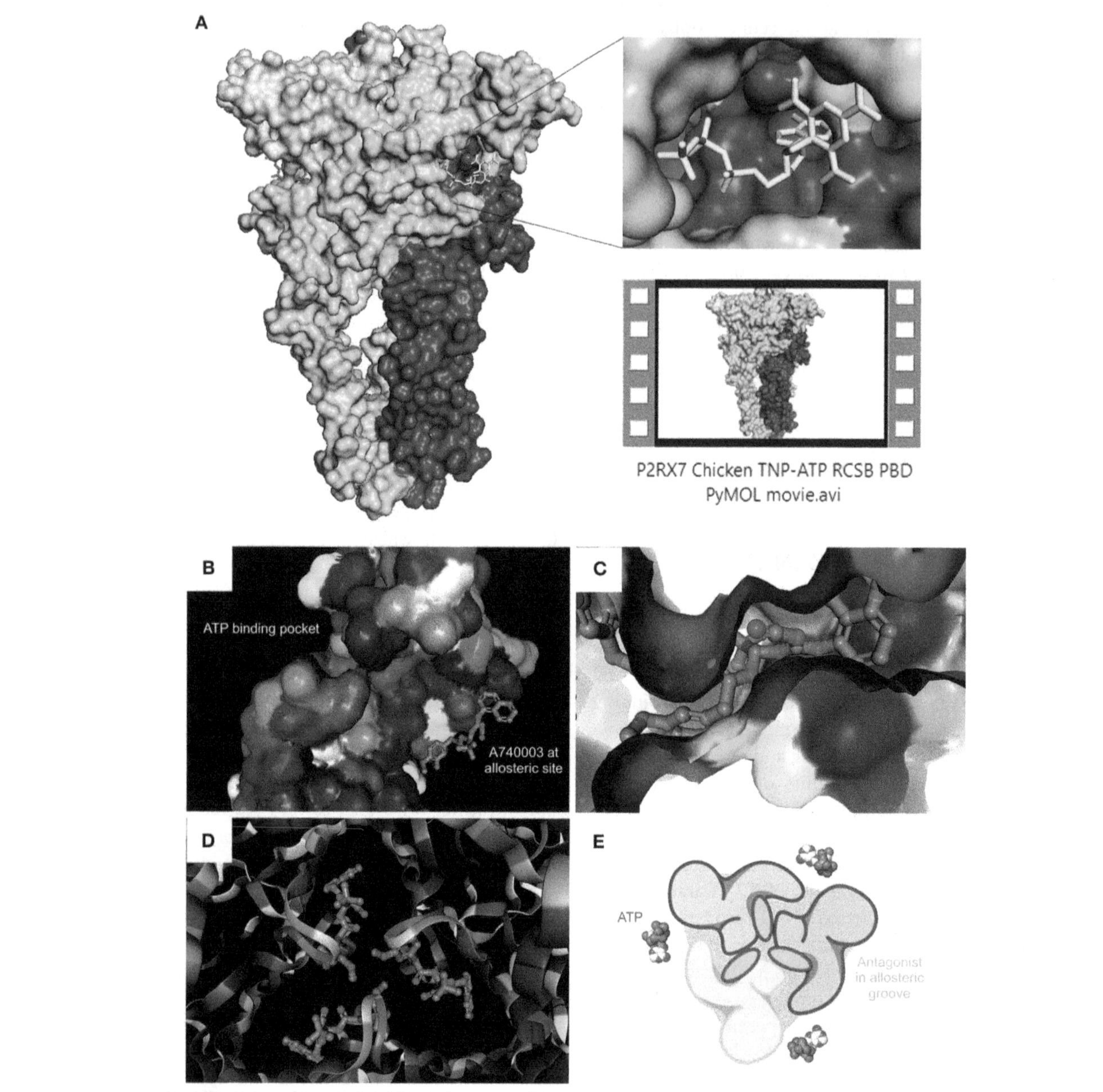

FIGURE 1 | Recent P2RX7 structural developments: the ATP binding pocket and the allosteric groove. **(A)** PyMOL (pymol.org) generated surface plot of P2RX7 trimer using RCSB PDB data file (rcsb.org) for chicken variant bound to the competitive antagonist TNP-ATP (structure 5XW6, 3.1A). ROI shows the ATP binding pocket (RHS, upper), PyMOL Video file gives structural overview of the trimer with detailed orientations of the ATP binding pocket and the central ion channel (see Supplementary Material **Video S1**). RCSB PDB generated images show location of the ATP binding pocket in relation to the newly discovered allosteric site on the monomer **(B)** and at the subunit interface of the trimer, forming an allosteric groove—here shown occupied by A740003 antagonist **(C)**. When imaged together from intracellular projection, the three allosteric grooves appear as a Shuriken, whose rotation is impeded by the allosteric antagonist A740003 **(D)**. **(E)** Cartoon representation of the relationship between the agonist binding site and the allosteric antagonist-binding groove. Adapted from Karasawa and Kawate (2016), with permission.

unquestionably facilitates massive membrane depolarization, dye permeability and, in some circumstances, cell death via mechanisms that might be cell-specific and even unique (e.g., pyroptosis, autosis etc.). However, the pore opening is reversible. Moreover, mechanism(s) behind these effects remained elusive. Two very mechanistically distinct hypotheses tried to explain the large pore phenomenon. One that P2RX7, under conditions of chronic eATP stimulation, recruits a secondary pore complex. The fact that P2RX7 expression alone in Xenopus oocytes proved insufficient to induce pore formation in these cells seemingly supported the role of either some accessory protein or other as yet unknown accessory mechanism (Petrou et al.,

1997), with pannexin1 (Panx1) channels being pointed out as the main candidate (Pelegrin and Surprenant, 2006). The second hypothesis is that the P2RX7 trimer can further change conformation resulting in ion channel to pore dilation (Browne et al., 2013). The LP-through-Panx1 theory is complex in its regulatory constitution, with multiple splice variants and cell-specific expression patterns to contend with (Ma et al., 2009). Moreover, there is evidence that the P2RX7 LP formation is retained in Panx1$^{-/-}$ cells (Qu et al., 2011; Hanley et al., 2012; Alberto et al., 2013) and that the P2RX7 trimer can form this LP structure alone (Browne et al., 2013; Karasawa et al., 2017). However, the existence of P2RX7 in two opening states was not supported by recent single-channel electrophysiological studies, which provided no evidence for dilation of the hP2X7R channel on sustained eATP stimulation (Pippel et al., 2017). Indeed, it was the discrepancy between the receptor activation data obtained by whole-cell vs. single-channel currents and via dye permeability, which triggered the notion that the LP must involve an additional molecular entity. Interestingly, a recent review seems to reconcile some of the seemingly contradictory findings (for a comprehensive discussion see Di Virgilio et al., 2018b). The authors argue that the model of channel-to-pore transition might have resulted from the different kinetics of fluorescence increases evoked by Ca^{2+} sensors in response to calcium influx (rapid) and the floresence from DNA dye binding (slow). Consequently, the LP formation may occur concomitantly with the opening of the ion channel and the two signals increasing over distinct time-scales. This model fits with recent data that the P2RX7 pore can dilate sufficiently to allow Yo-Pro permeation (Karasawa et al., 2017). However, as specific mutations (the nfP2RX7) or splicing affecting the C-terminus of P2RX7 abolish LP dye uptake but not ion channel functions, we may not have the full explanation yet. The picture should become clearer as we move closer to a complete 3-D crystal structure determination and understand the receptor interactome better. For instance, demonstration of cholesterol/membrane lipid-specific controls over pore dilation (Karasawa et al., 2017) could explain the inherent difficulties associated with successful patch-clamping involving the LP. The physical act of clamping a locality of the cell membrane may simply introduce sufficient rigidity to inhibit phospholipid movement in the vicinity of P2RX7. No doubt, this debate will continue, resulting in some ingenious technical development before the final conclusion is reached.

An additional level of complexity exists around the selectivity of the P2RX7 LP, which displays a preference for cations or anions under different physiological conditions and in different cell types as well as in individual cells within a clonal population: In P2RX7 transfected HEK293 cells, Lucifer Yellow (LY) uptake displays intracellular Ca^{2+} dependence at rat P2RX7, but not mouse P2RX7 expressed in Raw264.7 cells. In the same study, EtBr uptake showed no such dependence (Cankurtaran-Sayar et al., 2009). In macrophages, no such calcium dependence occurs, but distinct pathways do exist, as evidenced by preferential uptake of cationic or anionic dyes by individual cells <100 microns apart in the same dish (Schachter et al., 2008; Cankurtaran-Sayar et al., 2009). Our own studies have confirmed this uptake selectivity in dystrophic myoblast populations (**Figure 2**). Analysis of the fluorescent signal kinetics of LY vs. DNA binding dyes might be useful as the latter binds irreversibly and the difference in the dye uptake might be a reflection of cell health rather than the P2RX7 permeability function. Undoubtedly, understanding this mechanism might lead to tailored therapeutic approaches, with a particular scope in tumor cells.

Furthermore, irrespective of the mechanistic unknowns and controversies, the real ambiguity had always been the physiological relevance and function of this P2RX7 LP. The first demonstration of a functional link has been identification of a reciprocity between P2RX7 LP opening and autophagosome formation, where the one is indispensable for the other (Young et al., 2015). Given the recent progress in our understanding of the importance of autophagy-dependent processes in physiology and a range of human pathologies as diverse as neurological /neurodegenerative diseases (Alzheimer's, dementia, Parkinson's, and MLS), muscular dystrophies, infectious, lysosomal storage diseases, Crohn's, cancers and aging (Young et al., 2009, 2015; Rubinsztein et al., 2011; Nikoletopoulou et al., 2015; Qian et al., 2017), this link may suggest a potential for tuning autophagic responses in diverse human pathologies using P2RX7 modulation.

The relationship between pore formation and cell death is complex and also remains unclear; is pore formation a pre-requisite for P2RX7-dependent cell death? Given the controversies over the question whether the influx of ions through the channel is observed prior to the pore formation, we do not have a full answer. Working with these two facets involves independent conditions and very different experimental setups. The channel is mostly measured by electrophys and the LP by dye uptake. The sensitivity difference inherent to these methods is significant and generally, channel activity is recorded within seconds, whilst LP opening follows up to an hour later. Since no pharmacological antagonists truly specific to the LP has been identified, it is currently impossible to block the pore formation without blocking the channel. Hence, P2RX7-dependent death might be attributed to the channel without verifying pore functions (Kong et al., 2005). Whilst P2RX7-dependent, pore-independent cell death has been suggested in embryonic neural progenitor cells (Delarasse et al., 2009), this experiment was carried out using unusually high (2.5 mM) BzATP concentration. In contrast, P2RX7 activation with 100 μM BzATP was shown to induce differentiation in embryonic neural progenitor cells in N2-containing media, where pore formation and cell death were again not observed (Tsao et al., 2013). Yet, 300 μM has been shown to induce pore formation and cell death in adult neural progenitors in artificial cerebral spinal fluid (Messemer et al., 2013). This example illustrates difficulties in drawing conclusions around LP formation being a prerequisite for cell death as slightly different parameters will have a significant effect on experimental outcomes. Our own data suggest that serum content has a significant impact on the pore function (Young et al., 2017). This factor does not affect channel functions and is not always described in assay methodologies. The difference in P2RX7 receptor density on various cells and in the sensitivity of respective detection methods may also skew the analyses of

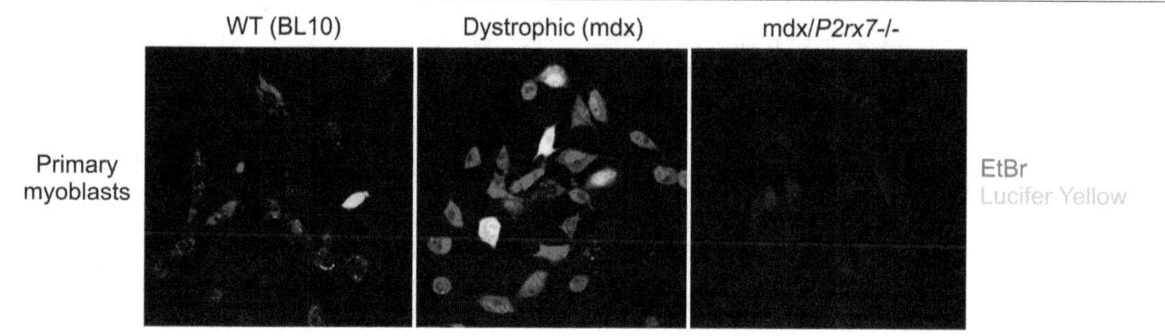

FIGURE 2 | Selective regulation of cationic and anionic dye permeation through the P2RX7 LP. Example of differences in P2RX7 LP permeation preferences to EtBr (cationic) and Lucifer Yellow (anionic) dyes in individual cells of a clonal population (Young and Gorecki, 2016): Compared to WT myoblasts **(Left)**, the dystrophic mdx myoblasts **(Center)** display upregulated P2RX7 expression and increased LP permeability in response to eATP (Young et al., 2015, 2017). The mdx/P2RX7$^{-/-}$ myoblasts **(Right)** show no dye uptake under these conditions, as expected. Note that the majority of the seemingly identical cells in this clonal population shows a clear preferential uptake of EtBr over LY upon the LP opening, which is considered to be a non-selective pore. The molecular mechanisms underlying this phenomenon are currently under investigation as this experiment illustrates the potential for diverse LP responses in heterogeneous and functionally plastic populations of e.g., immune cells *in vivo*.

channel and pore responses. Moreover, it is commonplace for one P2RX7 activation mode to be studied without the other. Hence, it is often difficult to make cross-study comparisons.

P2RX7 LOCALISATION, SIGNALING, INTERACTOME, AND REGULATION

P2RX7 is a membrane-spanning receptor. Targeted mutagenesis has implicated the C-terminal tail region in this receptor trafficking to the membrane (reviewed in Robinson and Murrell-Lagnado, 2013). Interestingly, nuclear P2RX7 localisation has also been reported (Atkinson et al., 2002), with suggested roles in modulating neuronal plasticity, albeit no follow-up studies supported this finding. The association of P2RX7 with lipid rafts has been demonstrated in various systems (Garcia-Marcos et al., 2006) and may be associated with palmitoylation of C-terminal cysteine residues (Gonnord et al., 2009), which is a reversible modification associated with membrane targeting. This is intriguing given the more recent demonstration of cholesterol-mediated inhibition of both P2RX7 LP (Karasawa et al., 2017) and channel (Murrell-Lagnado, 2017), cholesterol being a significant constituent of lipid rafts. The idea that P2RX7 is both targeted to and could be inhibited by lipid raft cholesterol, suggests an as yet un-characterized mechanism of spatial regulation through lipid raft targeting. Interestingly, multiple tumor types show upregulation of lipid rafts and cholesterol-depleting agents were shown to induce apoptosis in such cells (Li et al., 2006). The existence of a P2RX7-evoked cell death cascade silencing through cholesterol regulation in cancer is an interesting possibility.

In this context of cancer cell targeting, the 'non-functional' P2RX7 (nfP2RX7) (Slater et al., 2004) is the subject of numerous patents for epitope-specific antibody-based therapy for several cancer types (Gilbert et al., 2017). The nfP2RX7, in fact, retains the calcium channel functions, which are used by cancer cells to support its growth but lacks the ability to form the large pore and therefore not able to trigger cell death in the high eATP environment. This conformational change might be a specific mechanism controlling the potentially deleterious LP opening and allowing cancer cells expressing high P2RX7 levels to survive in the high eATP environment.

Furthermore, a feedback loop has been discovered, where sustained activation of P2RX7 with LP opening causes release of active MMP-2, which halts responses *via* the MMP-2-dependent receptor cleavage (Young et al., 2017). This mechanism operates in diverse cells, including macrophages, dystrophic myoblasts, P2RX7-transfected HEK293 and also in cancer cells. This tuning mechanism allows malignant cells to profit from P2RX7 channel activation eliciting proliferation, growth, migration, invasion and metabolic advantages, whilst avoiding cell death cascades associated with the LP. Moreover, MMP-2 is found in serum, where it displays complex regulation via TIMP expression/activity. Therefore, P2RX7 in organs with discontinuous capillaries, or in pathologies affecting capillary permeability (e.g., inflammation or tumor neo-vascularisation) may be under the regulatory control of MMP-2 cleavage balanced by TIMPs. CD44 has been reported to allosterically positively modulate P2RX7 activity by facilitating eATP binding through GAG chain interactions (Moura et al., 2015). CD44 itself was found to be a proteolytic target of MMP-2 (Young et al., 2017), suggesting that an additional levels of regulatory control may also exist. Given that MMP-2 inhibition can re-open the P2RX7 LP in cancer cells and effectively switch on the LP-associated cell death pathway, it might be possible to develop a new generation of cancer therapeutics promoting this P2RX7 LP formation (Young et al., 2017). Furthermore, as P2RX7 ablation eliminated gelatinase activity *in vivo,* P2RX7 antagonists could be a good alternative to highly toxic MMP inhibitors in treatments of inflammation and cancers.

Interestingly, non-eATP P2RX7 agonists also exist. NAD^+ is perhaps the best studied here: ADP-ribosyltransferase (ART) enzymes catalyze the transfer of ADP-ribose groups from NAD^+ to arginine residue 125 of the ecto-domain lying proximal to the P2RX7 ATP binding site (Seman et al., 2003). Ribosylations are covalent modifications and therefore constitutively activate P2RX7. However, this mode of P2RX7 activation appears to be species-specific, acting on mouse P2RX7 receptor variants, but not human. One rationale is that the Art2b gene encoding ART2.2 ADP-ribosyl transferase is differentially expressed between human and mouse; mice have two active copies of this gene, whereas in humans the transcript is translationally silenced by three premature stop codons (Haag et al., 1994). Moreover, this mechanism of activation is known to function in mouse T lymphocytes but not macrophages, the latter only display augmentation of eATP-induced receptor activation in the presence of NAD^+ (Hong et al., 2009). Therefore, this effect may also be cell or isoform specific. Mouse but not human has two N-terminal isoforms and the unique P2RX7k variant is prominent in mouse T lymphocytes and particularly sensitive to ADP-ribosylation (Rissiek et al., 2015). Therefore, it might be the mouse-specific P2RX7k isoform responding to NAD^+ stimulus. Indeed, in the Glaxo knockout, which retains the P2RX7k variant, receptor responses in T lymphocytes are retained (see P2X7 knockout section below). Finally, ADP-ribosyltransferase enzymes also display tissue specific expression patterns, which would also contribute to the regulation of NAD^+ P2RX7 signaling.

While other non-nucleotide agonists of P2RX7 have been reported, the mode of their receptor interaction has not been determined and may either represent competitive or allosteric agonist/modulation. The recent structural analyses seem to favor the latter, given the steric constraints of the ATP-binding pocket. The immunopeptides amyloid β (Sanz et al., 2009) and serum amyloid A (Elssner et al., 2004), along with LL-37 (Elssner et al., 2004), and polymyxin B (Ferrari et al., 2004) have all been implicated in activating/potentiating the P2RX7 channel function through direct interactions with the receptor extracellular loop region. Cytoplasmic agonists have also been postulated, although these are indirect in nature: LPS binding P2RX7 C-terminal tail was shown to lower the stimulus intensity required for channel gating through eATP release (Yang et al., 2015). Cytoplasmic levels of Alu-RNA were suggested to function in the same manner, yet without inducing eATP release (Fowler et al., 2014).

Numerous cell-specific downstream signaling pathways are linked with P2RX7 activation. Those associated with the release of inflammatory mediators: caspase-1, IL-1β, IL-6, and NLRP3/ASC activation/recruitment have already been described. P2RX7 is also a key modulator of various signaling cascades involved in many physiological processes, including PKC-MEK-ERK-FOS-JUN (Tsao et al., 2013), PI3K-AKT-mTOR (Bian et al., 2013), MyD88-NFKB (Liu et al., 2011), MMP-2/9-Dystroglycan-CD44 (Young et al., 2017), and Calcineurin-NFATc1 (Shiratori et al., 2010). These numerous cascades illustrate the diversity and complexity of P2RX7 signaling, with implications for cellular processes such as growth, proliferation, differentiation, metabolism, migration, invasion, autophagy and also cell death. Mechanisms of P2RX7-dependent cell death have been well documented and are numerous, including apoptosis (Zanovello et al., 1990) as well as several unique processes: aponecrosis (MacKenzie et al., 2001), necroptosis (Cullen et al., 2015), pyroptosis (de Gassart and Martinon, 2015), pseudo-apoptosis (Roger and Pelegrin, 2011), and autosis (Draganov et al., 2015). Autophagic cell death has also been identified (Young et al., 2015).

The P2RX7 interactome is just as diverse. This receptor has been suggested to directly interact with over 50 different binding partners, most of which have been identified by combinations of mass spectrometry, immunoprecipitation and immunoblotting. P2RX7 interactors include soluble, membrane-bound, peripheral, cytoskeletal and chaperone proteins (summarized in P2X7.co.uk). This diversity of proteins may reflect further spatial and temporal complexity. Soluble biglycan for example, a ubiquitous extracellular matrix (ECM) proteoglycan is responsible for coordinating the interaction of P2RX7, TLR4, and P2RX4, facilitating NLRP3 inflammasome formation and IL-1β release (Babelova et al., 2009). When proteolytically activated in the ECM, biglycan itself becomes a danger signal, with the capacity to orchestrate both sterile and infectious inflammation (Nastase et al., 2012). Interestingly, biglycan has been studied extensively in muscle disorders, where P2RX7 upregulation and role in both inflammatory and non-inflammatory processes has also been established (Young et al., 2012, 2013, 2015; Sinadinos et al., 2015). Thus, tissue- and cell-specific modalities, as well as expression, localization and activation of binding partners plus influence of inflammatory mediators, all play a role in P2RX7 signaling.

P2RX7 AGONISTS AND ANTAGONISTS: WHERE ARE WE?

As already explained, eATP is able to induce different gating characteristics depending on concentrations around the active site. Essentially, eATP $>100\,\mu M$ is sufficient to activate the channel and >100–$300\,\mu M$ and above are necessary to induce LP formation (Donnelly-Roberts et al., 2009). Endogenous eATP is subject to degradation by ubiquitous extracellular nucleotidases such as CD73 and CD39, as well as tissue-specific enzymes, such as α-sarcoglycan (adhalin) found in skeletal muscles (Betto et al., 1999). In this way, eATP concentrations in the extracellular space are tightly regulated, where high concentrations are quickly degraded to ADP, AMP and adenosine, which activate other P2X, P2Y, and P1 receptors, respectively. Importantly, activation of these different P1 and P2 receptors can have opposite effects to eATP stimulation, thus creating yet another level of homeostasis but is also confounding pharmacological studies. Moreover, conditions where surface nucleotidases become deregulated, such as in the case of loss of adhalin from the muscle sarcolemma in Duchenne and limb-girdle muscular dystrophies, result in elevated levels of eATP on the cell surface (Betto et al., 1999). In such conditions, changes in the receptor activity might be unrelated to its properties or expression levels. Therefore, P2RX7 specific and non-hydrolysable agonists would be useful tools for dissecting distinct P2RX7-specific downstream responses. While the competitive agonist benzoylated-ATP (BzATP) and non-hydrolysable sulfonated-ATP (ATPγS) display increased specificity and affinity over endogenous eATP, no true P2RX7-specific agonist has been identified so far. Hence, BzATP, with 10-30 times higher affinity for channel gating at the human P2RX7 receptor is the most widely used (Bianchi et al., 1999) despite its known activity at P2RX1 and P2RX3 and being metabolized to lower MW constituents (De Marchi et al., 2016). Species-specific differences in agonist specificity and sensitivity add an additional level of complexity to pharmacological studies (Hibell et al., 2000).

P2RX7 blockers are currently divided into two main mechanistic groups: one which binds orthosterically and competitively to the eATP binding pocket and another that binds allosterically to sites other than the eATP site and reduces ligand binding affinity. First generation P2RX7 antagonists were developed in the 1990s and can now be grouped according to their lack of specificity. Examples include Reactive Blue 2, Suramin (and its derivatives), Coomassie Brilliant Blue G (BBG), pyridoxal phosphate-6-azophenyl-2-4-disulfonic acid (PPADS), 1-N,O-bis(5-isoquinolinesulfonyl)-N-methyl-l-tyrosyl-4-phenylpiperazine (KN-62), and oxidized ATP (oATP), see Bartlett et al. for a review (Bartlett et al., 2014). Despite its "non-druggable" nature and lack of absolute specificity for P2RX7 and capacity for near-infra red fluorescence upon protein binding, BBG remains one of the most widely used and useful reagents as it is effective at human, mouse, rat, dog and guinea pig P2RX7. BBG also had triggered the initial interest in therapeutic applications by showing effectiveness in preventing eATP-induced cell death in murine models of spinal cord injury *in vivo* (Wang et al., 2004; Peng et al., 2009) and because of its blood-brain barrier (BBB) permeability. Indeed, despite its limitations, BBG has been used widely to block P2RX7 in various pathologies such as neuroexcitotoxicity (Carmo et al., 2014), graft-vs.-host disease (Geraghty et al., 2017) and muscular dystrophy (Young et al., 2012). However, as BBG is not a specific P2RX7 antagonist, also inhibiting P2RX4 and P2RX1 receptors, the pharmacological findings obtained with this antagonist have been confirmed using *p2rx7* KO models. Two of these are available and have been used in the bulk of studies: The GSK knockout carries a lacZ/Neo cassette insertion in exon 1 (Sikora et al., 1999; Chessell et al., 2005) and Pfizer's (available via JAX) has a Neo cassette insertion in exon 13 (Solle et al., 2001). Importantly, in both models, *P2rx7* gene escaped complete inactivation, retaining expression of some isoforms P2RX7k in Glaxo (Nicke et al., 2009) and P2RX7a and P2RX7b in Pfizer (Masin et al., 2012). Specifically, T cells and lymphocytes from the Glaxo KO have been shown to retain P2RX7 responses, including LP function (Taylor et al., 2009). As discussed above, this is due to the existence, in the mouse, of the P2RX7k variant, which is driven by an alternative promoter and its exon 1 escaping inactivation in the GSK model. This isoform, although expressed at low levels, displays faster activation kinetics and a lower threshold for channel gating in comparison to the wild-type P2RX7a variant (Nicke et al., 2009). The Pfizer KO mouse retains expression of the alternative C-terminal variants, however these have limited homomeric functionality and low expression levels in most if not all cell types. Hence, while the Pfizer model can be regarded as a functional knockout, studies using the GSK animal should be carefully re-considered and interpreted appropriately. Recently, new mouse models have been developed, including some allowing the conditional, cell-type specific *p2rx7* knockout. These mice should be an invaluable resource for deciphering the cell, tissue-specific and temporal effects of P2RX7 receptor activation and inhibition.

Other groups of functionally related molecules have also been shown to block P2RX7: Naturally-occurring plant compounds such as alkaloids (Shemon et al., 2004), synthetic enzyme inhibitors such as CAY10593 (phospholipase D blocker) (Pupovac et al., 2013), antipsychotics (Hempel et al., 2013) as well as various cations, such as Ca^{2+} and Mg^{2+} (Jiang, 2009). While the first-generation compounds such as oATP and BBG are still being used in some experimental paradigms, second-generation P2RX7 antagonists offer significantly increased specificity, albeit at significantly increased cost. This second generation antagonists began to emerge in 2006 with the development by Abbott Labs of disubstituted tetrazoles such as A438079 (Nelson et al., 2006) and cyanoguanidines such as A740003 (Honore et al., 2006). Interestingly, both classes were previously thought to act reversibly and competitively (Donnelly-Roberts and Jarvis, 2007). However, recent structural data contradicted this assumption by placing A74003 not in the ATP-binding pocket but acting via the newly identified allosteric, non-competitive site instead (Karasawa and Kawate, 2016). Intriguingly, A438079 binding analysis is not yet available while this compound appears to preferentially block the LP (Haanes et al., 2012). It would be therefore interesting to interrogate the newly available crystal structure to determine whether A438079 and A740003 share the same binding site as this information may help our understanding of the channel vs. pore functionality. Another important step has been the development of a stable, selective orally bioavailable, blood brain barrier permeable P2RX7 antagonists suitable for the treatment of a host of human pathologies. High-throughput screening has led to the identfication of Glaxo GSK314181A (Broom et al., 2008) and AstraZeneca AZ11645373 (Stokes et al., 2006, also see Mehta et al., 2014 and Syed and Kennedy, 2012 for extensive reviews (Syed and Kennedy, 2012; Mehta et al., 2014) followed by AZD9056, also from AstraZeneca (Keystone et al., 2012) and CE-224,535 from Pfizer (Stock et al., 2012). Since the development of these new drugs, pharmacological inhibition of P2RX7 has proven to be effective and well-tolerated treatment in multiple rodent models of inflammatory diseases including neurological, musculoskeletal as well as retinal, kidney, bladder, liver, lung, and skin-based inflammatory disorders (reviewed extensively in Bartlett et al., 2014, in models of stroke, brain trauma, hemorrhage and also in BBB integrity loss Zhao et al., 2016) as well as muscular dystrophy, cardiomyopathy, respiratory disorders, inflammatory bowel disease and cancer. Additionally to the inflammatory diseases or those with an obvious inflammatory component, P2RX7 drugs showed efficacy in Azlheimer's and psychiatric disorders such as mania, depression and also prion disease (reviewed in Bartlett et al., 2014; Savio et al., 2018).

Unfortunately, the precise localization of P2RX7 expression in the brain remains controversial due to non-specific antibody binding (Anderson and Nedergaard, 2006) with *p2rx7* KO mouse brains showing strong immunoreactivity (Sim et al., 2004). A recent progress in this area has been the development and initial characterization of a humanized P2RX7 mouse model, where hP2RX7 expression was localized to glutamatergic pyramidal neurons of the hippocampus, as well as to non-neuronal lineages including astrocytes, microglia, and oligodendrocytes (Metzger et al., 2017). Interestingly, in yet another model, the P2RX7_EGFP mice the receptor expression has been localized to the dentate gyrus granule cell layer (Jimenez-Pacheco et al., 2016). The existence of neuronal P2RX7 responses remains the topic of debate, with arguments for both the neuronal P2RX7 responses being an important pharmacological target (Miras-Portugal et al., 2017) but also suggesting that these responses are due to P2RX7 expression on astrocytes or microglia instead (Illes et al., 2017). Clearly, full understanding of the P2RX7 localisation in the brain remains elusive and would be required for the development of targeted therapeutic approaches for the variety of CNS diseases in which this receptor appears to play a role.

Despite these limitations, >70 patents for P2RX7 antagonists have been filed in the last few years, including for the use of A438079 in depression, anxiety and bipolar disorders, triazole-based drugs for CNS disorders and P2RX7 antagonists in epithelial cancers (from GSK, Abbott and Cleveland University Hospitals, respectively (Park and Kim, 2016). Moreover, trials have been conducted in relation to several inflammatory pathologies such as rheumatoid arthritis (Maini et al., 2006; Keystone et al., 2012), Crohn's (Eser et al., 2015), and basal cell carcinoma (Gilbert et al., 2017) to name but a few. Although AstraZeneca's AZD9056 trials were halted due to disappointing results, it's more recent application to Crohn's has been more promising. This suggests that P2RX7 inhibition may not be equally effective in various diseases with an inflammatory component and potentially that some drugs may show different efficacy in specific conditions. In this context, one remaining questions is whether selective targeting of the channel or the LP receptor functions would have more significant therapeutic effect. Another consideration is the impact of the P2RX7 polymorphisms, which are numerous and which have been demonstrated to impact various human disorders (Fuller et al., 2009). The benefit of the recent publication of the P2RX7 3-D crystal structure is that it will be possible to utilize it in the *in silico* high-throughput screening of chemical libraries and rational drug design. Structural prediction-based screening recently identified 3 novel competitive orthosteric antagonists. Intriguingly, one of these compounds was reported to specifically antagonize P2RX7 LP pore formation with no effect on the channel function (Caseley et al., 2016). Given that this drug binding to the eATP pocket affects LP only, it might provide some support for the hypothesis that the channel and pore are produced by the P2RX7 itself. However, while the publication focused on the therapeutic potential of this new "pore blocker" it did not consider this potentially distinguishing molecular mechanism.

Another example of the impact of the receptor crystal structure is the identification of the mechanism of action of AZT and other Nucleoside Reverse Transcriptase Inhibitors (NRTIs) at the P2RX7. These drugs have been shown previously to be able to block this receptor functions *in vitro* and to have therapeutic impact *in vivo*, in a number of mouse models of human diseases (Fowler et al., 2014). Molecular modeling showed that AZT and its derivatives occupy the same allosteric site as the canonical antagonists and also led to further work that proved AZT to be therapeutic in the mouse model of Duchenne muscular dystrophy (Al-Khalidi et al., 2018). AZT is a mainstay in the prevention of mother-to-child HIV transmission (Van Zyl et al., 2008). Consequently, there is extensive safety and pharmacokinetic data available following decades of AZT use in humans, also in children and neonates. Therefore, it is a good candidate for rapid re-purposing for treatment of human diseases requiring P2RX7 inhibition.

An exciting development in the P2RX7 targeting is a new class of antagonist—Multi-Target-Directed-Ligands (MTDLs), which permit the specific delivery of P2RX7 antagonists in a previously unattainably targeted manner. Specifically, dual NMDA-P2RX7 compounds were recently synthesized for targeting both the excitotoxicity-induced cell death as well as the P2RX7-dependent neuroinflammatory-induced cell death seen in Alzheimer's disease (Karoutzou et al., 2018). Such compounds represent an exciting and theoretically limitless combinatorial approach to P2RX7 inhibition.

With rational design-based drug screening set to replace classical approaches, the number of P2RX7 antagonists should increase further. Yet, for the rational clinical application of the existing as well as the new drugs, we still require a significant improvement of our basic understanding of underlying receptor physiology and pharmacology and of its involvement in various pathologies. Perhaps the holy grail of P2RX7 research remains the determination of the molecular mechanism of the channel vs. the LP opening (Karasawa et al., 2017) and also of the physiological and pathological importance of this phenomenon.

Cancer is the paragon of P2RX7's dual nature. P2RX7 is ubiquitously overexpressed in cancer (**Figure 3**). Yet, tumor cells appear to take advantage of the receptor responses, without succumbing to the LP-mediated cell death cascade activation, which would be fully expected given such significant overexpression in the presence of abundant eATP in the tumor environment (Young et al., 2017). Quite the reverse, tumor cells use this P2RX7 overexpression to their significant advantage though increases in growth, migration, the Warburg effect, VEGF production triggering tumor neo-angiogenesis and MMP release helping its invasion and metastasis (Young et al., 2017; reviewed by Di Virgilio, 2016). While many tumors expressed the "non-functional" P2RX7, there is evidence that the functional receptor can be expressed too. Only few loss-of function mutations have been identified in P2X7 expressed in various tumor types (**Figure 3**). Thus, the systemic administration of pharmacological P2RX7 blockers should have a potent anti-tumor effect by preventing the high jacking of this receptor by cancer cells. Interestingly, while this approach showed

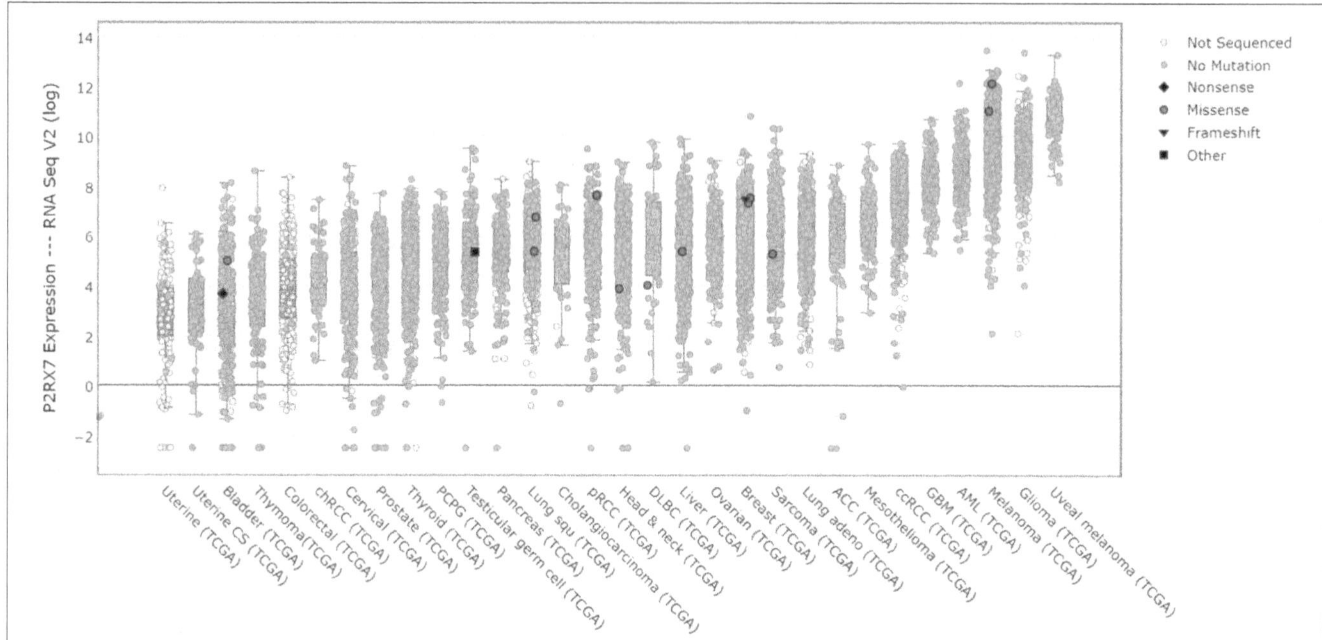

FIGURE 3 | P2RX7 expression is elevated in human cancers. cBioPortal (cbioportal.org) derived expression levels for P2RX7 multiple human cancer patient biopsies from TCGA data (cancergenome.nih.gov). Noticeable, across almost all tumor types, is the significant overexpression of P2RX7 and a paucity of detected mutations. This indicates that malignant cells express high levels of fully-functional receptors, which is an important consideration for drug treatment.

promise in some tumors, the effect was far from universal. The problem is that P2RX7 is a significant player in the immune response that, in turn, can inhibit growth of some tumors (reviewed by Di Virgilio, 2016). Indeed, there are indications that immune suppression following P2RX7 inhibition is a real and potentially significant drawback, as tumors in *p2rx7* KO mice show accelerated growth, increased tumor size and metastasis, recruitment and invasion, all of which reflects reduced immune cell activation (Adinolfi et al., 2015). Perhaps the appropriate metaphor for P2RX7 in cancer would be that of the sword and the shield, where the sword may be blunted through receptor blockade but at the expense of lowering the shield hand. Hence, a successful cancer treatment with P2RX7 antagonists should, ideally, selectively target cancer cells whilst leaving the host immune response unscathed. In addition, a treatment exploiting the overexpression of P2RX7 on tumor cells and turning it against the tumor is an appealing proposition. The aforementioned targeting of the "non-functional" P2RX7 with specific antibodies is one example currently in clinical trials. Another could be the development of positive modulators of P2RX7 LP formation or compounds which effectively upregulate or reinstate P2RX7 LP formation in tumor cells, which overexpress either functional or "non-functional" receptor variants. Such an approach abrogates any concerns over immune response dampening and potentially could even boost the anti-tumor responses as certain types of cell death trigger or potentiate immune responses.

In conclusion, recent progress in obtaining the receptor crystal structure, understanding the mechanism of action of structurally unrelated antagonists and in unraveling the feedback mechanism regulating its functions should result in a breakthrough in targeting P2RX7 in a host of human diseases.

AUTHOR CONTRIBUTIONS

CY and DG both made substantial, direct and intellectual contributions to the manuscript, and approved it for publication.

FUNDING

This work was supported by a VC's Early Career Fellowship, De Montfort University, Leicester to CY, the Research and Innovation Development Fund, University of Portsmouth to DG and Kosciuszko Programme (Ministry of National Defence, Poland) to DG.

ACKNOWLEDGMENTS

We would like to thank Prof Toshi Kawate, Cornell University for the kind permission to reproduce the P2RX7 allosteric groove cartoon and Prof Pedro Persechini, Federal University of Rio de Janeiro, for advice regarding LP permeation pathways.

REFERENCES

Adinolfi, E., Capece, M., Franceschini, A., Falzoni, S., Giuliani, A. L., Rotondo, A., et al. (2015). Accelerated tumor progression in mice lacking the ATP receptor P2X7. *Cancer Res.* 75, 635–644. doi: 10.1158/0008-5472.CAN-14-1259

Adinolfi, E., Pizzirani, C., Idzko, M., Panther, E., Norgauer, J., Di Virgilio, F., et al. (2005). P2X7 receptor: death or life? *Purinergic Signal.* 1, 219–227. doi: 10.1007/s11302-005-6322-x

Alberto, A. V., Faria, R. X., Couto, C. G., Ferreira, L. G., Souza, C. A., Teixeira, P. C. N., et al. (2013). Is pannexin the pore associated with the P2X7 receptor? *Naunyn Schmiedebergs. Arch. Pharmacol.* 386, 775–787. doi: 10.1007/s00210-013-0868-x

Al-Khalidi, R., Panicucci, C., Cox, P., Chira, N., Róg, J., Young, C. N. J., et al. (2018). Zidovudine ameliorates pathology in the mouse model of Duchenne muscular dystrophy via P2RX7 purinoceptor antagonism. *Acta Neuropathol. Commun.* 6:27. doi: 10.1186/s40478-018-0530-4

Amoroso, F., Falzoni, S., Adinolfi, E., Ferrari, D., and Di Virgilio, F. (2012). The P2X7 receptor is a key modulator of aerobic glycolysis. *Cell Death Dis.* 3:e370. doi: 10.1038/cddis.2012.105

Anderson, C. M., and Nedergaard, M. (2006). Emerging challenges of assigning P2X7 receptor function and immunoreactivity in neurons. *Trends Neurosci.* 29, 257–262. doi: 10.1016/j.tins.2006.03.003

Atkinson, L., Milligan, C. J., Buckley, N. J., and Deuchars, J. (2002). Purinergic receptors: An ATP-gated ion channel at the cell nucleus. *Nature* 420:42. doi: 10.1038/420042a

Babelova, A., Moreth, K., Tsalastra-Greul, W., Zeng-Brouwers, J., Eickelberg, O., Young, M. F., et al. (2009). Biglycan, a danger signal that activates the NLRP3 inflammasome via toll-like and P2X receptors. *J. Biol. Chem.* 284, 24035–24048. doi: 10.1074/jbc.M109.014266

Bartlett, R., Stokes, L., and Sluyter, R. (2014). The P2X7 receptor channel: recent developments and the use of P2X7 antagonists in models of disease. *Pharmacol. Rev.* 66, 638–675. doi: 10.1124/pr.113.008003

Betto, R., Senter, L., Ceoldo, S., Tarricone, E., Biral, D., and Salviati, G. (1999). Ecto-ATPase activity of α-sarcoglycan (adhalin). *J. Biol. Chem.* 274, 7907–7912. doi: 10.1074/jbc.274.12.7907

Bian, S., Sun, X., Bai, A., Zhang, C., Li, L., Enjyoji, K., et al. (2013). P2X7 integrates PI3K/AKT and AMPK-PRAS40-mTOR signaling pathways to mediate tumor cell death. *PLoS ONE* 8:e60184. doi: 10.1371/journal.pone.0060184

Bianchi, B. R., Lynch, K. J., Touma, E., Niforatos, W., Burgard, E. C., Alexander, K. M., et al. (1999). Pharmacological characterization of recombinant human and rat P2X receptor subtypes. *Eur. J. Pharmacol.* 376, 127–138. doi: 10.1016/S0014-2999(99)00350-7

Broom, D. C., Matson, D. J., Bradshaw, E., Buck, M. E., Meade, R., Coombs, S., et al. (2008). Characterization of N-(Adamantan-1-ylmethyl)-5-[(3R-aminopyrrolidin-1-yl)methyl]-2-chloro-benzamide, a P2X7 antagonist in animal models of pain and inflammation. *J. Pharmacol. Exp. Ther.* 327, 620–633. doi: 10.1124/jpet.108.141853

Browne, L. E., Compan, V., Bragg, L., and North, R. A. (2013). P2X7 Receptor channels allow direct permeation of nanometer-sized dyes. *J. Neurosci.* 33, 3557–3566. doi: 10.1523/JNEUROSCI.2235-12.2013

Burnstock, G., and Knight, G. E. (2004). Cellular distribution and functions of P2 receptor subtypes in different systems. *Int. Rev. Cytol.* 240, 31–304. doi: 10.1016/S0074-7696(04)40002-3

Burnstock, G., and Knight, G. E. (2017). The potential of P2X7 receptors as a therapeutic target, including inflammation and tumour progression. *Purinergic Signal.* 14, 1–18. doi: 10.1007/s11302-017-9593-0

Burnstock, G., and Verkhratsky, A. (2012). Evolution of P2X receptors. *Wiley Interdiscip. Rev. Membr. Transp. Signal.* 1, 188–200. doi: 10.1002/wmts.13

Cankurtaran-Sayar, S., Sayar, K., and Ugur, M. (2009). P2X7 receptor activates multiple selective dye-permeation pathways in RAW 264.7 and human embryonic kidney 293 cells. *Mol. Pharmacol.* 76, 1323–1332. doi: 10.1124/mol.109.059923

Carmo, M. R., Menezes, A. P., Nunes, A. C., Pliássova, A., Rolo, A. P., Palmeira, C. M., et al. (2014). The P2X7 receptor antagonist Brilliant Blue G attenuates contralateral rotations in a rat model of Parkinsonism through a combined control of synaptotoxicity, neurotoxicity and gliosis. *Neuropharmacology* 81, 145–152. doi: 10.1016/j.neuropharm.2014.01.045

Caseley, E. A., Muench, S. P., Fishwick, C. W., and Jiang, L. H. (2016). Structure-based identification and characterisation of structurally novel human P2X7 receptor antagonists. *Biochem. Pharmacol.* 116, 130–139. doi: 10.1016/j.bcp.2016.07.020

Cekic, C., and Linden, J. (2016). Purinergic regulation of the immune system. *Nat. Rev. Immunol.* 16, 177–192. doi: 10.1038/nri.2016.4

Chessell, I. P., Hatcher, J. P., Bountra, C., Michel, A. D., Hughes, J. P., Green, P., et al. (2005). Disruption of the P2X7 purinoceptor gene abolishes chronic inflammatory and neuropathic pain. *Pain* 114, 386–396. doi: 10.1016/j.pain.2005.01.002

Cockcroft, S., and Gomperts, B. D. (1980). The ATP4- receptor of rat mast cells. *Biochem. J.* 188, 789–98. doi: 10.1042/bj1880789

Cortés-Garcia, J. D., López-López, C., Cortez-Espinosa, N., García-Hernández, M. H., Guzmán-Flores, J. M., Layseca-Espinosa, E., et al. (2016). Evaluation of the expression and function of the P2X7 receptor and ART1 in human regulatory T-cell subsets. *Immunobiology* 221, 84–93. doi: 10.1016/j.imbio.2015.07.018

Csóka, B., Németh, Z. H., Törö, G., Idzko, M., Zech, A., Koscsó, B., et al. (2015). Extracellular ATP protects against sepsis through macrophage P2X7 purinergic receptors by enhancing intracellular bacterial killing. *FASEB J.* 29, 3626–3637. doi: 10.1096/fj.15-272450

Cullen, S. P., Kearney, C. J., Clancy, D. M., and Martin, S. J. (2015). Diverse activators of the NLRP3 inflammasome promote IL-1β secretion by triggering necrosis. *Cell Rep.* 11, 1535–1548. doi: 10.1016/j.celrep.2015.05.003

de Gassart, A., and Martinon, F. (2015). Pyroptosis: caspase-11 unlocks the gates of death. *Immunity* 43, 835–837. doi: 10.1016/j.immuni.2015.10.024

Delarasse, C., Gonnord, P., Galante, M., Auger, R., Daniel, H., Motta, I., et al. (2009). Neural progenitor cell death is induced by extracellular ATP via ligation of P2X7 receptor. *J. Neurochem.* 109, 846–857. doi: 10.1111/j.1471-4159.2009.06008.x

De Marchi, E., Orioli, E., Dal Ben, D., and Adinolfi, E. (2016). P2X7 receptor as a therapeutic target. *Adv. Protein Chem. Struct. Biol.* 39–79. doi: 10.1016/bs.apcsb.2015.11.004

Denlinger, L. C., Fisette, P. L., Sommer, J. A., Watters, J. J., Prabhu, U., Dubyak, G. R., et al. (2001). Cutting edge: the nucleotide receptor P2X7 contains multiple protein- and lipid-interaction motifs including a potential binding site for bacterial lipopolysaccharide. *J. Immunol.* 167, 1871–1876. doi: 10.4049/jimmunol.167.4.1871

Di Virgilio, F. (2000). Dr. Jekyll/Mr. Hyde: the dual role of extracellular ATP. *J. Auton. Nerv. Syst.* 81, 59–63. doi: 10.1016/S0165-1838(00)00114-4

Di Virgilio, F. (2016). P2RX7: a receptor with a split personality in inflammation and cancer. *Mol. Cell. Oncol.* 3:e1010937. doi: 10.1080/23723556.2015.1010937

Di Virgilio, F., Giuliani, A. L., Vultaggio-Poma, V., Falzoni, S., and Sarti, A. C. (2018a). Non-nucleotide agonists triggering P2X7 receptor activation and pore formation. *Front. Pharmacol.* 9:39. doi: 10.3389/fphar.2018.00039

Di Virgilio, F., Schmalzing, G., and Markwardt, F. (2018b). The elusive P2X7 macropore. *Trends Cell Biol.* 28, 392–404. doi: 10.1016/j.tcb.2018.01.005

Donnelly-Roberts, D. L., and Jarvis, M. F. (2007). Discovery of P2X7 receptor-selective antagonists offers new insights into P2X7 receptor function and indicates a role in chronic pain states. *Br. J. Pharmacol.* 151, 571–579. doi: 10.1038/sj.bjp.0707265

Donnelly-Roberts, D. L., Namovic, M. T., Han, P., and Jarvis, M. F. (2009). Mammalian P2X7 receptor pharmacology: comparison of recombinant mouse, rat and human P2X7 receptors. *Br. J. Pharmacol.* 157, 1203–1214. doi: 10.1111/j.1476-5381.2009.00233.x

Draganov, D., Gopalakrishna-Pillai, S., Chen, Y. R., Zuckerman, N., Moeller, S., Wang, C., et al. (2015). Modulation of P2X4/P2X7/Pannexin-1 sensitivity to extracellular ATP via Ivermectin induces a non-apoptotic and inflammatory form of cancer cell death. *Sci. Rep.* 5:16222. doi: 10.1038/srep16222

Dubyak, G. R. (2012). P2X7 receptor regulation of non-classical secretion from immune effector cells. *Cell. Microbiol.* 14, 1697–1706. doi: 10.1111/cmi.12001

Elssner, A., Duncan, M., Gavrilin, M., and Wewers, M. D. (2004). A novel P2X7 receptor activator, the human cathelicidin-derived peptide LL37, induces IL-1 processing and release. *J. Immunol.* 172, 4987–4994. doi: 10.4049/jimmunol.172.8.4987

Eser, A., Colombel, J. F., Rutgeerts, P., Vermeire, S., Vogelsang, H., Braddock, M., et al. (2015). Safety and efficacy of an oral inhibitor of the purinergic receptor P2X7 in adult patients with moderately to severely active crohn's disease. *Inflamm. Bowel Dis.* 21, 2247–2253. doi: 10.1097/MIB.0000000000000514

Feng, Y. H., Li, X., Zeng, R., and Gorodeski, G. I. (2006). Endogenously expressed truncated P2X7 receptor lacking the C-terminus is preferentially upregulated in epithelial cancer cells and fails to mediate ligand-induced pore formation and apoptosis. *Nucleosides Nucleotides Nucleic Acids* 25, 1271–1276. doi: 10.1080/15257770600890921

Ferrari, D., Pizzirani, C., Adinolfi, E., Forchap, S., Sitta, B., Turchet, L., et al. (2004). The antibiotic polymyxin b modulates P2X7 receptor function. *J. Immunol.* 173, 4652–4660. doi: 10.4049/jimmunol.173.7.4652

Figliuolo, V. R., Chaves, S. P., Savio, L. E. B., Thorstenberg, M. L. P., Machado Salles, É., Takiya, C. M., et al. (2017). The role of the P2X7 receptor in murine cutaneous leishmaniasis: aspects of inflammation and parasite control. *Purinergic Signal.* 13, 143–152. doi: 10.1007/s11302-016-9544-1

Fowler, B. J., Gelfand, B. D., Kim, Y., Kerur, N., Tarallo, V., Hirano, Y., et al. (2014). Nucleoside reverse transcriptase inhibitors possess intrinsic anti-inflammatory activity. *Science* 346, 1000–1003. doi: 10.1126/science.1261754

Fuller, S. J., Stokes, L., Skarratt, K. K., Gu, B. J., and Wiley, J. S. (2009). Genetics of the P2X7 receptor and human disease. *Purinergic Signal.* 5, 257–262. doi: 10.1007/s11302-009-9136-4

Garcia-Marcos, M., Pochet, S., Marino, A., and Dehaye, J. P. (2006). P2X7and phospholipid signalling: the search of the "missing link" in epithelial cells. *Cell. Signal.* 18, 2098–2104. doi: 10.1016/j.cellsig.2006.05.008.

Geraghty, N. J., Belfiore, L., Ly, D., Adhikary, S. R., Fuller, S. J., Varikatt, W., et al. (2017). The P2X7 receptor antagonist Brilliant Blue G reduces serum human interferon-gamma in a humanized mouse model of graft-versus-host disease. *Clin. Exp. Immunol.* 190, 79–95. doi: 10.1111/cei.13005

Gilbert, S. M., Gidley Baird, A., Glazer, S., Barden, J. A., Glazer, A., Teh, L. C., et al. (2017). A phase I clinical trial demonstrates that nfP2X7-targeted antibodies provide a novel, safe and tolerable topical therapy for basal cell carcinoma. *Br. J. Dermatol.* 177, 117–124. doi: 10.1111/bjd.15364

Gonnord, P., Delarasse, C., Auger, R., Benihoud, K., Prigent, M., Cuif, M. H., et al. (2009). Palmitoylation of the P2X7 receptor, an ATP-gated channel, controls its expression and association with lipid rafts. *FASEB J.* 23, 795–805. doi: 10.1096/fj.08-114637

Gu, B. J., and Wiley, J. S. (2006). Rapid ATP-induced release of matrix metalloproteinase 9 is mediated by the P2X7 receptor. *Blood* 107, 4946–4953. doi: 10.1182/blood-2005-07-2994

Haag, F., Koch-Nolte, F., Kühl, M., Lorenzen, S., and Thiele, H.-G. (1994). Premature stop codons inactivate the RT6 genes of the human and chimpanzee species. *J. Mol. Biol.* 243, 537–546. doi: 10.1006/jmbi.1994.1680

Haanes, K. A., Schwab, A., and Novak, I. (2012). The P2X7 receptor supports both life and death in fibrogenic pancreatic stellate cells. *PLoS ONE* 7:e51164. doi: 10.1371/journal.pone.0051164

Hanley, P. J., Kronlage, M., Kirschning, C., Del Rey, A., Di Virgilio, F., Leipziger, J., et al. (2012). Transient P2X 7 receptor activation triggers macrophage death independent of toll-like receptors 2 and 4, caspase-1, and pannexin-1 proteins. *J. Biol. Chem.* 287, 10650–10663. doi: 10.1074/jbc.M111.332676

Hattori, M., and Gouaux, E. (2012). Molecular mechanism of ATP binding and ion channel activation in P2X receptors. *Nature* 485, 207–212. doi: 10.1038/nature11010

He, Y., Taylor, N., Fourgeaud, L., and Bhattacharya, A. (2017). The role of microglial P2X7: modulation of cell death and cytokine release. *J. Neuroinflammation* 14:135. doi: 10.1186/s12974-017-0904-8

Hempel, C., Nörenberg, W., Sobottka, H., Urban, N., Nicke, A., Fischer, W., et al. (2013). The phenothiazine-class antipsychotic drugs prochlorperazine and trifluoperazine are potent allosteric modulators of the human P2X7 receptor. *Neuropharmacology* 75, 365–379. doi: 10.1016/j.neuropharm.2013.07.027

Hetherington, H. P., Spencer, D. D., Vaughan, J. T., and Pan, J. W. (2001). Quantitative 31P spectroscopic imaging of human brain at 4 Tesla: assessment of gray and white matter differences of phosphocreatine and ATP. *Magn. Reson. Med.* 45, 46–52. doi: 10.1002/1522-2594(200101)45:1<46::AID-MRM1008>3.0.CO;2-N

Hibell, A. D., Kidd, E. J., Chessell, I. P., Humphrey, P. P., and Michel, A. D. (2000). Apparent species differences in the kinetic properties of P2X(7) receptors. *Br. J. Pharmacol.* 130, 167–173. doi: 10.1038/sj.bjp.0703302

Hong, S., Schwarz, N., Brass, A., Seman, M., Haag, F., Koch-Nolte, F., et al. (2009). Differential regulation of P2X7 receptor activation by extracellular nicotinamide adenine dinucleotide and ecto-ADP-ribosyltransferases in murine macrophages and T cells. *J. Immunol.* 183, 578–592. doi: 10.4049/jimmunol.0900120

Honore, P., Donnelly-Roberts, D., Namovic, M. T., Hsieh, G., Zhu, C. Z., Mikusa, J. P., et al. (2006). A-740003 [N-(1-{[(cyanoimino)(5-quinolinylamino) methyl]amino}-2,2-dimethylpropyl)-2-(3,4-dimethoxyphenyl)acetamide], a novel and selective P2X7 receptor antagonist, dose-dependently reduces neuropathic pain in the rat. *J. Pharmacol. Exp. Ther.* 319, 1376–1385. doi: 10.1124/jpet.106.111559

Illes, P., Khan, T. M., and Rubini, P. (2017). Neuronal P2X7 receptors revisited: do they really exist? *J. Neurosci.* 37, 7049–7062. doi: 10.1523/JNEUROSCI.3103-16.2017

Jiang, L. H. (2009). Inhibition of P2X7 receptors by divalent cations: old action and new insight. *Eur. Biophys. J.* 38, 339–346. doi: 10.1007/s00249-008-0315-y

Jimenez-Pacheco, A., Diaz-Hernandez, M., Arribas-Blázquez, M., Sanz-Rodriguez, A., Olivos-Oré, L. A., Artalejo, A. R., et al. (2016). Transient P2X7 receptor antagonism produces lasting reductions in spontaneous seizures and gliosis in experimental temporal lobe epilepsy. *J. Neurosci.* 36, 5920–5932. doi: 10.1523/JNEUROSCI.4009-15.2016

Karasawa, A., and Kawate, T. (2016). Structural basis for subtype-specific inhibition of the P2X7 receptor. *Elife* 5:e22153. doi: 10.7554/eLife.22153

Karasawa, A., Michalski, K., Mikhelzon, P., and Kawate, T. (2017). The P2X7 receptor forms a dye-permeable pore independent of its intracellular domain but dependent on membrane lipid composition. *Elife* 6:e31186. doi: 10.7554/eLife.31186

Karmakar, M., Katsnelson, M. A., Dubyak, G. R., and Pearlman, E. (2016). Neutrophil P2X7receptors mediate NLRP3 inflammasome-dependent IL-1β secretion in response to ATP. *Nat. Commun.* 7:10555. doi: 10.1038/ncomms10555

Karoutzou, O., Kwak, S. H., Lee, S. D., Martínez-Falguera, D., Sureda, F. X., Vázquez, S., et al. (2018). Towards a novel class of multitarget-directed ligands: dual P2X7–NMDA receptor antagonists. *Molecules* 23:E230. doi: 10.3390/molecules23010230

Kasuya, G., Yamaura, T., Ma, X.-B., Nakamura, R., Takemoto, M., Nagumo, H., et al. (2017). Structural insights into the competitive inhibition of the ATP-gated P2X receptor channel. *Nat. Commun.* 8:876. doi: 10.1038/s41467-017-00887-9

Kawate, T., Michel, J. C., Birdsong, W. T., and Gouaux, E. (2009). Crystal structure of the ATP-gated P2X4ion channel in the closed state. *Nature* 460, 592–598. doi: 10.1038/nature08198

Keystone, E. C., Wang, M. M., Layton, M., Hollis, S., and McInnes, I. B. (2012). Clinical evaluation of the efficacy of the P2X7 purinergic receptor antagonist AZD9056 on the signs and symptoms of rheumatoid arthritis in patients with active disease despite treatment with methotrexate or sulphasalazine. *Ann. Rheum. Dis.* 71, 1630–1635. doi: 10.1136/annrheumdis-2011-143578

Kong, Q., Wang, M., Liao, Z., Camden, J. M., Yu, S., Simonyi, A., et al. (2005). P2X7 nucleotide receptors mediate caspase-8/9/3-dependent apoptosis in rat primary cortical neurons. *Purinergic Signal.* 1, 337–347. doi: 10.1007/s11302-005-7145-5

Li, M., Chang, T. H., Silberberg, S. D., and Swartz, K. J. (2008). Gating the pore of P2X receptor channels. *Nat. Neurosci.* 11, 883–887. doi: 10.1038/nn.2151

Li, Y. C., Park, M. J., Ye, S. K., Kim, C. W., and Kim, Y. N. (2006). Elevated levels of cholesterol-rich lipid rafts in cancer cells are correlated with apoptosis sensitivity induced by cholesterol-depleting agents. *Am. J. Pathol.* 168, 1107–1118. doi: 10.2353/ajpath.2006.050959

Liu, Y., Xiao, Y., and Li, Z. (2011). P2X7 receptor positively regulates MyD88-dependent NF-κB activation. *Cytokine* 55, 229–236. doi: 10.1016/j.cyto.2011.05.003.

Ma, W., Hui, H., Pelegrin, P., and Surprenant, A. (2009). Pharmacological characterization of Pannexin-1 currents expressed in mammalian cells. *J. Pharmacol. Exp. Ther.* 328, 409–418. doi: 10.1124/jpet.108.146365

MacKenzie, A., Wilson, H. L., Kiss-Toth, E., Dower, S. K., North, R. A., and Surprenant, A. (2001). Rapid secretion of interleukin-1β by microvesicle shedding. *Immunity* 15, 825–835. doi: 10.1016/S1074-7613(01)00229-1

Maini, R. N., Taylor, P. C., Szechinski, J., Pavelka, K., Bröll, J., Balint, G., et al. (2006). Double-blind randomized controlled clinical trial of the interleukin-6 receptor antagonist, tocilizumab, in European patients with rheumatoid arthritis who had an incomplete response to methotrexate. *Arthritis Rheum.* 54, 2817–2829. doi: 10.1002/art.22033

Mansoor, S. E., Lü, W., Oosterheert, W., Shekhar, M., Tajkhorshid, E., and Gouaux, E. (2016). X-ray structures define human P2X 3 receptor gating cycle and antagonist action. *Nature* 538, 66–71. doi: 10.1038/nature19367

Martel-Gallegos, G., Rosales-Saavedra, M. T., Reyes, J. P., Casas-Pruneda, G., Toro-Castillo, C., Pérez-Cornejo, P., et al. (2010). Human neutrophils do not express purinergic P2X7 receptors. *Purinergic Signal.* 6, 297–306. doi: 10.1007/s11302-010-9178-7

Masin, M., Young, C., Lim, K., Barnes, S. J., Xu, X. J., Marschall, V., et al. (2012). Expression, assembly and function of novel C-terminal truncated variants of the mouse P2X7 receptor: re-evaluation of P2X7 knockouts. *Br. J. Pharmacol.* 165, 978–993. doi: 10.1111/j.1476-5381.2011.01624.x

Massicot, F., Hache, G., David, L., Chen, D., Leuxe, C., Garnier-Legrand, L., et al. (2013). P2X7 cell death receptor activation and mitochondrial impairment in oxaliplatin-induced apoptosis and neuronal injury: cellular mechanisms and *in vivo* approach. *PLoS ONE* 8:e66830. doi: 10.1371/journal.pone.0066830

Mehta, N., Kaur, M., Singh, M., Chand, S., Vyas, B., Silakari, P., et al. (2014). Purinergic receptor P2X7: a novel target for anti-inflammatory therapy. *Bioorganic Med. Chem.* 22, 54–88. doi: 10.1016/j.bmc.2013.10.054

Messemer, N., Kunert, C., Grohmann, M., Sobottka, H., Nieber, K., Zimmermann, H., et al. (2013). P2X7 receptors at adult neural progenitor cells of the mouse subventricular zone. *Neuropharmacology* 73, 122–137. doi: 10.1016/j.neuropharm.2013.05.017

Metzger, M. W., Walser, S. M., Aprile-Garcia, F., Dedic, N., Chen, A., Holsboer, F., et al. (2017). Genetically dissecting P2rx7 expression within the central nervous system using conditional humanized mice. *Purinergic Signal.* 13, 153–170. doi: 10.1007/s11302-016-9546-z

Migita, K., Ozaki, T., Shimoyama, S., Yamada, J., Nikaido, Y., Furukawa, T., et al. (2016). HSP90 regulation of P2X7 receptor function requires an intact cytoplasmic C-terminus. *Mol. Pharmacol.* 90, 116–126. doi: 10.1124/mol.115.102988

Miras-Portugal, M. T., Sebastián-Serrano, Á., de Diego García, L., and Díaz-Hernández, M. (2017). Neuronal P2X7 receptor: involvement in neuronal physiology and pathology. *J. Neurosci.* 37, 7063–7072. doi: 10.1523/JNEUROSCI.3104-16.2017

Monif, M., Burnstock, G., and Williams, D. A. (2010). Microglia: proliferation and activation driven by the P2X7 receptor. *Int. J. Biochem. Cell Biol.* 42, 1753–1756. doi: 10.1016/j.biocel.2010.06.021

Morciano, G., Sarti, A. C., Marchi, S., Missiroli, S., Falzoni, S., Raffaghello, L., et al. (2017). Use of luciferase probes to measure ATP in living cells and animals. *Nat. Protoc.* 12, 1542–1562. doi: 10.1038/nprot.2017.052

Moura, G., Lucena, S., Lima, M., Nascimento, F., Gesteira, T., Nader, H., et al. (2015). Post-translational allosteric activation of the P2X7 receptor through glycosaminoglycan chains of CD44 proteoglycans. *Cell Death Discov.* 1:15005. doi: 10.1038/cddiscovery.2015.5

Munoz, F. M., Gao, R., Tian, Y., Henstenburg, B. A., Barrett, J. E., and Hu, H. (2017). Neuronal P2X7 receptor-induced reactive oxygen species production contributes to nociceptive behavior in mice. *Sci. Rep.* 7:3539. doi: 10.1038/s41598-017-03813-7

Murrell-Lagnado, R. D. (2017). Regulation of P2X purinergic receptor signaling by cholesterol. *Curr. Top. Membr.* 80, 211–232. doi: 10.1016/bs.ctm.2017.05.004

Nastase, M. V., Young, M. F., and Schaefer, L. (2012). Biglycan: a multivalent proteoglycan providing structure and signals. *J. Histochem. Cytochem.* 60, 963–975. doi: 10.1369/0022155412456380

Nelson, D. W., Gregg, R. J., Kort, M. E., Perez-Medrano, A., Voight, E. A., Wang, Y., et al. (2006). Structure-activity relationship studies on a series of novel, substituted 1-benzyl-5-phenyltetrazole P2X7 antagonists. *J. Med. Chem.* 49, 3659–3666. doi: 10.1021/jm051202e

Nicke, A., Kuan, Y. H., Masin, M., Rettinger, J., Marquez-Klaka, B., Bender, O., et al. (2009). A functional P2X7 splice variant with an alternative transmembrane domain 1 escapes gene inactivation in P2X7 knock-out mice. *J. Biol. Chem.* 284, 25813–25822. doi: 10.1074/jbc.M109.033134

Nikoletopoulou, V., Papandreou, M. E., and Tavernarakis, N. (2015). Autophagy in the physiology and pathology of the central nervous system. *Cell Death Differ.* 22, 398–407. doi: 10.1038/cdd.2014.204

Park, J. H., and Kim, Y. C. (2016). P2X7 receptor antagonists: a patent review (2010–2015). *Expert Opin. Ther. Pat.* 27, 257–267. doi: 10.1080/13543776.2017.1246538

Pelegrin, P., Barroso-Gutierrez, C., and Surprenant, A. (2008). P2X7 receptor differentially couples to distinct release pathways for IL-1 in mouse macrophage. *J. Immunol.* 180, 7147–7157. doi: 10.4049/jimmunol.180.11.7147

Pelegrin, P., and Surprenant, A. (2006). Pannexin-1 mediates large pore formation and interleukin-1beta release by the ATP-gated P2X7 receptor. *EMBO J.* 25, 5071–82. doi: 10.1038/sj.emboj.7601378

Pellegatti, P., Raffaghello, L., Bianchi, G., Piccardi, F., Pistoia, V., and Di Virgilio, F. (2008). Increased level of extracellular ATP at tumor sites: *in vivo* imaging with plasma membrane luciferase. *PLoS ONE* 3:e2599. doi: 10.1371/journal.pone.0002599

Peng, W., Cotrina, M. L., Han, X., Yu, H., Bekar, L., Blum, L., et al. (2009). Systemic administration of an antagonist of the ATP-sensitive receptor P2X7 improves recovery after spinal cord injury. *Proc. Natl. Acad. Sci.U.S.A.* 106, 12489–12493. doi: 10.1073/pnas.0902531106

Perregaux, D., and Gabel, C. A. (1994). Interleukin-1β maturation and release in response to ATP and nigericin. Evidence that potassium depletion mediated by these agents is a necessary and common feature of their activity. *J. Biol. Chem.* 269, 15195–15203.

Petrou, S., Ugur, M., Drummond, R. M., Singer, J. J., and Walsh, J. V. (1997). P2X7 purinoceptor expression in Xenopus oocytes is not sufficient to produce a pore-forming P2Z-like phenotype. *FEBS Lett.* 411, 339–345. doi: 10.1016/S0014-5793(97)00700-X

Pippel, A., Stolz, M., Woltersdorf, R., Kless, A., Schmalzing, G., and Markwardt, F. (2017). Localization of the gate and selectivity filter of the full-length P2X7 receptor. *Proc. Natl. Acad. Sci. U.S.A.* 144, E2156–E2165. doi: 10.1073/pnas.1610414114

Pupovac, A., Stokes, L., and Sluyter, R. (2013). CAY10593 inhibits the human P2X7 receptor independently of phospholipase D1 stimulation. *Purinergic Signal.* 9, 609–619. doi: 10.1007/s11302-013-9371-6

Qian, M., Fang, X., and Wang, X. (2017). Autophagy and inflammation. *Clin. Transl. Med.* 6:24. doi: 10.1186/s40169-017-0154-5

Qiu, Y., Li, W. H., Zhang, H. Q., Liu, Y., Tian, X. X., and Fang, W. G. (2014). P2X7 mediates ATP-driven invasiveness in prostate cancer cells. *PLoS ONE* 9:e114371. doi: 10.1371/journal.pone.0114371

Qu, Y., Misaghi, S., Newton, K., Gilmour, L. L., Louie, S., Cupp, J. E., et al. (2011). Pannexin-1 is required for ATP release during apoptosis but not for inflammasome activation. *J. Immunol.* 186, 6553–6561. doi: 10.4049/jimmunol.1100478

Rissiek, B., Haag, F., Boyer, O., Koch-Nolte, F., and Adriouch, S. (2015). P2X7 on mouse T cells: one channel, many functions. *Front. Immunol.* 6:204. doi: 10.3389/fimmu.2015.00204

Robinson, L. E., and Murrell-Lagnado, R. D. (2013). The trafficking and targeting of P2X receptors. *Front. Cell. Neurosci.* 7:233. doi: 10.3389/fncel.2013.00233

Roger, S., and Pelegrin, P. (2011). P2X7 receptor antagonism in the treatment of cancers. *Expert Opin. Investig. Drugs* 20, 875–880. doi: 10.1517/13543784.2011.583918

Rubinsztein, D. C., Mariño, G., and Kroemer, G. (2011). Autophagy and aging. *Cell* 146, 682–695. doi: 10.1016/j.cell.2011.07.030

Sanz, J. M., Chiozzi, P., Ferrari, D., Colaianna, M., Idzko, M., Falzoni, S., et al. (2009). Activation of microglia by amyloid {beta} requires P2X7 receptor expression. *J. Immunol.* 182, 4378–4385. doi: 10.4049/jimmunol.0803612

Savio, L. E. B., de Andrade Mello, P., da Silva, C. G., and Coutinho-Silva, R. (2018). The P2X7 receptor in inflammatory diseases: angel or demon? *Front. Pharmacol.* 9:52. doi: 10.3389/fphar.2018.00052

Schachter, J., Motta, A. P., de Souza Zamorano, A., da Silva-Souza, H. A., Guimarães, M. Z., and Persechini, P. M. (2008). ATP-induced P2X7-associated uptake of large molecules involves distinct mechanisms for cations and anions in macrophages. *J. Cell Sci.* 121, 3261–3270. doi: 10.1242/jcs.029991

Schenk, U., Frascoli, M., Proietti, M., Geffers, R., Traggiai, E., Buer, J., et al. (2011). ATP inhibits the generation and function of regulatory T cells through the activation of purinergic P2X receptors. *Sci. Signal.* 4:ra12. doi: 10.1126/scisignal.2001270

Seman, M., Adriouch, S., Scheuplein, F., Krebs, C., Freese, D., Glowacki, G., et al. (2003). NAD-induced T cell death: ADP-ribosylation of cell surface proteins by ART2 activates the cytolytic P2X7 purinoceptor. *Immunity* 19, 571–582. doi: 10.1016/S1074-7613(03)00266-8

Shemon, A. N., Sluyter, R., Conigrave, A. D., and Wiley, J. S. (2004). Chelerythrine and other benzophenanthridine alkaloids block the human P2X 7 receptor. *Br. J. Pharmacol.* 142, 1015–1019. doi: 10.1038/sj.bjp.0705868

Shiratori, M., Tozaki-Saitoh, H., Yoshitake, M., Tsuda, M., and Inoue, K. (2010). P2X7 receptor activation induces CXCL2 production in microglia through NFAT and PKC/MAPK pathways. *J. Neurochem.* 114, 810–819. doi: 10.1111/j.1471-4159.2010.06809.x

Sim, J. A., Young, M. T., Sung, H.-Y., North, R. A., and Surprenant, A. (2004). Reanalysis of P2X7 receptor expression in rodent brain. *J. Neurosci.* 24, 6307–6314. doi: 10.1523/JNEUROSCI.1469-04.2004

Sikora, A., Liu, J., Brosnan, C., Buell, G., Chessel, I., and Bloom, B. R. (1999). Cutting edge: purinergic signaling regulates radical-mediated bacterial killing mechanisms in macrophages through a P2X7-independent mechanism. *J. Immunol.* 163, 558–61.

Sinadinos, A., Young, C. N., Al-Khalidi, R., Teti, A., Kalinski, P., Mohamad, S., et al. (2015). P2RX7 purinoceptor: a therapeutic target for ameliorating the symptoms of duchenne muscular dystrophy. *PLoS Med.* 12:e1001888. doi: 10.1371/journal.pmed.1001888

Slater, M., Danieletto, S., Gidley-Baird, A., Teh, L. C., and Barden, J. A. (2004). Early prostate cancer detected using expression of non-functional cytolytic P2X7 receptors. *Histopathology* 44, 206–215. doi: 10.1111/j.0309-0167.2004.01798.x

Smart, M. L., Gu, B., Panchal, R. G., Wiley, J., Cromer, B., Williams, D. A., et al. (2003). P2X7 receptor cell surface expression and cytolytic pore formation are regulated by a distal C-terminal region. *J. Biol. Chem.* 278, 8853–8860. doi: 10.1074/jbc.M211094200

Solle, M., Labasi, J., Perregaux, D. G., Stam, E., Petrushova, N., Koller, B. H., et al. (2001). Altered cytokine production in mice lacking P2X(7) receptors. *J. Biol. Chem.* 276, 125–132. doi: 10.1074/jbc.M006781200

Sperlágh, B., Köfalvi, A., Deuchars, J., Atkinson, L., Milligan, C. J., Buckley, N. J., et al. (2002). Involvement of P2X7 receptors in the regulation of neurotransmitter release in the rat hippocampus. *J. Neurochem.* 81, 1196–211. doi: 10.1046/j.1471-4159.2002.00920.x

Stock, T. C., Bloom, B. J., Wei, N., Ishaq, S., Park, W., Wang, X., et al. (2012). Efficacy and safety of CE-224,535, an antagonist of P2X7 receptor, in treatment of patients with rheumatoid arthritis inadequately controlled by methotrexate. *J. Rheumatol.* 39, 720–727. doi: 10.3899/jrheum.110874

Stokes, L., Jiang, L. H., Alcaraz, L., Bent, J., Bowers, K., Fagura, M., et al. (2006). Characterization of a selective and potent antagonist of human P2X(7) receptors, AZ11645373. *Br. J. Pharmacol.* 149, 880–7. doi: 10.1038/sj.bjp.0706933

Surprenant, A., Rassendren, F., Kawashima, E., North, R. A., and Buell, G. (1996). The cytolytic P2Z receptor for extracellular ATP identified as a P2X receptor (P2X7). *Science* 272, 735–738. doi: 10.1126/science.272.5262.735

Syed, N. I. H., and Kennedy, C. (2012). Pharmacology of P2X receptors. *Wiley Interdiscip. Rev. Membr. Transp. Signal.* 1, 16–30. doi: 10.1002/wmts.1

Taylor, S. R. J., Gonzalez-Begne, M., Sojka, D. K., Richardson, J. C., Sheardown, S. A., Harrison, S. M., et al. (2009). Lymphocytes from P2X7-deficient mice exhibit enhanced P2X7 responses. *J. Leukoc. Biol.* 85, 978–986. doi: 10.1189/jlb.0408251

Tsao, H. K., Chiu, P. H., and Sun, S. H. (2013). PKC-dependent ERK phosphorylation is essential for P2X7 receptor-mediated neuronal differentiation of neural progenitor cells. *Cell Death Dis.* 4:e751. doi: 10.1038/cddis.2013.274

Ursu, D., Ebert, P., Langron, E., Ruble, C., Munsie, L., Zou, W., et al. (2014). Gain and loss of function of P2X7 receptors: mechanisms, pharmacology and relevance to diabetic neuropathic pain. *Mol. Pain* 10, 1–11. doi: 10.1186/1744-8069-10-37

Van Zyl, G. U., Claassen, M., Engelbrecht, S., Laten, J. D., Cotton, M. F., Theron, G. B., et al. (2008). Zidovudine with nevirapine for the prevention of HIV mother-to-child transmission reduces nevirapine resistance in mothers from the Western Cape, South Africa. *J. Med. Virol.* 80, 942–946. doi: 10.1002/jmv.21157

Virginio, C., Church, D., North, R. A., and Surprenant, A. (1997). Effects of divalent cations, protons and calmidazolium at the rat P2X7 receptor. *Neuropharmacology* 36, 1285–1294. doi: 10.1016/S0028-3908(97)00141-X

Wang, X., Arcuino, G., Takano, T., Lin, J., Peng, W. G., Wan, P., et al. (2004). P2X7 receptor inhibition improves recovery after spinal cord injury. *Nat. Med.* 10, 821–827. doi: 10.1038/nm1082

Yan, Z., Khadra, A., Li, S., Tomic, M., Sherman, A., and Stojilkovic, S. S. (2010). Experimental characterization and mathematical modeling of P2X7 receptor channel gating. *J. Neurosci.* 30, 14213–14224. doi: 10.1523/JNEUROSCI.2390-10.2010

Yang, D., He, Y., Muñoz-Planillo, R., Liu, Q., and Núñez, G. (2015). Caspase-11 requires the Pannexin-1 channel and the purinergic P2X7 pore to mediate pyroptosis and endotoxic shock. *Immunity* 43, 923–932. doi: 10.1016/j.immuni.2015.10.009

Young, A. R., Narita, M., Ferreira, M., Kirschner, K., Sadaie, M., Darot, J. F. J., et al. (2009). Autophagy mediates the mitotic senescence transition. *Genes Dev.* 23, 798–803. doi: 10.1101/gad.519709

Young, C. N., Brutkowski, W., Lien, C. F., Arkle, S., Lochmüller, H., Zabłocki, K., et al. (2012). P2X7 purinoceptor alterations in dystrophic mdx mouse muscles: relationship to pathology and potential target for treatment. *J. Cell. Mol. Med.* 16, 1026–1037. doi: 10.1111/j.1582-4934.2011.01397.x

Young, C. N. J., Chira, N., Róg, J., Al-Khalidi, R., Benard, M., Galas, L., et al. (2017). Sustained activation of P2X7 induces MMP-2-evoked cleavage and functional purinoceptor inhibition. *J. Mol. Cell Biol.* 10, 229–242. doi: 10.1093/jmcb/mjx030

Young, C. N. J., and Gorecki, D. C. (2016). "P2X7 in skeletal muscle disorders," in *Proceedings of the 1st UK-Italian Purine club meeting, 13-14th September 2016* (Bristol).

Young, C. N. J., Sinadinos, A., and Gorecki, D. C. (2013). P2X receptor signaling in skeletal muscle health and disease. *Wiley Interdiscip. Rev. Membr. Transp. Signal.* 2, 265–274. doi: 10.1002/wmts.96

Young, C. N., Sinadinos, A., Lefebvre, A., Chan, P., Arkle, S., Vaudry, D., et al. (2015). A novel mechanism of autophagic cell death in dystrophic muscle regulated by P2RX7 receptor large-pore formation and HSP90. *Autophagy* 11, 113–130. doi: 10.4161/15548627.2014.994402

Zanovello, P., Bronte, V., Rosato, A., Pizzo, P., and Di Virgilio, F. (1990). Responses of mouse lymphocytes to extracellular ATP. II. Extracellular ATP causes cell type-dependent lysis and DNA fragmentation. *J. Immunol.* 145, 1545–50.

Zhao, H., Zhang, X., Dai, Z., Feng, Y., Li, Q., Zhang, J. H., et al. (2016). P2X7 receptor suppression preserves blood-brain barrier through inhibiting RhoA activation after experimental intracerebral hemorrhage in rats. *Sci. Rep.* 6:23286. doi: 10.1038/srep23286

2

Drug Interactions with the Ca^{2+}-ATPase from Sarco(Endo)Plasmic Reticulum (SERCA)

Francesco Tadini-Buoninsegni [1], Serena Smeazzetto [1], Roberta Gualdani [2] and Maria Rosa Moncelli [1]*

[1] *Department of Chemistry "Ugo Schiff," University of Florence, Florence, Italy,* [2] *Laboratory of Cell Physiology, Institute of Neuroscience, Université Catholique de Louvain, Louvain-la-Neuve, Belgium*

***Correspondence:**
Francesco Tadini-Buoninsegni
francesco.tadini@unifi.it

The sarco(endo)plasmic reticulum Ca^{2+}-ATPase (SERCA) is an intracellular membrane transporter that utilizes the free energy provided by ATP hydrolysis for active transport of Ca^{2+} ions from the cytoplasm to the lumen of sarco(endo)plasmic reticulum. SERCA plays a fundamental role for cell calcium homeostasis and signaling in muscle cells and also in cells of other tissues. Because of its prominent role in many physiological processes, SERCA dysfunction is associated to diseases displaying various degrees of severity. SERCA transport activity can be inhibited by a variety of compounds with different chemical structures. Specific SERCA inhibitors were identified which have been instrumental in studies of the SERCA catalytic and transport mechanism. It has been proposed that SERCA inhibition may represent a novel therapeutic strategy to cure certain diseases by targeting SERCA activity in pathogens, parasites and cancer cells. Recently, novel small molecules have been developed that are able to stimulate SERCA activity. Such SERCA activators may also offer an innovative and promising therapeutic approach to treat diseases, such as heart failure, diabetes and metabolic disorders. In the present review the effects of pharmacologically relevant compounds on SERCA transport activity are presented. In particular, we will discuss the interaction of SERCA with specific inhibitors and activators that are potential therapeutic agents for different diseases.

Keywords: anticancer drug, antimalarial agent, drug-protein interaction, sarco(endo)plasmic reticulum Ca^{2+}-ATPase, SERCA activator, SERCA inhibitor, solid supported membrane

INTRODUCTION

P-type ATPases are membrane transporters that couple the energy provided by ATP hydrolysis to the active transport of various ions or phospholipids. These enzymes generate and maintain crucial electrochemical potential gradients across biological membranes (Kühlbrandt, 2004; Bublitz et al., 2011). During their enzymatic cycle P-type ATPases form a phosphorylated intermediate by interaction of ATP with a conserved aspartate residue at the catalytic domain.

The Ca^{2+}-ATPase from sarco(endo)plasmic reticulum (SERCA), belonging to the P_{IIA}-ATPase subfamily, is an intracellular membrane-associated protein of approximately 110 KDa which is involved in cell calcium signaling and homeostasis (Brini and Carafoli, 2009). In muscle cells this enzyme hydrolyzes one ATP molecule to transport two Ca^{2+} ions against their electrochemical potential gradient from the cytoplasm to the lumen of sarcoplasmic reticulum (SR) (Inesi and Tadini-Buoninsegni, 2014). SERCA therefore induces muscle relaxation by pumping back cytosolic calcium into the SR lumen. SERCA isoforms are involved in calcium signaling mechanisms for many biological functions, e.g., excitation-contraction coupling, excitation-secretion coupling, gene transcription, and apoptotic mechanisms. Because of its pivotal role, alterations in SERCA expression and impaired pump function have been related to several diseases, such as Brody's disease, Darier's disease, heart failure, cancer, and diabetes (Brini and Carafoli, 2009).

The SERCA enzyme is one of the best investigated membrane transporter. Its structure comprises three distinct cytoplasmic domains, i.e., the A (actuator), N (nucleotide binding), and P (phosphorylation) domains, and a transmembrane region of 10 helical segments (TM1–TM10) including the two Ca^{2+} binding sites. SERCA transport cycle is described by the E_1-E_2 scheme (de Meis and Vianna, 1979). If one starts at the E_1 state, the ATPase cycle (**Figure 1**) begins with high affinity binding of two Ca^{2+} ions derived from the cytosol, followed by phosphorylation of the enzyme by ATP and formation of a high energy $E_1{\sim}P$ state. During relaxation from the $E_1{\sim}P$ state to the lower energy E_2P state, Ca^{2+} ions are translocated across the membrane and released into the SR in exchange for luminal protons. Hydrolytic cleavage of the phosphoenzyme (dephosphorylation) is the final reaction step, which allows the enzyme to undergo a new transport cycle. High resolution crystal structures of various conformational states in the SERCA transport cycle were obtained, as described in detailed reviews (Toyoshima, 2008; Møller et al., 2010; Bublitz et al., 2013; Toyoshima and Cornelius, 2013).

In this short review we will focus our attention on the interaction of SERCA with specific inhibitors and activators that may represent potential therapeutic agents for different diseases. To investigate the effects of pharmacologically relevant compounds on SERCA transport activity, we employ an electrophysiological technique, which is discussed in the next section.

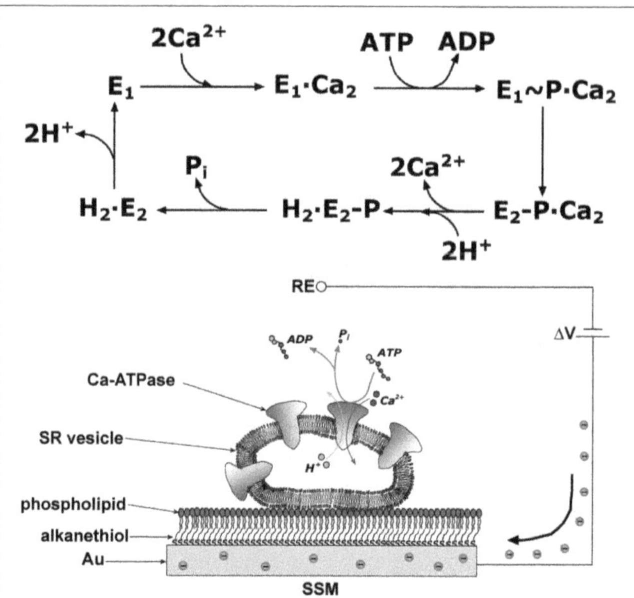

FIGURE 1 | Upper Panel: Schematic diagram of sequential reactions in the transport cycle of SERCA. **Lower Panel**: SR vesicle adsorbed on a SSM and subjected to an ATP concentration jump (not drawn to scale). If the ATP jump induces net charge displacement, a compensating current flows along the external circuit (the red spheres represent electrons) to keep constant the potential difference ΔV applied across the whole system. RE is the reference electrode. Reprinted from Tadini-Buoninsegni et al. (2008a) with permission from Elsevier.

DRUG INTERACTIONS INVESTIGATED BY ELECTROPHYSIOLOGY BASED ON SOLID SUPPORTED MEMBRANES

The ion transport mechanism of P-type ATPases, e.g., Na^+,K^+-ATPase, SERCA, and Cu^+-ATPases (ATP7A and ATP7B) (Pintschovius et al., 1999; Tadini-Buoninsegni et al., 2008a; Lewis et al., 2012; Inesi et al., 2014; Tadini-Buoninsegni and Smeazzetto, 2017), was investigated by an electrophysiological technique based on a solid supported membrane (SSM). In particular, SSM-based electrophysiology was useful to identify electrogenic steps and to assign rate constants to partial reactions in the transport cycle of P-type ATPases. In the case of Na^+,K^+-ATPase SSM-based electrophysiology provided a direct proof for the electrogenicity of Na^+ binding to the cytoplasmic side of the protein (Pintschovius et al., 1999). Also in the case of SERCA SSM-based electrophysiology was employed for a detailed characterization of the enzyme's transport cycle, especially as concerns Ca^{2+} binding and Ca^{2+}/H^+ exchange (Tadini-Buoninsegni et al., 2006; Liu et al., 2009).

This technique makes use of a hybrid alkanethiol/phospholipid bilayer supported by a gold electrode (SSM, **Figure 1**; Pintschovius and Fendler, 1999). The SSM is formed in two sequential self-assembly steps. First, an octadecanethiol monolayer is obtained which is covalently bound to the gold electrode via the sulfur atom. Then, a second phosphatidylcholine monolayer is formed on top of the thiol layer. Proteoliposomes, membrane fragments, or vesicles containing the ATPase are adsorbed on the SSM surface (**Figure 1**). Once adsorbed, the ATPase molecules are activated by a concentration jump of a specific substrate through fast solution exchange. By rapidly changing from a solution containing no substrate for the protein to one that contains a substrate, the protein is activated and a current transient is detected, which is related to charge displacement across the ATPase. The transient nature of the current signal is a consequence of the capacitively coupled system formed by the SSM and the membrane entities adsorbed on it (Schulz et al., 2008; Tadini-Buoninsegni and Bartolommei, 2016). In the case of SERCA,

Abbreviations: Br_2-TITU, 1,3-dibromo-2,4,6-tris(methyl-isothio-uronium) benzene; DBHQ, 2,5-di(tert-butyl)hydroquinone; CPA, cyclopiazonic acid; ER, endoplasmic reticulum; PLN, phospholamban; PSMA, prostate-specific membrane antigen; SR, sarcoplasmic reticulum; SERCA, sarco(endo)plasmic reticulum Ca^{2+}-ATPase; SSM, solid supported membrane; TG, thapsigargin.

an ATP concentration jump on SERCA-containing vesicles adsorbed on the SSM generates a current signal, that is related to an electrogenic event corresponding to translocation and release of bound Ca^{2+} upon phosphorylation by ATP within the first enzyme cycle (Tadini-Buoninsegni et al., 2006). Therefore, the SSM technique allows pre-steady state measurements of charge displacements within the first transport cycle of the ATPase, while steady-state currents are not measured.

SSM-based electrophysiology was successfully employed to investigate drug interactions with P-type ATPases. In this respect, the effects of various compounds of pharmacological interest on SERCA pumping activity were characterized by SSM-based current measurements (Tadini-Buoninsegni et al., 2008b, 2017; Bartolommei et al., 2011; Ferrandi et al., 2013; Sadafi et al., 2014). A molecular mechanism was proposed to explain the effect of each compound, and the reaction step and/or intermediate of the pump cycle affected by the drug was identified.

We point out that the SSM electrode combined with robotized instrumentation is an attractive tool for drug screening and development (Kelety et al., 2006). In this respect, high-throughput devices capable of performing automated measurements have been developed. For example, the SURFE^{2}R 96SE device (Nanion Technologies, Munich, Germany) is able to analyze 96 SSM sensors in a fully parallel mode allowing determination of the dose dependence of 100 compounds in <30 min (Bazzone et al., 2017).

PHARMACOLOGICAL INHIBITORS OF SERCA ACTIVITY

Various SERCA inhibitors with a variety of chemical structures are known (Michelangeli and East, 2011). These compounds represent a very useful tool in studies of the SERCA catalytic and transport mechanism. Using X-ray crystallography of SERCA-inhibitor complexes (Toyoshima and Nomura, 2002; Olesen et al., 2004; Obara et al., 2005; Moncoq et al., 2007; Laursen et al., 2009), distinct SERCA conformational states were determined at atomic resolution.

A very potent and highly selective inhibitor is thapsigargin (TG), a sesquiterpene lactone derived from the plant *Thapsia garganica* (Rasmussen et al., 1978). TG is the most widely employed SERCA inhibitor (Michelangeli and East, 2011) and can inhibit SERCA activity with an IC_{50} in the sub-nanomolar range (Sagara and Inesi, 1991). Other specific SERCA inhibitors are cyclopiazonic acid (CPA) (Seidler et al., 1989), a secondary metabolite from certain fungi, and the synthetic compound 2,5-di(tert-butyl)hydroquinone (DBHQ) (Moore et al., 1987). Mutational analysis and crystallographic data have shown that CPA and DBHQ occupy the same binding pocket at the cytoplasmic ends of the transmembrane helices TM1–TM4, while TG binds in a groove delimited by TM3, TM5, and TM7 (for a review see Yatime et al., 2009), where the residue Phe256 plays a fundamental role for both binding and inhibitory effect of TG (Xu et al., 2004). TG, CPA, and DBHQ (**Table 1**) affect SERCA transport activity in a similar way. These inhibitors bind to SERCA in a calcium-free E_2 conformation and stabilize a compact ATPase conformational state (dead-end state), preventing cytoplasmic calcium binding and catalytic activation (Inesi et al., 2005; Yatime et al., 2009; Michelangeli and East, 2011).

The inhibitory effects of TG, CPA, DBHQ, and1,3-dibromo-2,4,6-tris (methyl-isothio-uronium) benzene (Br_2-TITU), another SERCA inhibitor (Berman and Karlish, 2003), on Ca^{2+}-ATPase transport activity were also characterized by electrophysiological measurements on a SSM (Tadini-Buoninsegni et al., 2008b). In this study it was shown that Br_2-TITU displays an inhibitory mechanism different from that of TG, CPA, and DBHQ. In particular, it was demonstrated that the inhibitory effect of Br_2-TITU is related to kinetic interference with a conformational transition of the phosphorylated intermediate (E_1P-Ca_2 to E_2P transition).

It is noteworthy that TG-related prodrugs are being evaluated as anticancer drugs. Since TG will inhibit SERCA proteins regardless of the cell type thereby damaging intracellular calcium homeostasis not only in cancer cells but also in normal cells, its high cytotoxicity prevents direct use of TG as a general antitumor agent. However, a TG-based prodrug strategy was developed to overcome the above-mentioned limitation (Denmeade et al., 2012; Andersen et al., 2015; Doan et al., 2015; Cui et al., 2017). In particular, a prodrug, named mipsagargin, was obtained by conjugating a TG analog to a peptide that is targeted by prostate-specific membrane antigen (PSMA) (Denmeade et al., 2012; Andersen et al., 2015; Doan et al., 2015), which is overexpressed in prostate cancer cells and most tumor endothelial cells. This inactive and non-toxic prodrug becomes activated once it reaches tumor cells and the specific peptide sequence is cleaved by PSMA, thereby releasing the active cytotoxic TG analog. The prodrug mipsagargin can therefore be considered as a potential therapeutic agent for the treatment of various types of cancer, including prostate, breast and bladder cancers.

In the context of antitumor agents, SSM-based electrophysiology was employed to analyze the interaction of metal-based anticancer drugs with P-type ATPases, i.e., SERCA, Na^+,K^+-ATPase and Cu^+-ATPases (Sadafi et al., 2014; Tadini-Buoninsegni et al., 2014, 2017). In particular, the inhibitory effect of cisplatin (**Table 1**) on the transport activity of SERCA and Na^+,K^+-ATPase was very recently investigated (**Figure 2**) (Tadini-Buoninsegni et al., 2017). Cisplatin is a platinum-containing anticancer drug, which is widely employed as a chemotherapeutic agent against several tumors (Wang and Lippard, 2005). However, cisplatin administration causes inevitable adverse effects, which include nephrotoxicity, ototoxicity and neurotoxicity. We have shown that cisplatin is able to inhibit ATP-dependent cation translocation by SERCA and Na^+,K^+-ATPase with different degrees of potency (**Figure 2**). In particular, cisplatin was found to be a much stronger inhibitor of SERCA (IC_{50} of 1.3 μM) than of Na^+,K^+-ATPase (IC_{50} of 11.1 μM). We propose that cisplatin inhibition of SERCA and Na^+,K^+-ATPase activities may be relevant to the molecular mechanisms that underlie the various adverse effects of cisplatin and other platinum-containing anticancer drugs.

TABLE 1 | SERCA inhibitors and activators cited in the text.

	Compounds	Main properties and therapeutic applications	References
Inhibitors	Thapsigargin (TG)	Very potent and highly selective inhibitor. TG-related prodrugs as anticancer drugs.	Sagara and Inesi, 1991; Denmeade et al., 2012; Doan et al., 2015
	Cyclopiazonic acid (CPA)	Potent and specific inhibitor. Cardioprotective effect. CPA derivatives as antimalarial agents.	Seidler et al., 1989; Avellanal et al., 1998; Moncoq et al., 2007; Cardi et al., 2010
	2,5-di(tert-butyl)hydroquinone (DBHQ)	Specific inhibitor.	Moore et al., 1987; Obara et al., 2005
	1,3-dibromo-2,4,6-tris (methyl-isothio-uronium) benzene (Br_2-TITU)	SERCA and Na^+,K^+-ATPase inhibitor.	Berman and Karlish, 2003
	Cisplatin	Widely employed platinum-containing anticancer drug. SERCA and Na^+,K^+-ATPase inhibitor.	Wang and Lippard, 2005; Tadini-Buoninsegni et al., 2017
	Curcumin	Antioxidant, anti-inflammatory and anticancer effects. Antimalarial activity.	Bilmen et al., 2001; Reddy et al., 2005; Schaffer et al., 2015
Activators	Istaroxime	Cardiac drug with inotropic and lusotropic properties. Stimulatory effect on cardiac SERCA2a isoform. Therapeutic applications in acute and chronic heart failure.	Rocchetti et al., 2005; Micheletti et al., 2007; Gheorghiade et al., 2011; Ferrandi et al., 2013
	Pyridone derivative	Stimulatory effect on cardiac SERCA2a isoform. Potential therapeutic applications in heart failure.	Kaneko et al., 2017
	CDN1163	Allosteric SERCA activator. Potential pharmacological agent for diabetes and metabolic dysfunction.	Cornea et al., 2013; Gruber et al., 2014; Kang et al., 2016

As concerns other specific inhibitors of SERCA activity, CPA has been proposed to have therapeutic properties. In a study of the isolated rabbit heart CPA was found to have a cardioprotective effect on myocardial ischemia (Avellanal et al., 1998). The mechanism involved in CPA cardioprotection is not fully understood and could be partly attributed to a decreased SR calcium contribution to the calcium overload induced by ischemia.

It is noteworthy that CPA has been found to be a potent inhibitor of the SERCA ortholog PfATP6 of *Plasmodium falciparum* (Cardi et al., 2010; Arnou et al., 2011), the protozoan parasite causing malaria which is responsible for most malaria-related deaths globally. Considering that the parasite *P. falciparum* is becoming increasingly resistant to some of the most commonly used antimalarial drugs, PfATP6 has been validated as a potential and promising target for the development of new and effective antimalarials. PfATP6 and mammalian SERCA are characterized by a different pharmacological profile: compared to rabbit SERCA1a isoform from the skeletal muscle, PfATP6 is less sensitive to TG and DBHQ and exhibits a much higher affinity for CPA (Cardi et al., 2010; Arnou et al., 2011). Moreover, it was shown that PfATP6 is not inhibited by the widely employed antimalarial drug artemisinin (Cardi et al., 2010; Arnou et al., 2011), which was proposed to target PfATP6 (Eckstein-Ludwig et al., 2003). In a recent study, the interaction of CPA with PfATP6 and SERCA was characterized by molecular dynamics simulations (Di Marino et al., 2015). This study points to significant differences in the mode of CPA binding to the plasmodial and mammalian SERCA. These are useful information that can assist in the design and development of CPA derivatives, which are selective toward PfATP6 and with a reduced activity against mammalian SERCA. Besides PfATP6, the *P. falciparum* protein PfATP4, a P-type Na^+-ATPase in the plasma membrane of the parasite, has emerged as a potential antimalarial drug target and inhibition of this pump is also being considered as a possible treatment against malaria (Turner, 2016).

Among SERCA inhibitors of pharmacological interest, it is worth mentioning the polyphenolic compound curcumin (**Table 1**). Curcumin, which is obtained from the spice turmeric, is known for its antioxidant, anti-inflammatory and anticancer effects (Schaffer et al., 2015). It was reported that curcumin inhibits SERCA activity with an IC_{50} in the micromolar range (Bilmen et al., 2001; Dao et al., 2016) by stabilizing the E1 conformational state of SERCA and preventing ATP binding and ATP-dependent phosphoenzyme formation (Bilmen et al., 2001). In the search for new antimalarial agents, curcumin was shown to possess a remarkable antiplasmodial activity, as demonstrated by the inhibitory effects of curcumin on a chloroquine-resistant *P. falciparum* strain (Reddy et al., 2005). It was proposed that the PfATP6 protein could be a possible target for curcumin antimalarial action (Reddy et al., 2005). In a very recent study, selected curcumin analogs were synthesized and their antimalarial activity against different *P. falciparum* strains was evaluated (Dohutia et al., 2017). In particular, molecular docking was performed to investigate the interaction of these curcumin analogs with PfATP6. The results of this study may provide useful information for the development of curcumin derivatives which could serve as promising drug candidates against malaria.

PHARMACOLOGICAL STIMULATION OF SERCA ACTIVITY

Molecules that are able to stimulate SERCA activity have been recently identified (**Table 1**). A remarkable example

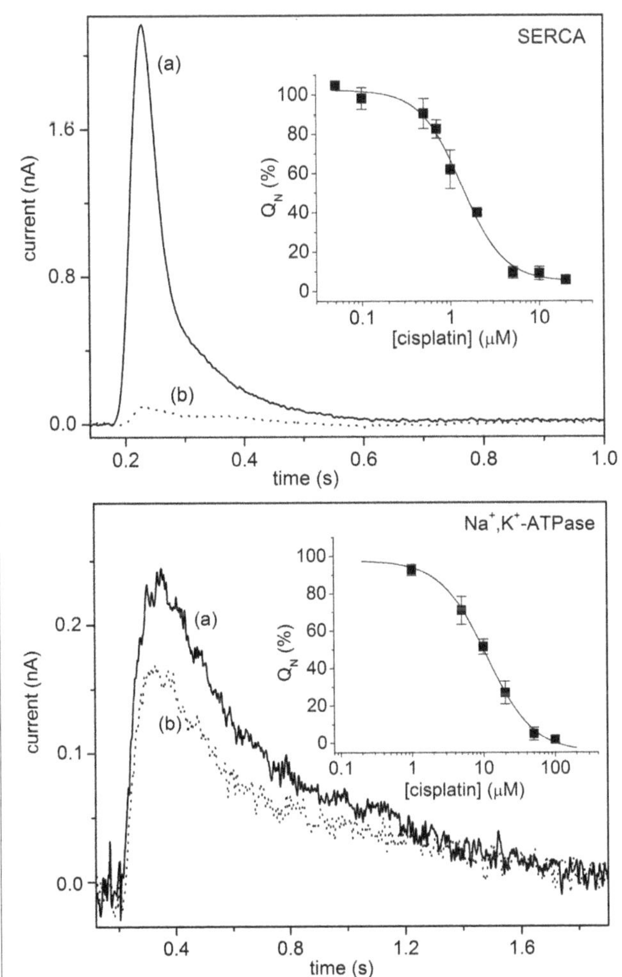

FIGURE 2 | Upper Panel: SERCA current signals induced by 100 μM ATP concentration jumps in the presence of 10 μM free Ca^{2+} and in the absence (control measurement, solid line, a) or in the presence of 5 μM cisplatin (dotted line, b). (*Inset*) Normalized charges (Q_N) related to ATP concentration jumps in the presence of Ca^{2+} ions as a function of cisplatin concentration. The charges are normalized with reference to the maximum charge attained in the absence of cisplatin (control measurement). The solid line represents the fitting curve to the ATP-induced charges ($IC_{50} = 1.3 \pm 0.1$ μM). The error bars represent S.E. of three independent measurements. **Lower Panel:** Na^+,K^+-ATPase current signals induced by 100 μM ATP concentration jumps in the presence of 80 mM NaCl and 50 mM KCl, and in the absence (control measurement, solid line, a) or in the presence of 5 μM cisplatin (dotted line, b). (*Inset*) Normalized charges (Q_N) related to ATP concentration jumps in the presence of Na^+ and K^+ ions as a function of cisplatin concentration. The charges are normalized with respect to the maximum charge measured in the absence of cisplatin (control measurement). The solid line represents the fitting curve to the ATP-induced charges ($IC_{50} = 11.1 \pm 0.8$ μM). The error bars represent S.E. of three independent measurements. Tadini-Buoninsegni et al. (2017)—Reproduced by permission of The Royal Society of Chemistry.

of SERCA activators is the drug istaroxime. Istaroxime is an innovative cardiac drug which combines inotropic (cardiomyocyte contraction) and lusotropic (cardiomyocyte relaxation) properties (Hasenfuss and Teerlink, 2011). Istaroxime has a double mechanism of action, i.e., it inhibits Na^+,K^+-ATPase activity and exerts a stimulatory effect on SERCA2a (Micheletti et al., 2002, 2007; Rocchetti et al., 2005, 2008), the SERCA isoform in the heart which is central to cardiac electrophysiological and mechanical function. Preclinical studies and clinical trials indicate that combining SERCA2a stimulation and Na^+,K^+-ATPase inhibition may increase contractility and facilitate active relaxation, improving both systolic and diastolic heart function (Gheorghiade et al., 2011). The stimulatory effect of istaroxime on SERCA activity was investigated by combining different experimental methods, including electrophysiological measurements on dog cardiac SR vesicles adsorbed to a SSM (Ferrandi et al., 2013). This study shows that istaroxime enhances SERCA2a activity, Ca^{2+} uptake, and Ca^{2+}-dependent charge movements into SR vesicles from healthy or failing dog hearts. It was proposed that istaroxime acts by displacing the regulatory protein phospholamban (PLN) from the SERCA2a/PLN complex, thereby removing the inhibitory effect of PLN on this complex. Displacement of PLN from SERCA2a may favor the SERCA2a conformational transition E_2 to E_1, thus accelerating Ca^{2+} cycling. Istaroxime with its unique mode of action may provide a new small-molecule therapeutics for the treatment of both acute and chronic heart failure.

Very recently, a pyridone derivative was reported to activate the SERCA2a isoform by attenuating the inhibitory effect of PLN (Kaneko et al., 2017). *In vitro* and *in vivo* experiments have demonstrated that the pyridone derivative stimulates the Ca^{2+}-dependent ATPase activity of cardiac SR vesicles, increases Ca^{2+} transients of isolated adult rat cardiomyocytes and accelerates contraction and relaxation of isolated perfused rat hearts. It was concluded that the pyridone derivative behaves like a SERCA2a activator, which binds and inhibits PLN, and enhances systolic and diastolic functions of the heart. The pyridone derivative is thus proposed as a novel lead compound for therapeutic applications in heart failure.

Impaired SERCA function leads to elevation of intracellular calcium concentration and alterations in calcium homeostasis, which trigger endoplasmic reticulum (ER) stress. ER stress is associated with a variety of common diseases (Oyadomari and Mori, 2004), including the metabolic syndrome and type 2 diabetes (Back and Kaufman, 2012). Pharmacological activation of SERCA can reduce ER stress and may therefore represent a novel strategy for the treatment of diabetes and metabolic disorders. A recent study (Kang et al., 2016) evaluated the metabolic effects of the quinoline-amide compound CDN1163, which is a novel SERCA activator (Cornea et al., 2013; Gruber et al., 2014). CDN1163 directly binds to the SERCA enzyme to activate Ca^{2+}-ATPase activity, probably via an allosteric mechanism (Cornea et al., 2013; Gruber et al., 2014). Kang et al. (2016) demonstrated that CDN1163 activation of the SERCA2b isoform from mouse liver reduces ER stress and improves mitochondrial efficiency and metabolic parameters in an animal model of insulin resistance and type 2 diabetes (*ob/ob* mice), suggesting that SERCA activators may represent promising pharmacological agents to treat diabetes and metabolic dysfunction. Finally, since defective SERCA is a significant cause of ER stress and neuron loss in Parkinson's disease, direct activation of SERCA by small-molecule drugs is currently explored as a viable strategy to develop a novel therapeutic approach to cure Parkinson's disease (Dahl, 2017).

CONCLUSIONS

SERCA plays an essential role in the maintenance of cellular calcium homeostasis and calcium pump malfunction is associated to severe disorders and several pathophysiological conditions. Therefore, the SERCA enzyme represents an important target for the development of new drugs. SERCA inhibitors have been identified as potential drug candidates against various diseases. As discussed above, inhibition of SERCA activity in cancer cells provides an alternative therapeutic approach to cure different types of cancer. Moreover, specific inhibitors targeting the SERCA ortholog PfATP6 in the parasite *P. falciparum* may serve as innovative and effective antimalarial agents. In addition, studies on novel SERCA activators indicate that pharmacological activation of SERCA may constitute a promising strategy for the treatment of heart failure and diabetes. Research effort is devoted to the synthesis of highly selective and potent drugs, that can target SERCA in a tissue-specific manner. As most tissue/cell types can express more than one SERCA isoform, it would be highly desirable, although very challenging, to develop isoform-specific drugs that can interact selectively with one SERCA isoform, leaving the other protein molecules intact (Yatime et al., 2009; Michelangeli and East, 2011).

AUTHOR CONTRIBUTIONS

FT-B: Wrote the manuscript and revised it critically for important intellectual content; SS, RG, and MM: Edited the manuscript and revised it critically for important intellectual content; SS: Helped FT-B in preparing the figures. All authors have read and agreed with the final version of the manuscript.

ACKNOWLEDGMENTS

The Italian Ministry of Education, University and Research (MIUR) and Ente Cassa di Risparmio di Firenze are gratefully acknowledged for support.

REFERENCES

Andersen, T. B., López, C. Q., Manczak, T., Martinez, K., and Simonsen, H. T. (2015). Thapsigargin-from *Thapsia* L. to mipsagargin. *Molecules* 20, 6113–6127. doi: 10.3390/molecules20046113

Arnou, B., Montigny, C., Morth, J. P., Nissen, P., Jaxel, C., Møller, J. V., et al. (2011). The *Plasmodium falciparum* Ca^{2+}-ATPase PfATP6: insensitive to artemisinin, but a potential drug target. *Biochem. Soc. Trans.* 39, 823–831. doi: 10.1042/BST0390823

Avellanal, M., Rodriguez, P., and Barrigon, S. (1998). Protective effects of cyclopiazonic acid on ischemia-reperfusion injury in rabbit hearts. *J. Cardiovasc. Pharmacol.* 32, 845–851. doi: 10.1097/00005344-199811000-00022

Back, S. H., and Kaufman, R. J. (2012). Endoplasmic reticulum stress and type 2 diabetes. *Annu. Rev. Biochem.* 81, 767–793. doi: 10.1146/annurev-biochem-072909-095555

Bartolommei, G., Tadini-Buoninsegni, F., Moncelli, M. R., Gemma, S., Camodeca, C., Butini, S., et al. (2011). The Ca^{2+}-ATPase (SERCA1) is inhibited by 4-aminoquinoline derivatives through interference with catalytic activation by Ca^{2+}, whereas the ATPase E_2 state remains functional. *J. Biol. Chem.* 286, 38383–38389. doi: 10.1074/jbc.M111.287276

Bazzone, A., Barthmes, M., and Fendler, K. (2017). SSM-based electrophysiology for transporter research. *Methods Enzymol.* 594, 31–83. doi: 10.1016/bs.mie.2017.05.008

Berman, M. C., and Karlish, S. J. (2003). Interaction of an aromatic dibromoisothiouronium derivative with the Ca^{2+}-ATPase of skeletal muscle sarcoplasmic reticulum. *Biochemistry* 42, 3556–3566. doi: 10.1021/bi026071n

Bilmen, J. G., Khan, S. Z., Javed, M. H., and Michelangeli, F. (2001). Inhibition of the SERCA Ca^{2+} pumps by curcumin. Curcumin putatively stabilizes the interaction between the nucleotide-binding and phosphorylation domains in the absence of ATP. *Eur. J. Biochem.* 268, 6318–6327. doi: 10.1046/j.0014-2956.2001.02589.x

Brini, M., and Carafoli, E. (2009). Calcium pumps in health and disease. *Physiol. Rev.* 89, 1341–1378. doi: 10.1152/physrev.00032.2008

Bublitz, M., Morth, J. P., and Nissen, P. (2011). P-type ATPases at a glance. *J. Cell Sci.* 124, 2515–2519. doi: 10.1242/jcs.088716

Bublitz, M., Musgaard, M., Poulsen, H., Thøgersen, L., Olesen, C., Schiøtt, B., et al. (2013). Ion pathways in the sarcoplasmic reticulum Ca^{2+}-ATPase. *J. Biol. Chem.* 288, 10759–10765. doi: 10.1074/jbc.R112.436550

Cardi, D., Pozza, A., Arnou, B., Marchal, E., Clausen, J. D., Andersen, J. P., et al. (2010). Purified E255L mutant SERCA1a and purified PfATP6 are sensitive to SERCA-type inhibitors but insensitive to artemisinins. *J. Biol. Chem.* 285, 26406–26416. doi: 10.1074/jbc.M109.090340

Cornea, R. L., Gruber, S. J., Lockamy, E. L., Muretta, J. M., Jin, D., Chen, J., et al. (2013). High-throughput FRET assay yields allosteric SERCA activators. *J. Biomol. Screen.* 18, 97–107. doi: 10.1177/1087057112456878

Cui, C., Merritt, R., Fu, L., and Pan, Z. (2017). Targeting calcium signaling in cancer therapy. *Acta Pharm. Sin. B* 7, 3–17. doi: 10.1016/j.apsb.2016.11.001

Dahl, R. (2017). A new target for Parkinson's disease: small molecule SERCA activator CDN1163 ameliorates dyskinesia in 6-OHDA-lesioned rats. *Bioorg. Med. Chem.* 25, 53–57. doi: 10.1016/j.bmc.2016.10.008

Dao, T. T., Sehgal, P., Tung, T. T., Møller, J. V., Nielsen, J., Palmgren, M., et al. (2016). Demethoxycurcumin is a potent inhibitor of P-Type ATPases from diverse kingdoms of life. *PLoS ONE* 11:e0163260. doi: 10.1371/journal.pone.0163260

de Meis, L., and Vianna, A. L. (1979). Energy interconversion by the Ca^{2+}-dependent ATPase of the sarcoplasmic reticulum. *Annu. Rev. Biochem.* 48, 275–292. doi: 10.1146/annurev.bi.48.070179.001423

Denmeade, S. R., Mhaka, A. M., Rosen, D. M., Brennen, W. N., Dalrymple, S., Dach, I., et al. (2012). Engineering a prostate-specific membrane antigen-activated tumor endothelial cell prodrug for cancer therapy. *Sci. Transl. Med.* 4:140ra86. doi: 10.1126/scitranslmed.3003886

Di Marino, D., D'Annessa, I., Coletta, A., Via, A., and Tramontano, A. (2015). Characterization of the differences in the cyclopiazonic acid binding mode to mammalian and *P. falciparum* Ca^{2+} pumps: a computational study. *Proteins* 83, 564–574. doi: 10.1002/prot.24734

Doan, N. T., Paulsen, E. S., Sehgal, P., Møller, J. V., Nissen, P., Denmeade, S. R., et al. (2015). Targeting thapsigargin towards tumors. *Steroids* 97, 2–7. doi: 10.1016/j.steroids.2014.07.009

Dohutia, C., Chetia, D., Gogoi, K., and Sarma, K. (2017). Design, *in silico* and *in vitro* evaluation of curcumin analogues against *Plasmodium falciparum*. *Exp. Parasitol.* 175, 51–58. doi: 10.1016/j.exppara.2017.02.006

Eckstein-Ludwig, U., Webb, R. J., Van Goethem, I. D., East, J. M., Lee, A. G., Kimura, M., et al. (2003). Artemisinins target the SERCA of *Plasmodium falciparum*. *Nature* 424, 957–961. doi: 10.1038/nature01813

Ferrandi, M., Barassi, P., Tadini-Buoninsegni, F., Bartolommei, G., Molinari, I., Tripodi, M. G., et al. (2013). Istaroxime stimulates SERCA2a and accelerates calcium cycling in heart failure by relieving phospholamban inhibition. *Br. J. Pharmacol.* 169, 1849–1861. doi: 10.1111/bph.12278

Gheorghiade, M., Ambrosy, A. P., Ferrandi, M., and Ferrari, P. (2011). Combining SERCA2a activation and Na-K ATPase inhibition: a promising new approach to managing acute heart failure syndromes with low cardiac output. *Discov. Med.* 12, 141–151.

Gruber, S. J., Cornea, R. L., Li, J., Peterson, K. C., Schaaf, T. M., Gillispie, G. D., et al. (2014). Discovery of enzyme modulators via high-throughput time-resolved FRET in living cells. *J. Biomol. Screen.* 19, 215–222. doi: 10.1177/1087057113510740

Hasenfuss, G., and Teerlink, J. R. (2011). Cardiac inotropes: current agents and future directions. *Eur. Heart J.* 32, 1838–1845. doi: 10.1093/eurheartj/ehr026

Inesi, G., Hua, S., Xu, C., Ma, H., Seth, M., Prasad, A. M., et al. (2005). Studies of Ca^{2+} ATPase (SERCA) inhibition. *J. Bioenerg. Biomembr.* 37, 365–368. doi: 10.1007/s10863-005-9472-1

Inesi, G., Pilankatta, R., and Tadini-Buoninsegni, F. (2014). Biochemical characterization of P-type copper ATPases. *Biochem. J.* 463, 167–176. doi: 10.1042/BJ20140741

Inesi, G., and Tadini-Buoninsegni, F. (2014). Ca^{2+}/H^{+} exchange, lumenal Ca^{2+} release and Ca^{2+}/ATP coupling ratios in the sarcoplasmic reticulum ATPase. *J. Cell Commun. Signal.* 8, 5–11. doi: 10.1007/s12079-013-0213-7

Kaneko, M., Yamamoto, H., Sakai, H., Kamada, Y., Tanaka, T., Fujiwara, S., et al. (2017). A pyridone derivative activates SERCA2a by attenuating the inhibitory effect of phospholamban. *Eur. J. Pharmacol.* 814, 1–8. doi: 10.1016/j.ejphar.2017.07.035

Kang, S., Dahl, R., Hsieh, W., Shin, A., Zsebo, K. M., Buettner, C., et al. (2016). Small molecular allosteric activator of the sarco/endoplasmic reticulum Ca^{2+}-ATPase (SERCA) attenuates diabetes and metabolic disorders. *J. Biol. Chem.* 291, 5185–5198. doi: 10.1074/jbc.M115.705012

Kelety, B., Diekert, K., Tobien, J., Watzke, N., Dörner, W., Obrdlik, P., et al. (2006). Transporter assays using solid supported membranes: a novel screening platform for drug discovery. *Assay Drug. Dev. Technol.* 4, 575–582. doi: 10.1089/adt.2006.4.575

Kühlbrandt, W. (2004). Biology, structure and mechanism of P-type ATPases. *Nat. Rev. Mol. Cell Biol.* 5, 282–295. doi: 10.1038/nrm1354

Laursen, M., Bublitz, M., Moncoq, K., Olesen, C., Møller, J. V., Young, H. S., et al. (2009). Cyclopiazonic acid is complexed to a divalent metal ion when bound to the sarcoplasmic reticulum Ca^{2+}-ATPase. *J. Biol. Chem.* 284, 13513–13518. doi: 10.1074/jbc.C900031200

Lewis, D., Pilankatta, R., Inesi, G., Bartolommei, G., Moncelli, M. R., and Tadini-Buoninsegni, F. (2012). Distinctive features of catalytic and transport mechanisms in mammalian sarco-endoplasmic reticulum Ca^{2+} ATPase (SERCA) and Cu^{+} (ATP7A/B) ATPases. *J. Biol. Chem.* 287, 32717–32727. doi: 10.1074/jbc.M112.373472

Liu, Y., Pilankatta, R., Lewis, D., Inesi, G., Tadini-Buoninsegni, F., Bartolommei, G., et al. (2009). High-yield heterologous expression of wild type and mutant Ca^{2+} ATPase: characterization of Ca^{2+} binding sites by charge transfer. *J. Mol. Biol.* 391, 858–871. doi: 10.1016/j.jmb.2009.06.044

Michelangeli, F., and East, J. M. (2011). A diversity of SERCA Ca^{2+} pump inhibitors. *Biochem. Soc. Trans.* 39, 789–797. doi: 10.1042/BST0390789

Micheletti, R., Mattera, G. G., Rocchetti, M., Schiavone, A., Loi, M. F., Zaza, A., et al. (2002). Pharmacological profile of the novel inotropic agent (E,Z)-3-((2-aminoethoxy)imino)androstane-6,17-dione hydrochloride (PST2744). *J. Pharmacol. Exp. Ther.* 303, 592–600. doi: 10.1124/jpet.102.038331

Micheletti, R., Palazzo, F., Barassi, P., Giacalone, G., Ferrandi, M., Schiavone, A., et al. (2007). Istaroxime, a stimulator of sarcoplasmic reticulum calcium adenosine triphosphatase isoform 2a activity, as a novel therapeutic approach to heart failure. *Am. J. Cardiol.* 99, 24A–32A. doi: 10.1016/j.amjcard.2006.09.003

Møller, J. V., Olesen, C., Winther, A. M., and Nissen, P. (2010). The sarcoplasmic Ca^{2+}-ATPase: design of a perfect chemi-osmotic pump. *Q. Rev. Biophys.* 43, 501–566. doi: 10.1017/S003358351000017X

Moncoq, K., Trieber, C. A., and Young, H. S. (2007). The molecular basis for cyclopiazonic acid inhibition of the sarcoplasmic reticulum calcium pump. *J. Biol. Chem.* 282, 9748–9757. doi: 10.1074/jbc.M611653200

Moore, G. A., McConkey, D. J., Kass, G. E., O'Brien, P. J., and Orrenius, S. (1987). 2,5-Di(tert-butyl)-1,4-benzohydroquinone–a novel inhibitor of liver microsomal Ca^{2+} sequestration. *FEBS Lett.* 224, 331–336. doi: 10.1016/0014-5793(87)80479-9

Obara, K., Miyashita, N., Xu, C., Toyoshima, I., Sugita, Y., Inesi, G., et al. (2005). Structural role of countertransport revealed in Ca^{2+} pump crystal structure in the absence of Ca^{2+}. *Proc. Natl. Acad. Sci. U.S.A.* 102, 14489–14496. doi: 10.1073/pnas.0506222102

Olesen, C., Sørensen, T. L., Nielsen, R. C., Møller, J. V., and Nissen, P. (2004). Dephosphorylation of the calcium pump coupled to counterion occlusion. *Science* 306, 2251–2255. doi: 10.1126/science.1106289

Oyadomari, S., and Mori, M. (2004). Roles of CHOP/GADD153 in endoplasmic reticulum stress. *Cell Death Differ.* 11, 381–389. doi: 10.1038/sj.cdd.4401373

Pintschovius, J., and Fendler, K. (1999). Charge translocation by the Na^{+}/K^{+}-ATPase investigated on solid supported membranes: rapid solution exchange with a new technique. *Biophys. J.* 76, 814–826. doi: 10.1016/S0006-3495(99)77245-0

Pintschovius, J., Fendler, K., and Bamberg, E. (1999). Charge translocation by the Na^{+}/K^{+}-ATPase investigated on solid supported membranes: cytoplasmic cation binding and release. *Biophys. J.* 76, 827–836. doi: 10.1016/S0006-3495(99)77246-2

Rasmussen, U., Brøogger Christensen, S., and Sandberg, F. (1978). Thapsigargine and thapsigargicine, two new histamine liberators from *Thapsia garganica* L. *Acta Pharm. Suec.* 15, 133–140.

Reddy, R. C., Vatsala, P. G., Keshamouni, V. G., Padmanaban, G., and Rangarajan, P. N. (2005). Curcumin for malaria therapy. *Biochem. Biophys. Res. Commun.* 326, 472–474. doi: 10.1016/j.bbrc.2004.11.051

Rocchetti, M., Alemanni, M., Mostacciuolo, G., Barassi, P., Altomare, C., Chisci, R., et al. (2008). Modulation of sarcoplasmic reticulum function by PST2744 [istaroxime; (E,Z)-3-((2-aminoethoxy)imino) androstane-6,17-dione hydrochloride)] in a pressure-overload heart failure model. *J. Pharmacol. Exp. Ther.* 326, 957–965. doi: 10.1124/jpet.108.138701

Rocchetti, M., Besana, A., Mostacciuolo, G., Micheletti, R., Ferrari, P., Sarkozi, S., et al. (2005). Modulation of sarcoplasmic reticulum function by Na^{+}/K^{+} pump inhibitors with different toxicity: digoxin and PST2744 [(E,Z)-3-((2-aminoethoxy)imino)androstane-6,17-dione hydrochloride]. *J. Pharmacol. Exp. Ther.* 313, 207–215. doi: 10.1124/jpet.104.077933

Sadafi, F. Z., Massai, L., Bartolommei, G., Moncelli, M. R., Messori, L., and Tadini-Buoninsegni, F. (2014). Anticancer ruthenium(III) complex KP1019 interferes with ATP-dependent Ca^{2+} translocation by sarco-endoplasmic reticulum Ca^{2+}-ATPase (SERCA). *ChemMedChem* 9, 1660–1664. doi: 10.1002/cmdc.201402128

Sagara, Y., and Inesi, G. (1991). Inhibition of the sarcoplasmic reticulum Ca^{2+} transport ATPase by thapsigargin at subnanomolar concentrations. *J. Biol. Chem.* 266, 13503–13506.

Schaffer, M., Schaffer, P. M., and Bar-Sela, G. (2015). An update on Curcuma as a functional food in the control of cancer and inflammation. *Curr. Opin. Clin. Nutr. Metab. Care.* 18, 605–611. doi: 10.1097/MCO.0000000000000227

Schulz, P., Garcia-Celma, J. J., and Fendler, K. (2008). SSM-based electrophysiology. *Methods* 46, 97–103. doi: 10.1016/j.ymeth.2008.07.002

Seidler, N. W., Jona, I., Vegh, M., and Martonosi, A. (1989). Cyclopiazonic acid is a specific inhibitor of the Ca^{2+}-ATPase of sarcoplasmic reticulum. *J. Biol. Chem.* 264, 17816–17823.

Tadini-Buoninsegni, F., and Bartolommei, G. (2016). Electrophysiological measurements on solid supported membranes. *Methods Mol. Biol.* 1377, 293–303. doi: 10.1007/978-1-4939-3179-8_26

Tadini-Buoninsegni, F., Bartolommei, G., Moncelli, M. R., and Fendler, K. (2008a). Charge transfer in P-type ATPases investigated on planar membranes. *Arch. Biochem. Biophys.* 476, 75–86. doi: 10.1016/j.abb.2008.02.031

Tadini-Buoninsegni, F., Bartolommei, G., Moncelli, M. R., Guidelli, R., and Inesi, G. (2006). Pre-steady state electrogenic events of Ca^{2+}/H^{+} exchange and transport by the Ca^{2+}-ATPase. *J. Biol. Chem.* 281, 37720–37727. doi: 10.1074/jbc.M606040200

Tadini-Buoninsegni, F., Bartolommei, G., Moncelli, M. R., Inesi, G., Galliani, A., Sinisi, M., et al. (2014). Translocation of platinum anticancer drugs by human copper ATPases ATP7A and ATP7B. *Angew. Chem. Int. Ed. Engl.* 53, 1297–1301. doi: 10.1002/anie.201307718

Tadini-Buoninsegni, F., Bartolommei, G., Moncelli, M. R., Tal, D. M., Lewis, D., and Inesi, G. (2008b). Effects of high-affinity inhibitors on partial reactions, charge movements, and conformational states of the Ca^{2+} transport ATPase (sarco-endoplasmic reticulum Ca^{2+} ATPase). *Mol. Pharmacol.* 73, 1134–1140. doi: 10.1124/mol.107.043745

Tadini-Buoninsegni, F., and Smeazzetto, S. (2017). Mechanisms of charge transfer in human copper ATPases ATP7A and ATP7B. *IUBMB Life* 69, 218–225. doi: 10.1002/iub.1603

Tadini-Buoninsegni, F., Sordi, G., Smeazzetto, S., Natile, G., and Arnesano, F. (2017). Effect of cisplatin on the transport activity of P_{II}-type ATPases. *Metallomics* 9, 960–968. doi: 10.1039/C7MT00100B

Toyoshima, C. (2008). Structural aspects of ion pumping by Ca^{2+}-ATPase of sarcoplasmic reticulum. *Arch. Biochem. Biophys.* 476, 3–11. doi: 10.1016/j.abb.2008.04.017

Toyoshima, C., and Cornelius, F. (2013). New crystal structures of PII-type ATPases: excitement continues. *Curr. Opin. Struct. Biol.* 23, 507–514. doi: 10.1016/j.sbi.2013.06.005

Toyoshima, C., and Nomura, H. (2002). Structural changes in the calcium pump accompanying the dissociation of calcium. *Nature* 418, 605–611. doi: 10.1038/nature00944

Turner, H. (2016). Spiroindolone NITD609 is a novel antimalarial drug that targets the P-type ATPase PfATP4. *Future Med. Chem.* 8, 227–238. doi: 10.4155/fmc.15.177

Wang, D., and Lippard, S. J. (2005). Cellular processing of platinum anticancer drugs. *Nat. Rev. Drug Discov.* 4, 307–320. doi: 10.1038/nrd1691

Xu, C., Ma, H., Inesi, G., Al-Shawi, M. K., and Toyoshima, C. (2004). Specific structural requirements for the inhibitory effect of thapsigargin on the Ca^{2+} ATPase SERCA. *J. Biol. Chem.* 279, 17973–17979. doi: 10.1074/jbc.M313263200

Yatime, L., Buch-Pedersen, M. J., Musgaard, M., Morth, J. P., Lund Winther, A. M., Pedersen, B. P., et al. (2009). P-type ATPases as drug targets: tools for medicine and science. *Biochim. Biophys. Acta* 1787, 207–220. doi: 10.1016/j.bbabio.2008.12.019

3

Ligand Screening Systems for Human Glucose Transporters as Tools in Drug Discovery

Sina Schmidl[1], Cristina V. Iancu[2], Jun-yong Choe[2] and Mislav Oreb[1*]*

[1] *Institute of Molecular Biosciences, Goethe University Frankfurt, Frankfurt am Main, Germany,* [2] *Department of Biochemistry and Molecular Biology, Rosalind Franklin University of Medicine and Science, North Chicago, IL, United States*

***Correspondence:**
Jun-yong Choe
junyong.choe@rosalindfranklin.edu
Mislav Oreb
m.oreb@bio.uni-frankfurt.de

Hexoses are the major source of energy and carbon skeletons for biosynthetic processes in all kingdoms of life. Their cellular uptake is mediated by specialized transporters, including glucose transporters (GLUT, SLC2 gene family). Malfunction or altered expression pattern of GLUTs in humans is associated with several widespread diseases including cancer, diabetes and severe metabolic disorders. Their high relevance in the medical area makes these transporters valuable drug targets and potential biomarkers. Nevertheless, the lack of a suitable high-throughput screening system has impeded the determination of compounds that would enable specific manipulation of GLUTs so far. Availability of structural data on several GLUTs enabled *in silico* ligand screening, though limited by the fact that only two major conformations of the transporters can be tested. Recently, convenient high-throughput microbial and cell-free screening systems have been developed. These remarkable achievements set the foundation for further and detailed elucidation of the molecular mechanisms of glucose transport and will also lead to great progress in the discovery of GLUT effectors as therapeutic agents. In this mini-review, we focus on recent efforts to identify potential GLUT-targeting drugs, based on a combination of structural biology and different assay systems.

Keywords: glucose transport, sugar transport inhibitors, screening system, sugar transport assays, drug discovery, hxt^0 strain

INTRODUCTION

In human cell membranes, glucose transporter family members (GLUT, gene family SLC2) facilitate the diffusion of glucose and related monosaccharides along the concentration gradient. The 14 GLUTs are grouped according to phylogenetic homology into 3 classes: class I with GLUT1-4 (all transport glucose, GLUT2 also transports fructose), class II with GLUT5, 7, 9, and 11 (all transport fructose and glucose except for GLUT5—a fructose-only transporter; GLUT9 also transports uric acid), and class III with GLUT6, 8, 10, 12, and 13 (all transport glucose, except for GLUT13, which is a myo-inositol/proton symporter) (Thorens and Mueckler, 2010; Mueckler and Thorens, 2013). Other GLUT substrates are galactose, mannose, glucosamine, and dehydroascorbic acid. GLUTs differ in transport capacity, substrate affinity and specificity, and tissue distribution; the latter reflects local physiological needs. Alterations in the function, localization or expression of GLUTs are associated with Mendelian disorders (Santer et al., 1997; Seidner et al., 1998), cancer (Thorens and Mueckler, 2010; Barron et al., 2016), diabetes (Elsas and Longo, 1992), obesity (Song and Wolfe, 2007), gout (George and Keenan, 2013), non-alcoholic fatty liver disease (Douard and Ferraris, 2013), and renal disease (Kawamura et al., 2011). Thus GLUTs are important subjects for medical research and show great potential as drug targets for the treatment of a number of these diseases for instance in cancer therapy. It is known that cancer cells show an increased expression of glucose transporters to meet their need for higher energy demand due to uncontrolled proliferation (Warburg, 1956; Cairns et al., 2011). A higher expression rate of several GLUTs has already been identified in various kinds of tumors (Szablewski, 2013). Most prominently, higher expression rates of GLUT1 have been found in most cancer tissues (Godoy et al., 2006) and studies indicate that this overexpression is an early event in the course of the disease (Rudlowski et al., 2003; Macheda et al., 2005). Various studies also related abnormal expression of other transporters, including GLUT4, GLUT6, GLUT7, GLUT8, GLUT11, and GLUT12, with the fast proliferation of cancer cells (Rogers et al., 2002; Godoy et al., 2006; McBrayer et al., 2012); GLUT5 was found in breast cancer tissue but was absent in normal breast tissue (Zamora-León et al., 1996). Metabolites which specifically modify the activity of certain GLUT isoforms would therefore be very valuable for cancer therapy which is furthermore encouraged by studies showing that cancer cells die faster than normal cells under glucose-limiting conditions (Liu et al., 2010).

Diabetes mellitus type 2 is another prominent example of a GLUT-related disease whereas GLUT4 is considered a key player in the pathogenesis of this disease. This transporter is predominantly expressed in adipose tissue, heart, and skeletal muscle and is stored in small vesicles in the cytoplasm until insulin triggers its translocation to the plasma membrane, where it mediates glucose uptake (Hajiaghaalipour et al., 2015). Diabetic type 2 cells show diminished expression of GLUT4 as well as impaired trafficking to the plasma membrane (Patel et al., 2006). Furthermore, a proper anchoring of GLUT2 at the surface of β-cells seems to be crucial for the physiological glucose-uptake in these cells which is in turn required for normal glucose-stimulated insulin secretion (Ohtsubo et al., 2005). Reduced stability of GLUT2 in the plasma membrane disrupts insulin secretion and therefore favors the development of type 2 diabetes (Ohtsubo et al., 2005). Substrates with the ability to modulate altered functions of GLUTs involved in the pathogenesis of diabetes might contribute to the therapy and diminish symptoms of diabetes type 2 patients.

Given the complex role that GLUTs play in different diseases the discovery of GLUT-selective is highly desirable. Recent advances in three-dimensional structure determination of GLUTs and their homologs (Sun et al., 2012; Iancu et al., 2013; Deng et al., 2014; Nomura et al., 2015) finally make structure-based drug design possible, as exemplified by two HIV integrase inhibitors Raltegravir and Elvitegravir (Williamson et al., 2012). In particular, *in silico* ligand screening studies have uncovered GLUT-specific inhibitors for the first time. In this mini-review article, we will summarize the current efforts to identify potential GLUT-targeting drugs, based on a combination of structural biology and different assay systems.

STRUCTURE-BASED DISCOVERY OF COMPOUNDS TARGETING GLUTs

GLUTs belong to the sugar porter family of the Major Facilitator Superfamily (MFS) proteins (Saier et al., 1999; www.tcdb.org), one of the largest and most ubiquitous protein families. As other MFS proteins, GLUTs have 12 transmembrane helices organized into two 6-helices domains (the N- and C-halves); a central polar cavity formed between the N- and C-domains contains the substrate binding site. GLUTs have an alternating access transport mechanism whereby the substrate cavity presents in turn to either the lumen (outward-facing conformation) or cytoplasm (inward-facing conformation). Crystal structures of GLUTs and their homologs have captured outward- and inward-facing conformations, in different ligation states (apo, with substrate or inhibitors), with the substrate cavity open (open conformation) to or partially shielded (occluded conformation) from solvent (Sun et al., 2012; Iancu et al., 2013; Deng et al., 2014; Nomura et al., 2015; Kapoor et al., 2016; see **Table 1**). Comparison of the crystal structures of GLUT1 inward-open conformation and GLUT3 outward-facing conformations (outward-occluded and –open), suggest that the alternating access mechanism involves a rigid-body rotation of the N-terminal half relative to the C-terminal half and rearrangements in the substrate interactions with residues mostly from the C-terminal domain (Deng et al., 2015). Ligand docking studies of substrate and inhibitors to different conformations of GLUT1, based on crystal structures of GLUT1, GLUT3 and the bacterial homolog XylE, show conformation-dependent variation in the number and location of the ligand binding sites: several potential glucose binding sites (three for the outward-open conformation, two for the outward-occluded conformation and one each for the inward-occluded and inward-open conformations) and, in the case of GLUT1 inhibitors, two maltose binding sites in the outward-facing conformation, and two sites for cytochalasin B in the outward-facing conformation (Lloyd et al., 2017). Obviously, structure-based ligand screening for GLUTs will need to employ all available conformations of a transporter.

Structure-based drug discovery relies on reliable 3D structures of a target protein, *in silico* ligand screening with libraries of small compounds, and assay systems to validate and characterize the ligand candidates. Subsequent rounds of chemical optimization, informed by structure-based design, may further increase the potency and specificity of the identified ligands (Sliwoski et al., 2014; Schreiber et al., 2015).

So far, *in silico* ligand screening has been reported for GLUT1, GLUT4, and GLUT5 (Mishra et al., 2015; George Thompson et al., 2016; Ung et al., 2016). This is a high-throughput ligand screening method in which millions of small compounds are assessed computationally for their ability to bind to a target structure (Colas et al., 2016). **Table 2** lists GLUT inhibitors with IC_{50} under 20 μM uncovered through *in silico* ligand screening studies. Human GLUT crystal structures were unavailable at the time of the initial virtual screening, so structural models were based on the crystal structures of bacterial GLUT homologs or

TABLE 1 | Crystal structures of GLUTs and their homologs.

Protein	Source	Conformation	PDB ID	References
Xylose/H^+ symporter	*Escherichia coli*	Outward-occluded	4GBY	Sun et al., 2012
			4GBZ	
			4GC0	
		Inward-open	4JA4	Quistgaard et al., 2013
			4JA3	
		Inward-open	4QIQ	Wisedchaisri et al., 2014
Glucose/H^+ symporter	*Staphylococcus epidermidis*	Inward-open	4LDS	Iancu et al., 2013
GLUT1	*Homo sapiens*	Inward-open	4PYP	Deng et al., 2014
		Inward-open	5EQI	Kapoor et al., 2016
			5EQG	
			5EGH	
GLUT3	*Homo sapiens*	Outward-occluded	4ZW9	Deng et al., 2015
		Outward-occluded	4ZWB	
		Outward-open	4ZWC	
		Outward-occluded	5C65	Pike et al., 2015
GLUT5	*Rattus*	Outward-facing	4YBQ	Nomura et al., 2015
	Bos taurus	Inward-open	4YB9	

other MFS proteins (**Table 2**) and represented either the inward-facing conformation (GLUT4 and GLUT5) or the outward-facing conformation (GLUT1). The number of molecules in the screen library varied: ~550,000 (Fragment Now and NCI-2007) for GLUT1, ~6 million (Chemnavigator) for GLUT5, and ~ 10 million (ZINC) for GLUT4. The number of resulting ligand candidates purchased and checked for activity against GLUTs was 17, 19, and 175, respectively, for GLUT4, GLUT1, and GLUT5. The transport assay systems were: GLUT1-expressing CHO cells, GLUT4-expressing HEK293 cells or multiple myeloma cell lines, and GLUT5 proteoliposomes. The studies identified eight GLUT1 inhibitors (including compounds A and B in **Table 2**), two GLUT4 inhibitors (compound E is a structural derivative of compound C, **Table 2**) and one GLUT5 inhibitor. Inhibitor selectivity was not established for GLUT1, but was determined at different extents for GLUT4 and GLUT5 inhibitors. Thus, compounds C and D (**Table 2**), seemed selective for GLUT4, compared to GLUT1, which is impressive given the extensive amino acid sequence conservation in the substrate binding cavity between these class I GLUTs. Compound F, did not affect the glucose transport of GLUT1, 2, 3 or 4, or the fructose transport of GLUT2, in proteoliposomes, proving to be a GLUT5-specific inhibitor. Mutagenesis studies on GLUT1, 5 and the bacterial GLUT homolog $GlcP_{Se}$ confirmed the predicted binding site of compound F in GLUT5 and identified His 387 of GLUT5 as a residue important in inhibitor selectivity. Nevertheless, whether compound F remains GLUT5-selective, compared to other class II GLUTs, in particular GLUT7, which has the equivalent of His 387, remains to be established. Subsequent chemical optimization has been done only for GLUT4 inhibitors so far. Based on compound E, Wei et al. performed SAR (structure–activity relationship) analysis and antagonist synthesis and found that compound E analogs decreased proliferation of the plasma cell malignancy multiple myeloma (Wei et al., 2017).

All the described *in silico* studies are a promising start for drug discovery efforts targeting GLUTs. Now that crystal structures for several human GLUTs are available, *in silico* studies for all GLUTs are possible. Furthermore, for the same GLUTs, inhibitors for the outward-facing and inward-facing conformations can be identified. To further establish the selectivity of the new inhibitors, GLUT-specific assay systems are required.

ASSAYS AND SCREENING SYSTEMS FOR GLUT ACTIVITY

In silico approaches usually yield a large number of compounds that need to be evaluated for their effect on hexose transport by GLUTs to select the best candidates for possible (pre)clinical trials. Thereby, an ideal assay system should be quick and inexpensive, but at the same time it must preserve the transporter's properties, e.g., in terms of transport kinetics.

In vitro (cell-free) systems offer the advantage of a strictly defined composition, which minimizes the risk of non-controllable interferences as often encountered in a complex cellular context. Thereby, studies of membrane proteins require the simulation of their native lipid environment. Different approaches have been tested with purified GLUTs to fulfill this task. Kraft et al. (2015) succeeded in producing milligram amounts of rat GLUT4 in mammalian HEK293 cells and were able to reconstitute correctly folded protein into detergent micelles, amphipols, nanodiscs and proteoliposomes. The latter are suitable for transport assays by constituting a two-compartment (outside/inside) system (Saier et al., 1999;

TABLE 2 | Leading probes for GLUTs from *in silico* ligand screening.

	Target protein	Template PDB ID	Screen library	Chemical IDs	Smiles	Synomyms	IC50 (μM)	References
A	GLUT1 Outward	4CGO (XylE)	Fragment Now, NCI-2007	PubChem CID: 417049	C1=CC=C(C(C=C1)C(C2=NC3C(=NC=NC3=O)N2)O	8-[hydroxy(phenyl) methyl]-5,9-dihydropurin-6-one	0.45	1
B	GLUT1 Outward	4CGO (XylE)	Fragment Now, NCI-2007	ZINC 17003013, PubChem CID: 250016, CAS: 13617-04-4	c1c2c(c(=O)[nH]n1)Sc3cn[nH]c(=O)c3S2	[1,4]dithiino[2,3-d:5,6-d']dipyridazine-1,6-diol	11.8	1
C	GLUT4 Inward	1PW4 (GlpT), 1PV6 (LacY), 2GFP (EmrD)	ZINC	ZINC 14974263, ChemBridge: 59900452	COc1ccccc1CCC(=O)N(Cc2ccncc2)Cc3cccc(c3)OCCc4ccc(cc4)F	N-{3-[2-(4-fluorophenyl)ethoxy]benzyl}-3-(2-methoxyphenyl) -N-(4-pyridinylmethyl)propanamide	18.9	2
D	GLUT4 Inward	1PW4 (GlpT), 1PV6 (LacY), 2GFP (EmrD)	ZINC	ZINC 11785066, ChemBridge: 27190707	C[NH+](Cc1cccc(c1)OC[C@@H]2CCCN(C2)C(=O)c3c4c([nH]n3)CCC4)Cc5ccc6c(c5)cccn6	N-methyl-1-(6-quino linyl)-N-(3-{[1-(1,4,5,6-tetrahydrocyclopenta[c]pyrazol-3-ylcarbonyl)-3-piperidinyl]methoxy}benzyl)methanamine	10.8	2
E	GLUT4 Inward	1PW4 1PV6, 2GFP	ZINC	ZINC 12152508, ChemBridge: 55751832	COc1ccc(cc1)C(=O)N(Cc2ccncc2)Cc3cccc(c3)OCCc4ccc(cc4)F	N-[[3-[2-(4-fluorophenyl)ethoxy]phenyl]methyl]-4-methoxy-N-(4-pyridyl methyl)benzamide	6.67	2
F	GLUT5 Inward	4LDS ($GlcP_{Se}$)	Chem Navigator	Structure_ID: 32283234, Enamine: Z31191163	[S](=O)(=O)(C)c1cc(c(cc1)Nc2cc3c(cc2)OCO3)[N+](=O)[O-]	N-[4-(methylsulfonyl)-2-nitrophenyl]-1,3-benzodioxol-5-amine, MSNBA	5.8	3

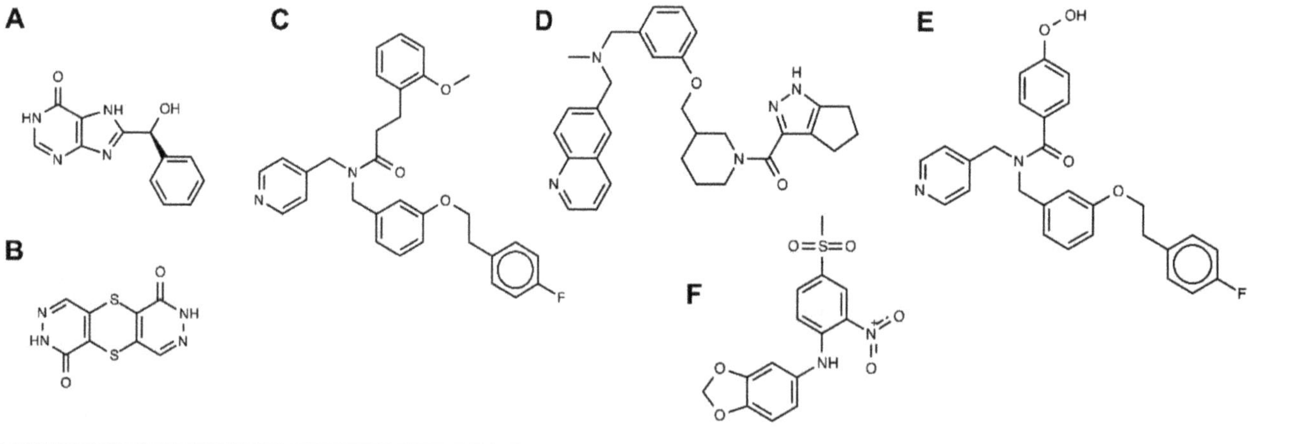

References: 1. Ung et al. (2016); 2. Mishra et al. (2015); 3. George Thompson et al. (2016).

Geertsma et al., 2008). By allowing lateral diffusion and the generation of a membrane curvature, this system best mimics the native surroundings of GLUTs compared to other *in vitro* systems (Kraft et al., 2015). A noteworthy advantage of proteoliposomes is the fact that parameters like the lipid composition or the degree of membrane curvature can be varied systematically. For instance, Hresko et al. (2016) could show that presence of anionic phospholipids in the proteoliposomes stabilized reconstituted GLUT3 and GLUT4 while conical lipids enhanced the transport rate. Besides considerable advantages, the liposome reconstitution approach also bears some drawbacks. First, for membrane reconstitution, a sufficient amount of purified protein is necessary. A general instability of membrane proteins outside of their native lipid environment and the shortcomings of most purification methods, concerning the purity or the yield of the target protein, makes the heterologous expression and purification of structurally and functionally stable protein time-, labor- and cost-intensive

(Geertsma et al., 2008; Kraft et al., 2015). Furthermore, many factors have to be taken into account and optimized for a successful membrane reconstitution, such as the application of a suitable (mild or harsh) detergent, its concentration as well as the protein-to-lipid ratio, protein-orientation and the choice for either synthetic lipids or lipid extracts (Geertsma et al., 2008) resulting in a complex handling. Nevertheless, progress has been made in the various fields of protein purification and stability (Kraft et al., 2015), improving the utility of proteoliposomes for transport assays. For instance, proteoliposomes were successfully used to assess the effect of inhibitors of GLUT1 (George Thompson et al., 2015) and GLUT5 (George Thompson et al., 2015, 2016).

As a complementary approach that avoids laborious protein purification and reconstitution procedures, different cell-based systems for assaying GLUTs have been employed.

Functional expression of membrane proteins in *Xenopus laevis* oocytes opened the gate for closer molecular characterization (Hediger et al., 1987). Early experiments on GLUT1-5 in this expression system already yielded valuable information about the kinetic properties, substrate selectivity and effective inhibitors of the transporters (Birnbaum, 1989; Gould and Lienhard, 1989; Keller et al., 1989; Kayano et al., 1990; Gould et al., 1991). The system was proven to be suitable for investigating GLUT functions, due to a low endogenous GLUT expression in frog oocytes (Gould and Lienhard, 1989). Additionally, the large size of these cells facilitates handling and allows their application for electrophysiological experiments (Long et al., 2018). However, not all GLUT isoforms integrate properly into the oocyte plasma membrane and calculating their abundancy in membrane is not trivial (Gould and Lienhard, 1989; Keller et al., 1989). Furthermore, *Xenopus laevis* oocytes might be too instable for the application in high-throughput screening assays (César-Razquin et al., 2015).

Investigations on GLUTs can also be performed by expression in human cell lines such as MCF-7 or Caco-2 cells as it has been shown for GLUT2 and GLUT5 (Mahraoui et al., 1994; Zamora-León et al., 1996; Lee et al., 2015). In these systems, parameters such as lipid composition, posttranslational modifications and protein trafficking are most likely identical to the native conditions, although some alterations in cultured cells are, at least principally, possible. However, mammalian cell lines endogenously express several GLUT isoforms with overlapping activity, making it difficult to establish unambiguously the GLUT member(s) targeted by a compound (Lee et al., 2015; Tripp et al., 2017).

More recently, efforts have concentrated on establishing a microbial system amenable to high-throughput screening of GLUT inhibitors. Due to the easy manipulation and short generation time, the yeast *Saccharomyces cerevisiae* provides a time-efficient, low-cost and versatile platform for this purpose (Tripp et al., 2017; Boles and Oreb, 2018). For exclusive uptake of hexoses via heterologously expressed GLUTs, all genes encoding endogenous transporters capable of hexose transport (*HXT1-17, GAL2* as well as the maltose transporter genes *AGT1, MPH2,* and *MPH3*) were deleted in the yeast strain background CEN.PK2-1C using the loxP-Cre recombinase system (Wieczorke et al., 1999). The resulting strain was named EBY.VW4000 and is unable to take up and grow on glucose or related hexoses as sole carbon source. The functional expression of human GLUTs in this hexose transporter deficient (hxt^0) yeast strain restores its ability to grow on glucose or fructose enabling compound screening for the particular human GLUT via simple cell growth assays (Wieczorke et al., 2002). Even though cell growth is the simplest parameter to determine the functionality of the transporters or potency of the inhibitors, compound screening is not limited to this method. For instance, yeast cells can be conveniently used for uptake assays of radiolabeled sugars, which allows for the determination of kinetic parameters of the transporters, including inhibitor constants (Maier et al., 2002; Tripp et al., 2017; Boles and Oreb, 2018).

However, the functional expression of human GLUTs in yeast cells require additional modifications either within the transporter or in the genome of the yeast strain. Whereas wildtype GLUT1, GLUT4 and GLUT5 (Kasahara and Kasahara, 1996, 1997; Wieczorke et al., 2002; Tripp et al., 2017) were not active in the hxt^0 strain, single point mutations in the transmembrane region 2 of GLUT1 and GLUT5 mediated their functional expression (Wieczorke et al., 2002; Tripp et al., 2017). Wild-type GLUT1 was active only in the hxt^0 strain that additionally acquired the *fgy1* (for functional expression of GLUT1 in yeast) mutation (Wieczorke et al., 2002). The affected gene encodes the Efr3 protein (Wieczorke and Boles, personal communication) that was later described as a scaffold for recruiting the Stt4 phosphatidylinositol-4-kinase to the plasma membrane and therefore necessary for normal phosphatidylinositol-4-phosphate levels in this compartment (Wu et al., 2014). The functional expression of GLUT4 required, in addition to *fgy1*, the *fgy4* mutation, that was later found to affect the *ERG4* gene (Boles et al., 2004), which encodes an enzyme involved in the last step of ergosterol biosynthesis. These observations suggest that the lipid composition of yeast membranes interferes with the functionality of GLUTs. Nevertheless, GLUT1, GLUT4 (Wieczorke et al., 2002), and GLUT5 (Tripp et al., 2017) expressed in yeast exhibited transport kinetic parameters comparable to those determined in liposomes or human cell lines and were responsive to established inhibitors of these transporters. Therefore, hxt^0 strains represent a convenient platform for screening approaches and characterization of human GLUTs in a high throughput manner. The discovery of specific effectors for one certain GLUT, which do not influence homologs of the same protein family, is challenging due to the high protein sequence similarity shared by the members of this family (George Thompson et al., 2015). Among existing screening systems, the microbial, high-throughput screening system is the most effective method to face this challenge. Its usage and expansion to other disease-relevant GLUTs will likely reveal new GLUT-specific effectors which might be of fundamental importance for clinical applications in the battle against widespread diseases like cancer or diabetes.

AUTHOR CONTRIBUTIONS

All authors listed have made a substantial, direct and intellectual contribution to the work, and approved it for publication.

FUNDING

This work was supported by the National Institutes of Health, Grant number R01-GM123103 (to JC and MO).

ACKNOWLEDGMENTS

We thank Eckhard Boles for helpful comments on the manuscript.

REFERENCES

Barron, C. C., Bilan, P. J., Tsakiridis, T., and Tsiani, E. (2016). Facilitative glucose transporters. Implications for cancer detection, prognosis and treatment. *Metabolism* 65, 124–139. doi: 10.1016/j.metabol.2015.10.007

Birnbaum, M. J. (1989). Identification of a novel gene encoding an insulin-responsive glucose transporter protein. *Cell* 57, 305–315. doi: 10.1016/0092-8674(89)90968-9

Boles, E., Dlugai, S., Mueller, G., and Voss, D. (2004). *Use of Saccharomyces Cerevisiae ERG4 Mutants for the Expression of Glucose Transporters From Mammals.* WO002004026907A3. Geneva: World Intellectual Property Organization.

Boles, E., and Oreb, M. (2018). A growth-based screening system for hexose transporters in yeast. *Methods Mol. Biol.* 1713, 123–135. doi: 10.1007/978-1-4939-7507-5_10

Cairns, R. A., Harris, I. S., and Mak, T. W. (2011). Regulation of cancer cell metabolism. *Nat. Rev. Cancer* 11, 85–95. doi: 10.1038/nrc2981

César-Razquin, A., Snijder, B., Frappier-Brinton, T., Isserlin, R., Gyimesi, G., Bai, X., et al. (2015). A call for systematic research on solute carriers. *Cell* 162, 478–487. doi: 10.1016/j.cell.2015.07.022

Colas, C., Ung, P. M.-U., and Schlessinger, A. (2016). SLC transporters. structure, function, and drug discovery. *Med. Chem. Comm.* 7, 1069–1081. doi: 10.1039/C6MD00005C

Deng, D., Xu, C., Sun, P., Wu, J., Yan, C., Hu, M., et al. (2014). Crystal structure of the human glucose transporter GLUT1. *Nature* 510, 121–125. doi: 10.1038/nature13306

Deng, D., Sun, P., Yan, C., Ke, M., Jiang, X., Xiong, L., et al. (2015). Molecular basis of ligand recognition and transport by glucose transporters. *Nature* 526, 391–396. doi: 10.1038/nature14655

Douard, V., and Ferraris, R. P. (2013). The role of fructose transporters in diseases linked to excessive fructose intake. *J. Physiol. (Lond).* 591, 401–414. doi: 10.1113/jphysiol.2011.215731

Elsas, L. J., and Longo, N. (1992). Glucose transporters. *Annu. Rev. Med.* 43, 377–393. doi: 10.1146/annurev.me.43.020192.002113

Geertsma, E. R., Nik Mahmood, N. A., Schuurman-Wolters, G. K., and Poolman, B. (2008). Membrane reconstitution of ABC transporters and assays of translocator function. *Nat. Protoc.* 3, 256–266. doi: 10.1038/nprot.2007.519

George, R. L., and Keenan, R. T. (2013). Genetics of hyperuricemia and gout. Implications for the present and future. *Curr. Rheumatol. Rep.* 15:309. doi: 10.1007/s11926-012-0309-8

George Thompson, A. M., Iancu, C. V., Nguyen, T. T., Kim, D., and Choe, J. Y. (2015). Inhibition of human GLUT1 and GLUT5 by plant carbohydrate products; insights into transport specificity. *Sci. Rep.* 5:12804. doi: 10.1038/srep12804

George Thompson, A. M., Ursu, O., Babkin, P., Iancu, C. V., Whang, A., Oprea, T. I., et al. (2016). Discovery of a specific inhibitor of human GLUT5 by virtual screening and *in vitro* transport evaluation. *Sci. Rep.* 6:160. doi: 10.1038/srep24240

Gould, G. W., Thomas, H. M., Jess, T. J., and Bell, G. I. (1991). Expression of human glucose transporters in *Xenopus* oocytes: kinetic characterization and substrate specificities of the erythrocyte, liver, and brain isoforms. *Biochemistry* 30, 5139–5145. doi: 10.1021/bi00235a004

Gould, G. W., and Lienhard, G. E. (1989). Expression of a functional glucose transporter in *Xenopus* oocytes. *Biochemistry* 28, 9447–9452. doi: 10.1021/bi00450a030

Godoy, A., Ulloa, V., Rodríguez, F., Reinicke, K., Yañez, A. J., GarcíaMde, L. et al. (2006). Differential subcellular distribution of glucose transporters GLUT1-6 and GLUT9 in human cancer. ultrastructural localization of GLUT1 and GLUT5 in breast tumor tissues. *J. Cell. Physiol.* 207, 614–627. doi: 10.1002/jcp.20606

Hajiaghaalipour, F., Khalilpourfarshbafi, M., and Arya, A. (2015). Modulation of glucose transporter protein by dietary flavonoids in type 2 diabetes mellitus. *Int. J. Biol. Sci.* 11, 508–524. doi: 10.7150/ijbs.11241

Hediger, M. A., Coady, M. J., Ikeda, T. S., and Wright, E. M. (1987). Expression cloning and cDNA sequencing of the Na^{+}/glucose co-transporter. *Nature* 330, 379–381. doi: 10.1038/330379a0

Hresko, R. C., Kraft, T. E., Quigley, A., Carpenter, E. P., and Hruz, P. W. (2016). Mammalian glucose transporter activity is dependent upon anionic and conical phospholipids. *J. Biol. Chem.* 291, 17271–17282. doi: 10.1074/jbc.M116.730168

Iancu, C. V., Zamoon, J., Woo, S. B., Aleshin, A., and Choe, J. Y. (2013). Crystal structure of a glucose/H^{+} symporter and its mechanism of action. *Proc. Natl. Acad. Sci. U.S.A.* 110, 17862–17867. doi: 10.1073/pnas.1311485110

Kapoor, K., Finer-Moore, J. S., Pedersen, B. P., Caboni, L., Waight, A., Hillig, R. C., et al. (2016). Mechanism of inhibition of human glucose transporter GLUT1 is conserved between cytochalasin B and phenylalanine amides. *Proc. Natl. Acad. Sci. U.S.A.* 113, 4711–4716. doi: 10.1073/pnas.1603735113

Kasahara, T., and Kasahara, M. (1996). Expression of the rat GLUT1 glucose transporter in the yeast *Saccharomyces cerevisiae*. *Biochem. J.* 315, 177–182. doi: 10.1042/bj3150177

Kasahara, T., and Kasahara, M. (1997). Characterization of rat Glut4 glucose transporter expressed in the yeast *Saccharomyces cerevisiae*: comparison with Glut1 glucose transporter. *Biochim. Biophys. Acta* 1324, 111–119. doi: 10.1016/S0005-2736(96)00217-9

Kawamura, Y., Matsuo, H., Chiba, T., Nagamori, S., Nakayama, A., Inoue, H., et al. (2011). Pathogenic GLUT9 mutations causing renal hypouricemia type 2 (RHUC2). *Nucleos. Nucleot. Nucl.* 30, 1105–1111. doi: 10.1080/15257770.2011.623685

Kayano, T., Burant, C. F., Fukumoto, H., Gould, G. W., Fan, Y. S., Eddy, R. L., et al. (1990). Human facilitative glucose transporters. *J. Biol. Chem.* 265, 13276-–13282.

Keller, K., Strube, M., and Mueckler, M. (1989). Functional expression of the human HepG2 and rat adipocyte glucose transporters in *Xenopus* Oocytes. *J. Biol. Chem.* 264, 18884–18889.

Kraft, T. E., Hresko, R. C., and Hruz, P. W. (2015). Expression, purification, and functional characterization of the insulin-responsive facilitative glucose transporter GLUT4. *Prot. Sci.* 24, 2008–2019. doi: 10.1002/pro.2812

Lee, Y., Lim, Y., and Kwon, O. (2015). Selected phytochemicals and culinary plant extracts inhibit fructose uptake in Caco-2 Cells. *Molecules* 20, 17393–17404. doi: 10.3390/molecules200917393

Liu, Y., Zhang, W., Cao, Y., Liu, Y., Bergmeier, S., and Chen, X. (2010). Small compound inhibitors of basal glucose transport inhibit cell proliferation and induce apoptosis in cancer cells via glucose-deprivation-like mechanisms. *Cancer Lett.* 298, 176–185. doi: 10.1016/j.canlet.2010.07.002

Lloyd, K. P., Ojelabi, O. A., De Zutter, J. K., and Carruthers, A. (2017). Reconciling contradictory findings: Glucose transporter 1 (GLUT1) functions as an oligomer of allosteric, alternating access transporters. *J. Biol. Chem.* 292, 21035–21046. doi: 10.1074/jbc.M117.815589

Long, W., O'Neill, D., and Cheeseman, C. I. (2018). GLUT characterization using frog *Xenopus laevis* Oocytes. *Methods Mol. Biol.* 1713, 45–55. doi: 10.1007/978-1-4939-7507-5_4

Macheda, M. L., Rogers, S., and Best, J. D. (2005). Molecular and cellular regulation of glucose transporter (GLUT) proteins in cancer. *J. Cell. Physiol.* 202, 654–662. doi: 10.1002/jcp.20166

Mahraoui, L., Takeda, J., Mesonero, J., Chantret, I., Dussaulx, E., Bell, G. I., et al. (1994). Regulation of expression of the human fructose transporter (GLUT5) by cyclic AMP. *Biochem. J.* 301, 169–175. doi: 10.1042/bj3010169

Maier, A., Völker, B., Boles, E., and Fuhrmann, G. F. (2002). Characterisation of glucose transport in *Saccharomyces cerevisiae* with plasma membrane vesicles (countertransport) and intact cells (initial uptake) with single Hxt1, Hxt2, Hxt3, Hxt4, Hxt6, Hxt7 or Gal2 transporters. *FEMS Yeast Res.* 2, 539–550. doi: 10.1111/j.1567-1364.2002.tb00121.x

McBrayer, S. K., Cheng, J. C., Singhal, S., Krett, N. L., Rosen, S. T., and Shanmugam, M. (2012). Multiple myeloma exhibits novel dependence on GLUT4, GLUT8, and GLUT11. Implications for glucose transporter-directed therapy. *Blood* 119, 4686–4697. doi: 10.1182/blood-2011-09-377846

Mishra, R. K., Wei, C., Hresko, R. C., Bajpai, R., Heitmeier, M., Matulis, S. M., et al. (2015). *In silico* modeling-based identification of glucose transporter 4 (GLUT4)-selective inhibitors for cancer therapy. *J. Biol. Chem.* 290, 14441–14453. doi: 10.1074/jbc.M114.628826

Mueckler, M., and Thorens, B. (2013). The SLC2 (GLUT) family of membrane transporters. *Mol. Aspects Med.* 34, 121–138. doi: 10.1016/j.mam.2012.07.001

Nomura, N., Verdon, G., Kang, H. J., Shimamura, T., Nomura, Y., Sonoda, Y., et al. (2015). Structure and mechanism of the mammalian fructose transporter GLUT5. *Nature* 526, 397–401. doi: 10.1038/nature14909

Ohtsubo, K., Takamatsu, S., Minowa, M. T., Yoshida, A., Takeuchi, M., and Marth, J. D. (2005). Dietary and genetic control of glucose transporter 2 glycosylation promotes insulin secretion in suppressing diabetes. *Cell* 123, 1307–1321. doi: 10.1016/j.cell.2005.09.041

Patel, N., Huang, C., and Klip, A. (2006). Cellular location of insulin-triggered signals and implications for glucose uptake. *Pflugers Arch.* 451, 499–510. doi: 10.1007/s00424-005-1475-6

Pike, A. C. W., Quigley, A., Chu, A., Tessitore, A., Xia, X., Mukhopadhyay, S., et al. (2015). *Structure of the Human Glucose Transporter GLUT3/SLC2A3.* Available online at: http://www.rcsb.org/structure/5C65

Quistgaard, E. M., Löw, C., Moberg, P., Trésaugues, L., and Nordlund, P. (2013). Structural basis for substrate transport in the GLUT-homology family of monosaccharide transporters. *Nat. Struct. Mol. Biol.* 20, 766–768. doi: 10.1038/nsmb.2569

Rogers, S., Macheda, M. L., Docherty, S. E., Carty, M. D., Henderson, M. A., Soeller, W. C., et al. (2002). Identification of a novel glucose transporter-like protein-GLUT-12. *Am. J. Physiol.* 282, 733–738. doi: 10.1152/ajpendo.2002.282.3.E733

Rudlowski, C., Becker, A. J., Schroder, W., Rath, W., Büttner, R., and Moser, M. (2003). GLUT1 messenger RNA and protein induction relates to the malignant transformation of cervical cancer. *Am. J. Clin. Pathol.* 120, 691–698. doi: 10.1309/4KYNQM5862JW2GD7

Saier, M. H., Beatty, J. T., Goffeau, A., Harley, K. T., Heijne, W. H., Huang, S. C., et al. (1999). The major facilitator superfamily. *J. Mol. Microbiol. Biotechnol.* 1, 257–279.

Santer, R., Schneppenheim, R., Dombrowski, A., Götze, H., Steinmann, B., and Schaub, J. (1997). Mutations in *GLUT2*, the gene for the liver-type glucose transporter, in patients with Fanconi-Bickel syndrome. *Nat. Genet.* 17, 324–326. doi: 10.1038/ng1197-324

Schreiber, S. L., Kotz, J. D., Li, M., Aubé, J., Austin, C. P., Reed, J. C., et al. (2015). Advancing biological understanding and therapeutics discovery with small-molecule probes. *Cell* 161, 1252–1265. doi: 10.1016/j.cell.2015.05.023

Seidner, G., Alvarez, M. G., Yeh, J. I., O'Driscoll, K. R., Klepper, J., Stump, T. S., et al. (1998). GLUT-1 deficiency syndrome caused by haploinsufficiency of the blood-brain barrier hexose carrier. *Nat. Genet.* 18, 188–191. doi: 10.1038/ng0298-188

Sliwoski, G., Kothiwale, S., Meiler, J., and Lowe, E. W. (2014). Computational methods in drug discovery. *Pharmacol. Rev.* 66, 334–395. doi: 10.1124/pr.112.007336

Song, D. H., and Wolfe, M. M. (2007). Glucose-dependent insulinotropic polypeptide and its role in obesity. *Curr. Opin. Endocrinol.* 14, 46–51. doi: 10.1097/MED.0b013e328011aa88

Sun, L., Zeng, X., Yan, C., Sun, X., Gong, X., Rao, Y., et al. (2012). Crystal structure of a bacterial homologue of glucose transporters GLUT1-4. *Nature* 490, 361–366. doi: 10.1038/nature11524

Szablewski, L. (2013). Expression of glucose transporters in cancers. *Biochim. Biophys. Acta* 1835, 164–169. doi: 10.1016/j.bbcan.2012.12.004

Thorens, B., and Mueckler, M. (2010). Glucose transporters in the 21st Century. *Am. J. Physiol. Endocrinol.* 298, E141–E145. doi: 10.1152/ajpendo.00712.2009

Tripp, J., Essl, C., Iancu, C. V., Boles, E., Choe, J. Y., and Oreb, M. (2017). Establishing a yeast-based screening system for discovery of human GLUT5 inhibitors and activators. *Sci. Re.* 7:124. doi: 10.1038/s41598-017-06262-4

Ung, P. M., Song, W., Cheng, L., Zhao, X., Hu, H., Chen, L., et al. (2016). Inhibitor discovery for the human GLUT1 from homology modeling and virtual screening. *ACS Chem. Biol.* 11, 1908–1916. doi: 10.1021/acschembio.6b00304

Warburg, O. (1956). On the origin of cancer cells. *Science* 3191, 309–314. doi: 10.1126/science.123.3191.309

Wei, C., Bajpai, R., Sharma, H., Heitmeier, M., Jain, A. D., Matulis, S. M., et al. (2017). Development of GLUT4-selective antagonists for multiple myeloma therapy. *Eur. J. Med. Chem.* 139, 573–586. doi: 10.1016/j.ejmech.2017.08.029

Wieczorke, R., Dlugai, S., Krampe, S., and Boles, E. (2002). Characterisation of mammalian GLUT glucose transporters in a heterologous yeast Expression system. *Cell. Physiol. Biochem.* 13, 123–134. doi: 10.1159/000071863

Wieczorke, R., Krampe, S., Weierstall, T., Freidel, K., Hollenberg, C. P., and Boles, E. (1999). Concurrent knock-out of at least 20 transporter genes is required to block uptake of hexoses in *Saccharomyces cerevisiae*. *FEBS Lett.* 464, 123–128. doi: 10.1016/S0014-5793(99)01698-1

Williamson, E. A., Damiani, L., Leitao, A., Hu, C., Hathaway, H., Oprea, T., et al. (2012). Targeting the transposase domain of the DNA repair component Metnase to enhance chemotherapy. *Cancer Res.* 72, 6200–6208. doi: 10.1158/0008-5472.CAN-12-0313

Wisedchaisri, G., Park, M. S., Iadanza, M. G., Zheng, H., and Gonen, T. (2014). Proton-coupled sugar transport in the prototypical major facilitator superfamily protein XylE. *Nat. Comm.* 5:4521. doi: 10.1038/ncomms5521

Wu, X., Chi, R. J., Baskin, J. M., Lucast, L., Burd, C. G., De Camilli, P., et al. (2014). Structural insights into assembly and regulation of the plasma membrane phosphatidylinositol 4-Kinase Complex. *Dev. Cell* 28, 19–29. doi: 10.1016/j.devcel.2013.11.012

Zamora-León, S. P., Golde, D. W., Concha, II., Rivas, C. I., Delgado-López, F., Baselga, J., et al. (1996). Expression of the fructose transporter GLUT5 in human breast cancer. *Proc. Natl. Acad. Sci. U.S.A.* 93, 1847–1852. doi: 10.1073/pnas.93.5.1847

4

Moving the Cellular Peptidome by Transporters

Rupert Abele [1*] *and Robert Tampé* [1,2*]

[1] *Institute of Biochemistry, Biocenter, Goethe University Frankfurt, Frankfurt, Germany,* [2] *Cluster of Excellence – Macromolecular Complexes, Goethe University Frankfurt, Frankfurt, Germany*

Correspondence:
Rupert Abele
abele@em.uni-frankfurt.de
Robert Tampé
tampe@em.uni-frankfurt.de

Living matter is defined by metastability, implying a tightly balanced synthesis and turnover of cellular components. The first step of eukaryotic protein degradation via the ubiquitin-proteasome system (UPS) leads to peptides, which are subsequently degraded to single amino acids by an armada of proteases. A small fraction of peptides, however, escapes further cytosolic destruction and is transported by ATP-binding cassette (ABC) transporters into the endoplasmic reticulum (ER) and lysosomes. The ER-resident heterodimeric transporter associated with antigen processing (TAP) is a crucial component in adaptive immunity for the transport and loading of peptides onto major histocompatibility complex class I (MHC I) molecules. Although the function of the lysosomal resident homodimeric TAPL-like (TAPL) remains, until today, only loosely defined, an involvement in immune defense is anticipated since it is highly expressed in dendritic cells and macrophages. Here, we compare the gene organization and the function of single domains of both peptide transporters. We highlight the structural organization, the modes of substrate binding and translocation as well as physiological functions of both organellar transporters.

Keywords: ABC transporter, antigen processing, antigen presentation, membrane proteins, viral immune escape, lysosome, endoplasmic reticulum

INTRODUCTION

In the life cycle of a cell, the proteome is metastable and dynamically shaped by synthesis, folding, modification, and degradation. Proteins are degraded when either being damaged, matched for a demanded life-time, and no longer used, or delivered as defective ribosomal products. The clearance of these proteins starts in the cytosol with hydrolysis to peptides of three to twenty residues in length predominately through the ubiquitin-proteasome system (UPS). Malfunction of this macromolecular degradation machinery is associated with neurodegenerative, autoimmune, and rheumatoid diseases, viral infections, and cancer (Schmidt and Finley, 2014). Most of the peptides generated by the UPS are processed within seconds to amino acids via cytosolic oligo- and aminopeptidases (Reits et al., 2003). Some of these peptides escape degradation to fulfill important functions (**Figure 1**). A well-studied example is the mating a-factor functioning as pheromone in yeast. The precursor of 36 amino acid length encoded by *MFA1* undergoes six consecutive steps of post-translational modification, yielding a mature 12-residue long a-factor, which is expelled to the external medium by the ATP-binding cassette (ABC) transporter Ste6 (Michaelis and Barrowman, 2012). In *Caenorhabditis elegans* mitochondrial unfolded stress response is signaled to the nucleus via peptides. In this process, mitochondrial proteins are degraded by ATP-dependent degradation machine ClpXP in the matrix and peptides are released to the cytosol most likely

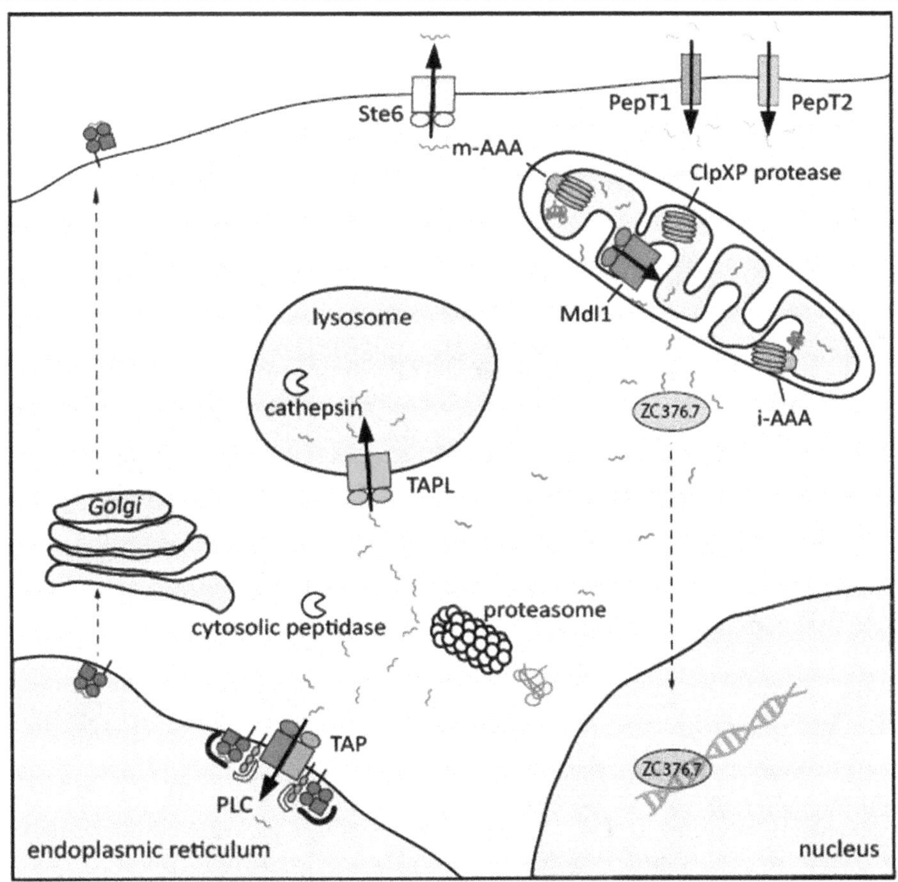

FIGURE 1 | Physiological role of eukaryotic peptide transporters. Peptide transporters are localized at different cellular membranes. At the plasma membrane of intestine and kidney cells, the secondary active transporters PepT1 and PepT2 import di- to tetramer peptides along a proton gradient. All peptide transporters belonging to the ABC superfamily are exporters. The peptide pheromone exporter Ste6 from *Saccharomyces cerevisiae* shuttles the mating a-factor into the extracellular space. Proteins in the matrix and inner membrane of mitochondria are degraded by the AAA+ proteases m-AAA and ClpXP and the resulting peptides are transported by Mdl1 in yeast, HAF-1 in *C. elegans*, and probably ABCB10 in human into the intermembrane space. Subsequently, the transcription factorZC376.7 (Atfs1) in *C. elegans*, the homolog of Atf5 in human, is activated and localized in the nucleus, where genes of the mitochondrial unfolded protein response are induced. Cytosolic proteins are degraded mainly by the proteasome. Peptides that escape further trimming by cytosolic peptidases are translocated by the heterodimeric ABC transporter associated with the antigen processing TAP into the ER, where these peptides are loaded onto MHC class I molecules to present the antigenic peptides on the cell surface to cytotoxic T-cells. The peptide transfer, editing, and proofreading is catalyzed by the peptide loading complex (PLC). In addition, cytosolic peptides are transported by TAPL to lysosomes for further processing by cathepsins.

by the ABC transporter HAF-1. Here, the peptides directly or indirectly bind to a transcription factor, which induces the expression of mitochondrial chaperones to cope with mitochondrial proteostasis (Haynes et al., 2010). The analysis of the mouse brain peptidome by mass spectrometry demonstrated that some intracellular peptides are enriched. It was therefore speculated that peptides can take over regulatory functions (Fricker, 2010).

The most well-studied and medically important function of cytosolic protein fragments is their role in building an adaptive immune response (**Figure 1**). Proteasomal degradation products are shuttled by the ABC transporter associated with antigen processing (TAP1/2, ABCB2/ABCB3) into the lumen of the endoplasmic reticulum (ER) where these peptides are loaded onto major histocompatibility complex class I (MHC I) molecules (Abele and Tampé, 2004; Parcej and Tampé, 2010; Blum et al., 2013). Peptide-MHC I complexes are subsequently transported to the cell surface in order to present the bits of the cellular proteome as metabolic snapshots to cytotoxic CD8^{+} T-lymphocytes. If the T-cell receptor recognizes antigenic "non-self" peptides in complex with MHC I as "self" component, virally or malignantly transformed cells will be destroyed (Gromme and Neefjes, 2002). Importantly, cytosolic peptides are also frequently found on MHC II molecules, which is an essential step in the negative selection during T-cell development to impede autoimmune response (Crotzer and Blum, 2010).

Different pathways seem to contribute to the delivery of cytosolic peptides to the lysosomes (**Figure 1**). Cytosolic proteins are typically delivered by macro-autophagy or by chaperone-mediated autophagy to lysosomes, where they are degraded by cathepsins (Crotzer and Blum, 2008). However, cytosolic peptides can also be transported directly into lysosomes and bound to MHC II without further processing. It was speculated that the transporter associated with antigen processing-like

(TAPL, ABCB9) is involved in this process (Dani et al., 2004). Here, we summarized some structural and mechanistic similarities but also a number of remarkable differences of these TAP-related peptide transporters.

THE DIVERSITY OF ORGANELLAR PEPTIDE TRANSPORTERS

Different classes of peptide transporters have evolved (**Figure 1**). All in common is a high substrate promiscuity. Peptides containing two to eight residues are transported by members belonging to the oligopeptide transporter and peptide transporter family (Gomolplitinant and Saier, 2011; Newstead, 2015). Both families belong to the Major Facilitator Superfamily of secondary active transporters, which are proton-dependent transport systems. Oligopeptide transporters, translocating peptides of three to eight amino acids in length, are found in bacteria, plants, and fungi. Di- and tripeptide transporters are also present in animals. Human PepT1 and PepT2 are found in the brush border membrane of the small intestine and at the renal epithelium in the kidney, respectively. Both transporters absorb or retain protein fragments in the body. Interestingly, PepT1 is the fast, low-affinity transporter while PepT2 shows slower transport rates paired with higher affinity (Brandsch, 2013).

Longer peptides are typically handled by ABC transporters, the largest family of primary active transporters. In bacteria, oligopeptides are complexed in the periplasm by a specific binding protein, which hands over the substrate to an ABC import system (Doeven et al., 2005). In eukaryotes, only oligopeptide ABC exporters are described. A vacuolar ATP dependent transporter was identified in plants, translocating peptides into the lumen of vacuoles (Ramos et al., 2011). Furthermore, peptide transporters with different intracellular localization exist in yeast, nematodes, and vertebrates (Herget and Tampé, 2007). In yeast, Mdl1 is located in the inner mitochondrial membrane and is proposed to transport degradation products of matrix or inner mitochondrial membrane proteins into the intermembrane space (Young et al., 2001).

The TAP family is composed of three half-transporters, TAP1 (ABCB2), TAP2 (ABCB3), and TAPL (ABCB9). Members of the TAP family are also found in *C. elegans* and in chordata but not in insects and crustaceans (**Figure 2**). TAP1 and TAP2 must pair to constitute a transport-competent complex, whereas TAPL forms homodimers (Powis et al., 1991; Leveson-Gower et al., 2004). Interestingly, HAF-4 and HAF-9 of *C. elegans* are orthologs of TAPL with a sequence identity of 38%. Both half-transporters are localized in large granules of intestinal cells. Loss-of-function mutants of either of these genes result in loss of these large non-acidic granules, accompanied by decreased brood size, extended defecation cycle, and slow growth (Kawai et al., 2009). HAF-4 and HAF-9 appear to form heterodimers and active heterodimers are essential for granule formation (Tanji et al., 2013).

In contrast to jawed vertebrates, which express TAP1, TAP2, and TAPL, only one member belonging to the TAP family was detected in agnatha (jawless vertebrates) and even in tunicates (Uinuk-ool et al., 2003; Ren et al., 2015). The half-transporter from the jawless vertebrate sea lamprey shows a higher sequence identity to human TAPL (52.4%) than to TAP1 (38.4%) and TAP2 (40.7%). Therefore, ABCB9 from agnatha can be regarded as the progenitor of the TAP family. Interestingly, TAP1 and TAP2 have evolved much faster than TAPL. Comparing the amino acid sequences from rat and mouse, the replacement rates in TAP1 and TAP2 are more than 10 times faster as in TAPL (Kobayashi et al., 2000).

In mammals, TAP and TAPL show a broad tissue distribution. TAP was found in nearly every nucleated cell. TAPL is also detected in all tissues examined (Bgee database: Bastian et al., 2008; The Human Protein Atlas: Uhlén et al., 2015) with high expression in the central nervous system and testis (Yamaguchi et al., 1999; Zhang et al., 2000; Mutch et al., 2004). Interestingly, TAPL is not found in monocytes but highly expressed in dendritic cells and macrophages implying a role in the immune response (Demirel et al., 2007).

PHYSIOLOGICAL FUNCTION

Although TAP and TAPL transport a similar range of peptides, their physiological functions are largely different. In the past, the paradigm was that MHC I presents peptides from endogenous antigens while MHC II displays peptides from exogenous antigens. Through analyzing the peptidome of MHC molecules it became evident that this sharp border is not correct. A quantitative amount of MHC II molecules is loaded with peptides from cytosolic origin (Stern and Santambrogio, 2016). Moreover, in professional antigen presenting cells a process called cross-presentation takes place, in which peptides of exogenous antigens are loaded on MHC I molecules (van Endert, 2016; Grotzke et al., 2017b). This pathway ensures the induction of an adaptive immune response to tumor antigens and antigens derived from pathogens, which does not infect dendritic cells. TAP is an essential machinery in delivering cytosolic peptides, mainly produced by the UPS, into the lumen of the ER for loading onto MHC I. Importantly, TAP is not only crucial for the classical MHC I presentation but also actively involved in the cross-presentation pathway. In the TAP-dependent cross-presentation, exogenous antigens are taken up by phagocytosis or receptor-mediated endocytosis. Subsequently, the antigen is transported from the phagosome or endosome into the cytosol putatively by Sec61 (Koopmann et al., 2000; Zehner et al., 2015; Grotzke et al., 2017a). In the cytosol, the antigen is proteasomally degraded and peptides are transported by TAP into the ER or phagosome/endosome for loading onto MHC I.

The importance of TAP in antigen presentation is highlighted in the Bare Lymphocyte Syndrome type I (BLS-I), a rare disease caused by TAP deficiency (Zimmer et al., 1998). Cells of BLS-I patients show a strong decreased cell surface expression of MHC I accompanied by a reduced number of $CD8^+$ T-cells.

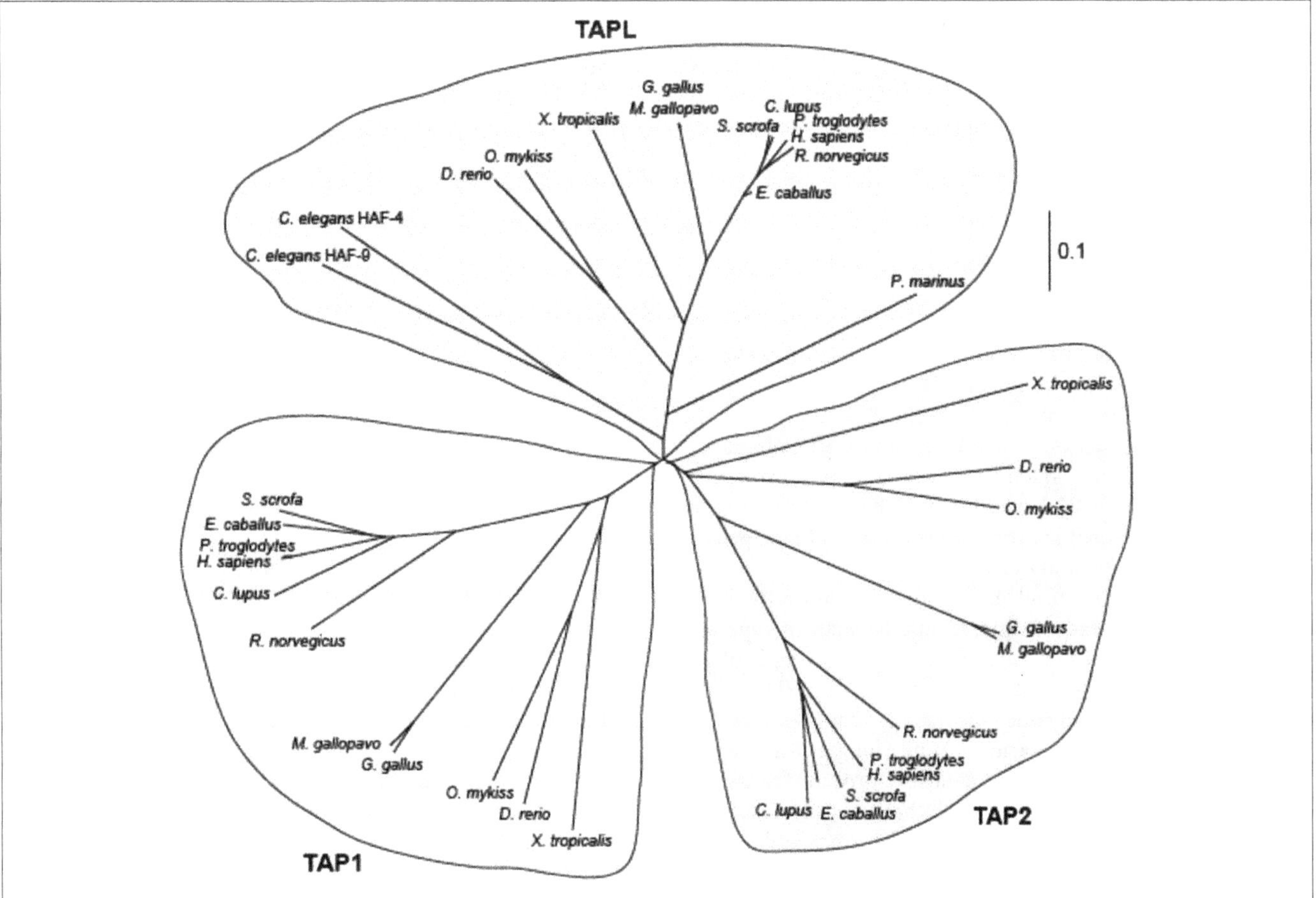

FIGURE 2 | Phylogenetic relationship of TAP and TAPL. Multiple sequence alignment of TAPL, TAP1, and TAP2 variants of human (*Homo sapiens*), chimpanzee (*Pan troglodytes*), horse (*Equus cabalus*), pig (*Sus scrofa*), dog (*Canis lupus*), rat (*Rattus norvegicus*), turkey (*Meleagris gallopavo*), chicken (*Gallus gallus*), trout (*Oncorhynchus mykiss*), zebrafisch (*Danio rerio*), western clawed frog (*Xenopus tropicalis*), sea lamprey (*Petromyzon marinus*), and roundworm (*Caenorhabditis elegans*) were performed with Clustal Omega (Sievers et al., 2011). An unrooted cladogram was drawn by Phylodendron (http://iubio.bio.indiana.edu/treeapp/). The bar indicates the evolutionary change rate. In the lower vertebrate lamprey and in the nematode *C. elegans* only homologs of TAPL are found. Longer branches of mammal and avian homologs reflect the higher evolutionary rate of TAP1 and TAP2 in comparison to TAPL.

BLS-I patients do not suffer from a prevalence of viral infections but instead show chronic necrotizing lesions in the lung and skin escorted by recurrent bacterial infections. Moreover, the key function of TAP is emphasized by the armada of viral factors inhibiting TAP (Mayerhofer and Tampé, 2015; van de Weijer et al., 2015). These viral immune evasins all derive from large DNA viruses belonging to the family of Herpesviridae or Poxviridae. Each viral factor has its own inhibition mechanism dealing with peptide binding, ATP binding, conformational changes, or proteasomal degradation of TAP (Mayerhofer and Tampé, 2015).

In addition to the effects on the formation of gut granules in *C. elegans*, the physiological function of TAPL remains loosely defined. Since TAPL is found in nearly all tissues, a housekeeping function can be assumed to protect the cytosol from accumulation of otherwise harmful peptides. However, TAPL may have a more specialized function in professional antigen-presenting cells, in which its expression is strongly upregulated (Demirel et al., 2007). There are alternative pathways of endogenous antigens for processing and loading on MHC II (Veerappan Ganesan and Eisenlohr, 2017). One of these pathways is proteasome dependent but TAP-independent (Dani et al., 2004; Miller et al., 2015; Thiele et al., 2015). Furthermore, the loading of MHC II occurs in the lysosomal compartment (Dani et al., 2004). Therefore, it can be speculated that TAPL is the translocation machinery in this process, which is supported by the interaction of TAPL with MHC II (Demirel et al., 2012).

There are several cross-presentation pathways for presenting exogenous antigens on MHC I. The main difference consists in the subcellular compartment of antigen degradation. In the vacuolar pathway, the endocytosed or phagocytosed antigen is transported to the endolysosomal system where the antigen is digested and loaded onto MHC I molecules. In the cytosolic pathway, the antigen is translocated to the cytosol for proteasomal degradation. Subsequently, antigenic peptides are transported into the ER or into phagosomes for MHC I loading. Although TAP is the main transport complex in this pathway, it was recently shown in mouse dendritic cells that a TAP-independent but ATP-consuming machinery exists for peptide loading of phagosomes (Merzougui et al., 2011; Lawand et al., 2016). Although the phagosomal localization and the peptide specificity of mouse TAPL still has to be evaluated, TAPL could possibly be this uncharacterized peptide transporter.

GENE ORGANIZATION

The genes coding for human TAP1 and TAP2 are localized in the MHC II locus of chromosome 6 and their expression is induced by IFN-γ (Deverson et al., 1990; Monaco et al., 1990; Spies et al., 1990; Trowsdale et al., 1990, 1991). In contrast, the *tapl* gene is found on chromosome 12, lacking any link to factors of the adaptive immune system. In addition, *tapl* expression is not affected by IFN-γ (Kobayashi et al., 2000). All three genes are composed of 11 coding exons whereas *tapl* and *tap2* possess an additional 5′-non-coding exon. Besides the flanking coding exons, the exon length of all three genes is identical with the exception of coding exon 9 with identical length in *tap2* and *tapl* but 3 bp elongated in *tap1*. Strikingly, the length of the introns is much longer for *tapl* than for *tap1* and *tap2* (Uinuk-ool et al., 2003). For TAP1 only one splice isoform has been reported. However, a short (748 amino acids, aa) and a long (808 aa) variant of human TAP1 is found in the database, probably caused by alternative translation start sites. TAP2 has two splice isoforms of 653 and 703 aa with different 3′-terminal exons and varying peptide specificity (Yan et al., 1999). In addition to several allelic variants with single amino acid substitutions, a short and a long allelic variant of TAP2 with 686 and 703 aa has been described (Colonna et al., 1992). However, the expression of these different TAP1 and TAP2 variants and the impact on antigen presentation is not studied in detail.

For TAPL, six splice isoforms have been assigned in the UniProt database. The splice variants 12A, 12B, and 12C differ in the 3′-terminal exon (Kobayashi et al., 2003). Isoform 12B and 12C are likely inactive in peptide transport since both variants lack the conserved H-loop being essential for ATP hydrolysis. Two additional isoforms are probably non-functional as they lack the coding exon 6 or 7, which comprises transmembrane helices (TM) 9 and 10, and the sequence connecting the transmembrane domain (TMD) with the nucleotide-binding domain (NBD) (Zhang et al., 2000). The sixth isoform of TAPL is characterized by the absence of almost the entire NBD. Biochemical and cell biological data are available only for isoform 12A, the longest reported version with 766 aa. The activity and physiological function of the other TAPL variants is not resolved and questionable.

DOMAIN ORGANIZATION OF TAP-RELATED TRANSPORTERS

All ABC transporters are modularly organized and consist of two NBDs and two TMDs. These domains are arranged either in the form of four polypeptides, one polypeptide, or as a fusion of two domains. In eukaryotes, only full transporters with all four domains in one polypeptide chain, or half-transporters composed of one TMD and one NBD, exist (Locher, 2016; Thomas and Tampé, 2018). TAP1, TAP2, and TAPL are half-transporters. TAPL forms a symmetric homodimer whereas TAP is composed of TAP1 and TAP2 and thus asymmetric (Powis et al., 1991; Leveson-Gower et al., 2004) (**Figure 3**). In addition to their conserved four-domain-architecture, termed coreTAP

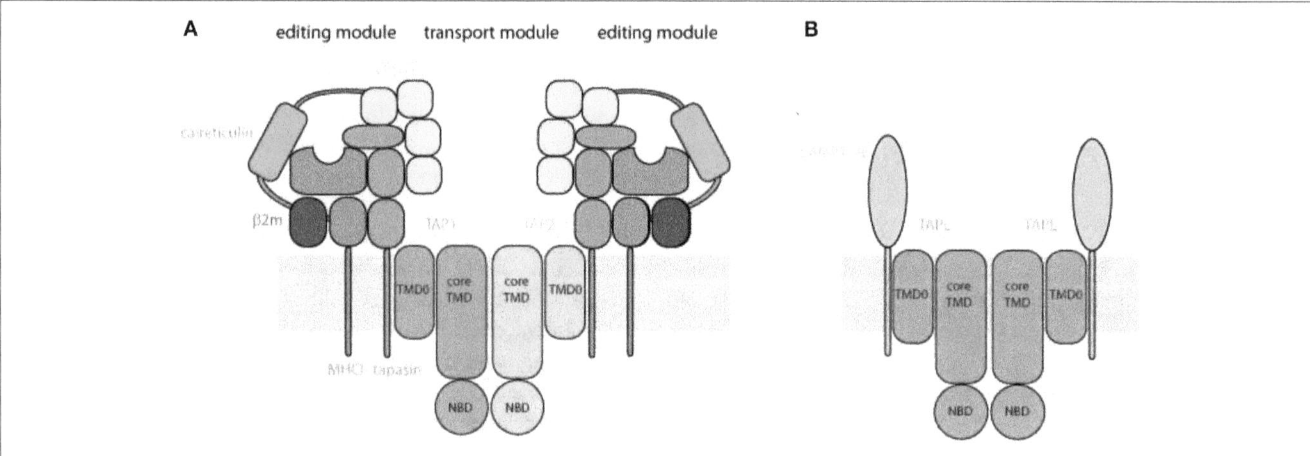

FIGURE 3 | Organization of the peptide transport machineries. **(A)** Architecture of the peptide loading complex. TAP composed of the half-transporter TAP1 and TAP2 forms the central translocation unit of the peptide loading complex. Each half-transporter consists of an N-terminal transmembrane domain (TMD) followed by a cytosolic nucleotide-binding domain (NBD). The core transporter, formed by the core TMDs, composed of 2 × 6 transmembrane helices and two NBDs, is fully active in peptide transport. The N-terminal TMD0s of TAP1 and TAP2, harboring four transmembrane helices each, interact with the transmembrane helix of tapasin. As central piece of the editing module, tapasin binds to ERp57, calreticulin and MHC I and destabilizes peptide MHC I interaction that only MHC I molecules loaded with high affinity peptides can shuttle to the cell surface. Depicted are two fully assembled editing modules, which can be found only transiently in cells. **(B)** TAPL forms a homodimeric transporter whereas the core transporter is composed of the 2 × 6 transmembrane helices and two NBDs. The four transmembrane helices comprising N-terminal TMD0 mediates lysosomal targeting as well as the interaction with LAMP1/2B. The stoichiometry between TAPL and LAMP1/2B is not solved.

and coreTAPL, each transporter subunit carries an extra N-terminal four-transmembrane helix domain named TMD0. For both complexes, the TMD0 is not required for peptide transport (Koch et al., 2004; Demirel et al., 2010). However, the TMD0s mediate the direct interaction with type I membrane proteins in different cellular compartments.

The TMD0s of TAP1 and TAP2 are essential for the assembly of the MHC I peptide-loading complex (PLC), composed of TAP1, TAP2, tapasin, MHC I, calreticulin, and ERp57, and consequently for efficient loading of MHC I molecules with antigenic peptides (Hulpke et al., 2012b) (**Figure 3A**). As illuminated by the cryo-EM structure of the human PLC, TAP as transport module is encircled by two editing modules (Blees et al., 2017). Tapasin as central factor of the editing module binds to MHC I, ERp57, and calreticulin, which spans as a clamp around the editing module and therefore seems to stabilize the subcomplex. Interestingly, the two editing modules are scaffolded by two tapasin molecules, which are stacked to each other via salt bridges. Tapasin comprises the editing function guaranteeing that only MHC I molecules loaded with stably bound, high-affinity peptides can leave the ER and are shuttled to the cell surface (Blees et al., 2017). The TMD0s of TAP1 and TAP2 interact independently from each other with the transmembrane helix of the MHC I specific chaperone tapasin (Hulpke et al., 2012a). For human TAP, the interaction between TAP and tapasin is mainly mediated by a salt bridge in the hydrophobic core of the ER membrane between a conserved aspartate in TM1 of each TAP subunit and a lysine of tapasin (Blees et al., 2015). Notably, an exchange of the conserved aspartate to lysine in TM1 of TAP1 or TAP2 abolished the PLC assembly, which was rescued by a double lysine-to-aspartate exchange. For rat TAP, however, this conserved aspartate in TAP2 can be exchanged to alanine without an effect on tapasin binding. In this case, leucine-rich areas in TM1 and TM2 of TAP2 seem to be important for tapasin binding (Rufer et al., 2015). Interestingly, tapasin interacts also with core TM9 of unassembled TAP1 which facilitates transporter stability and heterodimerization (Leonhardt et al., 2014). Hence tapasin may act as a dummy protein as found in the pre-B-cell receptor to guarantee correct folding of TAP1 which is a prerequisite for TAP2 assembly (Keusekotten et al., 2006).

In the case of TAPL, the TMD0 interacts with the lysosomal associated membrane proteins LAMP-1 and LAMP-2B but not with the splice variant LAMP-2A, which is the receptor for chaperone-mediated autophagy (**Figure 3B**). Remarkably, the interaction with LAMP-1 protects TAPL from lysosomal degradation and significantly increases its half-life (Demirel et al., 2012). Furthermore, the TMD0 of TAPL is essential and sufficient for lysosomal targeting of the complex. Solely expressed TMD0 is transported to lysosomes while coreTAPL traffics to the plasma membrane. Coexpression of both modules leads to their stable association and lysosomal localization (Demirel et al., 2010). The interaction with LAMP-1/2 has an impact neither on the lysosomal localization nor on the transport activity of TAPL (Demirel et al., 2012). Since TMD0 does not contain one of the conventional di-leucine or acidic-based lysosomal targeting motifs (Bonifacino and Traub, 2003), the targeting mechanism is currently unknown. In contrast, TAP retention in the ER is independent of its TMD0s. Unlike TAPL, coreTAP does not interact with the TMD0s (unpublished results).

CRYO-EM AND X-RAY STRUCTURES OF TAP-RELATED TRANSPORT SYSTEMS

In recent years, the ABC transporter field has experienced a revolution after reporting on the first high-resolution cryo-EM structure of an ABC transporter (**Figure 4A**) (Kim et al., 2015). The heterodimeric transporter TmrAB from *Thermus thermophilus* was selected from a structural genomic screen of TAP-related transporters. TmrAB was identified as a functional homolog of human TAP, complementing antigen processing and presentation in TAP-deficient cells isolated from BLS-I patients (Nöll et al., 2017). Despite the small complex size of 135 kDa and its pseudo-symmetric organization, cryo-EM revealed new insights into the asymmetric organization of TAP-related ABC transporters. Simultaneously, the X-ray structure of TmrAB in an apo, inward-facing conformation was determined at 2.7 Å resolution, providing atomistic details of peptide translocation complexes (Nöll et al., 2017) (**Figure 4C**).

The cryo-EM studies on TAP-related translocation complex TmrAB paved the way for numerous subsequent cryo-EM studies on ABC transporters, including human TAP (Oldham et al., 2016a,b), bovine MRP1 (Johnson and Chen, 2017, 2018), zebrafish and human CFTR (Liu et al., 2017; Zhang et al., 2017), ABCA1 (Qian et al., 2017), ABCG2 (Taylor et al., 2017), and SUR1 (Li et al., 2017; Martin et al., 2017a,b). To improve the resolution by cryo-EM, human TAP was arrested in a single conformation by the viral inhibitor ICP47, which has previously been shown to bind with high affinity to TAP (Ahn et al., 1996; Tomazin et al., 1996). By optimizing cryo-EM imaging and data processing, an average resolution of 4.0 Å was achieved in the core transport complex (**Figure 4B**), with higher resolution in TMDs, sufficient for registration of side chains, but at lower resolution in the NBDs, allowing the assignment of polypeptide backbone only (Oldham et al., 2016a). Due to their high flexibility, the TMD0s and the C-terminal part of the viral inhibitor comprising one-third of the complex could not be resolved.

The core translocation unit of TAP and also TmrAB resemble the structure of an inward-facing type I ABC exporter with 12 TMs where TM1-3 and 6 of one subunit and TM4/5 of the other subunit constitute one wing of the TMDs (Kim et al., 2015; Oldham et al., 2016a,b; Nöll et al., 2017). The NBDs are separated from each other but connected to the TMDs by cytosolic loops. In this ICP47-inhibited state, the interaction of the cytosolic loops is restricted to one NBD (ICL1 intra- and ICL2 intermolecular) and not both NBDs, as observed by disulfide crosslinking of TAP in ER membranes, when several conformations can be sampled (Oancea et al., 2009). The resolution of the NBDs, however, is not sufficient to allow detailed insights in the asymmetry of both TAP subunits. The first 55 residues of ICP47 form an α-helical hairpin structure and contact mainly TMs from TAP2 with an interface twice the average size of a binding

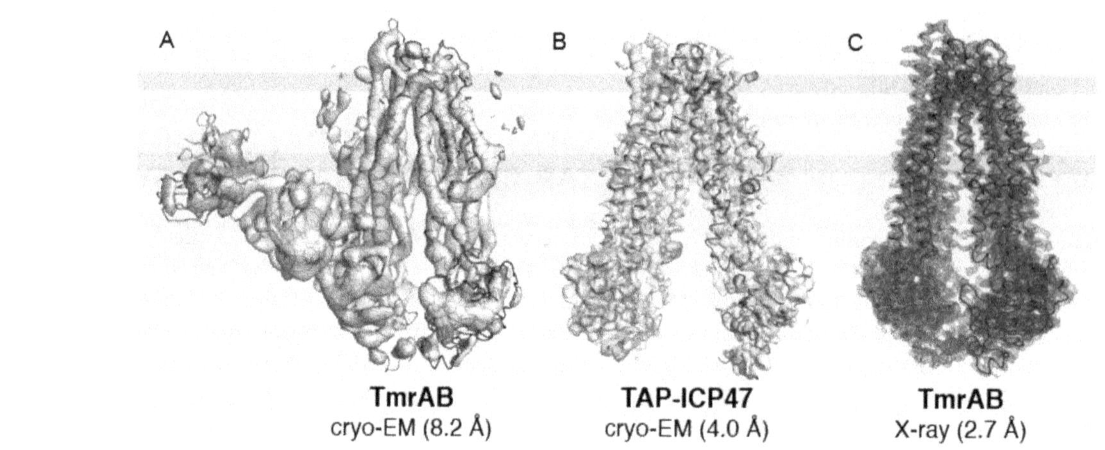

FIGURE 4 | Structures of TAP-related peptide transporters. **(A)** First high-resolution cryo-EM structure of an ABC transporter (Kim et al., 2015). The heterodimer TmrAB, a functional homolog of the TAP complex, was determined in an apo, inward-facing conformation in complex with a specific antibody fragment (EMD 6085. **(B)** Cryo-EM structure of human TAP in complex with ICP47 (EMD 8482; PDB 5U1D) at 4.0 Å (Oldham et al., 2016a). The N-terminal TMD0 of TAP1 and TAP2 and the C-terminal part of ICP47 are not visible due to their high flexibility. **(C)** X-ray structure of TmrAB at 2.7 Å resolution (PDB 5MKK) (Nöll et al., 2017). TmrAB and TAP1/2 are illustrated in light and dark magenta. The Fab fragment and ICP47 as fiducial marker or stabilizing factor are colored in yellow or green, respectively. The membrane border is indicated by thick gray lines.

interface, explaining the strong interaction and thermostability of the TAP complex (Herbring et al., 2016). The borders of the helical elements show a small deviation from the NMR structure of the active domain of ICP47 (residue 2–34) (Pfänder et al., 1999; Aisenbrey et al., 2006). The active domain has the same affinity as full-length ICP47 to inhibit peptide binding and transport, although the additional 21 residues resolved in the cryo-EM structure form close interactions with TM3 and cytosolic helix 1 of TAP2 (Galocha et al., 1997; Neumann et al., 1997). Although ICP47 interacts with TAP differently than antigenic peptides, the binding sites for the competitive inhibitor ICP47 and the peptides overlap at least partially, derived from a comparison of the ICP47-bound structure with biochemical data (Lehnert and Tampé, 2017). Remarkably, the inward-facing conformation of the ICP47-arrested TAP shows some distortion in the transmembrane region if compared to the X-ray structure of the TAP ortholog TmrAB. The lumenal gate is not closed, most likely induced by ICP47 binding, which leads to a strong bending of TM4/5 of TAP1 reflecting an altered cross-linking behavior (Lacaille and Androlewicz, 1998).

PEPTIDE BINDING

As for most ABC transporters, high-resolution structures with a bound substrate are still missing. Presently, the peptide-binding site of TAPL is not well-characterized because of the apparent micromolar peptide affinity (**Table 1**) (Wolters et al., 2005; Zhao et al., 2008). For TAP, molecular docking of peptides to homology models of TAP was performed to elucidate the peptide-binding site (Corradi et al., 2012; Geng et al., 2015; Lehnert et al., 2016). In all three studies, the binding site is localized in the transmembrane region. Depending on the template, and therefore on the opening of the TMD used to build the homology model of TAP, on the procedure to restrain the conformation of the peptide and on the method to dock the peptide, the conformation of the bound peptide as well as the exact localization within the TMD differ greatly. TAP inhibited by ICP47 is not the appropriate structure for docking experiments, since it shows obvious deviations in the TMD from other ABC transporters (see above). The conformation of the peptide has the strongest impact on the docking. Since, up to now, it has not been possible to dock a 9-mer peptide to the large cavity of TAP because of the high degree of freedom, all three studies had to cope with constraints concerning the peptide conformation. One study performed replica exchange simulations, in which the C_α of the N-terminal and C-terminal residue of the peptide were restrained to positively and negatively charged pockets assigned as binding sites for the N-terminal amino and the C-terminal carboxy group (Corradi et al., 2012). The peptide adopts an extended conformation. A second approach restrained the peptide in a β-hairpin conformation, which allowed docking in a position matching their crosslinking data (Geng et al., 2015).

Recently, the backbone structure of TAP-bound peptides was determined by dynamic nuclear polarization enhanced magic angle spinning solid-state NMR and subsequently used for molecular docking (Lehnert et al., 2016). This experimentally determined peptide structure adopts an extended conformation and perfectly agrees with pulsed EPR data, which showed for a similar peptide a distance of 2.5 nm of both termini (Herget et al., 2011). In the models by Corradi et al. and Lehnert et al. the binding pockets for the N- and C-terminus of the peptide

TABLE 1 | Characteristics of TAP-related transporters

	TAP1/2	TAPL
Localization	ER (phagosomes)[#] (endosomes)[#]	Lysosomes (non-acidic granules)
Core transport unit	Heterodimer (6 + 6 TMs)	Homodimer (6 + 6 TMs)
Interaction module	TMD0 (4 TMs)	TMD0 (4 TMs)
Interaction partner	TAPBR (tapasin)	LAMP-1, LAMP-2B
ATP-binding sites	Asymmetric	Symmetric
ATPase activity	Strictly coupled	Uncoupled
Substrate specificity	Peptides (8–16 aa) position 1-3 and Ω	Peptides (6–59 aa) position 1 and Ω
Peptide affinity	High-affinity (50 nM)	Low-affinity* (10 μM)
Trans-inhibition	Yes (16 μM)	Yes (1 mM)
Viral inhibitors	ICP47, US6, UL49.5, BNLF2a, CPXV012	

*[#]Antigen cross-presentation; *derived from K_m-value.*

are separated by 2.5 nm (Herget et al., 2011; Corradi et al., 2012; Lehnert et al., 2016; Lehnert and Tampé, 2017). The N-terminus of the peptide binds in both models to the same negatively charged pocket. However, in the model presented by Corradi et al. the peptide is aligned parallel to the membrane plane, whereas in the model of Lehnert et al. the peptide is more perpendicular to the membrane plane. Therefore, the C-termini of the extended peptides bind to different positively charged pockets. In the bent peptide structure modeled by Geng et al. there are no charged pockets within TAP involved in the binding of the N- and C-terminal group since they form a salt bridge by themselves (Geng et al., 2015). While the distance of the charged binding pockets perfectly fits with the minimal peptide length recognized by TAP, the binding site in the model of Geng et al. cannot explain the size restriction.

SPECIFICITY OF PEPTIDE TRANSPORTERS

TAP and TAPL are polypeptide ABC exporters, which move peptides out of the cytosol into the ER or into lysosomes, respectively. TAP prefers 8–16-mer peptides whereas TAPL displays a broader length window from 6 to 59-mer peptides with an optimum for 23-mer peptides (van Endert et al., 1994; Uebel et al., 1997; Wolters et al., 2005). The N-terminal amino group as well as the C-terminal carboxy group are involved in peptide binding since modifications of the termini interrupt peptide binding and transport. In initial experiments, using peptides composed of D-amino acids, the importance of side chains for substrate specificity was recognized. With combinatorial peptide libraries, the sequence specificity of both transporters was evaluated (Uebel et al., 1997; Zhao et al., 2008). For TAP, the first three N-terminal and the last C-terminal residues are relevant for peptide selection, whereas TAPL senses only the terminal residue on both ends. The selectivity pattern for TAP and TAPL is related: both favor basic and bulky residues and disfavor negatively charged side chains at their termini (Uebel et al., 1997; Zhao et al., 2008). Furthermore, for TAP a proline at position two and acidic residues at position three strongly interfere with peptide binding. Since peptides with a proline are found at position two on the peptide-recipient MHC I molecule, N-terminal trimming of the translocated peptides by ER-luminal peptidase ERAP-1 and-2 must occur (for review see van Endert, 2011). The sequence between both ends can be highly promiscuous for both transporters, and even large fluorophores or ε-amino linked polylysine chains with a mass equivalent to the unmodified peptide are tolerated at these positions (Grommé et al., 1997; Neumann and Tampé, 1999; Gorbulev et al., 2001). Although the peptide binding site seems to be large and flexible, TAP binds only one peptide as determined by fluorescence correlation spectroscopy (Herget et al., 2009). Whether TAPL as a homodimeric and therefore symmetric transporter binds more than one peptide is an open issue, however from existing transport studies any cooperativity in peptide binding can be excluded (Wolters et al., 2005; Zhao et al., 2008). The epitope RRYQKSTEL derived from histone 3.3 and fluorescently labeled derivatives were intensively used to study peptide binding and transport of TAP and TAPL. Based on its sequence, this peptide represents a good binder for both transporters. Interestingly, TAP binds this peptide with a 100-fold higher affinity as TAPL (**Table 1**). Peptide binding to TAP is a two-step process with a fast high-affinity association followed by a slow structural rearrangement of the transporter. Bound to TAP, the termini of the peptide feature a distance of 2.5 nm as revealed by pulsed EPR spectroscopy (Herget et al., 2011). This distance limits the size of the peptide to 8-mer peptides, which bind in an extended conformation discovered by solid-state NMR (Lehnert et al., 2016). Since longer peptides are restricted to the same distance, they have to adopt an extended kinked conformation in the binding pocket (Herget et al., 2011). Remarkably, the distance of the termini of MHC I bound peptides fits to that of TAP. It seems that not only in respect to sequence but also concerning the N- to C-terminal distance, MHC I and TAP has co-evolved and therefore TAP functions as a filter for MHC I. Taken together, TAPL recognizes a broader spectrum of peptides than TAP in respect to peptide length and sequence implying a more general function of the lysosomal transporter, respectively.

PEPTIDE TRANSLOCATION

TAP and TAPL export similar peptides out of the cytosol. Peptide transport is coupled with ATP hydrolysis since the non-hydrolysable ATP analog AMPPNP or mutations in the conserved sequences of the ATP binding site interfere with peptide translocation (Lapinski et al., 2001; Chen et al., 2004; Wolters et al., 2005; Perria et al., 2006; Demirel et al., 2007). Interestingly, mutation of the highly conserved aspartate of the D-loop of TAP1 to alanine turns TAP into a ligand-gated passive facilitator (Grossmann et al., 2014). The D-loop is localized in the interface between both NBDs and seems to be involved in communication between both ATP-binding sites. The ATP-binding site I of TAP formed by the Walker A/B motif of TAP1 and the C-loop of TAP2 shows strong deviation from the consensus sequences. This "degenerate" site has a strongly reduced ATP hydrolysis activity compared to the consensus site and is assumed to have a regulatory function not being directly involved in the energetics of peptide translocation (Lapinski et al., 2001; Chen et al., 2003). Interestingly, substituting the degenerate sequences by the consensus sequences creates a hyperactive transporter (Chen et al., 2004). TAP notably shows a direct coupling between peptide transport and ATP hydrolysis with no significant basal ATPase activity (Gorbulev et al., 2001; Grossmann et al., 2014). Moreover, there is a quality sensor since peptides, which bind to TAP but are not transported, do not stimulate ATPase activity (Gorbulev et al., 2001). Since TAPL has a high basal ATPase activity, a strong coupling between peptide binding, transport, and ATP hydrolysis is not expected (Zollmann et al., 2015).

Both transporters pump peptides against their concentration gradient as demonstrated by different techniques. Remarkably, TAPL accumulates peptides to an approximately 50-fold higher concentration than TAP. Both transporters do not reach the thermodynamic limit since they are inhibited in *trans*. This *trans* inhibition is comparable with product inhibition in classical enzyme kinetics. In the trans-inhibited state the transported peptide forces the transporter in the outward-facing conformation and therefore inhibits the conformational change to the inward-facing ground state. Subsequently, peptide transport and ATP hydrolysis are suppressed (Grossmann et al., 2014; Zollmann et al., 2015). The physiological meaning of this inhibition is an interesting point of discussion. In lysosomes, the peptides will be immediately degraded by the lysosomal proteases while in ER, the peptides will be bound to MHC class I and therefore removed from the pool of free peptides, or exported into the cytosol by an unresolved mechanism (Koopmann et al., 2000). The turnover rates of TAP and TAPL for peptide transport (k_{cat}) determined in proteoliposomes by classical ensemble experiments, averaging over all molecules, indicate a low transport rate with a k_{cat} of approximately 0.1 peptide/min (Zhao et al., 2008; Schölz et al., 2011; Grossmann et al., 2014). The amount of functional purified and reconstituted transporters can vary immensely and cannot be determined correctly by these ensemble experiments. Therefore, the single-molecule based method dual color fluorescence burst analysis was applied on TAPL transport (Zollmann et al., 2015), by which the accumulation of fluorescently labeled peptides in single liposomes is monitored in the confocal volume of a microscope. Thereby, active transporters can be separated from inactive ones. Remarkably, only approximately 10% of TAPL was active in transport after reconstitution. To the end, a transport rate of eight peptides per min was determined, which fits to ATP hydrolysis kinetics of other well-characterized ABC exporters such as MsbA and ABCC3 (Zehnpfennig et al., 2009; Kawai et al., 2011). It is worth mentioning that data on solute transport kinetics are limited since most of the eukaryotic ABC exporters translocate hydrophobic substances, which are intrinsically problematic to analyze. Furthermore, TAP as well as TAPL operate strictly unidirectional and the process is not reversible as for the F_0F_1 ATP-synthase, which functions as ATP hydrolase or synthase depending on the proton gradient (Grossmann et al., 2014; Zollmann et al., 2015).

PURIFICATION AND FUNCTIONAL RECONSTITUTION

A prerequisite for the detailed analysis of these transporters is their synthesis, purification, and functional reconstitution into liposomes. While there is no natural source with high expression found for TAPL, the B-lymphoma cell line Raji shows high endogenous expression suitable not only for cell biological but also for biochemical studies (Uebel et al., 1997; Gorbulev et al., 2001; Chen et al., 2003). Both transporters are stably and transiently expressed in mammalian cell lines (Demirel et al., 2012; Hinz et al., 2014). Moreover, good expression in *Spodoptera frugiperda* cells with the baculovirus expression system and even stably integrated in the genome in *Drosophila melanogaster* cells is reported (Meyer et al., 1994; van Endert et al., 1994; Schoenhals et al., 1999; Wolters et al., 2005). In baker's yeast only very small amounts of TAP were produced (Urlinger et al., 1997), whereas both transporters are expressed to a decent level in *Pichia pastoris*, high enough for biochemical and structural studies (Schölz et al., 2011; Parcej et al., 2013; Zollmann et al., 2015; Oldham et al., 2016a). For TAPL, a single step purification via His-tag was applied (Zhao et al., 2008), whereas the heterodimeric TAP complex is isolated in a two-step, orthogonal process using a His-tag and a streptavidin-binding-peptide tag to capture only heterodimeric complexes (Parcej et al., 2013). More recently, TAP was isolated by the viral inhibitor ICP47 ending with a thermostable, inhibited complex well-suited for single particle cryo-EM analyses of the native MHC I peptide loading complex (Herbring et al., 2016; Blees et al., 2017). Functional reconstitution is a prerequisite for mechanistic studies. A critical step is the detergent used for solubilization. Interestingly, TAPL is less dependent on the detergent since digitonin as well as n-dodecyl-β-D-maltoside (DDM) restores its activity (Zhao et al., 2008), whereas TAP is only functionally solubilized in digitonin and the steroid based glycol-diosgenin in the range of 80 different detergents tested (Herget et al., 2009; Lehnert et al., 2016). Digitonin solubilized TAP is enriched in phosphatidylethanolamine and phosphatidylinositol. Remarkably, TAP solubilized in DDM and therefore inactive could regain its activity if reconstituted in membranes rich in these phospholipids (Schölz et al., 2011).

AUTHOR CONTRIBUTIONS

All authors listed have made a substantial, direct and intellectual contribution to the work, and approved it for publication.

ACKNOWLEDGMENTS

The German Research Foundation (SFB 807 and AB 149 to RA and RT) supported this work. We thank Philipp Graab and Christoph Bock for the assistance in figure preparation. We are grateful to all members of the Institute of Biochemistry (Goethe University Frankfurt) for their helpful comments on the manuscript.

REFERENCES

Abele, R., and Tampé, R. (2004). The ABCs of immunology: structure and function of TAP, the transporter associated with antigen processing. *Physiology* 19, 216–224. doi: 10.1152/physiol.00002.2004

Ahn, K., Meyer, T. H., Uebel, S., Sempé, P., Djaballah, H., Yang, Y., et al. (1996). Molecular mechanism and species specificity of TAP inhibition by herpes simplex virus ICP47. *EMBO J.* 15, 3247–3255.

Aisenbrey, C., Sizun, C., Koch, J., Herget, M., Abele, R., Bechinger, B., et al. (2006). Structure and dynamics of membrane-associated ICP47, a viral inhibitor of the MHC I antigen-processing machinery. *J. Biol. Chem.* 281, 30365–30372. doi: 10.1074/jbc.M603000200

Bastian, F., Parmentier, G., Roux, J., Moretti, S., Laudet, V., and Robinson-Rechavi, M. (2008). "Bgee: Integrating and comparing heterogeneous transcriptome data among species," in *Data Integration in the Life Sciences, 5th International Workshop*, ed A. Bairoch (Berlin: Springer), 124–131.

Blees, A., Januliene, D., Hofmann, T., Koller, N., Schmidt, C., Trowitzsch, S., et al. (2017). Structure of the human MHC-I peptide-loading complex. *Nature* 551, 525–528. doi: 10.1038/nature24627

Blees, A., Reichel, K., Trowitzsch, S., Fisette, O., Bock, C., Abele, R., et al. (2015). Assembly of the MHC I peptide-loading complex determined by a conserved ionic lock-switch. *Sci. Rep.* 5:17341. doi: 10.1038/srep17341

Blum, J. S., Wearsch, P. A., and Cresswell, P. (2013). Pathways of antigen processing. *Annu. Rev. Immunol.* 31, 443–473. doi: 10.1146/annurev-immunol-032712-095910

Bonifacino, J. S., and Traub, L. M. (2003). Signals for sorting of transmembrane proteins to endosomes and lysosomes. *Annu. Rev. Biochem.* 72, 395–447. doi: 10.1146/annurev.biochem.72.121801.161800

Brandsch, M. (2013). Drug transport via the intestinal peptide transporter PepT1. *Curr. Opin. Pharmacol.* 13, 881–887. doi: 10.1016/j.coph.2013.08.004

Chen, M., Abele, R., and Tampé, R. (2003). Peptides induce ATP hydrolysis at both subunits of the transporter associated with antigen processing. *J. Biol. Chem.* 278, 29686–29692. doi: 10.1074/jbc.M302757200

Chen, M., Abele, R., and Tampé, R. (2004). Functional non-equivalence of ATP-binding cassette signature motifs in the transporter associated with antigen processing (TAP). *J. Biol. Chem.* 279, 46073–46081. doi: 10.1074/jbc.M404042200

Colonna, M., Bresnahan, M., Bahram, S., Strominger, J. L., and Spies, T. (1992). Allelic variants of the human putative peptide transporter involved in antigen processing. *Proc. Natl. Acad. Sci. U.S.A.* 89, 3932–3936. doi: 10.1073/pnas.89.9.3932

Corradi, V., Singh, G., and Tieleman, D. P. (2012). The human transporter associated with antigen processing: molecular models to describe peptide binding competent states. *J. Biol. Chem.* 287, 28099–28111. doi: 10.1074/jbc.M112.381251

Crotzer, V. L., and Blum, J. S. (2008). Cytosol to lysosome transport of intracellular antigens during immune surveillance. *Traffic* 9, 10–16. doi: 10.1111/j.1600-0854.2007.00664.x

Crotzer, V. L., and Blum, J. S. (2010). Autophagy and adaptive immunity. *Immunology* 131, 9–17. doi: 10.1111/j.1365-2567.2010.03321.x

Dani, A., Chaudhry, A., Mukherjee, P., Rajagopal, D., Bhatia, S., George, A., et al. (2004). The pathway for MHCII-mediated presentation of endogenous proteins involves peptide transport to the endo-lysosomal compartment. *J. Cell Sci.* 117, 4219–4230. doi: 10.1242/jcs.01288

Demirel, O., Bangert, I., Tampé, R., and Abele, R. (2010). Tuning the cellular trafficking of the lysosomal peptide transporter TAPL by its N-terminal domain. *Traffic* 11, 383–393. doi: 10.1111/j.1600-0854.2009.01021.x

Demirel, Ö., Jan, I., Wolters, D., Blanz, J., Saftig, P., Tampé, R., et al. (2012). The lysosomal polypeptide transporter TAPL is stabilized by interaction with LAMP-1 and LAMP-2. *J. Cell Sci.* 125, 4230–4240. doi: 10.1242/jcs.087346

Demirel, O., Waibler, Z., Kalinke, U., Grünebach, F., Appel, S., Brossart, P., et al. (2007). Identification of a lysosomal peptide transport system induced during dendritic cell development. *J. Biol. Chem.* 282, 37836–37843. doi: 10.1074/jbc.M708139200

Deverson, E. V., Gow, I. R., Coadwell, W. J., Monaco, J. J., Butcher, G. W., and Howard, J. C. (1990). MHC class II region encoding proteins related to the multidrug resistance family of transmembrane transporters. *Nature* 348, 738–741. doi: 10.1038/348738a0

Doeven, M. K., Kok, J., and Poolman, B. (2005). Specificity and selectivity determinants of peptide transport in *Lactococcus lactis* and other microorganisms. *Mol. Microbiol.* 57, 640–649. doi: 10.1111/j.1365-2958.2005.04698.x

Fricker, L. D. (2010). Analysis of mouse brain peptides using mass spectrometry-based peptidomics: implications for novel functions ranging from non-classical neuropeptides to microproteins. *Mol. Biosyst.* 6, 1355–1365. doi: 10.1039/c003317k

Galocha, B., Hill, A., Barnett, B. C., Dolan, A., Raimondi, A., Cook, R. F., et al. (1997). The active site of ICP47, a herpes simplex virus-encoded inhibitor of the major histocompatibility complex (MHC)-encoded peptide transporter associated with antigen processing (TAP), maps to the NH2-terminal 35 residues. *J. Exp. Med.* 185, 1565–1572. doi: 10.1084/jem.185.9.1565

Geng, J., Pogozheva, I. D., Mosberg, H. I., and Raghavan, M. (2015). Use of functional polymorphisms to elucidate the peptide binding site of TAP complexes. *J. Immunol.* 195, 3436–3448. doi: 10.4049/jimmunol.1500985

Gomolplitinant, K. M., and Saier, M. H. (2011). Evolution of the oligopeptide transporter family. *J. Membr. Biol.* 240, 89–110. doi: 10.1007/s00232-011-9347-9

Gorbulev, S., Abele, R., and Tampé, R. (2001). Allosteric crosstalk between peptide-binding, transport, and ATP hydrolysis of the ABC transporter TAP. *Proc. Natl. Acad. Sci. U.S.A.* 98, 3732–3737. doi: 10.1073/pnas.061467898

Grommé, M., van der Valk, R., Sliedregt, K., Vernie, L., Liskamp, R., Hämmerling, G., et al. (1997). The rational design of TAP inhibitors using peptide substrate modifications and peptidomimetics. *Eur. J. Immunol.* 27, 898–904. doi: 10.1002/eji.1830270415

Gromme, M., and Neefjes, J. (2002). Antigen degradation or presentation by MHC class I molecules via classical and non-classical pathways. *Mol. Immunol.* 39, 181–202. doi: 10.1016/S0161-5890(02)00101-3

Grossmann, N., Vakkasoglu, A. S., Hulpke, S., Abele, R., Gaudet, R., and Tampé, R. (2014). Mechanistic determinants of the directionality and energetics of active export by a heterodimeric ABC transporter. *Nat. Commun.* 5:5419. doi: 10.1038/ncomms6419

Grotzke, J. E., Kozik, P., Morel, J. D., Impens, F., Pietrosemoli, N., Cresswell, P., et al. (2017a). Sec61 blockade by mycolactone inhibits antigen cross-presentation independently of endosome-to-cytosol export. *Proc. Natl. Acad. Sci. U.S.A.* 114, E5910–E5919. doi: 10.1073/pnas.1705242114

Grotzke, J. E., Sengupta, D., Lu, Q., and Cresswell, P. (2017b). The ongoing saga of the mechanism(s) of MHC class I-restricted cross-presentation. *Curr. Opin. Immunol.* 46, 89–96. doi: 10.1016/j.coi.2017.03.015

Haynes, C. M., Yang, Y., Blais, S. P., Neubert, T. A., and Ron, D. (2010). The matrix peptide exporter HAF-1 signals a mitochondrial UPR by activating the transcription factor ZC376.7 in *C. elegans*. *Mol. Cell* 37, 529–540. doi: 10.1016/j.molcel.2010.01.015

Herbring, V., Bäucker, A., Trowitzsch, S., and Tampé, R. (2016). A dual inhibition mechanism of herpesviral ICP47 arresting a conformationally thermostable TAP complex. *Sci. Rep.* 6:36907. doi: 10.1038/srep36907

Herget, M., Baldauf, C., Schölz, C., Parcej, D., Wiesmüller, K. H., Tampé, R., et al. (2011). Conformation of peptides bound to the transporter associated with antigen processing (TAP). *Proc. Natl. Acad. Sci. U.S.A.* 108, 1349–1354. doi: 10.1073/pnas.1012355108

Herget, M., Kreissig, N., Kolbe, C., Schölz, C., Tampé, R., and Abele, R. (2009). Purification and reconstitution of the antigen transport complex TAP: a prerequisite for determination of peptide stoichiometry and ATP hydrolysis. *J. Biol. Chem.* 284, 33740–33749. doi: 10.1074/jbc.M109.047779

Herget, M., and Tampé, R. (2007). Intracellular peptide transporters in human–compartmentalization of the "peptidome". *Pflug. Arch.* 453, 591–600. doi: 10.1007/s00424-006-0083-4

Hinz, A., Jedamzick, J., Herbring, V., Fischbach, H., Hartmann, J., Parcej, D., et al. (2014). Assembly and function of the major histocompatibility complex (MHC) I peptide-loading complex are conserved across higher vertebrates. *J. Biol. Chem.* 289, 33109–33117. doi: 10.1074/jbc.M114.609263

Hulpke, S., Baldauf, C., and Tampé, R. (2012a). Molecular architecture of the MHC I peptide-loading complex: one tapasin molecule is essential and sufficient for antigen processing. *FASEB J.* 26, 5071–5080. doi: 10.1096/fj.12-217489

Hulpke, S., Tomioka, M., Kremmer, E., Ueda, K., Abele, R., and Tampé, R. (2012b). Direct evidence that the N-terminal extensions of the TAP complex act as autonomous interaction scaffolds for the assembly of the MHC I peptide-loading complex. *Cell. Mol. Life Sci.* 69, 3317–3327. doi: 10.1007/s00018-012-1005-6

Johnson, Z. L., and Chen, J. (2017). Structural basis of substrate recognition by the multidrug resistance Protein MRP1. *Cell* 168, 1075.e9–1085e9. doi: 10.1016/j.cell.2017.01.041

Johnson, Z. L., and Chen, J. (2018). ATP binding enables substrate release from multidrug resistance protein 1. *Cell* 172, 81.e10–89.e10. doi: 10.1016/j.cell.2017.12.005

Kawai, H., Tanji, T., Shiraishi, H., Yamada, M., Iijima, R., Inoue, T., et al. (2009). Normal formation of a subset of intestinal granules in *Caenorhabditis elegans* requires ATP-binding cassette transporters HAF-4 and HAF-9, which are highly homologous to human lysosomal peptide transporter TAP-like. *Mol. Biol. Cell* 20, 2979–2990. doi: 10.1091/mbc.E08-09-0912

Kawai, T., Caaveiro, J. M., Abe, R., Katagiri, T., and Tsumoto, K. (2011). Catalytic activity of MsbA reconstituted in nanodisc particles is modulated by remote interactions with the bilayer. *FEBS Lett.* 585, 3533–3537. doi: 10.1016/j.febslet.2011.10.015

Keusekotten, K., Leonhardt, R. M., Ehses, S., and Knittler, M. R. (2006). Biogenesis of functional antigenic peptide transporter TAP requires assembly of pre-existing TAP1 with newly synthesized TAP2. *J. Biol. Chem.* 281, 17545–17551. doi: 10.1074/jbc.M602360200

Kim, J., Wu, S., Tomasiak, T. M., Mergel, C., Winter, M. B., Stiller, S. B., et al. (2015). Subnanometre-resolution electron cryomicroscopy structure of a heterodimeric ABC exporter. *Nature* 517, 396–400. doi: 10.1038/nature 13872

Kobayashi, A., Hori, S., Suita, N., and Maeda, M. (2003). Gene organization of human transporter associated with antigen processing-like (TAPL, ABCB9): analysis of alternative splicing variants and promoter activity. *Biochem. Biophys. Res. Commun.* 309, 815–822. doi: 10.1016/j.bbrc.2003. 08.081

Kobayashi, A., Kasano, M., Maeda, T., Hori, S., Motojima, K., Suzuki, M., et al. (2000). A half-type ABC transporter TAPL is highly conserved between rodent and man, and the human gene is not responsive to interferon-gamma in contrast to TAP1 and TAP2. *J. Biochem.* 128, 711–718. doi: 10.1093/oxfordjournals.jbchem.a022805

Koch, J., Guntrum, R., Heintke, S., Kyritsis, C., and Tampé, R. (2004). Functional dissection of the transmembrane domains of the transporter associated with antigen processing (TAP). *J. Biol. Chem.* 279, 10142–10147. doi: 10.1074/jbc.M312816200

Koopmann, J. O., Albring, J., Hüter, E., Bulbuc, N., Spee, P., Neefjes, J., et al. (2000). Export of antigenic peptides from the endoplasmic reticulum intersects with retrograde protein translocation through the Sec61p channel. *Immunity* 13, 117–127. doi: 10.1016/S1074-7613(00)00013-3

Lacaille, V. G., and Androlewicz, M. J. (1998). Herpes simplex virus inhibitor ICP47 destabilizes the transporter associated with antigen processing (TAP) heterodimer. *J. Biol. Chem.* 273, 17386–17390. doi: 10.1074/jbc.273.28. 17386

Lapinski, P. E., Neubig, R. R., and Raghavan, M. (2001). Walker A lysine mutations of TAP1 and TAP2 interfere with peptide translocation but not peptide binding. *J. Biol. Chem.* 276, 7526–7533. doi: 10.1074/jbc.M009448200

Lawand, M., Abramova, A., Manceau, V., Springer, S., and van Endert, P. (2016). TAP-dependent and -independent peptide import into dendritic cell phagosomes. *J. Immunol.* 197, 3454–3463. doi: 10.4049/jimmunol.15 01925

Lehnert, E., Mao, J., Mehdipour, A. R., Hummer, G., Abele, R., Glaubitz, C., et al. (2016). Antigenic peptide recognition on the human ABC transporter TAP resolved by DNP-enhanced solid-state NMR spectroscopy. *J. Am. Chem. Soc.* 138, 13967–13974. doi: 10.1021/jacs.6b07426

Lehnert, E., and Tampé, R. (2017). Structure and dynamics of antigenic peptides in complex with TAP. *Front. Immunol.* 8:10. doi: 10.3389/fimmu.2017.00010

Leonhardt, R. M., Abrahimi, P., Mitchell, S. M., and Cresswell, P. (2014). Three tapasin docking sites in TAP cooperate to facilitate transporter stabilization and heterodimerization. *J. Immunol.* 192, 2480–2494. doi: 10.4049/jimmunol.1302637

Leveson-Gower, D. B., Michnick, S. W., and Ling, V. (2004). Detection of TAP family dimerizations by an *in vivo* assay in mammalian cells. *Biochemistry* 43, 14257–14264. doi: 10.1021/bi0491245

Li, N., Wu, J. X., Ding, D., Cheng, J., Gao, N., and Chen, L. (2017). Structure of a pancreatic ATP-sensitive potassium channel. *Cell* 168, 101.e10–110.e10. doi: 10.1016/j.cell.2016.12.028

Liu, F., Zhang, Z., Csanády, L., Gadsby, D. C., and Chen, J. (2017). Molecular structure of the human CFTR ion channel. *Cell* 169, 85.e.8–95.e8. doi: 10.1016/j.cell.2017.02.024

Locher, K. P. (2016). Mechanistic diversity in ATP-binding cassette (ABC) transporters. *Nat. Struct. Mol. Biol.* 23, 487–493. doi: 10.1038/nsmb.3216

Martin, G. M., Kandasamy, B., DiMaio, F., Yoshioka, C., and Shyng, S. L. (2017a). Anti-diabetic drug binding site in a mammalian KATP channel revealed by Cryo-EM. *Elife* 6:e31054. doi: 10.7554/eLife.31054

Martin, G. M., Yoshioka, C., Rex, E. A., Fay, J. F., Xie, Q., Whorton, M. R., et al. (2017b). Cryo-EM structure of the ATP-sensitive potassium channel illuminates mechanisms of assembly and gating. *Elife* 6:e24149. doi: 10.7554/eLife.24149

Mayerhofer, P. U., and Tampé, R. (2015). Antigen translocation machineries in adaptive immunity and viral immune evasion. *J. Mol. Biol.* 427, 1102–1118. doi: 10.1016/j.jmb.2014.09.006

Merzougui, N., Kratzer, R., Saveanu, L., and van Endert, P. (2011). A proteasome-dependent, TAP-independent pathway for cross-presentation of phagocytosed antigen. *EMBO Rep.* 12, 1257–1264. doi: 10.1038/embor.2011.203

Meyer, T. H., van Endert, P. M., Uebel, S., Ehring, B., and Tampé, R. (1994). Functional expression and purification of the ABC transporter complex associated with antigen processing (TAP) in insect cells. *FEBS Lett.* 351, 443–447. doi: 10.1016/0014-5793(94)00908-2

Michaelis, S., and Barrowman, J. (2012). Biogenesis of the Saccharomyces cerevisiae pheromone a-factor, from yeast mating to human disease. *Microbiol. Mol. Biol. Rev.* 76, 626–651. doi: 10.1128/MMBR.00010-12

Miller, M. A., Ganesan, A. P., Luckashenak, N., Mendonca, M., and Eisenlohr, L. C. (2015). Endogenous antigen processing drives the primary CD4+ T cell response to influenza. *Nat. Med.* 21, 1216–1222. doi: 10.1038/ nm.3958

Monaco, J. J., Cho, S., and Attaya, M. (1990). Transport protein genes in the murine MHC: possible implications for antigen processing. *Science* 250, 1723–1726. doi: 10.1126/science.2270487

Mutch, D. M., Anderle, P., Fiaux, M., Mansourian, R., Vidal, K., Wahli, W., et al. (2004). Regional variations in ABC transporter expression along the mouse intestinal tract. *Physiol. Genomics* 17, 11–20. doi: 10.1152/physiolgenomics.00150.2003

Neumann, L., Kraas, W., Uebel, S., Jung, G., and Tampé, R. (1997). The active domain of the herpes simplex virus protein ICP47: a potent inhibitor of the transporter associated with antigen processing. *J. Mol. Biol.* 272, 484–492. doi: 10.1006/jmbi.1997.1282

Neumann, L., and Tampé, R. (1999). Kinetic analysis of peptide binding to the TAP transport complex: evidence for structural rearrangements induced by substrate binding. *J. Mol. Biol.* 294, 1203–1213. doi: 10.1006/jmbi. 1999.3329

Newstead, S. (2015). Molecular insights into proton coupled peptide transport in the PTR family of oligopeptide transporters. *Biochim. Biophys. Acta* 1850, 488–499. doi: 10.1016/j.bbagen.2014.05.011

Nöll, A., Thomas, C., Herbring, V., Zollmann, T., Barth, K., Mehdipour, A. R., et al. (2017). Crystal structure and mechanistic basis of a functional homolog of the antigen transporter TAP. *Proc. Natl. Acad. Sci. U.S.A.* 114, E438–E447. doi: 10.1073/pnas.1620009114

Oancea, G., O'Mara, M. L., Bennett, W. F., Tieleman, D. P., Abele, R., and Tampé, R. (2009). Structural arrangement of the transmission interface in the antigen ABC transport complex TAP. *Proc. Natl. Acad. Sci. U.S.A.* 106, 5551–5556. doi: 10.1073/pnas.0811260106

Oldham, M. L., Grigorieff, N., and Chen, J. (2016a). Structure of the transporter associated with antigen processing trapped by herpes simplex virus. *Elife* 5:e21829. doi: 10.7554/eLife.21829

Oldham, M. L., Hite, R. K., Steffen, A. M., Damko, E., Li, Z., Walz, T., et al. (2016b). A mechanism of viral immune evasion revealed by cryo-EM analysis of the TAP transporter. *Nature* 529, 537–540. doi: 10.1038/nature16506

Parcej, D., Guntrum, R., Schmidt, S., Hinz, A., and Tampé, R. (2013). Multicolour fluorescence-detection size-exclusion chromatography for structural genomics of membrane multiprotein complexes. *PLoS ONE* 8:e67112. doi: 10.1371/journal.pone.0067112

Parcej, D., and Tampé, R. (2010). ABC proteins in antigen translocation and viral inhibition. *Nat. Chem. Biol.* 6, 572–580. doi: 10.1038/nchembio.410

Perria, C. L., Rajamanickam, V., Lapinski, P. E., and Raghavan, M. (2006). Catalytic site modifications of TAP1 and TAP2 and their functional consequences. *J. Biol. Chem.* 281, 39839–39851. doi: 10.1074/jbc.M6054 92200

Pfänder, R., Neumann, L., Zweckstetter, M., Seger, C., Holak, T. A., and Tampé, R. (1999). Structure of the active domain of the herpes simplex virus protein ICP47 in water/sodium dodecyl sulfate solution determined by nuclear magnetic resonance spectroscopy. *Biochemistry* 38, 13692–13698. doi: 10.1021/bi99 09647

Powis, S. J., Townsend, A. R., Deverson, E. V., Bastin, J., Butcher, G. W., and Howard, J. C. (1991). Restoration of antigen presentation to the mutant cell line RMA-S by an MHC-linked transporter. *Nature* 354, 528–531. doi: 10.1038/354528a0

Qian, H., Zhao, X., Cao, P., Lei, J., Yan, N., and Gong, X. (2017). Structure of the human lipid exporter ABCA1. *Cell* 169, 1228.e10–1239.e10. doi: 10.1016/j.cell.2017.05.020

Ramos, M. S., Abele, R., Nagy, R., Grotemeyer, M. S., Tampé, R., Rentsch, D., et al. (2011). Characterization of a transport activity for long-chain peptides in barley mesophyll vacuoles. *J. Exp. Bot.* 62, 2403–2410. doi: 10.1093/jxb/erq397

Reits, E., Griekspoor, A., Neijssen, J., Groothuis, T., Jalink, K., van Veelen, P., et al. (2003). Peptide diffusion, protection, and degradation in nuclear and cytoplasmic compartments before antigen presentation by MHC class I. *Immunity* 18, 97–108. doi: 10.1016/S1074-7613(02)00511-3

Ren, J., Chung-Davidson, Y. W., Yeh, C. Y., Scott, C., Brown, T., and Li, W. (2015). Genome-wide analysis of the ATP-binding cassette (ABC) transporter gene family in sea lamprey and Japanese lamprey. *BMC Genomics* 16:436. doi: 10.1186/s12864-015-1677-z

Rufer, E., Kägebein, D., Leonhardt, R. M., and Knittler, M. R. (2015). Hydrophobic interactions are key to drive the association of tapasin with peptide transporter subunit TAP2. *J. Immunol.* 195, 5482–5494. doi: 10.4049/jimmunol.15 00246

Schmidt, M., and Finley, D. (2014). Regulation of proteasome activity in health and disease. *Biochim. Biophys. Acta* 1843, 13–25. doi: 10.1016/j.bbamcr.2013. 08.012

Schoenhals, G. J., Krishna, R. M., Grandea, A. G. III, Spies, T., Peterson, P. A., Yang, Y., et al. (1999). Retention of empty MHC class I molecules by tapasin is essential to reconstitute antigen presentation in invertebrate cells. *EMBO J.* 18, 743–753. doi: 10.1093/emboj/18.3.743

Schölz, C., Parcej, D., Ejsing, C. S., Robenek, H., Urbatsch, I. L., and Tampé, R. (2011). Specific lipids modulate the transporter associated with antigen processing (TAP). *J. Biol. Chem.* 286, 13346–13356. doi: 10.1074/jbc.M110.216416

Sievers, F., Wilm, A., Dineen, D., Gibson T. J., Karplus, K., Li, W., Lopez, R., et al. (2011). Fast, scalable generation of high-quality protein multiple sequence alignments using Clustal Omega. *Mol. Syst. Biol.* 7:539. doi: 10.1038/msb.2011.75

Spies, T., Bresnahan, M., Bahram, S., Arnold, D., Blanck, G., Mellins, E., et al. (1990). A gene in the human major histocompatibility complex class II region controlling the class I antigen presentation pathway. *Nature* 348, 744–747. doi: 10.1038/348744a0

Stern, L. J., and Santambrogio, L. (2016). The melting pot of the MHC II peptidome. *Curr. Opin. Immunol.* 40, 70–77. doi: 10.1016/j.coi.2016. 03.004

Tanji, T., Nishikori, K., Shiraishi, H., Maeda, M., and Ohashi-Kobayashi, A. (2013). Co-operative function and mutual stabilization of the half ATP-binding cassette transporters HAF-4 and HAF-9 in *Caenorhabditis elegans*. *Biochem. J.* 452, 467–475. doi: 10.1042/BJ20130115

Taylor, N. M. I., Manolaridis, I., Jackson, S. M., Kowal, J., Stahlberg, H., and Locher, K. P. (2017). Structure of the human multidrug transporter ABCG2. *Nature* 546, 504–509. doi: 10.1038/nature22345

Thiele, F., Tao, S., Zhang, Y., Muschaweckh, A., Zollmann, T., Protzer, U., et al. (2015). Modified vaccinia virus Ankara-infected dendritic cells present CD4+ T-cell epitopes by endogenous major histocompatibility complex class II presentation pathways. *J. Virol.* 89, 2698–2709. doi: 10.1128/JVI.03 244-14

Thomas, C., and Tampé, R. (2018). Multifaceted structures and mechanisms of ABC transporters in health and disease. *Curr. Opin. Struct. Biol.* 51, 116–128. doi: 10.1016/j.sbi.2018.03.016

Tomazin, R., Hill, A. B., Jugovic, P., York, I., van Endert, P., Ploegh, H. L., et al. (1996). Stable binding of the herpes simplex virus ICP47 protein to the peptide binding site of TAP. *EMBO J.* 15, 3256–3266.

Trowsdale, J., Hanson, I., Mockridge, I., Beck, S., Townsend, A., and Kelly, A. (1990). Sequences encoded in the class II region of the MHC related to the 'ABC' superfamily of transporters. *Nature* 348, 741–744. doi: 10.1038/348741a0

Trowsdale, J., Ragoussis, J., and Campbell, R. D. (1991). Map of the human MHC. *Immunol. Today* 12, 443–446. doi: 10.1016/0167-5699(91)90017-N

Uebel, S., Kraas, W., Kienle, S., Wiesmüller, K. H., Jung, G., and Tampé, R. (1997). Recognition principle of the TAP transporter disclosed by combinatorial peptide libraries. *Proc. Natl. Acad. Sci. U.S.A.* 94, 8976–8981. doi: 10.1073/pnas.94.17.8976

Uhlén, M., Fagerberg, L., Hallström, B. M., Lindskog, C., Oksvold, P., Mardinoglu, A., et al. (2015). Proteomics. tissue-based map of the human proteome. *Science* 347:1260419. doi: 10.1126/science.1260419

Uinuk-ool, T. S., Mayer, W. E., Sato, A., Takezaki, N., Benyon, L., Cooper, M. D., et al. (2003). Identification and characterization of a TAP-family gene in the lamprey. *Immunogenetics* 55, 38–48. doi: 10.1007/s00251-003-0548-y

Urlinger, S., Kuchler, K., Meyer, T. H., Uebel, S., and Tampé, R. (1997). Intracellular location, complex formation, and function of the transporter associated with antigen processing in yeast. *Eur. J. Biochem.* 245, 266–272. doi: 10.1111/j.1432-1033.1997.00266.x

van de Weijer, M. L., Luteijn, R. D., and Wiertz, E. J. (2015). Viral immune evasion: lessons in MHC class I antigen presentation. *Semin. Immunol.* 27, 125–137. doi: 10.1016/j.smim.2015.03.010

van Endert, P. (2011). Post-proteasomal and proteasome-independent generation of MHC class I ligands. *Cell. Mol. Life Sci.* 68, 1553–1567. doi: 10.1007/s00018-011-0662-1

van Endert, P. (2016). Intracellular recycling and cross-presentation by MHC class I molecules. *Immunol. Rev.* 272, 80–96. doi: 10.1111/imr.12424

van Endert, P. M., Tampé, R., Meyer, T. H., Tisch, R., Bach, J. F., and McDevitt, H. O. (1994). A sequential model for peptide binding and transport by the transporters associated with antigen processing. *Immunity* 1, 491–500. doi: 10.1016/1074-7613(94)90091-4

Veerappan Ganesan, A. P., and Eisenlohr, L. C. (2017). The elucidation of non-classical MHC class II antigen processing through the study of viral antigens. *Curr. Opin. Virol.* 22, 71–76. doi: 10.1016/j.coviro.2016.11.009

Wolters, J. C., Abele, R., and Tampé, R. (2005). Selective and ATP-dependent translocation of peptides by the homodimeric ATP binding cassette transporter TAP-like (ABCB9). *J. Biol. Chem.* 280, 23631–23636. doi: 10.1074/jbc.M503231200

Yamaguchi, Y., Kasano, M., Terada, T., Sato, R., and Maeda, M. (1999). An ABC transporter homologous to TAP proteins. *FEBS Lett.* 457, 231–236. doi: 10.1016/S0014-5793(99)01042-X

Yan, G., Shi, L., and Faustman, D. (1999). Novel splicing of the human MHC-encoded peptide transporter confers unique properties. *J. Immunol.* 162, 852–859.

Young, L., Leonhard, K., Tatsuta, T., Trowsdale, J., and Langer, T. (2001). Role of the ABC transporter Mdl1 in peptide export from mitochondria. *Science* 291, 2135–2138. doi: 10.1126/science.1056957

Zehner, M., Marschall, A. L., Bos, E., Schloetel, J. G., Kreer, C., Fehrenschild, D., et al. (2015). The translocon protein Sec61 mediates antigen transport from endosomes in the cytosol for cross-presentation to CD8(+) T cells. *Immunity* 42, 850–863. doi: 10.1016/j.immuni.2015.04.008

Zehnpfennig, B., Urbatsch, I. L., and Galla, H. J. (2009). Functional reconstitution of human ABCC3 into proteoliposomes reveals a transport mechanism with positive cooperativity. *Biochemistry* 48, 4423–4430. doi: 10.1021/bi90 01908

Zhang, F., Zhang, W., Liu, L., Fisher, C. L., Hui, D., Childs, S., et al. (2000). Characterization of ABCB9, an ATP binding cassette protein associated with lysosomes. *J. Biol. Chem.* 275, 23287–23294. doi: 10.1074/jbc.M0018 19200

Zhang, Z., Liu, F., and Chen, J. (2017). Conformational Changes of CFTR upon Phosphorylation and ATP Binding. *Cell* 170, 483.e8–491.e8. doi: 10.1016/j.cell.2017.06.041

Zhao, C., Haase, W., Tampé, R., and Abele, R. (2008). Peptide specificity and lipid activation of the lysosomal transport complex ABCB9 (TAPL). *J. Biol. Chem.* 283, 17083–17091. doi: 10.1074/jbc.M801794200

Zimmer, J., Donato, L., Hanau, D., Cazenave, J. P., Tongio, M. M., Moretta, A., et al. (1998). Activity and phenotype of natural killer cells in peptide transporter (TAP)-deficient patients (type I bare lymphocyte syndrome). *J. Exp. Med.* 187, 117–122. doi: 10.1084/jem.187.1.117

Zollmann, T., Moiset, G., Tumulka, F., Tampé, R., Poolman, B., and Abele, R. (2015). Single liposome analysis of peptide translocation by the ABC transporter TAPL. *Proc. Natl. Acad. Sci. U.S.A.* 112, 2046–2051. doi: 10.1073/pnas.1418100112

5

Targeting Channels and Transporters in Protozoan Parasite Infections

*Anna Meier†, Holger Erler† and Eric Beitz**

Department of Pharmaceutical and Medicinal Chemistry, Christian-Albrechts-University of Kiel, Kiel, Germany

***Correspondence:**
Eric Beitz
ebeitz@pharmazie.uni-kiel.de

†These authors have contributed equally to this work.

Infectious diseases caused by pathogenic protozoa are among the most significant causes of death in humans. Therapeutic options are scarce and massively challenged by the emergence of resistant parasite strains. Many of the current anti-parasite drugs target soluble enzymes, generate unspecific oxidative stress, or act by an unresolved mechanism within the parasite. In recent years, collections of drug-like compounds derived from large-scale phenotypic screenings, such as the *malaria* or *pathogen box*, have been made available to researchers free of charge boosting the identification of novel promising targets. Remarkably, several of the compound hits have been found to inhibit membrane proteins at the periphery of the parasites, i.e., channels and transporters for ions and metabolites. In this review, we will focus on the progress made on targeting channels and transporters at different levels and the potential for use against infections with apicomplexan parasites mainly *Plasmodium* spp. (malaria) and *Toxoplasma gondii* (toxoplasmosis), with kinetoplastids *Trypanosoma brucei* (sleeping sickness), *Trypanosoma cruzi* (Chagas disease), and *Leishmania* ssp. (leishmaniasis), and the amoeba *Entamoeba histolytica* (amoebiasis).

Keywords: drug target, transport, infection, resistance, parasite, malaria, protozoa

HUMAN-PATHOGENIC PROTOZOA, CURRENT TREATMENT, RESISTANCE

Apicomplexa

With more than 200 million new infections per year, malaria-causing *Plasmodium* spp. are the most prominent parasites. The death toll of malaria is still >400,000 per year. About 90% of the cases occur in the WHO African Region and are caused almost exclusively by the species *Plasmodium falciparum*. In the subtropical zones outside of Africa, *Plasmodium vivax* is responsible for up to 64% of the cases. Ongoing efforts to eradicate malaria are hampered by the lack of effective antisera and the spreading of resistant strains against antimalarial treatment (WHO, 2017b). Hence, current research aims at identifying suitable epitopes for future immunization programs, and discovery of new drug targets to establish novel modes of antimalarial drug action.

The current first-line treatment of uncomplicated *P. falciparum* malaria is an oral artemisinin-based combination therapy (WHO, 2015). The mechanisms of how artemisinin and its derivatives, such as artesunate and artemether, attain antimalarial activity are thought to reside in generating oxidative stress by liberating reactive oxygen species from an internal peroxo-moiety, and in affecting a calcium ATPase (SERCA or PfATP6) of the sarcoplasmic-endoplasmic reticulum (Moore et al., 2011). The half-life of the fast-acting artemisinins is very short, typically around 1 h. To maintain this highly efficient therapeutic option in view of an increasing number of mutant parasite strains with varying degrees of resistance to the artemisinins (Jambou et al., 2005), these compounds are combined with drugs that exhibit longer half-lives (WHO, 2001; Kavishe et al., 2017). Patients infected with *P. vivax*, *Plasmodium ovale*, *Plasmodium malariae*, or *Plasmodium knowlesi* are equally treated with an artemisinin combination therapy or with chloroquine depending on the sensitivity of the infecting strain. For a number of decades, chloroquine was used for monotherapy until massive resistance occurred. Chloroquine accumulates in the parasite's digestive vacuole and interferes with heme-detoxification during hydrolysis of hemoglobin from the host (Slater, 1993; Thomé et al., 2013; WHO, 2015). For preventing relapse from dormant liver stages after infections with *P. vivax* or *P. ovale*, the use of primaquine is recommended (Fernando et al., 2011; Mikolajczak et al., 2015; Lalève et al., 2016). Complicated infections require rapid administration via intravenous or intramuscular injections of artesunate for at least 24 h followed by artemisinin-based combination therapy (Abiodun et al., 2013; WHO, 2015).

A malaria-related, tick-borne disease, babesiosis, normally occurs in livestock and domestic animals, and only occasionally emerges in humans. Most cases of human babesiosis are caused by *Babesia microti*. First-line treatment is a combination of the ubiquinone analog atovaquone and the antibiotic macrolide azithromycin (Krause et al., 2000).

Another apicomplexan parasite, *Toxoplasma gondii*, causes the food-borne disease toxoplasmosis. It is estimated that 30–50% of the world's population are infected with this parasite. It persists, often life-long, in the host in a dormant, cystic bradyzoite form. Although the infection usually occurs asymptomatic, it can evolve to a life-threating illness in immune-compromised patients. Infections of pregnant women can be transmitted to the fetus giving rise to spontaneous abortion or stillbirth (Flegr et al., 2014). Toxoplasmosis is treated with the dihydrofolate reductase inhibitor pyrimethamine or the antibiotic sulfadiazine. Second-line drugs are azithromycin, clarithromycin, atovaquone, dapsone, and cotrimoxazole. Due to side effects and ineffectiveness against the dormant bradyzoite form novel therapeutics are urgently needed (Petersen and Schmidt, 2003).

Kinetoplastids

Parasites of the phylum euglenozoa, i.e., the kinetoplastids, are the causative agents of various infections that are classified as neglected tropical diseases. Overall, it is estimated that one billion people in tropical and subtropical countries are affected. Infections with *Leishmania* spp. lead to cutaneous (*Leishmania major*, *Leishmania tropica*) mucocutaneous (*Leishmania braziliensis*), or visceral leishmaniasis (*Leishmania donovani*, *Leishmania infantum*), which is spread by sandflies. About 250,000 new cases are registered per year in 87 countries (WHO, 2017a). For treatment, sodium stibogluconate, amphotericin B, miltefosine, paromomycin, and pentamidine are used; yet, the therapy needs major improvement as it is characterized by high levels of toxicity for the patient. Further, resistance against the drugs, in particular to the pentavalent antimonial stibogluconate, strongly limits their usability (Loiseau and Bories, 2006; Ponte-Sucre et al., 2017).

Parasites of a related kinetoplastid species, *Trypanosoma*, cause life-threatening infections, i.e., human African trypanosomiasis or sleeping sickness (*Trypanosoma brucei*) and Chagas disease (*Trypanosoma cruzi*). Human African trypanosomiasis is spread by the tsetse fly in tropical Africa. Approximately 3,000 cases were reported in 2016 (WHO, 2016). In the first hemolytic stage, *T. brucei* replicates extracellularly in the host blood causing fever and joint pain among other symptoms. In the second, severe neurological stage of the disease, the parasite reaches the central nervous system. Patients suffer from disruption of the sleep-wake cycle and irreparable neurological damage. Parasites in the peripheral blood stream can be attacked by the drugs suramin and pentamidine. For the central nervous system form, only the mercurial melarsoprol and eflornithine are available (Brun et al., 2010). As in the case of leishmaniasis, modern, i.e., less toxic and more effective drugs are needed. *T. cruzi*-derived Chagas disease is prevalent in Latin-America claiming 14.000 deaths per year. An estimated 6 million people are infected by *T. cruzi* spread by the bug *Triatoma infestans* (also kissing bug or winchuka). As a treatment, the chemical radical-producing drug benznidazole and nifurtimox are available. With only two compounds at hand, limited success rates and severe side-effects, new drugs are required against this parasite (Castro et al., 2006).

Amoebae

The free-living amoebozoan parasite *Entamoeba histolytica* causes amoebiasis. With an estimated death toll of 40,000–100,000 per year, it ranges second behind *Plasmodium* infections (Stanley, 2003). The disease is most prevalent in but not restricted to the tropics when sanitation is poor. Although the majority of infections progress asymptomatically, a life-threatening amoebic colitis can manifest. *E. histolytica* forms hardy, infectious cysts that are ingested by the host via contaminated food or water. After reaching the colon, the cysts transform into trophozoites that are capable of invading the intestinal mucosa. When breaching the mucosa, trophozoites can disseminate, among others, to the liver and the central nervous system causing serious complications, i.e., amoebic abscesses (Shirley and Moonah, 2016). First line treatment is a combination of the antibiotics metronidazole and paromomycin. Alternative, second line treatments for metronidazole are other nitroimidazoles, e.g., tinidazole or ornidazole, and the broad-spectrum anti-parasitic nitazoxanide. Paromomycin can be substituted by diiodohydroxyquinoline and diloxanide, both drugs act by a so-far unresolved mechanism and may not be effective against all strains (McAuley and Juranek, 1992).

The severity of infections by protozoan parasites, the limited arsenal of drugs, often with hardly tolerable side effects, and the increasing resistance problem call for novel approaches. The scope of this review is, thus, to discuss the potential of channel and transport proteins as novel targets for anti-parasite chemotherapy in terms of druggability, selectivity, and proneness to resistance. There is considerably more data available from the malaria research field compared to the more neglected parasite-caused diseases. A major criterion for inclusion of a channel or transporter into this review was existing proof of principle involving first small-molecule inhibitors that exhibit anti-parasitic potency.

TARGETING TRANSPORT PROCESSES OF PARASITES AT DIFFERENT LEVELS

Transmembrane transporters and channels are usually classified based on their biophysical and biochemical properties, such as mechanism of transport and substrate selectivity. We decided to provide a pharmacological and pharmaceutical view on the topic and structured this manuscript based on the location of the transporter of interest and, accordingly, the site of action of a respective drug (**Figure 1**). We will approach the parasite from the outside, first hitting the host cell in the case of intracellular parasites. i. *Indirect targeting.* If it is possible to address infected host cells selectively by targeting transport proteins of the host cell plasma membrane this would leave the parasite little options for defending itself against the attack. Malaria parasites for instance are known to modify the functionality of red blood cell proteins and to integrate plasmodial membrane proteins into the erythrocyte membrane. ii. *Peripheral targeting.* Target proteins residing in a parasite's plasma membrane possibly can be inhibited from the outside. In this case and in *indirect* targeting, resistance mechanisms would be limited to changing the drug binding site of the target protein. iii. *Internal targeting.* For targeting transporters within a parasite, i.e., at organelles such as the digestive vacuole or mitochondria, respective drugs would need to enter the parasite's cytosol. In this case, the parasite has additional means to generate resistance, either by preventing uptake of the compound, by altering it chemically, or by pumping it out via efflux transporters. Hence, we will also address iv. *Targeting drug efflux transporters.*

Indirect Targeting—Channels and Transporters of the Infected Host Cell Membrane

It was recognized early on in malaria research that the transport of ions, amino acids, and other nutrients across the plasma membrane of infected red blood cells increases compared to uninfected cells. This way, the parasite actively adapts the ionic environment inside the erythrocyte to its needs and ensures access to nutrients from the host blood. Over the years, it has become evident that such new permeability pathways (NPP) are not only due to infection-dependent alteration of the host membrane proteins but also to export of *Plasmodium*-derived proteins and integration into the host cell membrane (Overman, 1947; Ginsburg et al., 1985; Desai et al., 2000; Huber et al., 2002). Proteins at the erythrocyte plasma membrane pose attractive targeting sites as the respective inhibitor compounds would not be in direct contact with the parasite. Interference by the parasite with drug action would be restricted to alteration of the protein resulting from gene mutations, whereas other means, such as expedited drug export or metabolism would not be applicable. It remains to be shown, however, whether this *indirect* approach can reliably kill parasites (Cohn et al., 2003). The efficiency of compounds that indirectly target parasites is summarized in **Table 1**.

Plasmodial Surface Anion Channel

One extensively studied type of conductivity of the red blood cell membrane that is brought about upon infection is derived from the plasmodial surface anion channel (PSAC; **Figure 1**). Despite a still elusive protein identity, permeability for various substrates, such as sugars, amino acids, nucleosides, and inorganic anions and cations, has been attributed to this voltage-dependent channel (Ginsburg et al., 1985; Kirk and Horner, 1995; Upston and Gero, 1995; Saliba et al., 1998; Hill et al., 2007). PSAC seems to transport the mentioned substrates via two different routes within the protein or protein complex. One path is said to be used primarily for alanine and sorbitol uptake and can be blocked by furosemide, whereas the other one conducts mainly proline and the unnatural substrate phenyltrimethylammonium (PhTMA). The latter path is sensitive to so-called PSAC residual transport inhibitors, abbreviated as PRT (Alkhalil et al., 2004; Pain et al., 2016). Based on this finding, full blockade of PSAC may require a combination of a PRT inhibitor plus a furosemide derivative. For example, PRT1-20 alone (**Table 1**) yielded an IC_{50} on *P. falciparum* growth of 5 μM; in combination with furosemide it was 10 times lower (Pain et al., 2016). Toward identification of the PSAC protein or regulators thereof, the finding could become helpful that certain parasite strains are susceptible to one particular group of PSAC inhibitors. This pointed to two genes, CLAG3.1 and CLAG3.2 (cytoadherence linked asexual protein) of which only one appears to be active at a time. Mutations in the genes led to modified PSAC activity. Further, epigenetic regulation of the CLAG3 genes was suggested to modulate PSAC (Sharma et al., 2013; Nguitragool et al., 2014). To illustrate this, ISPA-28 (**Table 1**), an isolate-specific PSAC antagonist, exhibited an IC_{50} of 56 nM against the *P. falciparum* Dd2 strain and 43 μM against the HB3 strain, i.e., a value higher by three orders of magnitude. When the CLAG3 gene of the Dd2 strain was transferred to the HB3 strain, it showed the same nanomolar susceptibility (Nguitragool et al., 2011, 2014). Clearly, identification of the true nature of the PSAC protein and/or components as well as expression or reconstitution in a heterologous or artificial system would be highly appreciated for in-depth structure-function analyses, inhibitor screening and development.

Host Ion Channels

Besides the parasite-derived PSAC, host encoded transport proteins of the erythrocyte may be exploited as drug targets if their functionality changes with infection. Oxidative stress was shown to alter potassium and chloride conductance of infected red blood cells (Staines et al., 2001; Huber et al., 2004). However, specific inhibitors are yet to be found to determine their potential as anti-parasite drugs.

There is evidence that in the liver-stage, *Plasmodium berghei* infection leads to a sevenfold increase in chloride conductance of the host's volume-regulated anion channel, VRAC, as found using a human hepatoma cell line (**Figure 1**; Prudêncio et al., 2009). Conductivity was inhibited by tamoxifen, and

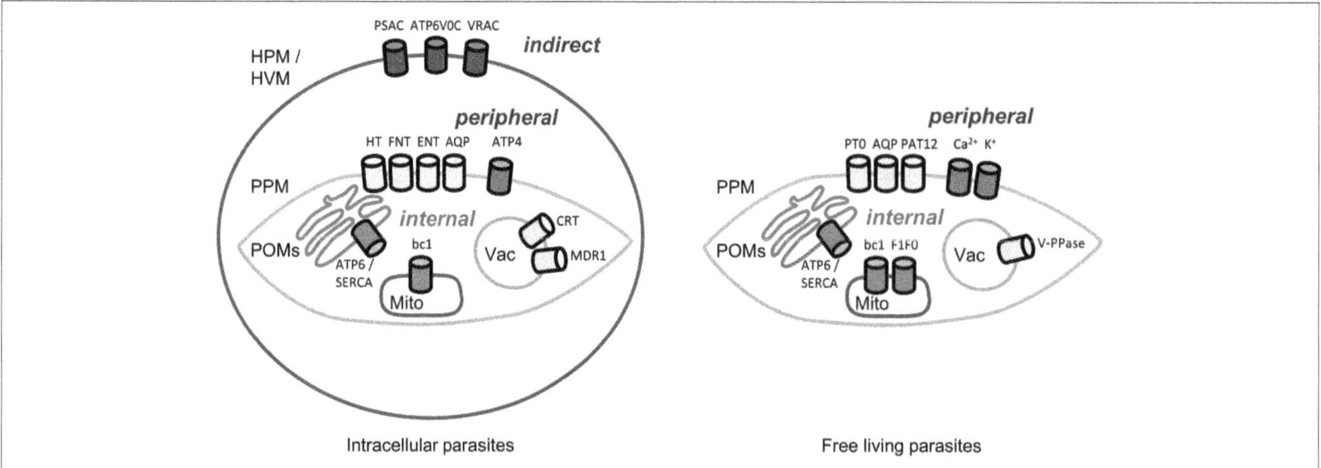

FIGURE 1 | Channels and transporters of parasites as targets for *indirect*, *peripheral*, and *internal* therapeutic attacks. HPM, host plasma membrane; HVM, host vacuolar membrane; PPM, parasite plasma membrane; POMs, parasite organelle membranes; Mito, mitochondrion; Vac, vacuole. Abbreviations of the channel and transporter proteins are explained in the text.

mefloquine at single-digit micromolar concentrations (**Table 1**). The underlying mechanism of channel activation by the parasite, the effect of estrogen receptor modulators on VRAC conductivity, and, ultimately, whether indirect targeting of VRAC would be suitable for malarial therapy of the liver stage is not clear at this time. With the system and compounds at hand further investigations will be possible that may shed some light on the phenomenon.

Host V-Type Proton ATPase

In the search of new drug targets against *L. donovani*, Muylder et al. chose a strategy of host-directed therapy. The amastigote form of the parasite develops primarily inside phagocytic cells and is inert to digesting enzymes. A screening assay using a human macrophage cell line infected with *L. donovani* yielded one hit compound, a μ-opioid receptor antagonist naloxonazine (de Muylder et al., 2011; **Table 1**). It turned out that naloxonazine upregulates expression of the V-type proton ATPase subunit C, ATP6V0C. This upregulation was linked to an increase in the volume of intracellular acidic vacuoles suggesting an *indirect* effect on *Leishmania* amastigotes through host cell vacuolar remodeling (de Muylder et al., 2016). How such a therapy would be tolerated by the host and whether the parasites will find ways to adapt to the remodeled vacuoles is not known.

Host Nutrient Channels and Transporters

We describe two examples illustrating that nutrient transport of the host cell affects growth of *P. berghei* parasites, i.e., in the blood-stage depending on the glycerol permeability of an aquaporin (Liu et al., 2007), and in the liver-stage via arginine transport (Meireles et al., 2017). Aquaporin-9 knockout mice lack a functional glycerol channel in their erythrocytes. In this environment, *P. berghei*, grew considerably slower compared to wildtype erythrocytes, and infected AQP9-null mice survived longer. The authors attribute the effect to reduced glycerol levels in the parasite impeding glyceroplipid biosynthesis for the build-up of membranes during growth. Similarly, knockdown of the arginine-transporting SLC7A2 of the solute carrier family decreased intra-hepatic growth and multiplication of *P. berghei* parasites *in vivo* and *ex vivo* (Meireles et al., 2017). A sufficient supply of arginine is required for the vital polyamine synthesis of the parasites. Today, glycerol or arginine transport-modulating small molecules have not been found and/or tested.

Together, although an *indirect* approach holds strong potential against parasite infections, several gaps in basic knowledge need to be filled with regard to the identity of the involved transport proteins, selectivity of inhibitors, and susceptibility/adaptability of the parasites.

Peripheral Targeting—Channels and Transporters of the Parasite Plasma Membrane

The substrate spectrum of the parasite-induced new permeation pathways at the host cell membrane is broad. Transport proteins at the parasite's plasma membrane (**Figure 1**), in turn, appear much more specific. These membrane proteins facilitate the uptake of the main energy source, glucose, and precursors for biosynthesis, such as nucleosides for DNA/RNA, or glycerol for glycerolipids. Equally vital is the efficient release of waste molecules derived from energy metabolism, e.g., lactic acid, or from protein degradation, i.e., ammonia and urea. Nutrient and metabolite transport often depends on transmembrane ion gradients, e.g., of protons or sodium, generated by ATPases and is further modulated by ion channels. Efficiency data on compounds for peripheral parastite targeting are displayed in **Table 2**.

Targeting Peripheral Nutrient and Metabolite Transporters

Considering their significance for survival, it seems quite surprising that plasmodia rely on a single hexose transporter, HT,

TABLE 1 | Efficiency of compounds for *indirect* targeting.

Target	Parasite species	Compound name	Effect on protein	Effect on parasite	Cell stage *in vitro*	Effect *in vivo*	Host species	Reference
PSAC	*P. falciparum*	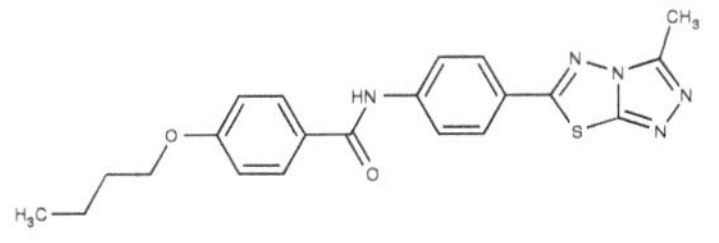 PRT1-20	–	IC_{50} 5 μM	Trophozoites	–	Human	Pain et al., 2016
		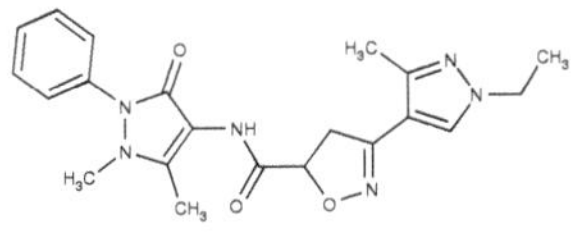 ISPA-28	–	IC_{50} 0.06 μM	Trophozoites	–	Human	Nguitragool et al., 2011
VRAC (host)	*P. berghei*	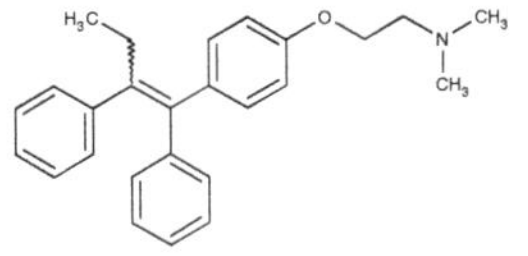 Tamoxifen	IC_{50} 4 μM	–	Liver-stage	–	Human	Prudêncio et al., 2009
		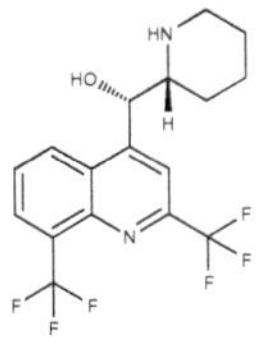 Mefloquine	IC_{50} 2 μM	–	Liver-stage	–	Human	Prudêncio et al., 2009
ATP6V0C (host)	*L. donovani*	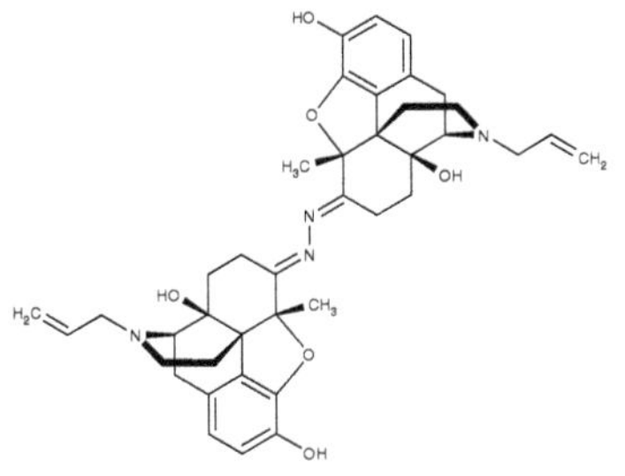 Naloxonazine	–	IC_{50} 3.5 μM	Amastigotes (Intracellular)	–	Human	de Muylder et al., 2011

and a single lactic acid transporter, the latter being a member of the microbial formate-nitrite-transporter family, FNT. Both transporters are present at the plasma membrane and both have been validated as novel antimalarial drug targets using cultured parasites.

Glucose transporters

Soon after the identification of HT, first weak glucose-analog inhibitors were described (Krishna and Woodrow, 1999; Woodrow et al., 1999; Joet et al., 2003). One of these compounds, C3361 (**Table 2**), yielded K_i-values in the μM range on glucose transport of *Plasmodium berghei, Plasmodium falciparum, Plasmodium yoelii, Plasmodium vivax, Plasmodium knowlesi, Babesia bovis,* and *T. gondii* (Joet et al., 2003; Blume et al., 2011). C3361 was not only active in the blood-stage but also inhibited parasite development in the liver-stage of *P. berghei* with an IC_{50} of 11 μM (Slavic et al., 2011). The vector stages, however, were much less susceptible, and a transmission block required 1 mM. Interestingly, C3361 failed to inhibit growth of the related apicomplexan *Babesia* parasites suggesting an alternative glucose transport pathway. In fact, the *B. bovis* genome contains two putative hexose transporter genes, of which only one has been characterized so-far (Derbyshire et al., 2008). Knockout of the homologous *Toxoplasma* glucose transporter, GT, led to moderate growth inhibition. Apparently, it is dispensable for the survival of the parasite. A search for alternative transporters in *Toxoplasma* produced three more putative sugar transporters of which one was found to be located at the plasma membrane. Yet, a knockout failed to effect parasite growth. Contrary to plasmodia, *Toxoplasma* seems not to rely exclusively on glucose as an energy source. It is discussed that glutamine can

TABLE 2 | Efficiency of compounds for *peripheral* targeting.

Target	Parasite species	Compound name	Effect on protein	Effect on parasite	Cell stage *in vitro*	Effect *in vivo*	Host species	Reference
HT	*Plasmodium* spp.	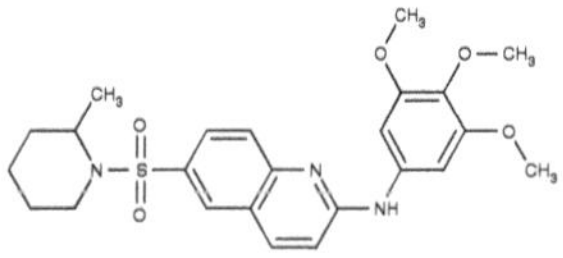 TCMDC-125163	IC_{50} 39 nM	IC_{50} 1.24 μM	Trophozoites	–	–	Ortiz et al., 2015
		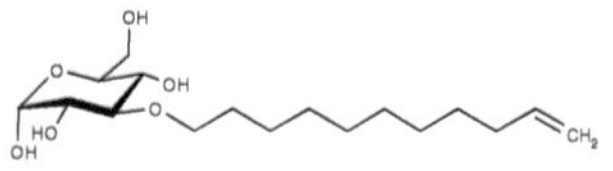 C3361	K_i 8.6–53 μM	IC_{50} 15–16 μM	Trophozoites	–	–	Joet et al., 2003; Blume et al., 2011
			–	IC_{50} 11 μM	Liver-stage	–	Human	Slavic et al., 2011
HT1	*B. bovis*		K_i 4.1 μM	No inhibition at 100 μM	Trophozoites	–	–	de Muylder et al., 2011
GT1	*T. gondii*		K_i 82 μM	No inhibition at 200 μM	Tachyzoites	–	–	Blume et al., 2011
FNT	*P. falciparum*	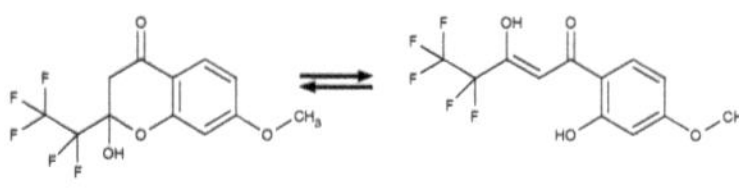 MMV007839	IC_{50} 0.02–0.17 μM	IC_{50} 0.14 μM	Trophozoites	–	–	Golldack et al., 2017; Hapuarachchi et al., 2017
		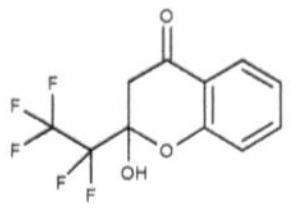 MMV000972	IC_{50} 0.05–0.17 μM	IC_{50} 1.70 μM	Trophozoites	–	–	
PTO	*T. brucei*	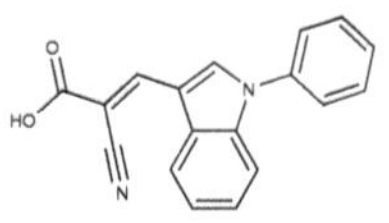 UK5099	Inhibition at 250 μM	–	–	–	–	Sanchez, 2013
PAT12	*T.cruzi*	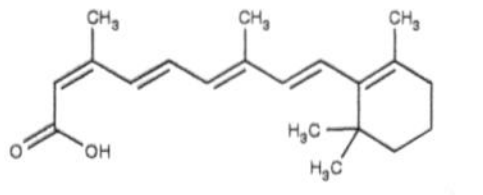 Isotretinoin	–	IC_{50} 0.13 μM	Epimastigotes	–	–	Reigada et al., 2017
				IC_{50} 30.6 μM	Trypomastigotes	–	–	
ENT1	*Plasmodium* spp.	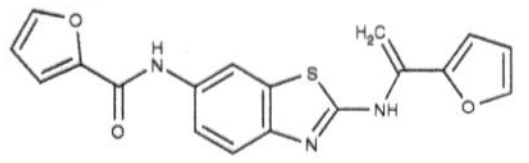 ChemBridge 9001893; 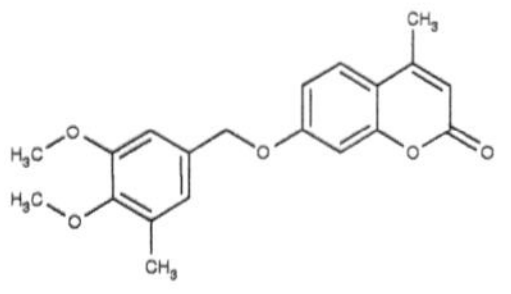 ChemBridge 6946484	IC_{50} 2.5–30 nM	IC_{50} 3–55 μM	Trophozoites	–	–	Frame et al., 2015b

(Continued)

TABLE 2 | Continued

Target	Parasite species	Compound name	Effect on protein	Effect on parasite	Cell stage *in vitro*	Effect *in vivo*	Host species	Reference
ATP4	*P. falciparum*	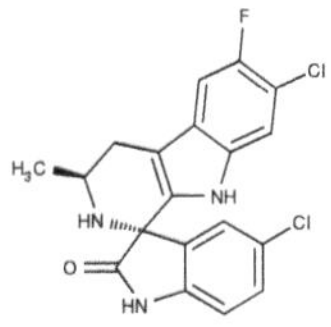 Cipargamin	–	IC_{50} 0.5–1.4 nM	Trophozoites	Clearance with 3-day dosing, 30 mg per day	Human	Rottmann et al., 2010; Spillman and Kirk, 2015
		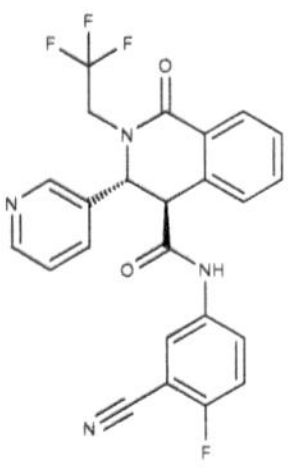 SJ733	–	IC_{50} 30 μM	Trophozoites	–	–	Spillman and Kirk, 2015
Calcium channels	*Leishmania* spp.	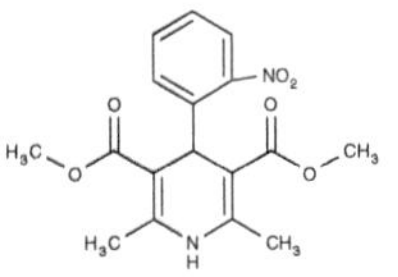 1,4-dihydropyridines (e.g., Nifedipine)	–	IC_{50} 2.6–181 μM	Promastigotes/ Amastigotes	–	–	Tempone et al., 2009
	Trypanosoma spp.		–		Trypomastigotes	–	–	Reimão et al., 2010, 2011
	A. castellanii	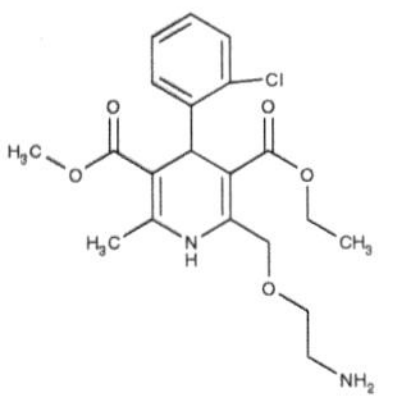 Amlodipine	–	Large inhibition at 1.2 μM	Trophozoites	–	–	Baig et al., 2013
	L. infantum	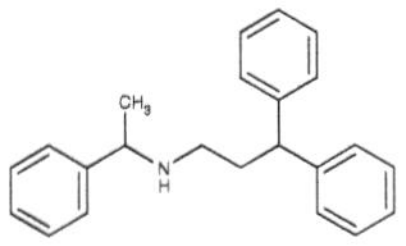 Non-dihydropyridines (e.g., fendiline)	–	IC_{50} 2–16 μM	Promastigotes	–	–	Reimão et al., 2016
	T. cruzi		–		Epimastigotes	–	–	Reimão et al., 2016
K1/K2	*T. brucei*	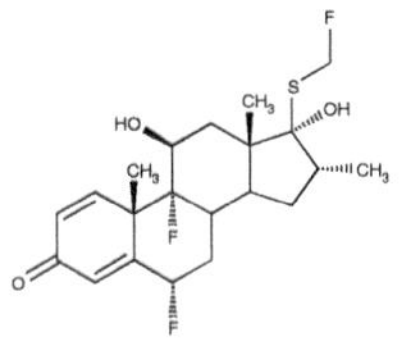 Fluticasone	IC_{50} 0.7 μM	–	–	–	–	Schmidt et al., 2017

be used as a potent alternative energy source (Blume et al., 2009).

More recent screenings for inhibitors of the plasmodial HT using the Tres Cantos antimalarial compound set (TCAMS) and the malaria box led to the discovery of nanomolar inhibitors, e.g., TCMDC-125163 (**Table 2**) has an IC_{50} of 39 nM for heterologously expressed HT, 3.2 μM for the human red blood cell glucose transporter GLUT1, and an EC_{50} of 1.24 μM for growth of cultured *P. falciparum* parasites. Binding of the identified compounds occurred mostly non-competitive with glucose and, hence, likely to a site different from the glucose binding pocket (Ortiz et al., 2015).

Lactate and pyruvate transporters

The end products of glucose-based energy metabolism are lactic acid in plasmodia, and pyruvic acid in trypanosomes. In order to prevent detrimental acidification of the cytosol and inhibition of the metabolic pathway by accumulating product, such molecules need to be swiftly released from the cells. Lactate transport in living *P. falciparum* parasites was experimentally shown in the early 1990s (Kanaani and Ginsburg, 1991). It took until 2015 that the responsible transporter was identified by our and Kiaran Kirk's group (Marchetti et al., 2015; Wu et al., 2015). The protein is structurally and in terms of transport mechanism unrelated to human lactate transporters from the monocarboxylate transporter family (MCT). Instead, the plasmodial lactic acid transporter is a member of the microbial formate-nitrite transporter family, FNT. Besides L-lactate, it transports D-lactate, as well as formate, acetate and pyruvate by a proton cotransport mechanism (Wiechert and Beitz, 2017; Wiechert et al., 2017).

Screening of the malaria box yielded two compounds, MMV007839 and MMV000972 (**Table 2**), that efficiently block PfFNT at nanomolar concentrations (Spangenberg et al., 2013; Golldack et al., 2017). *In vitro* selection of a resistant *P. falciparum* strain helped to locate the binding site at the intracellular face of the transporter. The compounds, thus, need to enter the parasite where they assume a lactate substrate-like form carrying a negative charge for efficient binding. Transport across consecutive membranes that shield the parasite is achieved by a cyclic hemiketal form that is neutral and lipophilic, see **Table 2** (Golldack et al., 2017). FNTs are absent in humans, however, some other protozoan parasites carry single or multiple copies of FNT genes, e.g., *Babesia* spp., *T. gondii*, and *E. histolytica*, representing putative targets. Kinetoplastids, in turn, do not encode FNTs in their genomes, raising the question of how monocarboxylate transport is achieved in these organisms. In *T. brucei*, a high-affinity pyruvate transporter, TbPT0, was recently discovered that is more related to polytopic proteins from plants than to mammalian MCTs (Sanchez, 2013). This transporter at the plasma membrane plus two additional mitochondrial pyruvate transporters of *T. brucei* were found to be inhibitable by the pyruvate-reminiscent compound UK5099 (Štáfková et al., 2016; **Table 2**).

Nucleobase and nucleoside transporters

Apart from nutrients and metabolites of energy metabolism, precursors, and components of biosynthetic pathways are typical substrates of parasite transporters. In this sense, a group of transporters found at the plasma membrane of plasmodia imports nucleobases and nucleosides. Four *P. falciparum* genes encode equilibrative nucleoside transporters, ENT1–4 of which ENT1 seems to provide the major uptake route (Downie et al., 2006, 2008, 2010; Frame et al., 2012, 2015a). Small molecule inhibitors were found by high throughput screening, e.g., ChemBridge no. 9001893 and 8946464 (**Table 2**), that inhibited the *P. falciparum* PfENT1 with IC_{50} values in the low nanomolar range. Efficiency was similar with the *P. vivax* and *P. berghei* ENT1 proteins (Arora et al., 2016; Deniskin et al., 2016). The compounds were less potent, however, in parasite cultures with EC_{50}-values from 0.8 to 6.5 μM (Frame et al., 2015b).

Aquaporin solute channels

Plasmodium and *Toxoplasma* parasites express a single aquaglyceroporin channel, AQP, at the plasma membrane (Hansen et al., 2002; Pavlovic-Djuranovic et al., 2006). These AQPs conduct water and small, uncharged solutes that are relevant in glycerolipid biosynthesis (glycerol), protein degradation (urea, ammonia), and oxidative stress (hydrogen peroxide) (Hansen et al., 2002; Beitz et al., 2004; Zeuthen et al., 2006; Wu et al., 2010; Wree et al., 2011; Almasalmeh et al., 2014). Small, drug-like inhibitors for apicomplexan AQPs are missing (Song et al., 2012), but their potential as drug targets is underscored by a *P. berghei* PbAQP knockout strain that exhibited strongly reduced growth, virulence, and progression through the liver stage (Promeneur et al., 2007, 2018). *T. brucei* expresses three AQPs of which TbAQP2 is a key factor for the uptake of the anti-trypanosomal drug pentamidine (Uzcategui et al., 2004; Song et al., 2016). The *L. major* AQP facilitates uptake of antimonite into the parasite released from the anti-leishmanial drug stibogluconate (Mukhopadhyay and Beitz, 2010; Mukhopadhyay et al., 2011).

Drug repurposing/polyamine transporters

An attempt to repurpose already used drugs revealed that retinoids, an established class for the pharmacotherapy of severe acne, target parasitic nutrient transporters. Initially, retinoic acid and retinol acetate were shown to inhibit the growth of *L. donovani* (Mukhopadhyay and Madhubala, 1994). More specifically, isotretinoin (**Table 2**) was found to block a polyamine transporter, PAT12, when adding to cultures of *T. cruzi* epimastigotes. *In vitro* growth of emerging trypomastigotes and epimastigotes was inhibited with IC_{50} values of 0.13 and 30.6 μM, respectively. PAT12 is a member of the polyamine and amino acid transporter family, AAAP, for which isotretinoin displayed activity as a multi-target inhibitor (Reigada et al., 2017). This shows that repurposing is a valid tool and can promote research in the field of neglected diseases.

Targeting Peripheral Ion Transporters and Channels

The establishment and maintenance of ion gradients across the parasite plasma membrane is vital for the membrane potential, osmotic balance, as well as for driving transport processes. P-type ATPases are single protein units that convert energy from ATP hydrolysis into cation transport (Weiner and Kooij, 2016). ATP4 of *P. falciparum* was recently shown to act as a sodium pump at the plasma membrane (Dyer et al., 1996; Spillman et al., 2013). There is evidence that sodium export by ATP4 is coupled to proton import. Whether cell death upon blockade of ATP4 occurs due to cytosol acidification, osmotic swelling, collapse of the electrochemical potential, or a combination thereof is unknown (Spillman et al., 2013; Spillman and Kirk, 2015). For whatever reason, blocking of ATP4 is lethal for malaria parasites rendering ATP4 a most attractive novel drug target. Analysis of the 400 malaria box compounds yielded the surprisingly high number of 28 hits, which further underscores the central role of ATP4 for parasite viability.

ATP4/P-type sodium ATPase

Two previously identified ATP4 inhibitors already entered the clinical trial stage. The clinical candidate cipargamin with a spiroindolone scaffold (**Table 2**) is thought to bind to the transport path of ATP4 from the intracellular entry site as deduced from *in vitro* selection of resistance mutations (Spillman and Kirk, 2015). Growth of sensitive *P. falciparum* strains was inhibited with IC_{50}-values in the range of 0.5–1.4 nM. Application of a single 100 mg kg^{-1} dose in an *in vivo* mouse model study killed all *P. berghei* parasites. In human trials, a 3-day dosing regime with 30 mg per day led to parasite clearance (Rottmann et al., 2010; White et al., 2014). Cipargamin exhibited low toxicity in humans, high oral bioavailability and suitable half-life. Other related ATP4-inhibiting spiroindolones have been found to be similarly potent (Spillman et al., 2013). The second promising candidate undergoing a clinical trial is the dihydroisoquinolone SJ733 (Jiménez-Díaz et al., 2014; **Table 2**). It shows more distant structure similarities to cipargamin with the 5-membered heterocycle of the indolone moiety replaced by a 6-membered ring (Jiménez-Díaz et al., 2014; Spillman and Kirk, 2015; Crawford et al., 2017). Although resistance mutations were selectable *in vitro* by sub-lethal concentrations, ATP4 inhibitors, when dosed properly, might prove advantageous against the rise of resistant strains in the clinic due to their fast acting property.

Drug repurposing/calcium channels

Drug repurposing approaches aim at ion channels at the plasma membrane of kinetoplastids. Several established 1,4-dihydropyridine calcium channel blockers used for the treatment of hypertension in humans were tested on various *Leishmania* and *Trypanosoma* species. Nifedipine, amlodipine, bepridil, nimodipine, and others showed weak effects *in vitro* with IC_{50}-values in the micromolar range (Maya et al., 2000; Tempone et al., 2009; Reimão et al., 2010, 2011). Amlodipine and lacidipine administered in four weekly single doses of 10 mg kg^{-1} reduced the parasite burden of *L. donovani*-infected BALB/c mice by 75–85% (Palit and Ali, 2008). Amlodipine was also tested for activity against cultured amoebae of *Acanthamoeba castellanii* and largely inhibited growth at 1.2 μM (Baig et al., 2013). The non-dihydropyridine calcium channel blockers fendiline, mibrefadil, and lidoflazine inhibited *in vitro* growth of *L. infantum* promastigotes and *T. cruzi* epimastigotes with IC_{50}-values from 2–16 μM (Reimão et al., 2016). Verapamil, however, failed to inhibit growth of *L. donovani* promastigotes, but seemed to reverse the resistance against stibogluconate by an unknown mechanism (Neal et al., 1989; Valiathan et al., 2006). Although being calcium channel blockers in humans, the target in the tested parasites remains to be established.

Drug repurposing/potassium channels

Recently, a screening by the National Center for Advancing Translational Sciences Small Molecule Resource identified fluticasone, an established corticosteroid for the treatment of asthma, to inhibit the *T. brucei* potassium channels TbK1 and TbK2. The proteins were localized to the parasite's plasma membrane and electrophysiologically characterized in *Xenopus* oocytes (Steinmann et al., 2015). Fluticasone was found to inhibit the TbK1/TbK2-mediated currents at an IC_{50} of 0.7 μM (Schmidt et al., 2017).

Internal Targeting—Channels and Transporters of Parasite Organelle Membranes

Drugs that need to enter the parasite's cytosol encounter several more challenges than compounds acting from the outside. Diffusional uptake across the plasma membrane requires high lipophilicity, small molecule size, and absence of charged moieties. Alternatively, compounds can be shuttled into the cell by a more active type of transport via endogenous channels and transporters. This route is taken for instance by antimonite released from stibogluconate in *Leishmania* therapy or by pentamidine against trypanosomes. In both cases, resistance mutations of a transporting aquaglyceroporin efficiently prevent the drugs from entering the parasites. Another factor is the metabolic stability of the drug within the parasite cell. This area is not well studied, yet it is conceivable that inactivation by chemical modification may well occur in a similar fashion as in the host cells, which detoxify xenobiotics e.g., by oxidation and conjugation reactions. Finally, drugs that actually made it to the site of action in a functional form may be pumped out of the parasite cell by drug resistance transporters. The prominent example is the chloroquine resistance transporter, CRT. **Table 3** gives an overview on the new developments of compound targeting channels and transporters of internal organelle membranes.

Despite these challenges, all currently used drugs in anti-parasite therapy act at internal sites. It remains to be seen how a shift to *peripheral* or even *indirect* attacks will affect resistance formation.

Artemisinins/Sarcoplasmic P-type Calcium ATPase SERCA/ATP6

Artemisinin (**Table 3**) and derivatives are the most important antimalarials today. The molecules contain a peroxo moiety. It is discussed that $iron^{II}$ from heme when released from hemoglobin during degradation in the digestive vacuole chemically activates the artemisinins producing reactive oxygen species that damage proteins more or less specifically inside the mitochondria

(Asawamahasakda et al., 1994; Moore et al., 2011) or at other sites in the cell including DNA as a target. Evidence further points to a P-type calcium ATPase, SERCA, or ATP6, at the sarcoplasmic endoplasmic reticulum as one of the affected proteins (Eckstein-Ludwig et al., 2003; Naik et al., 2011; Abiodun et al., 2013; Pulcini et al., 2013; Krishna et al., 2014; Nunes et al., 2016). However, there is a mismatch of artemisinin efficiency on the parasites and on heterologously expressed ATP6. In *P. falciparum* cultures, IC_{50}-values were 11 and 13 nM tested on a chloroquine resistant (K1) and a sensitive (NF54) strain, respectively (del Pilar Crespo et al., 2008). The artemisinins also showed some potency on several other protozoan parasites, i.e., *T. gondii* (Berens et al., 1998; Jones-Brando et al., 2006; Hencken et al., 2010), *T. brucei*, *T. cruzi*, *L. donovani*, *L. major* (Yang and Liew, 1993; Mishina et al., 2007), and *Babesia gibsoni* (Iguchi et al., 2015) yielding EC_{50}-values from 0.36 to 120 μM. For *Leishmania* spp., artemisinin exhibited *in vivo* activity in infected hamster and BALB/c mice models (Ma et al., 2004; Sen et al., 2010; Ghaffarifar et al., 2015). *Naegleria fowleri*, a problematic, cyst-forming amoeba, has been shown to be sensitive to artemisinin *in vitro* (Cooke et al., 1987), whereas treatment failed in a mouse model (Gupta et al., 1995). Purified recombinant *P. falciparum* ATP6, however, could not be directly inhibited by artemisinin or derivatives (Cardi et al., 2010; Arnou et al., 2011), and full inhibition of yeast expressed SERCA of *T. gondii* required high concentrations of 10 μM (Nagamune et al., 2007). The small molecule arterolane (**Table 3**) has a different scaffold than the artemisinins but equally contains a peroxo group and, thus, should be capable of releasing reactive oxygen species. When tested on *P. falciparum* ATP6 expressed in *Xenopus* oocytes it was found to be clearly less potent than artemisinin with a K_i-value of 7.7 μM; yet, parasite growth was inhibited a very low IC_{50} of 1.5 nM similar to artemisinin. These mixed results show that ATP6/SERCA is probably not the main target of the artemisinins.

Still, parasite SERCA/ATP6 seems to hold potential as a therapeutic target, because thapsigargin (**Table 3**), a plant sesquiterpene lactone and general SERCA inhibitor, killed cultured chloroquine resistant and sensitive *P. falciparum* parasites with IC_{50} of 246 and 298 nM (del Pilar Crespo et al., 2008; Abiodun et al., 2013). Thapsigargin further inhibited growth of *T. gondii*, *Trypanosoma* spp., *L. donovani*, *E. invadens*, and *Neospora canium* with EC_{50}-values in the range of 0.5–39 μM (Kim et al., 2002; Mishina et al., 2007; Martínez-Higuera et al., 2015). Yeast expressed *T. gondii* SERCA was fully inhibited by thapsigargin at 1 μM (Nagamune et al., 2007).

Atovaquone/Mitochondrial Cytochrome bc1 Complex

A key function of mitochondria in general is the build-up of a steep proton gradient across the inner mitochondrial membrane, which is used to drive ATP synthesis by the F-type ATPase, or ATP synthase. To this end, the inner membrane harbors a cytochrome bc1 complex. The bc1 proteins use ubiquinone, also called coenzyme Q, as a redox cofactor in electron transfer reactions (Q-cycle), which free four protons that are transported to the intermembrane space in the process (Crofts et al., 1999a,b; Crofts, 2004).

The drug atovaquone (**Table 3**), a ubiquinone analog and cytochrome bc1 complex inhibitor, is in use against malaria, toxoplasmosis and babesiosis for many years. It interferes with ubiquinone cofactor binding to the Q_0 site as shown by manifesting resistance mutations in this region of the protein (Fry and Pudney, 1992; Srivastava et al., 1999; McFadden et al., 2000; Kessl et al., 2007; Vallières et al., 2012; Siregar et al., 2015). Combination of atovaquone with proguanil lowers the IC_{50} from 2 nM to 400 pM probably by a synergistic mechanism as proguanil destroys the mitochondrial membrane potential in the presence of an electron transport inhibitor (Srivastava and Vaidya, 1999). Several resistant strains have formed during the use of atovaquone (Hutchinson et al., 1996; Painter et al., 2007; da Cruz et al., 2012). Since the cytochrome bc1 complex is common to mitochondria of all species is was possible to inhibit the growth of other parasites as well. Potency against *T. gondii* was sub-micromolar *in vitro*, i.e., tachyzoites in human foreskin fibroplasts, and *in vivo* using a mouse model with IC_{50}-values of 0.14 and 0.85 μM, respectively (Doggett et al., 2012). Similarly, atovaquone acted on *Babesia* spp. *in vitro* and *in vivo* in hamsters (Hughes and Oz, 1995; Wittner et al., 1996; Matsuu et al., 2008). In dog and human studies, combination with the antibiotic azithromycin turned out to be positive (Krause et al., 2000; Birkenheuer et al., 2004; Di Cicco et al., 2012; Checa et al., 2017). Treatment of *L. donovani* infections in a mouse model were less successful resulting only in a 30% lower parasite burden (Croft et al., 1992).

A related hydroxynaphthoquinone compound, buparvaquone (**Table 3**), is used for the treatment of theileriosis in cattle (McHardy et al., 1985; Minami et al., 1985; Muraguri et al., 1999; Mhadhbi et al., 2010), and horses (Zaugg and Lane, 1989). Anti-leishmanial activity was evaluated *in vitro* for *L. donovani*, *Leishmania aethiopica*, *L. major*, *Leishmania amazonensis*, *Leishmania mexicana*, *Leishmania panamensis*, *L. infantum*, *Leishmania chagasi*, *L. braziliensis*, and *L. tropica* promastigotes and amastigotes resulting in IC_{50}-values of 0.001–5.495 μM (Mäntylä et al., 2004a,b; Reimão et al., 2012; Jamal et al., 2015). Animal models showed that the *in vivo* efficiency was higher when prodrugs of buparvaquone were applied (Croft et al., 1992; Garnier et al., 2007) or when a nanoliposomal drug preparation was used (da Costa-Silva et al., 2017).

In the search for alternative chemical scaffolds, decoquinate (**Table 3**), a 4-oxo-quinoline, was tested. However, the overall structure is still similar to ubiquinone. The compound is in use in veterinary medicine against coccidia (Miner and Jensen, 1976; Ricketts and Pfefferkorn, 1993). When tested against blood-stage as well as liver-stage *P. falciparum*, in either case nanomolar IC_{50} values were found at low host cell toxicity (da Cruz et al., 2012). Another potent inhibitor of the cytochrome bc1 complex with good selectivity for *P. falciparum* is the dihydroacridinedione WR249685 (**Table 3**), which has an IC_{50} of 3 nM on the *in vitro* growth of the parasites (Biagini et al., 2008). Screening of the TCAMS library for cytochrome bc1 complex inhibition yielded one efficient compound, TCMDC-135546 (**Table 3**), with an IC_{50} of 22 nM on parasite growth (Raphemot et al., 2015). Naphthoquinone esters were derived from the anticancer drug rhinacanthin and showed low nanomolar IC_{50}-values on the

TABLE 3 | Efficiency of compounds for *internal* targeting.

Target	Parasite species	Compound name	Effect on protein	Effect on parasite	Cell stage *in vitro*	Effect *in vivo*	Host species	Reference
ATP6/SERCA	*P. falciparum*	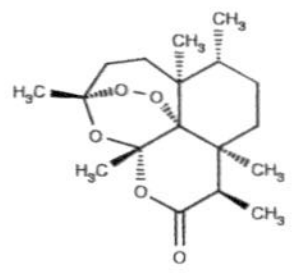 Artemisinin	–	IC_{50} 11 – 13 nM	Trophozoites	–	–	del Pilar Crespo et al., 2008
	T. gondii		Inhibition at 10 μM	IC_{50} 0.36–8 μM	Tachyzoites	–	–	Berens et al., 1998; Jones-Brando et al., 2006; Nagamune et al., 2007; Hencken et al., 2010
	Trypanosoma spp.		–	IC_{50} 13–20 μM	Trypomastigotes/ Epimastigotes	–	–	Yang and Liew, 1993; Mishina et al., 2007; Sen et al., 2010
	Leishmania spp.		–	IC_{50} 0.75–120 μM	Promastigotes/ Amastigotes	Reduction of parasite burden with oral dose of 10 mg kg^{-1}	Mouse/Hamster	
	B. gibsoni		–	IC_{50} 2.2 μM	Trophozoites	–	–	Iguchi et al., 2015
	P. falciparum	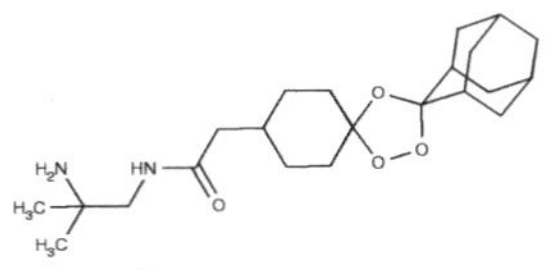 Arterolane	K_i 7.7 μM	IC_{50} 1.5 nM	Trophozoites	–	–	Abiodun et al., 2013
	P. falciparum	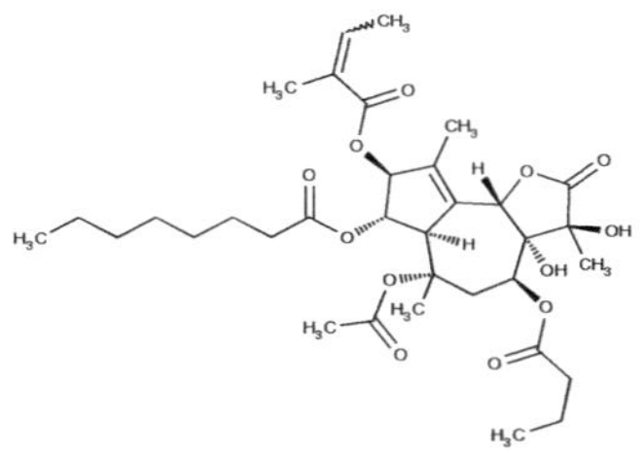 Thapsigargin	–	IC_{50} 0.25– 0.30 μM	Trophozoites	–	–	del Pilar Crespo et al., 2008; Abiodun et al., 2013
	T. gondii		Inhibition at 1 μM	–	–	–	–	Nagamune et al., 2007
	Trypanosoma spp.		–	IC_{50} 30–34 μM	Trypomastigotes/ Epimastigotes	–	–	Mishina et al., 2007
	L. donovani		–	28.1 μM	Promastigotes	–	–	Mishina et al., 2007
	E. invadens		–	Inhibition of encystation at 0.5 μM	Trophozoites	–	–	Martínez-Higuera et al., 2015
	N. canium		–	Growth Inhibition at 0.1 μg ml^{-1}	Tachyzoites	–	–	Kim et al., 2002

(Continued)

TABLE 3 | Continued

Target	Parasite species	Compound name	Effect on protein	Effect on parasite	Cell stage *in vitro*	Effect *in vivo*	Host species	Reference
Cytochrome bc_1 complex	*P. falciparum*	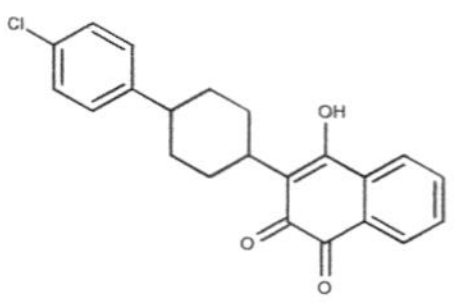 Atovaquone	IC_{50} 0.2 nM	IC_{50} 2 nM	Trophozoites	–	–	da Cruz et al., 2012
	T. gondii		–	IC_{50} 0.1–0.5 μM	Tachyzoites	IC_{50} 0.14–0.85 μM	Mouse	Doggett et al., 2012
	Babesia spp.		–	IC_{50} 94 nM	Trophozoites	Effective at dose of 100 mg kg^{-1} d^{-1}	Hamster	Hughes and Oz, 1995; Wittner et al., 1996; Matsuu et al., 2008
			–	–	–	Effective at dose of 1500 mg d^{-1} plus azithromycin 500 mg on day 1 and 250 mg per day thereafter	Human	Krause et al., 2000
	L. donovani		–	–	–	30 % reduction of parasite burden with 100 mg kg^{-1} for 5 days	Mouse	Croft et al., 1992
	Theileria spp.	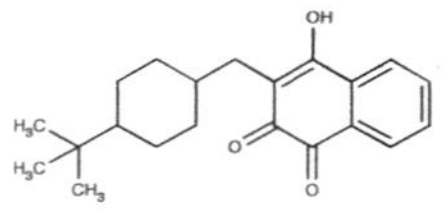 Buparvaquone	–	–	–	Effective at 2.5–6 mg kg^{-1}	Cattle, Horse	McHardy et al., 1985; Zaugg and Lane, 1989; Muraguri et al., 1999; Mhadhbi et al., 2010
	Leishmania spp.		–	IC_{50} 0.001–5.495 μM	Promastigotes/ Amastigotes	60% reduction of parasite burden with 100 mg kg^{-1} for 5 days	Mouse	Croft et al., 1992; Mäntylä et al., 2004a; Reimão et al., 2012; Jamal et al., 2015
	P. falciparum	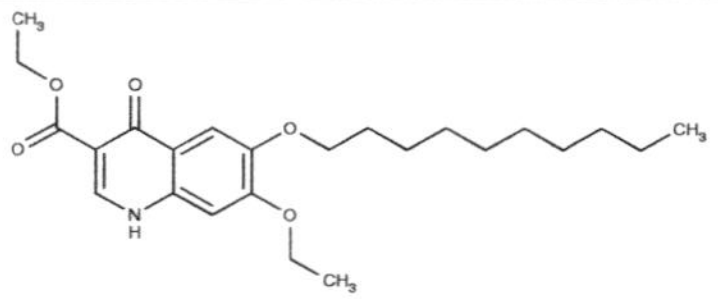 Decoquinate	IC_{50} 2 nM	IC_{50} 2.6–36 nM	Trophozoites	–	–	da Cruz et al., 2012

(Continued)

TABLE 3 | Continued

Target	Parasite species	Compound name	Effect on protein	Effect on parasite	Cell stage *in vitro*	Effect *in vivo*	Host species	Reference
	P. falciparum	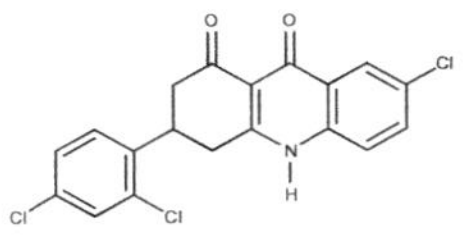 WR249685	–	IC_{50} 3 nM	Trophozoites	–	–	Biagini et al., 2008
	P. falciparum	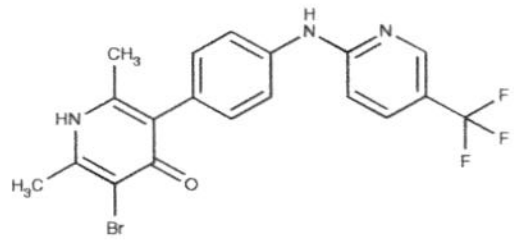 TCMDC-135546	–	IC_{50} 22 nM	Trophozoites	–	–	Raphemot et al., 2015
Mitochondrial F1F0 ATPase	*T. brucei*	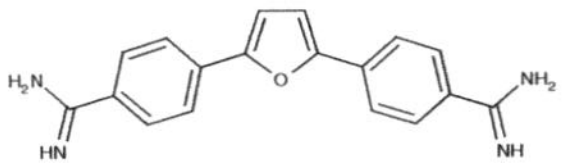 Furamidine (DB75)	Inhibition at 10 μM	IC_{50} 4.5 nM	Trypomastigotes	Effective as pentamidine at 3 mg kg^{-1} d^{-1}, for 7 days	Gerbil	Steck et al., 1982; Ismail et al., 2003; Lanteri et al., 2008
		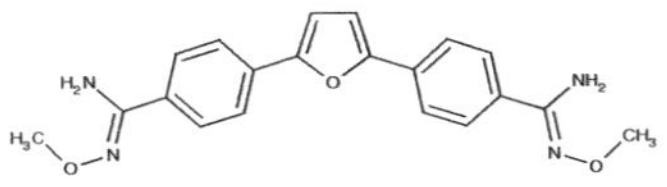 Pafuramidine (DB289)	–	IC_{50} 14.6 μM	Trypomastigotes	Effective at a dose of 400 mg kg^{-1} p.o.	Mouse	Ansede et al., 2004
		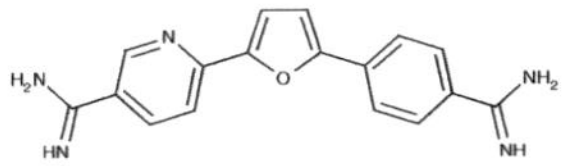 DB820	–	IC_{50} 7.9–141 nM	Trypomastigotes	Effective at 10 mg kg^{-1} i.p.	Mouse	Wenzler et al., 2009
		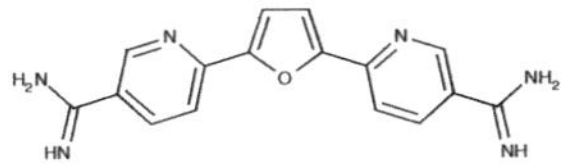 DB829	–	IC_{50} 20–346 nM	Trypomastigotes	Effective at 10 mg kg^{-1} i.p.	Mouse	Wenzler et al., 2009

(Continued)

TABLE 3 | Continued

Target	Parasite species	Compound name	Effect on protein	Effect on parasite	Cell stage *in vitro*	Effect *in vivo*	Host species	Reference
Mitochondrial choline transporter	*P. falciparum*	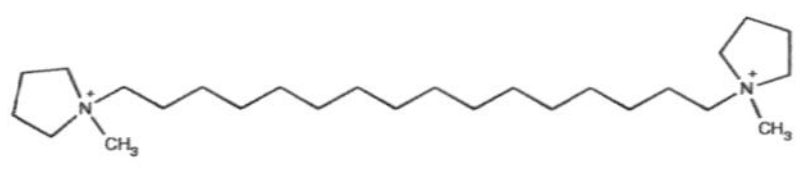 G25	–	–	–	–	–	Wengelnik et al., 2002; Biagini et al., 2004
	T. brucei		–	EC_{98} 0.16 μM	Trypomastigotes	–	–	de Macêdo et al., 2015
VPPase VP1	*T. gondii*	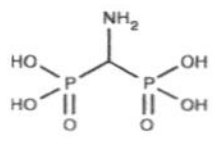 AMDP	IC_{50} 0.9 μM	Inhibition at 5–10 μM	–	–	–	Drozdowicz et al., 2003
CRT	*P. falciparum*	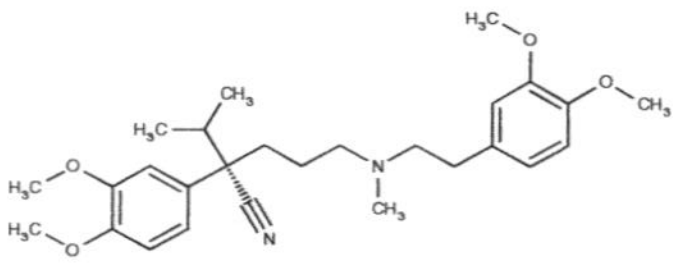 Verapamil	IC_{50} 30 μM	–	–	–	–	Ye and van Dyke, 1994
		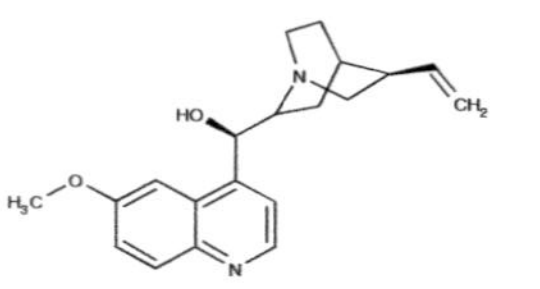 Quinine	IC_{50} 48 μM	–	–	–	–	Martin et al., 2009
		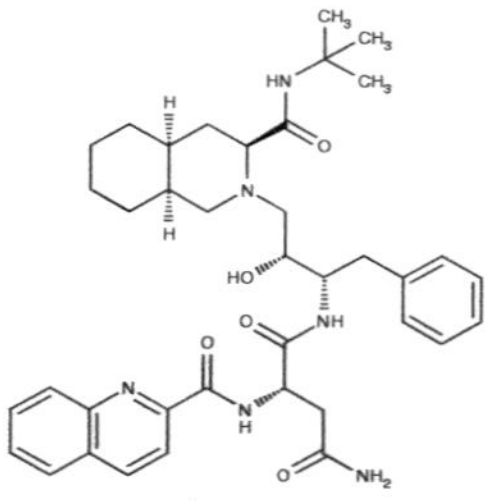 Saquinavir	IC_{50} 13 μM	–	–	–	–	Martin et al., 2012

(Continued)

TABLE 3 | Continued

Target	Parasite species	Compound name	Effect on protein	Effect on parasite	Cell stage *in vitro*	Effect *in vivo*	Host species	Reference
		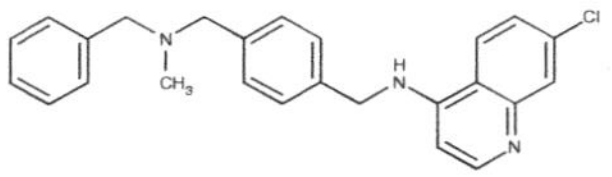 Dibemethin 6a	IC_{50} 69 μM	IC_{50} 26 nM	Trophozoites	–	–	Zishiri et al., 2011
MDR1	*P. falciparum*	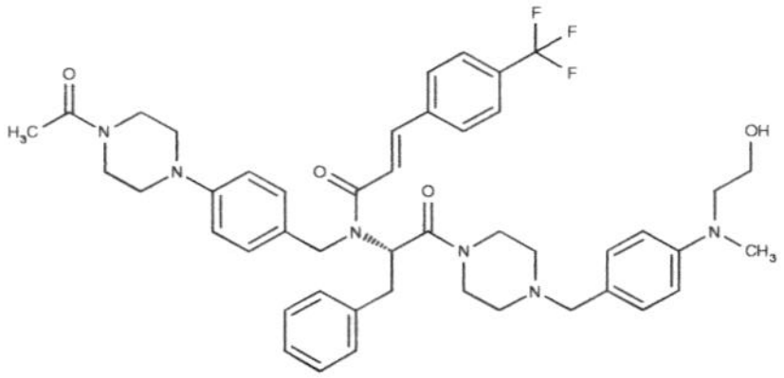 ACT-213615	–	IC_{50} 4 nM	Trophozoites	ED_{90} 8.4 mg kg^{-1} as effective as chloroquine	Mouse	Brunner et al., 2012, 2013
		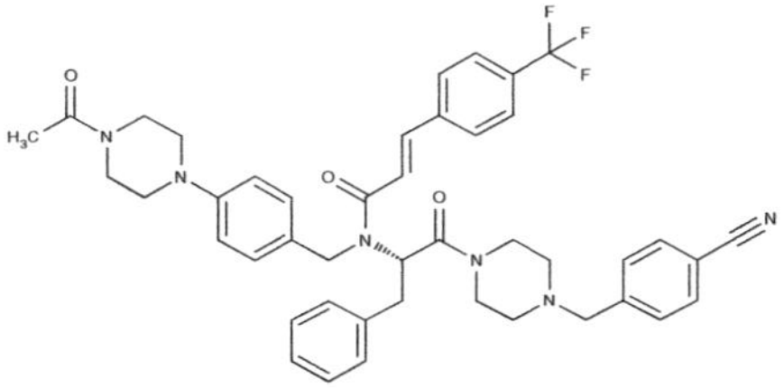 ACT-451840	–	IC_{50} 4 nM	Gametocytes	IC_{50} 2.7 ng ml^{-1} (3.6 nM)	Human	Krause et al., 2016; Le Bihan et al., 2016; Ng et al., 2016

growth of *P. falciparum*. Notably, the molecules seem to bind to the Q_i ubiquinone site of cytochrome bc1 rather than Q_0 as the above-mentioned compounds (Kongkathip et al., 2010). In a diversity oriented synthesis approach, macrolactame derivatives were generated that yielded nanomolar EC_{50}-values and are thought to target the Q_i site as well (Comer et al., 2014; Lukens et al., 2015). Finally, more compounds were derived from endochin, an experimental antimalarial of the 1940s, with the aim to improve solubility and metabolic stability in the host. Such compounds were found not to inhibit the human cytochrome bc1 complex but to very efficiently target the Q_i site of the cytochrome bc1 complex of *falciparum* and *vivax* plasmodia from various clinical field isolates as well as *T. gondii* and *Babesia microti* (Doggett et al., 2012; Nilsen et al., 2013; Lawres et al., 2016). *Leishmania* spp., however, were much less susceptible to this type of inhibitors with IC_{50}-values in the micromolar range (Ortiz et al., 2016).

Diamidines/Mitochondrial ATP Synthase

Similar to the artemisinins in plasmodia, the mode of diamidine action, e.g., pentamidine, in trypanosomes is not fully resolved. Screening of an diamidine library yielded furamidine (**Table 3**) and related compounds that act comparably to pentamidine against *T. brucei* parasites in mice and rhesus monkeys (Rane et al., 1976; Steck et al., 1982). Further, a prodrug of furamidine, DB289 (**Table 3**), with better oral availability was developed (Ismail et al., 2003; Ansede et al., 2004). Regarding transporter targeting, it was found that the F1F0-ATPase, i.e., the mitochondrial proton gradient-driven ATP synthase, was inhibited at concentrations around 10 μM and caused a collapse of the mitochondrial membrane potential. The efficiency of diamidines on the growth of trypanosomes, however, is clearly lower, i.e., in the submicromolar range, indicating that ATP synthase is not the main target. It was also suggested that the compounds inhibit other ATPases (Lanteri et al., 2008). DB289 entered phase III clinical trials as the first orally available drug against blood stage human African trypanosomiasis. However, due to manifestation of delayed renal insufficiency in a number of recipients, further development was terminated (Harrill et al., 2012). Two related aza analogs of furamidine (DB820, CPD0801) are still followed up on as they have shown efficiency against *T. brucei* in a mouse model of second stage trypanosomiasis (Wenzler et al., 2009; Ward et al., 2011).

G25/Mitochondrial Choline Transport

The notion that a choline-related compound, named G25 (**Table 3**) carrying two quaternary ammonium moieties spaced by a 16-carbon linker, efficiently kills malaria parasites led to the idea that choline transport might be a valid antimalarial target (Wengelnik et al., 2002; Biagini et al., 2004). Besides *P. falciparum*, also *T. brucei* and *L. mexicana* turned out to be sensitive to G25 (Ibrahim et al., 2011). The mode of action remains unclear. Besides the notion that these compounds inhibit choline transport, it was reported that the mitochondrial structure and function of trypanosomes was affected (Ibrahim et al., 2011; Macêdo et al., 2013). An RNA interference approach in the blood stream form of *T. brucei* hinted at the involvement of a member of a mitochondrial carrier protein family, TbMCP14, which is unrelated to mammalian carriers (Schumann Burkard et al., 2011; de Macêdo et al., 2015).

Aminomethylenediphosphonate/Vacuolar-Type Inorganic Pyrophosphatase

Vacuolar-type pyrophosphatases, V-PPases, seem to be absent in vertebrates, yet have vital functions in protozoan energy conservation and membrane transport. Accordingly, they may represent suitable drug targets (Rodrigues et al., 2000; Drozdowicz et al., 2003). Yeast-expressed V-PPase from *T. gondii*, TgVP1, was inhibitable by aminomethylenediphosphonate, AMDP (**Table 3**), with an IC_{50} of 0.9 μM. The presence of V-PPases has also been shown in *P. falciparum* and *T. cruzi* (Urbina et al., 1999; McIntosh et al., 2001). Anti-parasitic, drug-like molecules targeting V-PPases are yet to be found.

Targeting Drug Efflux Transporters

Drug resistance due to expedited export of the compounds is a key factor in pharmacotherapy not only of anti-infectives but in general. The loss of drug action may be reversed by inhibition of the responsible efflux transporter.

Verapamil, (Dimeric) Quinine, Saquinavir/Digestive Vacuole Chloroquine Resistance Transporter

The discovery of chloroquine was a breakthrough in malaria therapy. It acts by inhibiting heme detoxification in the form of polymerized hemozoin in the digestive vacuole (Foley and Tilley, 1997). Promoted by monotherapeutic use and widespread underdosing in eradication programs, however, resistant *P. falciparum* strains were selected over the years rendering chloroquine largely useless today (Wellems et al., 1991; Waller et al., 2003). Resistance mutations were found in one particular gene of unknown function at that time. It turned out that the mutations resulted in a gain-of-function transporter shuttling chloroquine out of the digestive vacuole at a strongly increased rate (Fidock et al., 2000; Lakshmanan et al., 2005). The physiological role of the chloroquine-resistance-transporter, CRT, is still elusive. However, a variety of amino acids, polyamines and peptides have been found to be CRT substrates (Juge et al., 2015). Several attempts have been undertaken to block CRT with the aim to reverse chloroquine resistance. The calcium channel blocker verapamil (**Table 3**) was shown to inhibit CRT expressed in *Xenopus* oocytes with an IC_{50} of 30 μM (Ye and van Dyke, 1988, 1994; Tanabe et al., 1989). In the same system, quinine, a natural product and chloroquine analog, yielded an IC_{50} of 48 μM (Martin et al., 2009), and the antiretroviral drug saquinavir was effective at 13 μM (Martin et al., 2012). Chemical synthesis of dimeric quinines lowered the IC_{50} to 1 μM on CRT-expressing oocytes and efficiently inhibited parasite growth in the nanomolar range (Hrycyna et al., 2014).

The resistance reversing effect of verapamil cannot be exploited in humans, because the required dose would be too high to be tolerable (Ye and van Dyke, 1988). One approach was to develop a drug-like compound with dual functionality, i.e., blockade of hemozoin formation plus inhibition of CRT (Burgess et al., 2006; Kelly et al., 2009). The obtained dibemethin derivates (**Table 3**) showed IC_{50} values of 26 nM on parasite growth, yet potency on the isolated CRT protein was only 69 μM. Bioavailability appeared sufficient after oral administration in mice (Zishiri et al., 2011).

ACT-213615, ACT-451840/Digestive Vacuole Multidrug Resistance Transporter 1

Based on similarity to human multidrug resistance transporters in terms of sequence and function another transporter of the digestive vacuole of malaria parasites was termed multidrug resistance transporter 1, MDR1 (Foote et al., 1989; Cowman et al., 1991). MDR1 transport is directed into the digestive vacuole. This way, mefloquine, artemisinin, and artesunate are thought to be trapped by compartmentalization preventing the drugs from hitting their target in the sarcoplasmic endoplasmic reticulum (Reed et al., 2000; Pickard et al., 2003; Price et al., 2004; Rohrbach et al., 2006). Resistance was increased in strains with multiple copies of the *pfmdr1* gene (Cowman et al., 1994; Pickard et al., 2003). For quinine in turn, it is required that MDR1 is functional to deliver the compound to its site of action inside the digestive vacuole. Therefore, a transport decreasing N1042D mutation of MDR1 was made responsible for quinine resistance (Rohrbach et al., 2006). Apart from transport of antimalarial drugs, MDR1 appears to be vital for the malaria parasite, because in cell viability screening and subsequent analyses, two small-molecule compounds were found to target MDR1. ACT-213615 (**Table 3**) is proposed to inhibit either PfMDR1 directly or a regulating protein upstream of it yielding an EC_{50} value of 4 nM on parasite growth (Brunner et al., 2012, 2013). The second, highly related compound, ACT-451840 (**Table 3**), was even more potent and a single nucleotide polymorphism in the MDR1 gene was identified that turned out to be responsible for resistance against the compound. The compound was well tolerated in first clinical trials, however, none of the eight tested subjects could be completely freed from parasites (Krause et al., 2016; Le Bihan et al., 2016; Ng et al., 2016). The physiological substrates and function of MDR1 remain to be established.

CONCLUSION

The identification of anti-parasitic targets at the parasite's plasma membrane or even at host membranes opens up options for *peripheral* or *indirect* therapeutic attacks (**Figure 1**). This approach holds the potential to limit resistance formation because the only remaining line of defense is mutational modification of the drug binding site at the target protein. It is thinkable that massive upregulation of target protein expression may also reduce efficiency, yet at high energetic cost for the parasite.

Still, most currently addressed targets are located inside the parasite. Here, specificity must be taken into account. Drugs affecting vital functions by hitting multiple targets, e.g., the artemisinins by eliciting oxidative stress, are hard to defend by the parasite at the various target sites. However, several ways exist to interfere with drug action by acting directly on the molecular entity. Drug uptake can be prevented if transporters are required to deliver the compound to the cytosol, e.g., pentamidine via TbAQP2. The drug can be chemically modified or compartmentalized, e.g., artesunate transport into the digestive vacuole by MDR1. Finally, the compound can be shuttled out to keep the concentration below a harmful level, e.g., chloroquine via CRT. Drug metabolism and transport issues cannot be fully appreciated beforehand. Hence, in the search for potent anti-infectives against parasites and bacteria alike, phenotypic screenings have proven more successful than specific approaches in designing inhibitors for a selected target protein.

The ideal anti-parasitic drug compound should i. reach the site of action independent of parasite transport proteins, ii. be specific for the parasite but not necessarily for a single target protein, iii. act fast, iv. be metabolically stable, and v. be safe for the patient. Meeting such demands and circumventing the influence by the parasite may be eased by addressing parasite-specific proteins at the periphery.

AUTHOR CONTRIBUTIONS

AM, HE, and EB jointly wrote the manuscript and prepared the figures.

FUNDING

This work was funded by the Deutsche Forschungsgemeinschaft (Be2253/7-1 and Be2253/8-1).

REFERENCES

Abiodun, O. O., Brun, R., and Wittlin, S. (2013). *In vitro* interaction of artemisinin derivatives or the fully synthetic peroxidic anti-malarial OZ277 with thapsigargin in *Plasmodium falciparum* strains. *Malar. J.* 12:43. doi: 10.1186/1475-2875-12-43

Alkhalil, A., Cohn, J. V., Wagner, M. A., Cabrera, J. S., Rajapandi, T., and Desai, S. A. (2004). *Plasmodium falciparum* likely encodes the principal anion channel on infected human erythrocytes. *Blood* 104, 4279–4286. doi: 10.1182/blood-2004-05-2047

Almasalmeh, A., Krenc, D., Wu, B., and Beitz, E. (2014). Structural determinants of the hydrogen peroxide permeability of aquaporins. *FEBS J.* 281, 647–656. doi: 10.1111/febs.12653

Ansede, J. H., Anbazhagan, M., Brun, R., Easterbrook, J. D., Hall, J. E., and Boykin, D. W. (2004). O-alkoxyamidine prodrugs of furamidine: *in vitro* transport and microsomal metabolism as indicators of *in vivo* efficacy in a mouse model of *Trypanosoma brucei rhodesiense* infection. *J. Med. Chem.* 47, 4335–4338. doi: 10.1021/jm030604o

Arnou, B., Montigny, C., Morth, J. P., Nissen, P., Jaxel, C., Møller, J. V., et al. (2011). The *Plasmodium falciparum* Ca^{2+}-ATPase PfATP6: insensitive to artemisinin, but a potential drug target. *Biochem. Soc. Trans.* 39, 823–831. doi: 10.1042/BST0390823

Arora, A., Deniskin, R., Sosa, Y., Nishtala, S. N., Henrich, P. P., Kumar, T. R. S., et al. (2016). Substrate and inhibitor specificity of the *Plasmodium berghei* equilibrative nucleoside transporter type 1. *Mol. Pharmacol.* 89, 678–685. doi: 10.1124/mol.115.101386

Asawamahasakda, W., Ittarat, I., Pu, Y. M., Ziffer, H., and Meshnick, S. R. (1994). Reaction of antimalarial endoperoxides with specific parasite proteins. *Antimicrob. Agents Chemother.* 38, 1854–1858. doi: 10.1128/AAC.38.8.1854

Baig, A. M., Iqbal, J., and Khan, N. A. (2013). *In vitro* efficacies of clinically available drugs against growth and viability of an *Acanthamoeba castellanii* keratitis isolate belonging to the T4 genotype. *Antimicrob. Agents Chemother.* 57, 3561–3567. doi: 10.1128/AAC.00299-13

Beitz, E., Pavlovic-Djuranovic, S., Yasui, M., Agre, P., and Schultz, J.E. (2004). Molecular dissection of water and glycerol permeability of the aquaglyceroporin from *Plasmodium falciparum* by mutational analysis. *Proc Natl Acad Sci U.S.A.* 101, 1153–1158. doi: 10.1073/pnas.0307295101

Berens, R. L., Krug, E. C., Nash, P. B., and Curiel, T. J. (1998). Selection and characterization of *Toxoplasma gondii* mutants resistant to artemisinin. *J. Infect. Dis.* 177, 1128–1131. doi: 10.1086/517411

Biagini, G. A., Pasini, E. M., Hughes, R., Koning, H. P., de Vial, H. J., O'Neill, P. M., et al. (2004). Characterization of the choline carrier of *Plasmodium falciparum*: a route for the selective delivery of novel antimalarial drugs. *Blood* 104, 3372–3377. doi: 10.1182/blood-2004-03-1084

Biagini, G. A., Fisher, N., Berry, N., Stocks, P. A., Meunier, B., Williams, D. P., et al. (2008). Acridinediones: selective and potent inhibitors of the malaria parasite mitochondrial bc1 complex. *Mol. Pharmacol.* 73, 1347–1355. doi: 10.1124/mol.108.045120

Birkenheuer, A. J., Levy, M. G., and Breitschwerdt, E. B. (2004). Efficacy of combined atovaquone and azithromycin for therapy of chronic *Babesia gibsoni* (Asian genotype) infections in dogs. *J. Vet. Intern. Med.* 18, 494–498. doi: 10.1111/j.1939-1676.2004.tb02573.x

Blume, M., Rodriguez-Contreras, D., Landfear, S., Fleige, T., Soldati-Favre, D., Lucius, R., et al. (2009). Host-derived glucose and its transporter in the obligate intracellular pathogen *Toxoplasma gondii* are dispensable by glutaminolysis. *Proc. Natl. Acad. Sci. U.S.A.* 106, 12998–13003. doi: 10.1073/pnas.0903831106

Blume, M., Hliscs, M., Rodriguez-Contreras, D., Sanchez, M., Landfear, S., Lucius, R., et al. (2011). A constitutive pan-hexose permease for the *Plasmodium* life cycle and transgenic models for screening of antimalarial sugar analogs. *FASEB J.* 25, 1218–1229. doi: 10.1096/fj.10-173278

Brun, R., Blum, J., Chappuis, F., and Burri, C. (2010). Human African trypanosomiasis. *Lancet* 375, 148–159. doi: 10.1016/S0140-6736(09)60829-1

Brunner, R., Aissaoui, H., Boss, C., Bozdech, Z., Brun, R., Corminboeuf, O., et al. (2012). Identification of a new chemical class of antimalarials. *J. Infect. Dis.* 206, 735–743. doi: 10.1093/infdis/jis418

Brunner, R., Ng, C. L., Aissaoui, H., Akabas, M. H., Boss, C., Brun, R., et al. (2013). UV-triggered affinity capture identifies interactions between the *Plasmodium falciparum* multidrug resistance protein 1 (PfMDR1) and antimalarial agents in live parasitized cells. *J. Biol. Chem.* 288, 22576–22583. doi: 10.1074/jbc.M113.453159

Burgess, S. J., Selzer, A., Kelly, J. X., Smilkstein, M. J., Riscoe, M. K., and Peyton, D. H. (2006). A chloroquine-like molecule designed to reverse resistance in *Plasmodium falciparum*. *J. Med. Chem.* 49, 5623–5625. doi: 10.1021/jm060399n

Cardi, D., Pozza, A., Arnou, B., Marchal, E., Clausen, J. D., Andersen, J. P., et al. (2010). Purified E255L mutant SERCA1a and purified PfATP6 are sensitive to SERCA-type inhibitors but insensitive to artemisinins. *J. Biol. Chem.* 285, 26406–26416. doi: 10.1074/jbc.M109.090340

Castro, J. A., de Mecca, M. M., and Bartel, L. C. (2006). Toxic side effects of drugs used to treat Chagas' disease (American trypanosomiasis). *Hum. Exp. Toxicol.* 25, 471–479. doi: 10.1191/0960327106het653oa

Checa, R., Montoya, A., Ortega, N., González-Fraga, J. L., Bartolomé, A., Gálvez, R., et al. (2017). Efficacy, safety and tolerance of imidocarb dipropionate versus atovaquone or buparvaquone plus azithromycin used to treat sick dogs naturally infected with the *Babesia microti*-like piroplasm. *Parasit. Vectors* 10, 145. doi: 10.1186/s13071-017-2049-0

Cohn, J. V., Alkhalil, A., Wagner, M. A., Rajapandi, T., and Desai, S. A. (2003). Extracellular lysines on the plasmodial surface anion channel involved in Na^+ exclusion. *Mol. Biochem. Parasitol.* 132, 27–34. doi: 10.1016/j.molbiopara.2003.08.001

Comer, E., Beaudoin, J. A., Kato, N., Fitzgerald, M. E., Heidebrecht, R. W., Lee, M. D., et al. (2014). Diversity-oriented synthesis-facilitated medicinal chemistry: Toward the development of novel antimalarial agents. *J. Med. Chem.* 57, 8496–8502. doi: 10.1021/jm500994n

Cooke, D. W., Lallinger, G. J., and Durack, D. T. (1987). *In vitro* sensitivity of *Naegleria fowleri* to qinghaosu and dihydroqinghaosu. *J. Parasitol.* 73, 411. doi: 10.2307/3282098

Cowman, A. F., Karcz, S., Galatis, D., and Culvenor, J. G. (1991). A P-glycoprotein homologue of *Plasmodium falciparum* is localized on the digestive vacuole. *J. Cell Biol.* 113, 1033–1042. doi: 10.1083/jcb.113.5.1033

Cowman, A. F., Galatis, D., and Thompson, J. K. (1994). Selection for mefloquine resistance in *Plasmodium falciparum* is linked to amplification of the pfmdr1 gene and cross-resistance to halofantrine and quinine. *Proc. Natl. Acad. Sci. U.S.A.* 91, 1143–1147. doi: 10.1073/pnas.91.3.1143

Crawford, E. D., Quan, J., Horst, J. A., Ebert, D., Wu, W., and DeRisi, J. L. (2017). Plasmid-free CRISPR/Cas9 genome editing in *Plasmodium falciparum* confirms mutations conferring resistance to the dihydroisoquinolone clinical candidate SJ733. *PLoS ONE* 12:e0178163. doi: 10.1371/journal.pone.0178163

Croft, S. L., Hogg, J., Gutteridge, W. E., Hudson, A. T., and Randall, A. W. (1992). The activity of hydroxynaphthoquinones against *Leishmania donovani*. *J. Antimicrob. Chemother.* 30, 827–832. doi: 10.1093/jac/30.6.827

Crofts, A. R., Barquera, B., Gennis, R. B., Kuras, R., Guergova-Kuras, M., and Berry, E. A. (1999a). Mechanism of ubiquinol oxidation by the bc1 complex: different domains of the quinol binding pocket and their role in the mechanism and binding of inhibitors. *Biochemistry* 38, 15807–15826. doi: 10.1021/bi990962m

Crofts, A. R., Guergova-Kuras, M., Huang, L., Kuras, R., Zhang, Z., and Berry, E. A. (1999b). Mechanism of ubiquinol oxidation by the bc1 complex: role of the iron sulfur protein and its mobility. *Biochemistry* 38, 15791–15806. doi: 10.1021/bi990961u

Crofts, A. R. (2004). The cytochrome bc1 complex: function in the context of structure. *Annu. Rev. Physiol.* 66, 689–733. doi: 10.1146/annurev.physiol.66.032102.150251

da Costa-Silva, T. A., Galisteo, A. J., Lindoso, J. A. L., Barbosa, L. R. S., and Tempone, A. G. (2017). Nanoliposomal buparvaquone immunomodulates *Leishmania infantum*-infected macrophages and is highly effective in a murine model. *Antimicrob. Agents Chemother.* 61:e02297-16. doi: 10.1128/AAC.02297-16

da Cruz, F. P., Martin, C., Buchholz, K., Lafuente-Monasterio, M. J., Rodrigues, T., Sönnichsen, B., et al. (2012). Drug screen targeted at *Plasmodium* liver stages identifies a potent multistage antimalarial drug. *J. Infect. Dis.* 205, 1278–1286. doi: 10.1093/infdis/jis184

de Macêdo, J. P., Schumann Burkard, G., Niemann, M., Barrett, M. P., Vial, H., Mäser, P., et al. (2015). An atypical mitochondrial carrier that mediates drug action in *Trypanosoma brucei*. *PLoS Pathog.* 11:e1004875. doi: 10.1371/journal.ppat.1004875

de Muylder, G., Ang, K. K. H., Chen, S., Arkin, M. R., Engel, J. C., and McKerrow, J. H. (2011). A screen against *Leishmania* intracellular amastigotes: comparison to a promastigote screen and identification of a host cell-specific hit. *PLoS Negl. Trop. Dis.* 5:e1253. doi: 10.1371/journal.pntd.0001253

de Muylder, G., Vanhollebeke, B., Caljon, G., Wolfe, A. R., McKerrow, J., and Dujardin, J.-C. (2016). Naloxonazine, an amastigote-specific compound, affects *Leishmania* parasites through modulation of host-encoded functions. *PLoS Negl. Trop. Dis.* 10:e0005234. doi: 10.1371/journal.pntd.0005234

del Pilar Crespo, M., Avery, T. D., Hanssen, E., Fox, E., Robinson, T. V., Valente, P., et al. (2008). Artemisinin and a series of novel endoperoxide antimalarials exert early effects on digestive vacuole morphology. *Antimicrob. Agents Chemother.* 52, 98–109. doi: 10.1128/AAC.00609-07

Deniskin, R., Frame, I. J., Sosa, Y., and Akabas, M. H. (2016). Targeting the *Plasmodium vivax* equilibrative nucleoside transporter 1 (PvENT1) for antimalarial drug development. *Int. J. Parasitol. Drugs Drug Resist.* 6, 1–11. doi: 10.1016/j.ijpddr.2015.11.003

Derbyshire, E. T., Franssen, F. J., de Vries, E., Morin, C., Woodrow, C. J., Krishna, S., et al. (2008). Identification, expression and characterisation of a *Babesia bovis* hexose transporter. *Mol. Biochem. Parasitol.* 161, 124–129. doi: 10.1016/j.molbiopara.2008.06.010

Desai, S. A., Bezrukov, S. M., and Zimmerberg, J. (2000). A voltage-dependent channel involved in nutrient uptake by red blood cells infected with the malaria parasite. *Nature* 406, 1001–1005. doi: 10.1038/35023000

Di Cicco, M. F., Downey, M. E., Beeler, E., Marr, H., Cyrog, P., Kidd, L., et al. (2012). Re-emergence of Babesia conradae and effective treatment of infected dogs with atovaquone and azithromycin. *Vet. Parasitol.* 187, 23–27. doi: 10.1016/j.vetpar.2012.01.006

Doggett, J. S., Nilsen, A., Forquer, I., Wegmann, K. W., Jones-Brando, L., Yolken, R. H., et al. (2012). Endochin-like quinolones are highly efficacious against acute and latent experimental toxoplasmosis. *Proc. Natl. Acad. Sci. U.S.A.* 109, 15936–15941. doi: 10.1073/pnas.1208069109

Downie, M. J., Saliba, K. J., Howitt, S. M., Bröer, S., and Kirk, K. (2006). Transport of nucleosides across the *Plasmodium falciparum* parasite plasma membrane has characteristics of PfENT1. *Mol. Microbiol.* 60, 738–748. doi: 10.1111/j.1365-2958.2006.05125.x

Downie, M. J., Saliba, K. J., Bröer, S., Howitt, S. M., and Kirk, K. (2008). Purine nucleobase transport in the intraerythrocytic malaria parasite. *Int. J. Parasitol.* 38, 203–209. doi: 10.1016/j.ijpara.2007.07.005

Downie, M. J., El Bissati, K., Bobenchik, A. M., Nic Lochlainn, L., Amerik, A., Zufferey, R., et al. (2010). PfNT2, a permease of the equilibrative nucleoside transporter family in the endoplasmic reticulum of *Plasmodium falciparum*. *J. Biol. Chem.* 285, 20827–20833. doi: 10.1074/jbc.M110.118489

Drozdowicz, Y. M., Shaw, M., Nishi, M., Striepen, B., Liwinski, H. A., Roos, D. S., et al. (2003). Isolation and characterization of TgVP1, a type I vacuolar H^+-translocating pyrophosphatase from *Toxoplasma gondii*. the dynamics of its subcellular localization and the cellular effects of a diphosphonate inhibitor. *J. Biol. Chem.* 278, 1075–1085. doi: 10.1074/jbc.M209436200

Dyer, M., Jackson, M., McWhinney, C., Zhao, G., and Mikkelsen, R. (1996). Analysis of a cation-transporting ATPase of *Plasmodium falciparum*. *Mol. Biochem. Parasitol.* 78, 1–12. doi: 10.1016/S0166-6851(96)02593-5

Eckstein-Ludwig, U., Webb, R. J., van Goethem, I. D. A., East, J. M., Lee, A. G., Kimura, M., et al. (2003). Artemisinins target the SERCA of *Plasmodium falciparum*. *Nature* 424, 957–961. doi: 10.1038/nature01813

Fernando, D., Rodrigo, C., and Rajapakse, S. (2011). Primaquine in vivax malaria: an update and review on management issues. *Malar. J.* 10, 351. doi: 10.1186/1475-2875-10-351

Fidock, D. A., Nomura, T., Talley, A. K., Cooper, R. A., Dzekunov, S. M., Ferdig, M. T., et al. (2000). Mutations in the *P. falciparum* digestive vacuole transmembrane protein PfCRT and evidence for their role in chloroquine resistance. *Mol. Cell* 6, 861–871. doi: 10.1016/S1097-2765(05)00077-8

Flegr, J., Prandota, J., Sovičková, M., and Israili, Z. H. (2014). Toxoplasmosis—a global threat. correlation of latent toxoplasmosis with specific disease burden in a set of 88 countries. *PLoS ONE* 9:e90203. doi: 10.1371/journal.pone.0090203

Foley, M., and Tilley, L. (1997). Quinoline antimalarials: mechanisms of action and resistance. *Int. J. Parasitol.* 27, 231–240. doi: 10.1016/S0020-7519(96)00152-X

Foote, S. J., Thompson, J. K., Cowman, A. F., and Kemp, D. J. (1989). Amplification of the multidrug resistance gene in some chloroquine-resistant isolates of *P. falciparum*. *Cell* 57, 921–930. doi: 10.1016/0092-8674(89)90330-9

Frame, I. J., Deniskin, R., Arora, A., and Akabas, M. H. (2015a). Purine import into malaria parasites as a target for antimalarial drug development. *Ann. N.Y. Acad. Sci.* 1342, 19–28. doi: 10.1111/nyas.12568

Frame, I. J., Deniskin, R., Rinderspacher, A., Katz, F., Deng, S.-X., Moir, R. D., et al. (2015b). Yeast-based high-throughput screen identifies *Plasmodium falciparum* equilibrative nucleoside transporter 1 inhibitors that kill malaria parasites. *ACS Chem. Biol.* 10, 775–783. doi: 10.1021/cb500981y

Frame, I. J., Merino, E. F., Schramm, V. L., Cassera, M. B., Akabas, M. H. (2012). Malaria parasite type 4 equilibrative nucleoside transporters (ENT4) are purine transporters with distinct substrate specificity. *Biochem. J.* 446, 179–190. doi: 10.1042/BJ20112220

Fry, M., and Pudney, M. (1992). Site of action of the antimalarial hydroxynaphthoquinone, 2-trans-4-(4′-chlorophenyl) cyclohexyl-3-hydroxy-1,4-naphthoquinone (566C80). *Biochem. Pharmacol.* 43, 1545–1553.

Garnier, T., Mäntylä, A., Järvinen, T., Lawrence, J., Brown, M., and Croft, S. L. (2007). *In vivo* studies on the antileishmanial activity of buparvaquone and its prodrugs. *J. Antimicrob. Chemother.* 60, 802–810. doi: 10.1093/jac/dkm303

Ghaffarifar, F., Esavand Heydari, F., Dalimi, A., Hassan, Z. M., Delavari, M., and Mikaeiloo, H. (2015). Evaluation of apoptotic and antileishmanial activities of artemisinin on promastigotes and BALB/C mice infected with *Leishmania major*. *Iran. J. Parasitol.* 10, 258–267.

Ginsburg, H., Kutner, S., Krugliak, M., and Ioav Cabantchik, Z. (1985). Characterization of permeation pathways appearing in the host membrane of *Plasmodium falciparum* infected red blood cells. *Mol. Biochem. Parasitol.* 14, 313–322. doi: 10.1016/0166-6851(85)90059-3

Golldack, A., Henke, B., Bergmann, B., Wiechert, M. I., Erler, H., Blancke Soares, A., et al. (2017). Substrate-analogous inhibitors exert antimalarial action by targeting the *Plasmodium* lactate transporter PfFNT at nanomolar scale. *PLoS Pathog.* 13, e1006172. doi: 10.1371/journal.ppat.1006172

Gupta, S., Ghosh, P. K., Dutta, G. P., and Vishwakarma, R. A. (1995). *In vivo* study of artemisinin and its derivatives against primary amebic meningoencephalitis caused by *Naegleria fowleri*. *J. Parasitol.* 81, 1012–1013. doi: 10.2307/3284060

Hansen, M., Kun, J. F. J., Schultz, J. E., and Beitz, E. (2002). A single, bi-functional aquaglyceroporin in blood-stage *Plasmodium falciparum* malaria parasites. *J. Biol. Chem.* 277, 4874–4882. doi: 10.1074/jbc.M110683200

Hapuarachchi, S. V., Cobbold, S. A., Shafik, S. H., Dennis, A. S. M., McConville, M. J., Martin, R. E., et al. (2017). The malaria parasite's lactate transporter PfFNT is the target of antiplasmodial compounds identified in whole cell phenotypic screens. *PLoS Pathog.* 13:e1006180. doi: 10.1371/journal.ppat.1006180

Harrill, A. H., Desmet, K. D., Wolf, K. K., Bridges, A. S., Eaddy, J. S., Kurtz, C. L., et al. (2012). A mouse diversity panel approach reveals the potential for clinical kidney injury due to DB289 not predicted by classical rodent models. *Toxicol. Sci.* 130, 416–426. doi: 10.1093/toxsci/kfs238

Hencken, C. P., Jones-Brando, L., Bordón, C., Stohler, R., Mott, B. T., Yolken, R., et al. (2010). Thiazole, oxadiazole, and carboxamide derivatives of artemisinin are highly selective and potent inhibitors of *Toxoplasma gondii*. *J. Med. Chem.* 53, 3594–3601. doi: 10.1021/jm901857d

Hill, D. A., Pillai, A. D., Nawaz, F., Hayton, K., Doan, L., Lisk, G., et al. (2007). A blasticidin S-resistant *Plasmodium falciparum* mutant with a defective plasmodial surface anion channel. *Proc. Natl. Acad. Sci. U.S.A.* 104, 1063–1068. doi: 10.1073/pnas.0610353104

Hrycyna, C. A., Summers, R. L., Lehane, A. M., Pires, M. M., Namanja, H., Bohn, K., et al. (2014). Quinine dimers are potent inhibitors of the *Plasmodium falciparum* chloroquine resistance transporter and are active against quinoline-resistant *P. falciparum*. *ACS Chem. Biol.* 9, 722–730. doi: 10.1021/cb4008953

Huber, S. M., Uhlemann, A.-C., Gamper, N. L., Duranton, C., Kremsner, P. G., and Lang, F. (2002). *Plasmodium falciparum* activates endogenous Cl^- channels of human erythrocytes by membrane oxidation. *EMBO J.* 21, 22–30. doi: 10.1093/emboj/21.1.22

Huber, S. M., Duranton, C., Henke, G., van de Sand, C., Heussler, V., Shumilina, E., et al. (2004). *Plasmodium* induces swelling-activated ClC-2 anion channels in the host erythrocyte. *J. Biol. Chem.* 279, 41444–41452. doi: 10.1074/jbc.M407618200

Hughes, W. T., and Oz, H. S. (1995). Successful prevention and treatment of babesiosis with atovaquone. *J. Infect. Dis.* 172, 1042–1046. doi: 10.1093/infdis/172.4.1042

Hutchinson, D. B., Viravan, C., Kyle, D. E., Looareesuwan, S., Canfield, C. J., and Webster, H. K. (1996). Clinical studies of atovaquone, alone or in combination with other antimalarial drugs, for treatment of acute uncomplicated malaria in Thailand. *Am. J. Trop. Med. Hyg.* 54, 62–66. doi: 10.4269/ajtmh.1996.54.62

Ibrahim, H. M. S., Al-Salabi, M. I., El Sabbagh, N., Quashie, N. B., Alkhaldi, A. A. M., Escale, R., et al. (2011). Symmetrical choline-derived dications display strong anti-kinetoplastid activity. *J. Antimicrob. Chemother.* 66, 111–125. doi: 10.1093/jac/dkq401

Iguchi, A., Matsuu, A., Matsuyama, K., and Hikasa, Y. (2015). The efficacy of artemisinin, artemether, and lumefantrine against *Babesia gibsoni in vitro*. *Parasitol. Int.* 64, 190–193. doi: 10.1016/j.parint.2014.12.006

Ismail, M. A., Brun, R., Easterbrook, J. D., Tanious, F. A., Wilson, W. D., and Boykin, D. W. (2003). Synthesis and antiprotozoal activity of aza-analogues of furamidine. *J. Med. Chem.* 46, 4761–4769. doi: 10.1021/jm0302602

Jamal, Q., Khan, N. H., Wahid, S., Awan, M. M., Sutherland, C., and Shah, A. (2015). *In-vitro* sensitivity of Pakistani *Leishmania tropica* field isolate against buparvaquone in comparison to standard anti-leishmanial drugs. *Exp. Parasitol.* 154, 93–97. doi: 10.1016/j.exppara.2015.04.017

Jambou, R., Legrand, E., Niang, M., Khim, N., Lim, P., Volney, B., et al. (2005). Resistance of *Plasmodium falciparum* field isolates to *in-vitro* artemether and point mutations of the SERCA-type PfATPase6. *Lancet* 366, 1960–1963. doi: 10.1016/S0140-6736(05)67787-2

Jiménez-Díaz, M. B., Ebert, D., Salinas, Y., Pradhan, A., Lehane, A. M., Myrand-Lapierre, M.-E., et al. (2014). (+)-SJ733, a clinical candidate for malaria that acts through ATP4 to induce rapid host-mediated clearance of *Plasmodium*. *Proc. Natl. Acad. Sci. U.S.A.* 111, E5455–E5462. doi: 10.1073/pnas.1414221111

Joet, T., Eckstein-Ludwig, U., Morin, C., and Krishna, S. (2003). Validation of the hexose transporter of *Plasmodium falciparum* as a novel drug target. *Proc. Natl. Acad. Sci. U.S.A.* 100, 7476–7479. doi: 10.1073/pnas.1330865100

Jones-Brando, L., D'Angelo, J., Posner, G. H., and Yolken, R. (2006). *In vitro* inhibition of *Toxoplasma gondii* by four new derivatives of artemisinin. *Antimicrob. Agents Chemother.* 50, 4206–4208. doi: 10.1128/AAC.00793-06

Juge, N., Moriyama, S., Miyaji, T., Kawakami, M., Iwai, H., Fukui, T., et al. (2015). *Plasmodium falciparum* chloroquine resistance transporter is a H^+-coupled polyspecific nutrient and drug exporter. *Proc. Natl. Acad. Sci. U.S.A.* 112, 3356–3361. doi: 10.1073/pnas.1417102112

Kanaani, J., and Ginsburg, H. (1991). Transport of lactate in *Plasmodium falciparum*-infected human erythrocytes. *J. Cell. Physiol.* 149, 469–476. doi: 10.1002/jcp.1041490316

Kavishe, R. A., Koenderink, J. B., and Alifrangis, M. (2017). Oxidative stress in malaria and artemisinin combination therapy: pros and cons. *FEBS J.* 284, 2579–2591. doi: 10.1111/febs.14097

Kelly, J. X., Smilkstein, M. J., Brun, R., Wittlin, S., Cooper, R. A., Lane, K. D., et al. (2009). Discovery of dual function acridones as a new antimalarial chemotype. *Nature* 459, 270–273. doi: 10.1038/nature07937

Kessl, J. J., Meshnick, S. R., and Trumpower, B. L. (2007). Modeling the molecular basis of atovaquone resistance in parasites and pathogenic fungi. *Trends Parasitol.* 23, 494–501. doi: 10.1016/j.pt.2007.08.004

Kim, J.-T., Park, J.-Y., Seo, H.-S., Oh, H.-G., Noh, J.-W., Kim, J.-H., et al. (2002). *In vitro* antiprotozoal effects of artemisinin on *Neospora caninum*. *Vet. Parasitol.* 103, 53–63. doi: 10.1016/S0304-4017(01)00580-5

Kirk, K., and Horner, H. A. (1995). In search of a selective inhibitor of the induced transport of small solutes in *Plasmodium falciparum*-infected erythrocytes: effects of arylaminobenzoates. *Biochem. J.* 311, 761–768. doi: 10.1042/bj3110761

Kongkathip, N., Pradidphol, N., Hasitapan, K., Grigg, R., Kao, W.-C., Hunte, C., et al. (2010). Transforming rhinacanthin analogues from potent anticancer agents into potent antimalarial agents. *J. Med. Chem.* 53, 1211–1221. doi: 10.1021/jm901545z

Krause, P. J., Lepore, T., Sikand, V. K., Gadbaw, J., Burke, G., Telford, S. R., et al. (2000). Atovaquone and azithromycin for the treatment of babesiosis. *New Engl. J. Med.* 343, 1454–1458. doi: 10.1056/NEJM200011163432004

Krause, A., Dingemanse, J., Mathis, A., Marquart, L., Möhrle, J. J., and McCarthy, J. S. (2016). Pharmacokinetic/pharmacodynamic modelling of the antimalarial effect of Actelion-451840 in an induced blood stage malaria study in healthy subjects. *Br. J. Clin. Pharmacol.* 82, 412–421. doi: 10.1111/bcp.12962

Krishna, S., and Woodrow, C. J. (1999). Expression of parasite transporters in Xenopus oocytes. *Novartis Found. Symp.* 226, 126–139.

Krishna, S., Pulcini, S., Moore, C. M., Teo, B. H.-Y., and Staines, H. M. (2014). Pumped up: reflections on PfATP6 as the target for artemisinins. *Trends Pharmacol. Sci.* 35, 4–11. doi: 10.1016/j.tips.2013.10.007

Lakshmanan, V., Bray, P. G., Verdier-Pinard, D., Johnson, D. J., Horrocks, P., Muhle, R. A., et al. (2005). A critical role for PfCRT K76T in *Plasmodium falciparum* verapamil-reversible chloroquine resistance. *EMBO J.* 24, 2294–2305. doi: 10.1038/sj.emboj.7600681

Lalève, A., Vallières, C., Golinelli-Cohen, M.-P., Bouton, C., Song, Z., Pawlik, G., et al. (2016). The antimalarial drug primaquine targets Fe-S cluster proteins and yeast respiratory growth. *Redox Biol.* 7, 21–29. doi: 10.1016/j.redox.2015.10.008

Lanteri, C. A., Tidwell, R. R., and Meshnick, S. R. (2008). The mitochondrion is a site of trypanocidal action of the aromatic diamidine DB75 in bloodstream forms of *Trypanosoma brucei*. *Antimicrob. Agents Chemother.* 52, 875–882. doi: 10.1128/AAC.00642-07

Lawres, L. A., Garg, A., Kumar, V., Bruzual, I., Forquer, I. P., Renard, I., et al. (2016). Radical cure of experimental babesiosis in immunodeficient mice using a combination of an endochin-like quinolone and atovaquone. *J. Exp. Med.* 213, 1307–1318. doi: 10.1084/jem.20151519

Le Bihan, A., de Kanter, R., Angulo-Barturen, I., Binkert, C., Boss, C., Brun, R., et al. (2016). Characterization of novel antimalarial compound ACT-451840: preclinical assessment of activity and dose-efficacy modeling. *PLoS Med.* 13, e1002138. doi: 10.1371/journal.pmed.1002138

Liu, Y., Promeneur, D., Rojek, A., Kumar, N., Frøkiaer, J., Nielsen, S., et al. (2007). Aquaporin 9 is the major pathway for glycerol uptake by mouse erythrocytes, with implications for malarial virulence. *Proc. Natl. Acad. Sci. U.S.A.* 104, 12560–12564. doi: 10.1073/pnas.0705313104

Loiseau, P. M., and Bories, C. (2006). Mechanisms of drug action and drug resistance in *Leishmania* as basis for therapeutic target identification and design of antileishmanial modulators. *Curr. Top. Med. Chem.* 6, 539–550. doi: 10.2174/156802606776743165

Lukens, A. K., Heidebrecht, R. W., Mulrooney, C., Beaudoin, J. A., Comer, E., Duvall, J. R., et al. (2015). Diversity-oriented synthesis probe targets *Plasmodium falciparum* cytochrome b ubiquinone reduction site and synergizes with oxidation site inhibitors. *J. Infect. Dis.* 211, 1097–1103. doi: 10.1093/infdis/jiu565

Ma, Y., Lu, D.-M., Lu, X.-J., Liao, L., and Hu, X.-S. (2004). Activity of dihydroartemisinin against *Leishmania donovani* both *in vitro* and *vivo*. *Chin. Med. J.* 117, 1271–1273.

Macêdo, J. P., Schmidt, R. S., Mäser, P., Rentsch, D., Vial, H. J., Sigel, E., et al. (2013). Characterization of choline uptake in *Trypanosoma brucei* procyclic and bloodstream forms. *Mol. Biochem. Parasitol.* 190, 16–22. doi: 10.1016/j.molbiopara.2013.05.007

Mäntylä, A., Garnier, T., Rautio, J., Nevalainen, T., Vepsälainen, J., Koskinen, A., et al. (2004a). Synthesis, *in vitro* evaluation, and antileishmanial activity of water-soluble prodrugs of buparvaquone. *J. Med. Chem.* 47, 188–195. doi: 10.1021/jm030868a

Mäntylä, A., Rautio, J., Nevalainen, T., Vepsälainen, J., Juvonen, R., Kendrick, H., et al. (2004b). Synthesis and antileishmanial activity of novel buparvaquone oxime derivatives. *Bioorg. Med. Chem.* 12, 3497–3502. doi: 10.1016/j.bmc.2004.04.032

Marchetti, R. V., Lehane, A. M., Shafik, S. H., Winterberg, M., Martin, R. E., and Kirk, K. (2015). A lactate and formate transporter in the intraerythrocytic malaria parasite, *Plasmodium falciparum*. *Nat. Commun.* 6:6721. doi: 10.1038/ncomms7721

Martin, R. E., Marchetti, R. V., Cowan, A. I., Howitt, S. M., Bröer, S., and Kirk, K. (2009). Chloroquine transport via the malaria parasite's chloroquine resistance transporter. *Science* 325, 1680–1682. doi: 10.1126/science.1175667

Martin, R. E., Butterworth, A. S., Gardiner, D. L., Kirk, K., McCarthy, J. S., and Skinner-Adams, T. S. (2012). Saquinavir inhibits the malaria parasite's chloroquine resistance transporter. *Antimicrob. Agents Chemother.* 56, 2283–2289. doi: 10.1128/AAC.00166-12

Martínez-Higuera, A., Herrera-Martínez, M., Chávez-Munguía, B., Valle-Solís, M., Muñiz-Lino, M. A., Cázares-Apátiga, J., et al. (2015). *Entamoeba invadens*: Identification of a SERCA protein and effect of SERCA inhibitors on encystation. *Microb. Pathog.* 89, 18–26. doi: 10.1016/j.micpath.2015.08.016

Matsuu, A., Yamasaki, M., Xuan, X., Ikadai, H., and Hikasa, Y. (2008). *In vitro* evaluation of the growth inhibitory activities of 15 drugs against *Babesia gibsoni* (Aomori strain). *Vet. Parasitol.* 157, 1–8. doi: 10.1016/j.vetpar.2008.07.023

Maya, J. D., Morello, A., Repetto, Y., Tellez, R., Rodriguez, A., Zelada, U., et al. (2000). Effects of 3-chloro-phenyl-1,4-dihydropyridine derivatives on *Trypanosome cruzi* epimastigotes. *Comp. Biochem. Physiol. C* 125, 103–109. doi: 10.1016/S0742-8413(99)00096-1

McAuley, J. B., and Juranek, D. D. (1992). Luminal agents in the treatment of amebiasis. *Clin. Infect. Dis.* 14, 1161–1162. doi: 10.1093/clinids/14.5.1161

McFadden, D. C., Tomavo, S., Berry, E. A., and Boothroyd, J. C. (2000). Characterization of cytochrome b from *Toxoplasma gondii* and Q(o) domain mutations as a mechanism of atovaquone-resistance. *Mol. Biochem. Parasitol.* 108, 1–12. doi: 10.1016/S0166-6851(00)00184-5

McHardy, N., Wekesa, L. S., Hudson, A. T., and Randall, A. W. (1985). Antitheilerial activity of BW720C (buparvaquone): a comparison with parvaquone. *Res. Vet. Sci.* 39, 29–33.

McIntosh, M. T., Drozdowicz, Y. M., Laroiya, K., Rea, P. A., and Vaidya, A. B. (2001). Two classes of plant-like vacuolar-type H^+-pyrophosphatases in malaria parasites. *Mol. Biochem. Parasitol.* 114, 183–195. doi: 10.1016/S0166-6851(01)00251-1

Meireles, P., Mendes, A.M., Aroeira, R.I., Mounce, B.C., Vignuzzi, M., Staines, H.M., et al. (2017). Uptake and metabolism of arginine impact *Plasmodium* development in the liver. *Sci. Rep.* 7:4072. doi: 10.1038/s41598-017-04424-y

Mhadhbi, M., Naouach, A., Boumiza, A., Chaabani, M. F., BenAbderazzak, S., and Darghouth, M. A. (2010). *In vivo* evidence for the resistance of *Theileria annulata* to buparvaquone. *Vet. Parasitol.* 169, 241–247. doi: 10.1016/j.vetpar.2010.01.013

Mikolajczak, S. A., Vaughan, A. M., Kangwanrangsan, N., Roobsoong, W., Fishbaugher, M., Yimamnuaychok, N., et al. (2015). *Plasmodium vivax* liver stage development and hypnozoite persistence in human liver-chimeric mice. *Cell Host Microbe* 17, 526–535. doi: 10.1016/j.chom.2015.02.011

Minami, T., Nakano, T., Shimizu, S., Shimura, K., Fujinaga, T., and Ito, S. (1985). Efficacy of naphthoquinones and imidocarb dipropionate on *Theileria sergenti* infections in splenectomized calves. *Jpn. J. Vet. Sci.* 47, 297–300. doi: 10.1292/jvms1939.47.297

Miner, M. L., and Jensen, J. B. (1976). Decoquinate in the control of experimentally induced coccidiosis of calves. *Am. J. Vet. Res.* 37, 1043–1045.

Mishina, Y. V., Krishna, S., Haynes, R. K., and Meade, J. C. (2007). Artemisinins inhibit *Trypanosoma cruzi* and *Trypanosoma brucei rhodesiense in vitro* growth. *Antimicrob. Agents Chemother.* 51, 1852–1854. doi: 10.1128/AAC.01544-06

Moore, C. M., Hoey, E. M., Trudgett, A., and Timson, D. J. (2011). Artemisinins act through at least two targets in a yeast model. *FEMS Yeast Res.* 11, 233–237. doi: 10.1111/j.1567-1364.2010.00706.x

Mukhopadhyay, R., and Beitz, E. (2010). Metalloid transport by aquaglyceroporins: consequences in the treatment of human diseases. *Adv. Exp. Med. Biol.* 679, 57–69. doi: 10.1007/978-1-4419-6315-4_5

Mukhopadhyay, R., and Madhubala, R. (1994). Effect of antioxidants on the growth and polyamine levels of *Leishmania donovani*. *Biochem. Pharmacol.* 47, 611–615. doi: 10.1016/0006-2952(94)90122-8

Mukhopadhyay, R., Mandal, G., Atluri, V. S. R., Figarella, K., Uzcategui, N.L., Zhou, Y., et al. (2011). The role of alanine 163 in solute permeability of *Leishmania major* aquaglyceroporin LmAQP1. *Mol. Biochem. Parasitol.* 175, 83–90. doi: 10.1016/j.molbiopara.2010.09.007

Muraguri, G. R., Kiara, H. K., and McHardy, N. (1999). Treatment of East Coast fever: a comparison of parvaquone and buparvaquone. *Vet. Parasitol.* 87, 25–37. doi: 10.1016/S0304-4017(99)00154-5

Nagamune, K., Beatty, W. L., and Sibley, L. D. (2007). Artemisinin induces calcium-dependent protein secretion in the protozoan parasite *Toxoplasma gondii*. *Eukaryotic Cell* 6, 2147–2156. doi: 10.1128/EC.00262-07

Naik, P. K., Srivastava, M., Bajaj, P., Jain, S., Dubey, A., Ranjan, P., et al. (2011). The binding modes and binding affinities of artemisinin derivatives with *Plasmodium falciparum* Ca^{2+}-ATPase (PfATP6). *J. Mol. Model.* 17, 333–357. doi: 10.1007/s00894-010-0726-4

Neal, R. A., van Bueren, J., McCoy, N. G., and Iwobi, M. (1989). Reversal of drug resistance in *Trypanosoma cruzi* and *Leishmania donovani* by verapamil. *Trans. R. Soc. Trop. Med. Hyg.* 83, 197–198. doi: 10.1016/0035-9203(89)90642-1

Ng, C. L., Siciliano, G., Lee, M. C. S., Almeida, M. J., de, Corey, V. C., Bopp, S. E., et al. (2016). CRISPR-Cas9-modified pfmdr1 protects *Plasmodium falciparum* asexual blood stages and gametocytes against a class of piperazine-containing compounds but potentiates artemisinin-based combination therapy partner drugs. *Mol. Microbiol.* 101, 381–393. doi: 10.1111/mmi.13397

Nguitragool, W., Bokhari, A. A. B., Pillai, A. D., Rayavara, K., Sharma, P., Turpin, B., et al. (2011). Malaria parasite clag3 genes determine channel-mediated nutrient uptake by infected red blood cells. *Cell* 145, 665–677. doi: 10.1016/j.cell.2011.05.002

Nguitragool, W., Rayavara, K., and Desai, S. A. (2014). Proteolysis at a specific extracellular residue implicates integral membrane CLAG3 in malaria parasite nutrient channels. *PLoS ONE* 9:e93759. doi: 10.1371/journal.pone.0093759

Nilsen, A., LaCrue, A. N., White, K. L., Forquer, I. P., Cross, R. M., Marfurt, J., et al. (2013). Quinolone-3-diarylethers: a new class of antimalarial drug. *Sci. Transl. Med.* 5, 177ra37. doi: 10.1126/scitranslmed.3005029

Nunes, R. R., Costa, M. D. S., Santos, B. D. R., Fonseca, A. L. D., Ferreira, L. S., Chagas, R. C. R., et al. (2016). Successful application of virtual screening and molecular dynamics simulations against antimalarial molecular targets. *Mem. Inst. Oswaldo Cruz* 111, 721–730. doi: 10.1590/0074-02760160207

Ortiz, D., Guiguemde, W. A., Johnson, A., Elya, C., Anderson, J., Clark, J., et al. (2015). Identification of selective inhibitors of the *Plasmodium falciparum* hexose transporter PfHT by screening focused libraries of anti-malarial compounds. *PLoS ONE* 10:e0123598. doi: 10.1371/journal.pone.0123598

Ortiz, D., Forquer, I., Boitz, J., Soysa, R., Elya, C., Fulwiler, A., et al. (2016). Targeting the cytochrome bc1 complex of *Leishmania* parasites for discovery of novel drugs. *Antimicrob. Agents Chemother.* 60, 4972–4982. doi: 10.1128/AAC.00850-16

Overman, R. R. (1947). Reversible cellular permeability alterations in disease. *in vivo* studies on sodium, potassium and chloride concentrations in erythrocytes of the malarious monkey. *Am. J. Physiol.* 152, 113–121. doi: 10.1152/ajplegacy.1947.152.1.113

Pain, M., Fuller, A. W., Basore, K., Pillai, A. D., Solomon, T., Bokhari, A. A. B., et al. (2016). Synergistic malaria parasite killing by two types of plasmodial surface anion channel Inhibitors. *PLoS ONE* 11:e0149214. doi: 10.1371/journal.pone.0149214

Painter, H. J., Morrisey, J. M., Mather, M. W., and Vaidya, A. B. (2007). Specific role of mitochondrial electron transport in blood-stage *Plasmodium falciparum*. *Nature* 446, 88–91. doi: 10.1038/nature05572

Palit, P., and Ali, N. (2008). Oral therapy with amlodipine and lacidipine, 1,4-dihydropyridine derivatives showing activity against experimental visceral leishmaniasis. *Antimicrob. Agents Chemother.* 52, 374–377. doi: 10.1128/AAC.00522-07

Pavlovic-Djuranovic, S., Kun, J. F. J., Schultz, J. E., and Beitz, E. (2006). Dihydroxyacetone and methylglyoxal as permeants of the *Plasmodium* aquaglyceroporin inhibit parasite proliferation. *Biochim. Biophys. Acta* 1758, 1012–1017. doi: 10.1016/j.bbamem.2005.12.002

Petersen, E., and Schmidt, D. R. (2003). Sulfadiazine and pyrimethamine in the postnatal treatment of congenital toxoplasmosis: what are the options? *Expert Rev. Anti Infect. Ther.* 1, 175–182. doi: 10.1586/14787210.1.1.175

Pickard, A. L., Wongsrichanalai, C., Purfield, A., Kamwendo, D., Emery, K., Zalewski, C., et al. (2003). Resistance to antimalarials in Southeast Asia and genetic polymorphisms in pfmdr1. *Antimicrob. Agents Chemother.* 47, 2418–2423. doi: 10.1128/AAC.47.8.2418-2423.2003

Ponte-Sucre, A., Gamarro, F., Dujardin, J.-C., Barrett, M. P., López-Vélez, R., García-Hernández, R., et al. (2017). Drug resistance and treatment failure in leishmaniasis: a 21st century challenge. *PLoS Negl. Trop. Dis.* 11:e0006052. doi: 10.1371/journal.pntd.0006052

Price, R. N., Uhlemann, A.-C., Brockman, A., McGready, R., Ashley, E., Phaipun, L., et al. (2004). Mefloquine resistance in *Plasmodium falciparum* and increased pfmdr1 gene copy number. *Lancet* 364, 438–447. doi: 10.1016/S0140-6736(04)16767-6

Promeneur, D., Liu, Y., Maciel, J., Agre, P., King, L. S., and Kumar, N. (2007). Aquaglyceroporin PbAQP during intraerythrocytic development of the malaria parasite *Plasmodium berghei*. *Proc. Natl. Acad. Sci. U.S.A.* 104, 2211–2216. doi: 10.1073/pnas.0610843104

Promeneur, D., Mlambo, G., Agre, P., and Coppens, I. (2018). Aquaglyceroporin PbAQP is required for efficient progression through the liver stage of *Plasmodium* infection. *Sci. Rep.* 8:655. doi: 10.1038/s41598-017-18987-3

Prudêncio, M., Derbyshire, E.T., Marques, C.A., Krishna, S., Mota, M.M., and Staines, H.M. (2009). *Plasmodium berghei*-infection induces volume-regulated anion channel-like activity in human hepatoma cells. *Cell. Microbiol.* 11, 1492–1501. doi: 10.1111/j.1462-5822.2009.01342.x

Pulcini, S., Staines, H. M., Pittman, J. K., Slavic, K., Doerig, C., Halbert, J., et al. (2013). Expression in yeast links field polymorphisms in PfATP6 to *in vitro* artemisinin resistance and identifies new inhibitor classes. *J. Infect. Dis.* 208, 468–478. doi: 10.1093/infdis/jit171

Rane, L., Rane, D. S., and Kinnamon, K. E. (1976). Screening large numbers of compounds in a model based on mortality of *Trypanosoma rhodesiense* infected mice. *Am. J. Trop. Med. Hyg.* 25, 395–400. doi: 10.4269/ajtmh.1976.25.395

Raphemot, R., Lafuente-Monasterio, M. J., Gamo-Benito, F. J., Clardy, J., and Derbyshire, E. R. (2015). Discovery of dual-stage malaria inhibitors with new targets. *Antimicrob. Agents Chemother.* 60, 1430–1437. doi: 10.1128/AAC.02110-15

Reed, M. B., Saliba, K. J., Caruana, S. R., Kirk, K., and Cowman, A. F. (2000). Pgh1 modulates sensitivity and resistance to multiple antimalarials in *Plasmodium falciparum*. *Nature* 403, 906–909. doi: 10.1038/35002615

Reigada, C., Valera-Vera, E. A., Sayé, M., Errasti, A. E., Avila, C. C., Miranda, M. R., et al. (2017). Trypanocidal effect of isotretinoin through the inhibition of polyamine and amino acid transporters in *Trypanosoma cruzi*. *PLoS Negl. Trop. Dis.* 11:e0005472. doi: 10.1371/journal.pntd.0005472

Reimão, J. Q., Scotti, M. T., and Tempone, A. G. (2010). Anti-leishmanial and anti-trypanosomal activities of 1,4-dihydropyridines: *In vitro* evaluation and structure-activity relationship study. *Bioorg. Med. Chem.* 18, 8044–8053. doi: 10.1016/j.bmc.2010.09.015

Reimão, J. Q., Colombo, F. A., Pereira-Chioccola, V. L., and Tempone, A. G. (2011). *In vitro* and experimental therapeutic studies of the calcium channel blocker bepridil: detection of viable *Leishmania (L.) chagasi* by real-time PCR. *Exp. Parasitol.* 128, 111–115. doi: 10.1016/j.exppara.2011.02.021

Reimão, J. Q., Colombo, F. A., Pereira-Chioccola, V. L., and Tempone, A. G. (2012). Effectiveness of liposomal buparvaquone in an experimental hamster model of *Leishmania (L.) infantum* chagasi. *Exp. Parasitol.* 130, 195–199. doi: 10.1016/j.exppara.2012.01.010

Reimão, J. Q., Mesquita, J. T., Ferreira, D. D., and Tempone, A. G. (2016). Investigation of calcium channel blockers as antiprotozoal agents and their interference in the metabolism of *Leishmania (L.) infantum*. *Evid. Based Complement. Alternat. Med.* 2016:1523691. doi: 10.1155/2016/1523691

Ricketts, A. P., and Pfefferkorn, E. R. (1993). *Toxoplasma gondii*: Susceptibility and development of resistance to anticoccidial drugs *in vitro*. *Antimicrob. Agents Chemother.* 37, 2358–2363. doi: 10.1128/AAC.37.11.2358

Rodrigues, C. O., Scott, D. A., Bailey, B. N., Souza, W., de Benchimol, M., Moreno, B., et al. (2000). Vacuolar proton pyrophosphatase activity and pyrophosphate (PPi) in *Toxoplasma gondii* as possible chemotherapeutic targets. *Biochem. J.* 349, 737–745. doi: 10.1042/bj3490737

Rohrbach, P., Sanchez, C. P., Hayton, K., Friedrich, O., Patel, J., Sidhu, A. B. S., et al. (2006). Genetic linkage of pfmdrl with food vacuolar solute import in *Plasmodium falciparum*. *EMBO J.* 25, 3000–3011. doi: 10.1038/sj.emboj.7601203

Rottmann, M., McNamara, C., Yeung, B. K. S., Lee, M. C. S., Zou, B., Russell, B., et al. (2010). Spiroindolones, a potent compound class for the treatment of malaria. *Science* 329, 1175–1180. doi: 10.1126/science.1193225

Saliba, K. J., Horner, H. A., and Kirk, K. (1998). Transport and metabolism of the essential vitamin pantothenic acid in human erythrocytes infected with the malaria parasite *Plasmodium falciparum*. *J. Biol. Chem.* 273, 10190–10195. doi: 10.1074/jbc.273.17.10190

Sanchez, M. A. (2013). Molecular identification and characterization of an essential pyruvate transporter from *Trypanosoma brucei*. *J. Biol. Chem.* 288, 14428–14437. doi: 10.1074/jbc.M113.473157

Schmidt, R. S., Macêdo, J. P., Steinmann, M. E., Salgado, A. G., Bütikofer, P., Sigel, E., et al. (2017). Transporters of *Trypanosoma brucei*: phylogeny, physiology, pharmacology. *FEBS J.* doi: 10.1111/febs.14302. [Epub ahead of print].

Schumann Burkard, G., Jutzi, P., and Roditi, I. (2011). Genome-wide RNAi screens in bloodstream form trypanosomes identify drug transporters. *Mol. Biochem. Parasitol.* 175, 91–94. doi: 10.1016/j.molbiopara.2010.09.002

Sen, R., Ganguly, S., Saha, P., and Chatterjee, M. (2010). Efficacy of artemisinin in experimental visceral leishmaniasis. *Int. J. Antimicrob. Agents* 36, 43–49. doi: 10.1016/j.ijantimicag.2010.03.008

Sharma, P., Wollenberg, K., Sellers, M., Zainabadi, K., Galinsky, K., Moss, E., et al. (2013). An epigenetic antimalarial resistance mechanism involving parasite genes linked to nutrient uptake. *J. Biol. Chem.* 288, 19429–19440. doi: 10.1074/jbc.M113.468371

Shirley, D.-A., and Moonah, S. (2016). Fulminant amebic colitis after corticosteroid therapy: a systematic review. *PLoS Negl. Trop. Dis.* 10:e0004879. doi: 10.1371/journal.pntd.0004879

Siregar, J. E., Kurisu, G., Kobayashi, T., Matsuzaki, M., Sakamoto, K., Mi-Ichi, F., et al. (2015). Direct evidence for the atovaquone action on the *Plasmodium* cytochrome bcl complex. *Parasitol. Int.* 64, 295–300. doi: 10.1016/j.parint.2014.09.011

Slater, A. F.G. (1993). Chloroquine: mechanism of drug action and resistance in *Plasmodium falciparum*. *Pharmacol. Ther.* 57, 203–235. doi: 10.1016/0163-7258(93)90056-J

Slavic, K., Delves, M. J., Prudêncio, M., Talman, A. M., Straschil, U., Derbyshire, E. T., et al. (2011). Use of a selective inhibitor to define the chemotherapeutic potential of the plasmodial hexose transporter in different stages of the parasite's life cycle. *Antimicrob. Agents Chemother.* 55,2824–2830. doi: 10.1128/AAC.01739-10

Song, J., Almasalmeh, A., Krenc, D., and Beitz, E. (2012). Molar concentrations of sorbitol and polyethylene glycol inhibit the *Plasmodium* aquaglyceroporin but not that of *E. coli:* involvement of the channel vestibules. *Biochim. Biophys. Acta* 1818, 1218–1224. doi: 10.1016/j.bbamem.2012.01.025

Song, J., Baker, N., Rothert, M., Henke, B., Jeacock, L., Horn, D., et al. (2016). Pentamidine is not a permeant but a nanomolar inhibitor of the *Trypanosoma brucei* aquaglyceroporin-2. *PLoS Pathog.* 12:e1005436. doi: 10.1371/journal.ppat.1005436

Spangenberg, T., Burrows, J. N., Kowalczyk, P., McDonald, S., Wells, T. N. C., and Willis, P. (2013). The open access malaria box: a drug discovery catalyst for neglected diseases. *PLoS ONE* 8:e62906. doi: 10.1371/journal.pone.0062906

Spillman, N. J., Allen, R. J. W., McNamara, C. W., Yeung, B. K. S., Winzeler, E. A., Diagana, T. T., et al. (2013). Na^+ regulation in the malaria parasite *Plasmodium falciparum* involves the cation ATPase PfATP4 and is a target of the spiroindolone antimalarials. *Cell Host Microbe* 13, 227–237. doi: 10.1016/j.chom.2012.12.006

Spillman, N. J., and Kirk, K. (2015). The malaria parasite cation ATPase PfATP4 and its role in the mechanism of action of a new arsenal of antimalarial drugs. *Int. J. Parasitol. Drugs Drug Resist.* 5, 149–162. doi: 10.1016/j.ijpddr.2015.07.001

Srivastava, I. K., and Vaidya, A. B. (1999). A mechanism for the synergistic antimalarial action of atovaquone and proguanil. *Antimicrob. Agents Chemother.* 43, 1334–1339.

Srivastava, I. K., Morrisey, J. M., Darrouzet, E., Daldal, F., and Vaidya, A. B. (1999). Resistance mutations reveal the atovaquone-binding domain of cytochrome b in malaria parasites. *Mol. Microbiol.* 33, 704–711. doi: 10.1046/j.1365-2958.1999.01515.x

Šťáfková, J., Mach, J., Biran, M., Verner, Z., Bringaud, F., and Tachezy, J. (2016). Mitochondrial pyruvate carrier in *Trypanosoma brucei*. *Mol. Microbiol.* 100, 442–456. doi: 10.1111/mmi.13325

Staines, H. M., Ellory, J. C., and Kirk, K. (2001). Perturbation of the pump-leak balance for Na^+ and K^+ in malaria-infected erythrocytes. *Am. J. Physiol.* 280, C1576–C1587. doi: 10.1152/ajpcell.2001.280.6.C1576

Stanley, S. L. (2003). Amoebiasis. *Lancet* 361, 1025–1034. doi: 10.1016/S0140-6736(03)12830-9

Steck, E. A., Kinnamon, K. E., Davidson, D. E., Duxbury, R. E., Johnson, A. J., and Masters, R. E. (1982). *Trypanosoma rhodesiense*: Evaluation of the antitrypanosomal action of 2,5-bis(4-guanylphenyl)furan dihydrochloride. *Exp. Parasitol.* 53, 133–144. doi: 10.1016/0014-4894(82)90099-6

Steinmann, M. E., González-Salgado, A., Bütikofer, P., Mäser, P., and Sigel, E. (2015). A heteromeric potassium channel involved in the modulation of the plasma membrane potential is essential for the survival of African trypanosomes. *FASEB J.* 29, 3228–3237. doi: 10.1096/fj.15-271353

Tanabe, K., Izumo, A., Kato, M., Miki, A., and Doi, S. (1989). Stage dependent inhibition of *Plasmodiun falciparum falciparum* by potent Ca^{2+} and calmodulin modulators. *J. Protozool.* 36, 139–143. doi: 10.1111/j.1550-7408.1989.tb01060.x

Tempone, A. G., Taniwaki, N. N., and Reimão, J. Q. (2009). Antileishmanial activity and ultrastructural alterations of *Leishmania (L.) chagasi* treated with the calcium channel blocker nimodipine. *Parasitol. Res.* 105, 499–505. doi: 10.1007/s00436-009-1427-8

Thomé, R., Lopes, S. C. P., Costa, F. T. M., and Verinaud, L. (2013). Chloroquine: modes of action of an undervalued drug. *Immunol. Lett.* 153, 50–57. doi: 10.1016/j.imlet.2013.07.004

Upston, J. M., and Gero, A. M. (1995). Parasite-induced permeation of nucleosides in *Plasmodium falciparum* malaria. *Biochim. Biophys. Acta* 1236, 249–258. doi: 10.1016/0005-2736(95)00055-8

Urbina, J. A., Moreno, B., Vierkotter, S., Oldfield, E., Payares, G., Sanoja, C., et al. (1999). *Trypanosoma cruzi* contains major pyrophosphate stores, and its growth *in vitro* and *in vivo* is blocked by pyrophosphate analogs. *J. Biol. Chem.* 274, 33609–33615. doi: 10.1074/jbc.274.47.33609

Uzcategui, N.L., Szallies, A., Pavlovic-Djuranovic, S., Palmada, M., Figarella, K., Boehmer, C., et al. (2004). Cloning, heterologous expression and characterization of three aquaglyceroporins from *Trypanosoma brucei*. *J. Biol. Chem.* 279, 42669–42676. doi: 10.1074/jbc.M404518200

Valiathan, R., Dubey, M. L., Mahajan, R. C., and Malla, N. (2006). *Leishmania donovani*: effect of verapamil on *in vitro* susceptibility of promastigote and amastigote stages of Indian clinical isolates to sodium stibogluconate. *Exp. Parasitol.* 114, 103–108. doi: 10.1016/j.exppara.2006.02.015

Vallières, C., Fisher, N., Antoine, T., Al-Helal, M., Stocks, P., Berry, N. G., et al. (2012). HDQ, a potent inhibitor of *Plasmodium falciparum* proliferation, binds to the quinone reduction site of the cytochrome bc1 complex. *Antimicrob. Agents Chemother.* 56, 3739–3747. doi: 10.1128/AAC.00486-12

Waller, K. L., Muhle, R. A., Ursos, L. M., Horrocks, P., Verdier-Pinard, D., Sidhu, A. B. S., et al. (2003). Chloroquine resistance modulated *in vitro* by expression levels of the *Plasmodium falciparum* chloroquine resistance transporter. *J. Biol. Chem.* 278, 33593–33601. doi: 10.1074/jbc.M302215200

Ward, C. P., Wong, P. E., Burchmore, R. J., de Koning, H. P., and Barrett, M. P. (2011). Trypanocidal furamidine analogues: influence of pyridine nitrogens on trypanocidal activity, transport kinetics, and resistance patterns. *Antimicrob. Agents Chemother.* 55, 2352–2361. doi: 10.1128/AAC.01551-10

Weiner, J., and Kooij, T. W. A. (2016). Phylogenetic profiles of all membrane transport proteins of the malaria parasite highlight new drug targets. *Microb Cell* 3, 511–521. doi: 10.15698/mic2016.10.534

Wellems, T. E., Walker-Jonah, A., and Panton, L. J. (1991). Genetic mapping of the chloroquine-resistance locus on *Plasmodium falciparum* chromosome 7. *Proc. Natl. Acad. Sci. U.S.A.* 88, 3382–3386. doi: 10.1073/pnas.88.8.3382

Wengelnik, K., Vidal, V., Ancelin, M. L., Cathiard, A.-M., Morgat, J. L., Kocken, C. H., et al. (2002). A class of potent antimalarials and their specific accumulation in infected erythrocytes. *Science* 295, 1311–1314. doi: 10.1126/science.1067236

Wenzler, T., Boykin, D. W., Ismail, M. A., Hall, J. E., Tidwell, R. R., and Brun, R. (2009). New treatment option for second-stage African sleeping sickness: *In vitro* and *in vivo* efficacy of aza analogs of DB289. *Antimicrob. Agents Chemother.* 53, 4185–4192. doi: 10.1128/AAC.00225-09

White, N. J., Pukrittayakamee, S., Phyo, A. P., Rueangweerayut, R., Nosten, F., Jittamala, P., et al. (2014). Spiroindolone KAE609 for *falciparum* and *vivax* malaria. *New Engl. J. Med.* 371, 403–410. doi: 10.1056/NEJMoa1315860

WHO (2001). *Antimalarial Drug Combination Therapy: Report of a WHO Technical Consultation.*

WHO (2015). *Guidelines for the Treatment of Malaria.* Geneva: World Health Organization.

WHO (2016). *Report of the Second WHO Stakeholders Meeting on Gambiense Human African Trypanosomiasis Elimination*, Geneva, 21–23.

WHO (2017a). Global leishmaniasis update, 2006–2015: a turning point in leishmaniasis surveillance, weekly epidemiological record. *Relevé Épidémiologique Hebdomadaire* 92, 557–572.

WHO (2017b). *World Malaria Report 2017.* Geneva: World Health Organization.

Wiechert, M. I., and Beitz, E. (2017). Mechanism of formate-nitrite transporters by dielectric shift of substrate acidity. *EMBO J.* 36, 949–958. doi: 10.15252/embj.201695776

Wiechert, M., Erler, H., Golldack, A., and Beitz, E. (2017). A widened substrate selectivity filter of eukaryotic formate-nitrite transporters enables high-level lactate conductance. *FEBS J.* 284, 2663–2673. doi: 10.1111/febs.14117

Wittner, M., Lederman, J., Tanowitz, H. B., Rosenbaum, G. S., and Weiss, L. M. (1996). Atovaquone in the treatment of *Babesia microti* infections in hamsters. *Am. J. Trop. Med. Hyg.* 55, 219–222. doi: 10.4269/ajtmh.1996.55.219

Woodrow, C. J., Penny, J. I., and Krishna, S. (1999). Intraerythrocytic *Plasmodium falciparum* expresses a high affinity facilitative hexose transporter. *J. Biol. Chem.* 274, 7272–7277. doi: 10.1074/jbc.274.11.7272

Wree, D., Wu, B., Zeuthen, T., and Beitz, E. (2011). Requirement for asparagine in the aquaporin NPA signature motifs for cation exclusion. *FEBS J.* 278, 740–748. doi: 10.1111/j.1742-4658.2010.07993.x

Wu, B., Song, J., and Beitz, E. (2010). Novel channel-enzyme fusion proteins confer arsenate resistance. *J. Biol. Chem.* 285, 40081–40087. doi: 10.1074/jbc.M110.184457

Wu, B., Rambow, J., Bock, S., Holm-Bertelsen, J., Wiechert, M. I., Soares, A. B., et al. (2015). Identity of a *Plasmodium* lactate/H^+ symporter structurally unrelated to human transporters. *Nat. Commun.* 6, 6284. doi: 10.1038/ncomms7284

Yang, D. M., and Liew, F. Y. (1993). Effects of qinghaosu (artemisinin) and its derivatives on experimental cutaneous leishmaniasis. *Parasitology* 106(Pt 1), 7–11. doi: 10.1017/S0031182000074758

Ye, Z., and van Dyke, K. (1988). Reversal of chloroquine resistance in *falciparum* malaria independent of calcium channels. *Biochem. Biophys. Res. Commun.* 155, 476–481. doi: 10.1016/S0006-291X(88)81111-2

Ye, Z., and van Dyke, K. (1994). Reversal of chloroquine resistance in *falciparum* malaria by some calcium channel inhibitors and optical isomers is independent of calcium channel blockade. *Drug Chem. Toxicol.* 17, 149–162. doi: 10.3109/01480549409014308

Zaugg, J. L., and Lane, V. M. (1989). Evaluations of buparvaquone as a treatment for equine babesiosis (*Babesia equi*). *Am. J. Vet. Res.* 50, 782–785.

Zeuthen, T., Wu, B., Pavlovic-Djuranovic, S., Holm, L. M., Uzcategui, N. L., Duszenko, M., et al. (2006). Ammonia permeability of the aquaglyceroporins from *Plasmodium falciparum*, *Toxoplasma gondii* and *Trypansoma brucei*. *Mol. Microbiol.* 61, 1598–1608. doi: 10.1111/j.1365-2958.2006.05325.x

Zishiri, V. K., Joshi, M. C., Hunter, R., Chibale, K., Smith, P. J., Summers, R. L., et al. (2011). Quinoline antimalarials containing a dibemethin group are active against chloroquinone-resistant *Plasmodium falciparum* and inhibit chloroquine transport via the *P. falciparum* chloroquine-resistance transporter (PfCRT). *J. Med. Chem.* 54, 6956–6968. doi: 10.1021/jm2009698

6

The Emerging Role of microRNAs in Aquaporin Regulation

André Gomes[1,2], Inês V. da Silva[1,2], Cecília M. P. Rodrigues[1,2], Rui E. Castro[1,2] and Graça Soveral[1,2*]*

[1] *Research Institute for Medicines (iMed.ULisboa), Faculty of Pharmacy, Universidade de Lisboa, Lisbon, Portugal,*
[2] *Department Bioquimica e Biologia Humana, Faculty of Pharmacy, Universidade de Lisboa, Lisbon, Portugal*

***Correspondence:**
Graça Soveral
gsoveral@ff.ulisboa.pt
Rui E. Castro
ruieduardocastro@ff.ulisboa.pt

Aquaporins (AQPs) are membrane channels widely distributed in human tissues. AQPs are essential for water and energy homeostasis being involved in a broad range of pathophysiological processes such as edema, brain injury, glaucoma, nephrogenic diabetes insipidus, salivary and lacrimal gland dysfunction, cancer, obesity and related metabolic complications. Compelling evidence indicates that AQPs are targets for therapeutic intervention with potential broad application. Nevertheless, efficient AQP modulators have been difficult to find due to either lack of selectivity and stability, or associated toxicity that hamper *in vivo* studies. MicroRNAs (miRNAs) are naturally occurring small non-coding RNAs that regulate post-transcriptional gene expression and are involved in several diseases. Recent identification of miRNAs as endogenous modulators of AQP expression provides an alternative approach to target these proteins and opens new perspectives for therapeutic applications. This mini-review compiles the current knowledge of miRNA interaction with AQPs highlighting miRNA potential for regulation of AQP-based disorders.

Keywords: aquaporin, miRNA, gene expression regulation, post-transcriptional modulation, membrane proteins, permeability, disease

INTRODUCTION

Aquaporins (AQPs) are membrane channels that facilitate diffusion of water and small molecules (e.g., glycerol) through cell membranes driven by osmotic or solute gradients. The 13 isoforms (AQP0-12) expressed in mammals are crucial for water homeostasis and energy balance, which in turn influence survival and adaptation of living organisms. AQPs participate in many physiological processes such as renal water absorption, brain water homeostasis, skin hydration, intestinal permeability, cell proliferation, migration and angiogenesis, and oxidative stress response (Verkman, 2012; Pelagalli et al., 2016; Rodrigues et al., 2016). This suggests that their role may go far beyond the simple facilitation of membrane permeability. Indeed, over the years the importance of AQPs in health and disease has gained the attention of several research groups around the world; there is now compelling evidence that aquaporins are drug targets with potential broad application (Soveral et al., 2016). Modulators of AQPs expression or function with high selectivity and low side-toxicity are anticipated to have high value for the treatment of AQP-related disorders such as edema, brain injury, glaucoma, nephrogenic diabetes insipidus, salivary and lacrimal gland dysfunction, cancer and obesity, among others (Verkman et al., 2014; Soveral et al., 2016).

Although several potential AQP modulators have been reported and patented for use in diagnostic and therapeutics (Beitz et al., 2015; Soveral and Casini, 2017), their lack of selectivity and toxic side effects has hampered application in clinical trials. In addition, the protein structural conformation with channel pore access restrictions renders the molecule difficult to target and has slowed the progress of AQP drug discovery (Verkman et al., 2014; Madeira et al., 2016).

The recent recognition of AQP targeting by microRNAs (miRNAs) has opened new avenues for drug development. Here, we summarize updated information on the role of miRNAs in AQP-selective regulation and discuss their usefulness to tailor specific AQP-based therapeutics.

OVERVIEW OF miRNA BIOGENESIS AND FUNCTION

miRNAs are small, single-stranded non-coding RNAs with important functions in the post-transcriptional control of gene expression (Ha and Kim, 2014; Christopher et al., 2016; Vishnoi and Rani, 2017). In humans, miRNA biogenesis follows a multi-step process depicted in **Figure 1**. miRNAs are firstly transcribed in the nucleus by RNA polymerase II (Pol II) as long primary transcripts (pri-miRNAs), exhibiting a double-stranded hairpin loop structure (Ha and Kim, 2014). This stem loop is then cropped by nuclear RNase III Drosha to release a small hairpin-shaped RNA of ~65 nucleotides in length (pre-miRNA). Next, the pre-miRNA is exported to the cytoplasm through a nuclear pore complex comprising protein exportin 5 and further processed by RNase III endonuclease DICER near the terminal loop, liberating a small ~22 nucleotides in length RNA duplex. This duplex is then loaded into the miRNA-induced silencing complex (miRISC), unwounded, and the mature miRNA transferred to Argonaute (AGO) proteins within the complex. Following its assembly in the miRISC, the miRNA will target one or multiple mRNAs, leading to translational repression or, in particular cases, to mRNA degradation (Pereira et al., 2013; Ha and Kim, 2014; Vishnoi and Rani, 2017). Of note, miRNAs may also act as transcriptional or splicing regulators, within the nucleus (Hwang et al., 2007), and be involved in genetic exchange with adjacent cells, through exosomes (Valadi et al., 2007). Approximately 60% of protein-coding genes are influenced by miRNAs (Friedman et al., 2009) that play crucial roles in several biological processes, including control of cell cycle and differentiation, proliferation and metabolism. As such, miRNA deregulation is being increasingly associated with several human pathologies.

miRNAs might embody prospective therapeutic targets. We have recently shown that miR-21 is systematically increased in animal models and in human patients with steatohepatitis, thus contributing for disease pathogenesis. In contrast, miR-21 abrogation significantly improved steatosis, inflammation and fibrosis, as well as overall lipid and cholesterol metabolism (Rodrigues et al., 2017). Other studies have similarly shown that miRNA functional manipulation *in vivo* can impact on metabolic phenotypes and even reverse the course of insulin resistance and diabetes (Sethupathy, 2016). These results suggest that miRNA-based therapies may become a viable strategy for treating a broad range of disorders such as cancer and cardiovascular disease, among others (van Rooij and Kauppinen, 2014; Adams et al., 2017). Further, in oncology the aim is to downregulate or block the function of oncogenic miRNAs and/or upregulate expression of tumor suppressor miRNAs, for which different miRNA-targeting strategies have been proposed (as reviewed in Ling et al., 2013; Li and Rana, 2014; Robb et al., 2017). Replacement of tumor suppressor miRNAs typically involves the introduction of synthetic miRNA mimics or miRNA expression vectors. In this regard, a synthetic miRNA mimic based on the sequence of the miR-15/16 family is being evaluated in a clinical trial to treat patients with malignant pleural mesothelioma and advanced non-small cell lung cancer (van Zandwijk et al., 2017). As for inhibition of oncogenic miRNAs overexpressed in cancer, the top approaches being investigated include expression vectors (miRNA sponges), small-molecule inhibitors and antisense oligonucleotides (ASOs or antagomiRs) (Robb et al., 2017). Miravirsen (Santaris Pharma A/S) is a typical example of the later, inhibiting miR-122 function in the liver that is essential for the replication of the hepatitis C virus (HCV). A Phase II clinical trial showed that miravirsen is able to reduce HCV RNA levels in patients (Janssen et al., 2013).

In parallel with therapeutic targeting, circulating miRNA patterns are associated with metabolic, neurodegenerative and infectious pathologies (Keller et al., 2015; Mirra et al., 2015, 2018; Verma et al., 2016), making miRNAs attractive disease biomarkers and allowing the prospective implementation of personalized therapies (Mirra et al., 2018). Nonetheless, the use of miRNAs as either therapeutic targets or disease biomarkers still requires extensive optimization and validation.

AQUAPORIN TARGETING BY miRNAS

The discovery of miRNAs as endogenous modulators of AQPs offers a potential therapeutic approach for the regulation AQP-related disorders. Below, we address the current knowledge of miRNA interaction with AQP isoforms and the potential advantage for AQP-related pathologies (**Table 1**).

AQPs are specialized water and/or glycerol channels expressed in various tissues including the kidney, lung, gastrointestinal tract, brain, adipose tissue and liver (Verkman, 2012) and are implicated in water imbalance disorders, such as edema.

AQP1 and AQP4 are associated with cerebral edema (Griesdale and Honey, 2004; Zador et al., 2007), and their modulation may improve the outcome of cerebral disorders such as cytotoxic and vasogenic edema, stroke and traumatic brain injury (Papadopoulos and Verkman, 2007; Zador et al., 2007). Interestingly, miRNA deregulation has also been reported in cerebral ischemia (Koutsis et al., 2013; Ouyang et al., 2013; Di et al., 2014), a condition that can induce cerebral edema (Marmarou, 2007). miR-320a was reported to inhibit *AQP1* and *AQP4* gene expression both *in vitro* and *in vivo* in a cerebral ischemia rat model (Sepramaniam et al., 2010), whereas anti-miR-320a upregulated *AQP1* and *AQP4* expression with

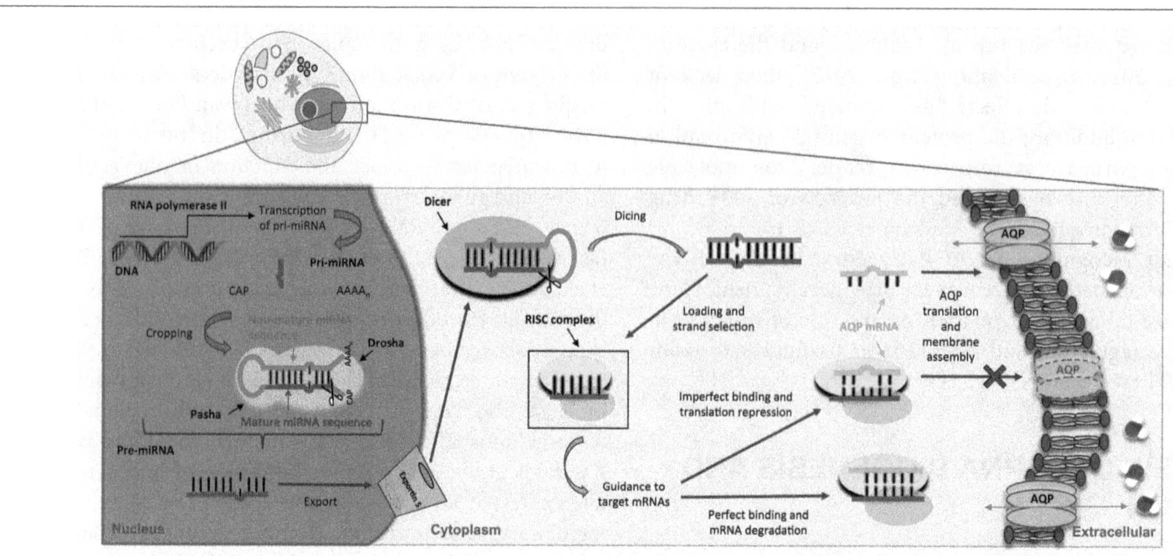

FIGURE 1 | miRNA biogenesis and mode of action. miRNA biogenesis embodies a multistep process catalyzed by specific RNA polymerases. miRNAs are initially transcribed as a long, capped and polyadenylated pri-miRNA, cropped by the Drosha complex into a hairpin pre-miRNA. Following translocation to the cytoplasm by Exportin-5, the pre-miRNA is further processed by the Dicer complex, generating a ~22-nucleotide mature miRNA–miRNA duplex. The guide strand is then selected by the Argonaute protein and integrated into an RNA-induced silencing complex (RISC) to form the miRNA–RISC. This will act on target mRNAs, including aquaporin (AQP) mRNAs, by binding to the 3′-UTR and leading to translational inhibition or mRNA degradation (see text for more details).

consequent reduction of infarct volume (Sepramaniam et al., 2010). The inhibitory effect of miR-320a on *AQP4* expression was also confirmed in astrocyte primary cultures from brain tissue of epileptic rats (Song et al., 2015), a condition that may induce cytotoxic cerebral edema. In addition, in a rat model of spinal cord edema, downregulation of *AQP1* at the blood–spinal cord barrier by miR-320a showed to positively affect spinal cord edema after ischemia reperfusion injury (Li et al., 2016). These findings suggest that miR-320a can be used as modulator of AQP1 and AQP4 in cerebral and spinal cord edema.

Further studies identified miR-130a as a transcriptional repressor of *AQP4* M1 isoform in human astrocytes (Sepramaniam et al., 2012). This transcript shows higher expression and function in the human brain under ischemic conditions compared to *AQP4* M23 (Hirt et al., 2009). Modulation of miR-130a and subsequent influence on *AQP4* M1 gene and protein expression may be used to reduce cerebral infarct and promote ischemic recovery (Sepramaniam et al., 2012). Additionally, *AQP4* down-regulation by miR-145 (Zheng et al., 2017a), miR-130b (Zheng et al., 2017b) and miR-29b (Wang et al., 2015) revealed the protecting role of these miRNAs against ischemic stroke. A recent study demonstrated that *AQP4* silencing in rat astrocyte primary cultures was associated with an increase of miR-224 and miR-19a expression, and this could be a molecular mechanism responsible for decreased astrocyte connectivity and water mobility in the brain (Jullienne et al., 2018).

AQP1 is also expressed in the lung alveolar epithelia and plays an important role in lung fluid transport and alveolar fluid clearance (King et al., 1996). Increased alveolar capillary membrane permeability, apoptosis of alveolar epithelial cells, inflammation and edema are characteristics of acute lung injury. In a mouse model of lipopolysaccharide-induced acute lung injury, miR-126-5p was down-regulated while AQP1 and epithelial sodium channel (ENaC) protein expression was reduced in alveolar type II cells (Tang et al., 2016). AQP1 and ENaC reduction was attenuated when miR-126-5p was overexpressed, suggesting that miR-126-5p may ameliorate dysfunction of alveolar fluid clearance by maintaining the activity of both AQP1 and ENaC. An opposite effect was promoted by miR-144-3p in acute lung injury mice and in a lung epithelial carcinoma cell line, where AQP1 mRNA and protein expression were both decreased when miR-144-3p was overexpressed, reducing lung epithelial cell apoptosis (Li et al., 2018).

AQP1 plays an important role in cell migration, angiogenesis, wound healing and tumor growth (Saadoun et al., 2002a; Tomita et al., 2017). It is highly expressed in cancer tissues and often associated with worse prognosis (Papadopoulos and Saadoun, 2015). miR-320 was shown to negatively regulate AQP1 expression and to reduce cell proliferation, migration, and invasion of breast cancer cells (Luo et al., 2018). The role of AQP1 in angiogenesis, fibrosis and portal hypertension in cirrhotic mice has been investigated in AQP1 knockout mice, which showed reduced angiogenesis and fibrosis. The osmotically sensitive miR-666 and miR-708 are decreased in cirrhosis and were found to regulate AQP1 expression, suggesting its modulation as a therapeutic strategy in chronic liver disease (Huebert et al., 2011).

AQP2 is expressed in kidney collecting duct epithelial cells where the high transepithelial water permeability accounts for fluid retention and urine concentration. Water reabsorption via

TABLE 1 | Interaction of different miRNAs with AQPs in several pathophysiological conditions.

Gene	miRNA	Tissue	Disease/condition	References
AQP1	29a	Colon	IBS	Chao et al., 2017
	126-5p	Lung	Acute lung injury	Tang et al., 2016
	144-3p	Lung	Acute lung injury	Li et al., 2018
	320a	Brain	Cerebral ischemia	Sepramaniam et al., 2010
		Spinal cord	Spinal cord edema	Li et al., 2016
	320	Breast	Breast cancer	Luo et al., 2018
	666	Liver	Cirrhosis	Huebert et al., 2011
	708	Liver	Cirrhosis	Huebert et al., 2011
AQP2	32	Kidney	Water reabsorption	Kim et al., 2015
	137	Kidney	Water reabsorption	Kim et al., 2015; Ranieri et al., 2018
AQP3	1	Epidermis	Wound healing	Banerjee and Sen, 2015
	29a	Colon	IBS	Chao et al., 2017
	124	Liver	HCC	Chen et al., 2018
	185-5p	Epidermis	SCC	Ratovitski, 2013
	874	Stomach	GC	Jiang et al., 2014
		Intestine	Intestinal ischemic injury	Zhi et al., 2014
		Pancreas	PDAC	Huang et al., 2017
AQP4	19a	Brain	Astrocyte connectivity	Jullienne et al., 2018
	29b	Brain	Cerebral ischemia	Wang et al., 2015
	130a	Brain	Cerebral ischemia	Sepramaniam et al., 2012
		Brain	AD	Zhang et al., 2017
	130b	Brain	Cerebral ischemia	Zheng et al., 2017b
	145	Brain	Cerebral ischemia	Zheng et al., 2017a
	203	Lung	Asthma	Jardim et al., 2012
	224	Brain	Astrocyte connectivity	Jullienne et al., 2018
	320a	Brain	Cerebral ischemia	Sepramaniam et al., 2010
		Brain	Epilepsy	Song et al., 2015
		Brain	Glioma	Xiong et al., 2018
AQP5	21	Gallbladder	Gallbladder carcinoma	Sekine et al., 2013
	96	Lung	Sepsis	Zhang et al., 2014; Rump and Adamzik, 2018
	330	Lung	Sepsis	Zhang et al., 2014; Rump and Adamzik, 2018
AQP8	16	Colon	Ulcerative colitis	Min et al., 2013
	29a	Colon	IBS	Chao et al., 2017
	195	Colon	Ulcerative colitis	Min et al., 2013
	330	Colon	Ulcerative colitis	Min et al., 2013
	424	Colon	Ulcerative colitis	Min et al., 2013
	612	Colon	Ulcerative colitis	Min et al., 2013
AQP9	22	Liver	Diabetes	Karolina et al., 2014
	23a	Liver	Diabetes	Karolina et al., 2014

AD, Alzheimer's disease; HCC, hepatocellular carcinoma; IBS, irritable bowel syndrome; GC, gastric cancer; PDAC, pancreatic ductal adenocarcinoma; SCC, squamous cell carcinoma.

AQP2 is controlled by vasopressin, which triggers AQP2 trafficking to the apical plasma membrane (short-term regulation) or increases transcription of *AQP2* gene (long-term regulation) (Nielsen et al., 2000). Two AQP2-targeting miRNAs, miR-32 and miR-137, were reported to decrease *AQP2* expression in kidney collecting duct cells independently of vasopressin regulation (Kim et al., 2015). *AQP2* targeting by miR-137 has recently been correlated with impaired response to vasopressin and reduction of urine concentration via the calcium-sensing receptor (CaSR). Once activated by high external calcium, CaSR promotes the synthesis of miRNA-137 and increases AQP2 ubiquitination and proteasomal degradation resulting in reduced AQP2 mRNA translation (Ranieri et al., 2018).

AQP3 is expressed in epidermal keratinocytes acting as a skin-hydration protein due to its ability to increase glycerol cellular content (Hara and Verkman, 2003). However, AQP3 is aberrantly expressed in different tumors (Papadopoulos and Saadoun, 2015) and its suppression has been proposed as a potential tool to reduce epidermal cell migration, proliferation and tumorigenicity (Hara-Chikuma and Verkman, 2008). AQP3-targeting by miRNAs resulted in decreased cell differentiation in different cancers, such as in squamous cell carcinoma by miR-185-5p (Ratovitski, 2013), gastric adenocarcinoma (Jiang et al., 2014) and pancreatic ductal adenocarcinoma (Huang et al., 2017) by miR-874, and hepatocellular carcinoma by miR-124 (Chen et al., 2018). In addition, miR-1 was proposed to indirectly target AQP3 impairing keratinocyte migration (Banerjee and Sen, 2015).

AQP3 has also an established role in transepithelial water transport in the colon, along with AQP1 and AQP8 (Laforenza, 2012; Zhao et al., 2016). Altered water secretion or absorption in the colon is linked to gut disorders such as irritable bowel syndrome (IBS), where increased intestinal permeability due to disruption of intestinal tight junctions contributes to diarrhea and abdominal pain. It has been reported that *AQP3* silencing leads to impairment of intestinal barrier integrity possibly by increasing paracellular permeability via an opening of the tight junction complex (Zhang et al., 2011) where miR-874 is involved through AQP3 targeting (Zhi et al., 2014; Su et al., 2016). Analysis of intestinal tissue samples from patients with IBS revealed that miR-29 reduces the expression of critical signaling molecules involved in the regulation of intestinal permeability (Zhou et al., 2015). The finding that AQP1, AQP3 and AQP8 are down-regulated by miR-29a in rat colon tissues, and increased by anti-miR-29a (Chao et al., 2017) unveils a potential tool to restore intestinal permeability via miR-29 blockage and AQP up-regulation.

AQP4 is mainly expressed in the brain with a polarized distribution in the perivascular endfeet of astrocytes. There is strong evidence that AQP4 mislocalization contributes to the excessive accumulation of amyloid-β in brain found in Alzheimer's disease (AD) (Yang et al., 2012). In a recent study, miR-130a restored AQP4 polarity by repressing the transcriptional activity of *AQP4* M1 decreasing the *AQP4* M1/M23 ratio (Zhang et al., 2017), thus protecting against AD. In addition to normal astrocytes, AQP4 is also expressed in human astrocytomas where the level of expression correlates with tumor aggressiveness (Saadoun et al., 2002b; Verkman et al., 2014). In glioma cells, miR-320a overexpression down-regulates AQP4 and diminishes cell invasion and migration, suggesting it could be used as a therapeutic target to suppress the aggressive capacity of this tumor (Xiong et al., 2018). Interestingly, AQP4 was found to be up-regulated in bronchial epithelial cells from asthmatic donors, following down-regulation of miR-203, together with pro-inflammatory genes (Jardim et al., 2012). The role of AQP4 in asthma is not clear, but since the progression of asthma usually includes edema, a contribution to fluid clearance cannot be ruled out.

AQP5 is a selective water channel important for saliva production and airway fluid clearance (Song and Verkman, 2001; Delporte et al., 2016). In the lung of rats after LPS-induced sepsis, decreased AQP5 gene and protein expression correlates with up-regulation of miR-96 and miR-330 and establishment of pulmonary edema (Zhang et al., 2014). AQP5 is also involved in cell proliferation, migration and invasion (Papadopoulos and Saadoun, 2015; Direito et al., 2016). AQP5 up-regulation in different cancer tissues together with markers of cancer progression suggests its involvement in cancer signaling pathways and highlights its potential as promising target for cancer therapy (Direito et al., 2016, 2017). *AQP5* expression in gallbladder carcinoma was regulated by miR-21 and correlated with early-stage tumor progression with favorable prognosis (Sekine et al., 2013), suggesting novel potential drug targets for this malignancy.

AQP8 is expressed in the epithelial cells of the intestine (Laforenza, 2012). In colon samples of ulcerative colitis patients, AQP8 mRNA and protein were found three-fold decreased. A search for candidate target miRNAs revealed miR-16, miR-195, miR-424, miR-612, and miR-330 as putative down-regulators of AQP8 expression (Min et al., 2013).

AQP7 and AQP9 transport glycerol in addition to water (aquaglyceroporins) and are involved in fat metabolism in the adipose and liver tissues (Hibuse et al., 2006; Madeira et al., 2015). In fasting conditions, when triglyceride lipolysis occurs, AQP7 facilitates glycerol efflux from adipose tissue into the circulation, which is taken up in the liver via AQP9 to be used for gluconeogenesis (Rodriguez et al., 2011). AQP7 and AQP9 coordinated function is crucial for energy homeostasis and deregulation has been implicated in obesity and diabetes (Rodriguez et al., 2014; da Silva and Soveral, 2017). Selective modulation of AQP7 and AQP9 may constitute a promising approach for controlling obesity and metabolic-related disorders (da Silva et al., 2018). Among the candidate miRNA regulators of adipogenesis and gluconeogenesis, miR-22 and miR-23a showed to reduce *AQP9* expression in liver cells, suggesting a potential application for glycaemia control in diabetic patients (Karolina et al., 2014).

FINAL REMARKS

The wide distribution of the various AQP-isoforms in mammalian tissues and their implication in a broad range of pathophysiological conditions makes AQPs exciting drug targets for novel therapies. Yet, with the exception of a few small molecules, no modulators of AQPs are available for *in vivo* use (Soveral and Casini, 2017). The recent discovery of miRNAs as endogenous regulators of AQP expression highlights an alternative and indirect approach to selectively target AQPs through modulation of signal transduction pathways. Moreover, since miRNA-targeting oligonucleotides can be chemically modified to enhance their pharmacokinetic/pharmacodynamic properties, targeting of mRNA expression by miRNAs typically leads to faster and longer-lasting responses comparing with protein inhibition by conventional targeted therapy. Further, the ability of miRNAs to target different genes simultaneously, as it is the case for miR-320a that targets both AQP1 and AQP4, or mi29a interacting with both AQP1 and AQP3, makes another compelling point toward the development of novel AQP-targeting therapies through modulation of miRNA function. However, there are still major challenges related with miRNA application, including *in vitro* validation of *in silico* predicted miRNAs, achievement of efficient up- or down-regulation, assessment of the therapeutic effect in the most appropriate cell model and evaluation of potential off-target effects that could impair their use. Indeed, due to very small sizes, the chance that an anti-miRNA will interact with an endogenous mRNA is rather high. In addition, a hairpin RNA structure generates different miRNAs from each strand, which may bind to different mRNAs and exhibit opposite functions. Nevertheless, the possibility of using miRNAs alone or in combined therapy with other chemical or biological drugs to modulate specific AQP proteins involved in disease provides new clues for AQP-based therapeutics.

AUTHOR CONTRIBUTIONS

GS and RC conception and design of research; IdS and AG prepared figures; AG and IdS drafted the manuscript; GS, RC, and CR edited and revised manuscript; AG, IdS, CR, RC, and GS approved final version of manuscript.

ACKNOWLEDGMENTS

This work was supported by Fundação para a Ciência e Tecnologia, Portugal (UID/DTP/04138/2013 to iMed.ULisboa).

REFERENCES

Adams, B. D., Parsons, C., Walker, L., Zhang, W. C., and Slack, F. J. (2017). Targeting noncoding RNAs in disease. *J. Clin. Invest.* 127, 761–771. doi: 10.1172/JCI84424

Banerjee, J., and Sen, C. K. (2015). microRNA and wound healing. *Adv. Exp. Med. Biol.* 888, 291–305. doi: 10.1007/978-3-319-22671-2_15

Beitz, E., Golldack, A., Rothert, M., and von Bulow, J. (2015). Challenges and achievements in the therapeutic modulation of aquaporin functionality. *Pharmacol. Ther.* 155, 22–35. doi: 10.1016/j.pharmthera.2015.08.002

Chao, G., Wang, Y., Zhang, S., Yang, W., Ni, Z., and Zheng, X. (2017). MicroRNA-29a increased the intestinal membrane permeability of colonic epithelial cells in irritable bowel syndrome rats. *Oncotarget* 8, 85828–85837. doi: 10.18632/oncotarget.20687

Chen, G., Shi, Y., Liu, M., and Sun, J. (2018). circHIPK3 regulates cell proliferation and migration by sponging miR-124 and regulating AQP3 expression in hepatocellular carcinoma. *Cell Death Dis.* 9:175. doi: 10.1038/s41419-017-0204-3

Christopher, A. F., Kaur, R. P., Kaur, G., Kaur, A., Gupta, V., and Bansal, P. (2016). MicroRNA therapeutics: discovering novel targets and developing specific therapy. *Perspect. Clin. Res.* 7, 68–74. doi: 10.4103/2229-3485.179431

da Silva, I. V., Rodrigues, J. S., Rebelo, I., Miranda, J. P. G., and Soveral, G. (2018). Revisiting the metabolic syndrome: the emerging role of aquaglyceroporins. *Cell. Mol. Life Sci.* 75, 1973–1988. doi: 10.1007/s00018-018-2781-4

da Silva, I. V., and Soveral, G. (2017). Aquaporins in Obesity. *Adv. Exp. Med. Biol.* 969, 227–238. doi: 10.1007/978-94-024-1057-0_15

Delporte, C., Bryla, A., and Perret, J. (2016). Aquaporins in salivary glands: from basic research to clinical applications. *Int. J. Mol. Sci.* 17:E166. doi: 10.3390/ijms17020166

Di, Y., Lei, Y., Yu, F., Changfeng, F., Song, W., and Xuming, M. (2014). MicroRNAs expression and function in cerebral ischemia reperfusion injury. *J. Mol. Neurosci.* 53, 242–250. doi: 10.1007/s12031-014-0293-8

Direito, I., Madeira, A., Brito, M. A., and Soveral, G. (2016). Aquaporin-5: from structure to function and dysfunction in cancer. *Cell. Mol. Life Sci.* 73, 1623–1640. doi: 10.1007/s00018-016-2142-0

Direito, I., Paulino, J., Vigia, E., Brito, M. A., and Soveral, G. (2017). Differential expression of aquaporin-3 and aquaporin-5 in pancreatic ductal adenocarcinoma. *J. Surg. Oncol.* 115, 980–996. doi: 10.1002/jso.24605

Friedman, R. C., Farh, K. K., Burge, C. B., and Bartel, D. P. (2009). Most mammalian mRNAs are conserved targets of microRNAs. *Genome Res.* 19, 92–105. doi: 10.1101/gr.082701.108

Griesdale, D. E., and Honey, C. R. (2004). Aquaporins and brain edema. *Surg. Neurol.* 61, 418–421. doi: 10.1016/j.surneu.2003.10.047

Ha, M., and Kim, V. N. (2014). Regulation of microRNA biogenesis. *Nat. Rev. Mol. Cell Biol.* 15, 509–524. doi: 10.1038/nrm3838

Hara, M., and Verkman, A. S. (2003). Glycerol replacement corrects defective skin hydration, elasticity, and barrier function in aquaporin-3-deficient mice. *Proc. Natl. Acad. Sci. U.S.A.* 100, 7360–7365. doi: 10.1073/pnas.1230416100.

Hara-Chikuma, M., and Verkman, A. S. (2008). Prevention of skin tumorigenesis and impairment of epidermal cell proliferation by targeted aquaporin-3 gene disruption. *Mol. Cell. Biol.* 28, 326–332. doi: 10.1128/MCB.01482-07

Hibuse, T., Maeda, N., Nagasawa, A., and Funahashi, T. (2006). Aquaporins and glycerol metabolism. *Biochim. Biophys. Acta* 1758, 1004–1011. doi: 10.1016/j.bbamem.2006.01.008.

Hirt, L., Ternon, B., Price, M., Mastour, N., Brunet, J. F., and Badaut, J. (2009). Protective role of early aquaporin 4 induction against postischemic edema formation. *J. Cereb. Blood Flow Metab.* 29, 423–433. doi: 10.1038/jcbfm.2008.133

Huang, X., Huang, L., and Shao, M. (2017). Aquaporin 3 facilitates tumor growth in pancreatic cancer by modulating mTOR signaling. *Biochem. Biophys. Res. Commun.* 486, 1097–1102. doi: 10.1016/j.bbrc.2017.03.168.

Huebert, R. C., Jagavelu, K., Hendrickson, H. I., Vasdev, M. M., Arab, J. P., Splinter, P. L., et al. (2011). Aquaporin-1 promotes angiogenesis, fibrosis, and portal hypertension through mechanisms dependent on osmotically sensitive microRNAs. *Am. J. Pathol.* 179, 1851–1860. doi: 10.1016/j.ajpath.2011.06.045

Hwang, H. W., Wentzel, E. A., and Mendell, J. T. (2007). A hexanucleotide element directs microRNA nuclear import. *Science* 315, 97–100. doi: 10.1126/science.1136235

Janssen, H. L., Reesink, H. W., Lawitz, E. J., Zeuzem, S., Rodriguez-Torres, M., Patel, K., et al. (2013). Treatment of HCV infection by targeting microRNA. *N. Engl. J. Med.* 368, 1685–1694. doi: 10.1056/NEJMoa1209026

Jardim, M. J., Dailey, L., Silbajoris, R., and Diaz-Sanchez, D. (2012). Distinct microRNA expression in human airway cells of asthmatic donors identifies a novel asthma-associated gene. *Am. J. Respir. Cell Mol. Biol.* 47, 536–542. doi: 10.1165/rcmb.2011-0160OC

Jiang, B., Li, Z., Zhang, W., Wang, H., Zhi, X., Feng, J., et al. (2014). miR-874 Inhibits cell proliferation, migration and invasion through targeting aquaporin-3 in gastric cancer. *J. Gastroenterol.* 49, 1011–1025. doi: 10.1007/s00535-013-0851-9

Jullienne, A., Fukuda, A. M., Ichkova, A., Nishiyama, N., Aussudre, J., Obenaus, A., et al. (2018). Modulating the water channel AQP4 alters miRNA expression, astrocyte connectivity and water diffusion in the rodent brain. *Sci. Rep.* 8:4186. doi: 10.1038/s41598-018-22268-y

Karolina, D. S., Armugam, A., Sepramaniam, S., Pek, S. L. T., Wong, M. T. K., Lim, S. C., et al. (2014). miR-22 and miR-23a control glycerol-dependent gluconeogenesis by regulating aquaporin 9 expression. *Metabolomics* S2:002. doi: 10.4172/2153-0769.S2-002

Keller, A., Leidinger, P., Meese, E., Haas, J., Backes, C., Rasche, L., et al. (2015). Next-generation sequencing identifies altered whole blood microRNAs in neuromyelitis optica spectrum disorder which may permit discrimination from multiple sclerosis. *J. Neuroinflammation* 12:196. doi: 10.1186/s12974-015-0418-1

Kim, J. E., Jung, H. J., Lee, Y. J., and Kwon, T. H. (2015). Vasopressin-regulated miRNAs and AQP2-targeting miRNAs in kidney collecting duct cells. *Am. J. Physiol. Renal Physiol.* 308, F749–764. doi: 10.1152/ajprenal.00334.2014

King, L. S., Nielsen, S., and Agre, P. (1996). Aquaporin-1 water channel protein in lung: ontogeny, steroid-induced expression, and distribution in rat. *J. Clin. Invest.* 97, 2183–2191. doi: 10.1172/JCI118659

Koutsis, G., Siasos, G., and Spengos, K. (2013). The emerging role of microRNA in stroke. *Curr. Top. Med. Chem.* 13, 1573–1588. doi: 10.2174/15680266113139990106

Laforenza, U. (2012). Water channel proteins in the gastrointestinal tract. *Mol. Aspects Med.* 33, 642–650. doi: 10.1016/j.mam.2012.03.001

Li, H., Shi, H., Gao, M., Ma, N., and Sun, R. (2018). Long non-coding RNA CASC2 improved acute lung injury by regulating miR-144-3p/AQP1 axis to reduce lung epithelial cell apoptosis. *Cell Biosci.* 8:15. doi: 10.1186/s13578-018-0205-7

Li, X. Q., Fang, B., Tan, W. F., Wang, Z. L., Sun, X. J., Zhang, Z. L., et al. (2016). miR-320a affects spinal cord edema through negatively regulating aquaporin-1 of blood-spinal cord barrier during bimodal stage after ischemia reperfusion injury in rats. *BMC Neurosci.* 17:10. doi: 10.1186/s12868-016-0243-1

Li, Z., and Rana, T. M. (2014). Therapeutic targeting of microRNAs: current status and future challenges. *Nat. Rev. Drug Discov.* 13, 622–638. doi: 10.1038/nrd4359

Ling, H., Fabbri, M., and Calin, G. A. (2013). MicroRNAs and other non-coding RNAs as targets for anticancer drug development. *Nat. Rev. Drug Discov.* 12, 847–865. doi: 10.1038/nrd4140

Luo, L., Yang, R., Zhao, S., Chen, Y., Hong, S., Wang, K., et al. (2018). Decreased miR-320 expression is associated with breast cancer progression, cell migration, and invasiveness via targeting Aquaporin 1. *Acta Biochim. Biophys. Sin.* 50, 473–480. doi: 10.1093/abbs/gmy023

Madeira, A., Moura, T. F., and Soveral, G. (2015). Aquaglyceroporins: implications in adipose biology and obesity. *Cell. Mol. Life Sci.* 72, 759–771. doi: 10.1007/s00018-014-1773-2

Madeira, A., Moura, T. F., and Soveral, G. (2016). Detecting aquaporin function and regulation. *Front Chem.* 4:3. doi: 10.3389/fchem.2016.00003

Marmarou, A. (2007). A review of progress in understanding the pathophysiology and treatment of brain edema. *Neurosurg. Focus* 22:E1. doi: 10.3171/foc.2007.22.5.2

Min, M., Peng, L. H., Sun, G., Guo, M. Z., Qiu, Z. W., and Yang, Y. S. (2013). Aquaporin 8 expression is reduced and regulated by microRNAs in patients with ulcerative colitis. *Chin. Med. J.* 126, 1532–1537. doi: 10.3760/cma.j.issn.0366-6999.20122989

Mirra, P., Nigro, C., Prevenzano, I., Leone, A., Raciti, G. A., Formisano, P., et al. (2018). The destiny of glucose from a microRNA perspective. *Front. Endocrinol.* 9:46. doi: 10.3389/fendo.2018.00046

Mirra, P., Raciti, G. A., Nigro, C., Fiory, F., D'Esposito, V., Formisano, P., et al. (2015). Circulating miRNAs as intercellular messengers, potential biomarkers and therapeutic targets for Type 2 diabetes. *Epigenomics* 7, 653–667. doi: 10.2217/epi.15.18

Nielsen, S., Kwon, T. H., Frokiaer, J., and Knepper, M. A. (2000). Key roles of renal aquaporins in water balance and water-balance disorders. *News Physiol. Sci.* 15, 136–143. doi: 10.1152/physiologyonline.2000.15.3.136

Ouyang, Y. B., Stary, C. M., Yang, G. Y., and Giffard, R. (2013). microRNAs: innovative targets for cerebral ischemia and stroke. *Curr. Drug Targets* 14, 90–101. doi: 10.2174/1389450111314010010

Papadopoulos, M. C., and Saadoun, S. (2015). Key roles of aquaporins in tumor biology. *Biochim. Biophys. Acta* 1848(10 Pt B), 2576–2583. doi: 10.1016/j.bbamem.2014.09.001

Papadopoulos, M. C., and Verkman, A. S. (2007). Aquaporin-4 and brain edema. *Pediatr. Nephrol.* 22, 778–784. doi: 10.1007/s00467-006-0411-0

Pelagalli, A., Squillacioti, C., Mirabella, N., and Meli, R. (2016). Aquaporins in health and disease: an overview focusing on the gut of different species. *Int. J. Mol. Sci.* 17:E1213. doi: 10.3390/ijms17081213

Pereira, D. M., Rodrigues, P. M., Borralho, P. M., and Rodrigues, C. M. (2013). Delivering the promise of miRNA cancer therapeutics. *Drug Discov. Today* 18, 282–289. doi: 10.1016/j.drudis.2012.10.002

Ranieri, M., Zahedi, K., Tamma, G., Centrone, M., Di Mise, A., Soleimani, M., et al. (2018). CaSR signaling down-regulates AQP2 expression via a novel microRNA pathway in pendrin and NaCl cotransporter knockout mice. *FASEB J.* 32, 2148–2159. doi: 10.1096/fj.201700412RR

Ratovitski, E. A. (2013). Phospho-DeltaNp63alpha regulates AQP3, ALOX12B, CASP14 and CLDN1 expression through transcription and microRNA modulation. *FEBS Lett.* 587, 3581–3586. doi: 10.1016/j.febslet.2013.09.023

Robb, T., Reid, G., and Blenkiron, C. (2017). Exploiting microRNAs as cancer therapeutics. *Target. Oncol.* 12, 163–178. doi: 10.1007/s11523-017-0476-7

Rodrigues, C., Mosca, A. F., Martins, A. P., Nobre, T., Prista, C., Antunes, F., et al. (2016). Rat aquaporin-5 Is pH-gated induced by phosphorylation and is implicated in oxidative stress. *Int. J. Mol. Sci.* 17:2090. doi: 10.3390/ijms17122090

Rodrigues, P. M., Afonso, M. B., Simao, A. L., Carvalho, C. C., Trindade, A., Duarte, A., et al. (2017). miR-21 ablation and obeticholic acid ameliorate nonalcoholic steatohepatitis in mice. *Cell Death Dis.* 8:e2748. doi: 10.1038/cddis.2017.172

Rodriguez, A., Catalan, V., Gomez-Ambrosi, J., Garcia-Navarro, S., Rotellar, F., Valenti, V., et al. (2011). Insulin- and leptin-mediated control of aquaglyceroporins in human adipocytes and hepatocytes is mediated via the PI3K/Akt/mTOR signaling cascade. *J. Clin. Endocrinol. Metab.* 96, E586–E597. doi: 10.1210/jc.2010-1408

Rodriguez, A., Gena, P., Mendez-Gimenez, L., Rosito, A., Valenti, V., Rotellar, F., et al. (2014). Reduced hepatic aquaporin-9 and glycerol permeability are related to insulin resistance in non-alcoholic fatty liver disease. *Int. J. Obes.* 38, 1213–1220. doi: 10.1038/ijo.2013.234

Rump, K., and Adamzik, M. (2018). Function of aquaporins in sepsis: a systematic review. *Cell Biosci.* 8:10. doi: 10.1186/s13578-018-0211-9

Saadoun, S., Papadopoulos, M. C., Davies, D. C., Bell, B. A., and Krishna, S. (2002a). Increased aquaporin 1 water channel expression in human brain tumours. *Br. J. Cancer* 87, 621–623. doi: 10.1038/sj.bjc.6600512

Saadoun, S., Papadopoulos, M. C., Davies, D. C., Krishna, S., and Bell, B. A. (2002b). Aquaporin-4 expression is increased in oedematous human brain tumours. *J. Neurol. Neurosurg. Psychiatry* 72, 262–265. doi: 10.1136/jnnp.72.2.262

Sekine, S., Shimada, Y., Nagata, T., Sawada, S., Yoshioka, I., Matsui, K., et al. (2013). Role of aquaporin-5 in gallbladder carcinoma. *Eur. Surg. Res.* 51, 108–117. doi: 10.1159/000355675

Sepramaniam, S., Armugam, A., Lim, K. Y., Karolina, D. S., Swaminathan, P., Tan, J. R., et al. (2010). MicroRNA 320a functions as a novel endogenous modulator of aquaporins 1 and 4 as well as a potential therapeutic target in cerebral ischemia. *J. Biol. Chem.* 285, 29223–29230. doi: 10.1074/jbc.M110.144576

Sepramaniam, S., Ying, L. K., Armugam, A., Wintour, E. M., and Jeyaseelan, K. (2012). MicroRNA-130a represses transcriptional activity of aquaporin 4 M1 promoter. *J. Biol. Chem.* 287, 12006–12015. doi: 10.1074/jbc.M111.280701

Sethupathy, P. (2016). The promise and challenge of therapeutic microrna silencing in diabetes and metabolic diseases. *Curr. Diab. Rep.* 16:52. doi: 10.1007/s11892-016-0745-3

Song, Y. C., Li, W. J., and Li, L. Z. (2015). Regulatory effect of miRNA 320a on expression of aquaporin 4 in brain tissue of epileptic rats. *Asian Pac. J. Trop. Med.* 8, 807–812. doi: 10.1016/j.apjtm.2015.09.006

Song, Y., and Verkman, A. S. (2001). Aquaporin-5 dependent fluid secretion in airway submucosal glands. *J. Biol. Chem.* 276, 41288–41292. doi: 10.1074/jbc.M107257200

Soveral, G., and Casini, A. (2017). Aquaporin modulators: a patent review (2010-2015). *Expert Opin. Ther. Pat.* 27, 49–62. doi: 10.1080/13543776.2017.1236085

Soveral, G., Nielsen, S., and Casini, A. (2016). *Aquaporins in Health and Disease: New Molecular Targets for Drug Discovery.* Boca Raton, FL: CRC Press; Taylor & Francis Group.

Su, Z., Zhi, X., Zhang, Q., Yang, L., Xu, H., and Xu, Z. (2016). LncRNA H19 functions as a competing endogenous RNA to regulate AQP3 expression by sponging miR-874 in the intestinal barrier. *FEBS Lett.* 590, 1354–1364. doi: 10.1002/1873-3468.12171

Tang, R., Pei, L., Bai, T., and Wang, J. (2016). Down-regulation of microRNA-126-5p contributes to overexpression of VEGFA in lipopolysaccharide-induced acute lung injury. *Biotechnol. Lett.* 38, 1277–1284. doi: 10.1007/s10529-016-2107-2

Tomita, Y., Dorward, H., Yool, A. J., Smith, E., Townsend, A. R., Price, T. J., et al. (2017). Role of aquaporin 1 signalling in cancer development and progression. *Int. J. Mol. Sci.* 18:299. doi: 10.3390/ijms18020299

Valadi, H., Ekstrom, K., Bossios, A., Sjostrand, M., Lee, J. J., and Lotvall, J. O. (2007). Exosome-mediated transfer of mRNAs and microRNAs is a novel mechanism of genetic exchange between cells. *Nat. Cell Biol.* 9, 654–659. doi: 10.1038/ncb1596

van Rooij, E., and Kauppinen, S. (2014). Development of microRNA therapeutics is coming of age. *EMBO Mol. Med.* 6, 851–864. doi: 10.15252/emmm.201100899

van Zandwijk, N., Pavlakis, N., Kao, S. C., Linton, A., Boyer, M. J., Clarke, S., et al. (2017). Safety and activity of microRNA-loaded minicells in patients with recurrent malignant pleural mesothelioma: a first-in-man, phase 1, open-label, dose-escalation study. *Lancet Oncol.* 18, 1386–1396. doi: 10.1016/S1470-204530621-6

Verkman, A. S. (2012). Aquaporins in clinical medicine. *Annu. Rev. Med.* 63, 303–316. doi: 10.1146/annurev-med-043010-193843

Verkman, A. S., Anderson, M. O., and Papadopoulos, M. C. (2014). Aquaporins: important but elusive drug targets. *Nat. Rev. Drug Discov.* 13, 259–277. doi: 10.1038/nrd4226

Verma, P., Pandey, R. K., Prajapati, P., and Prajapati, V. K. (2016). Circulating MicroRNAs: potential and emerging biomarkers for diagnosis of human infectious diseases. *Front. Microbiol.* 7:1274. doi: 10.3389/fmicb.2016.01274

Vishnoi, A., and Rani, S. (2017). MiRNA biogenesis and regulation of diseases: an overview. *Methods Mol. Biol.* 1509, 1–10. doi: 10.1007/978-1-4939-6524-3_1

Wang, Y., Huang, J., Ma, Y., Tang, G., Liu, Y., Chen, X., et al. (2015). MicroRNA-29b is a therapeutic target in cerebral ischemia associated with aquaporin 4. *J. Cereb. Blood Flow Metab.* 35, 1977–1984. doi: 10.1038/jcbfm.2015.156

Xiong, W., Ran, J., Jiang, R., Guo, P., Shi, X., Li, H., et al. (2018). miRNA-320a inhibits glioma cell invasion and migration by directly targeting aquaporin 4. *Oncol. Rep.* 39, 1939–1947. doi: 10.3892/or.2018.6274

Yang, W., Wu, Q., Yuan, C., Gao, J., Xiao, M., Gu, M., et al. (2012). Aquaporin-4 mediates astrocyte response to beta-amyloid. *Mol. Cell. Neurosci.* 49, 406–414. doi: 10.1016/j.mcn.2012.02.002

Zador, Z., Bloch, O., Yao, X., and Manley, G. T. (2007). Aquaporins: role in cerebral edema and brain water balance. *Prog. Brain Res.* 161, 185–194. doi: 10.1016/S0079-612361012-1

Zhang, J., Zhan, Z., Li, X., Xing, A., Jiang, C., Chen, Y., et al. (2017). Intermittent fasting protects against alzheimer's disease possible through restoring aquaporin-4 polarity. *Front. Mol. Neurosci.* 10:395. doi: 10.3389/fnmol.2017.00395

Zhang, W., Xu, Y., Chen, Z., Xu, Z., and Xu, H. (2011). Knockdown of aquaporin 3 is involved in intestinal barrier integrity impairment. *FEBS Lett.* 585, 3113–3119. doi: 10.1016/j.febslet.2011.08.045

Zhang, Y., Chen, M., Zhang, Y., Peng, P., Li, J., and Xin, X. (2014). miR-96 and miR-330 overexpressed and targeted AQP5 in lipopolysaccharide-induced rat lung damage of disseminated intravascular coagulation. *Blood Coagul. Fibrinolysis* 25, 731–737. doi: 10.1097/MBC.0000000000000133

Zhao, G. X., Dong, P. P., Peng, R., Li, J., Zhang, D. Y., Wang, J. Y., et al. (2016). Expression, localization and possible functions of aquaporins 3 and 8 in rat digestive system. *Biotech. Histochem.* 91, 269–276. doi: 10.3109/10520295.2016.1144079

Zheng, L., Cheng, W., Wang, X., Yang, Z., Zhou, X., and Pan, C. (2017a). Overexpression of MicroRNA-145 ameliorates astrocyte injury by targeting aquaporin 4 in cerebral ischemic stroke. *Biomed Res. Int.* 2017:9530951. doi: 10.1155/2017/9530951

Zheng, Y., Wang, L., Chen, M., Pei, A., Xie, L., and Zhu, S. (2017b). Upregulation of miR-130b protects against cerebral ischemic injury by targeting water channel protein aquaporin 4 (AQP4). *Am. J. Transl. Res.* 9, 3452–3461.

Zhi, X., Tao, J., Li, Z., Jiang, B., Feng, J., Yang, L., et al. (2014). MiR-874 promotes intestinal barrier dysfunction through targeting AQP3 following intestinal ischemic injury. *FEBS Lett.* 588, 757–763. doi: 10.1016/j.febslet.2014.01.022

Zhou, Q., Costinean, S., Croce, C. M., Brasier, A. R., Merwat, S., Larson, S. A., et al. (2015). MicroRNA 29 targets nuclear factor-kappaB-repressing factor and Claudin 1 to increase intestinal permeability. *Gastroenterology* 148, 158–169.e8. doi: 10.1053/j.gastro.2014.09.037

7

Pancreatic Aquaporin-7: A Novel Target for Anti-Diabetic Drugs?

Leire Méndez-Giménez[1,2], Silvia Ezquerro[1,2], Inês V. da Silva[3], Graça Soveral[3], Gema Frühbeck[1,2,4] and Amaia Rodríguez[1,2]*

[1] Metabolic Research Laboratory, University of Navarra, Pamplona, Spain, [2] CIBER Fisiopatología de la Obesidad y Nutrición, Instituto de Salud Carlos III, Madrid, Spain, [3] Faculty of Pharmacy, Research Institute for Medicines (iMed.ULisboa), Universidade de Lisboa, Lisboa, Portugal, [4] Department of Endocrinology and Nutrition, Clínica Universidad de Navarra, Pamplona, Spain

***Correspondence:**
Amaia Rodríguez
arodmur@unav.es

Aquaporins comprise a family of 13 members of water channels (AQP0-12) that facilitate a rapid transport of water across cell membranes. In some cases, these pores are also permeated by small solutes, particularly glycerol, urea or nitric oxide, among other solutes. Several aquaporins have been identified in the pancreas, an exocrine and endocrine organ that plays an essential role in the onset of insulin resistance and type 2 diabetes. The exocrine pancreas, which accounts for 90% of the total pancreas, secretes daily large volumes of a near-isotonic fluid containing digestive enzymes into the duodenum. AQP1, AQP5, and AQP8 contribute to fluid secretion especially from ductal cells, whereas AQP12 allows the proper maturation and exocytosis of secretory granules in acinar cells of the exocrine pancreas. The endocrine pancreas (10% of the total pancreatic cells) is composed by the islets of Langerhans, which are distributed in α, β, δ, ε, and pancreatic polypeptide (PP) cells that secrete glucagon, insulin, somatostatin, ghrelin and PP, respectively. AQP7, an aquaglyceroporin permeated by water and glycerol, is expressed in pancreatic β-cells and murine studies have confirmed its participation in insulin secretion, triacylglycerol synthesis and proliferation of these endocrine cells. In this regard, transgenic AQP7-knockout mice develop adult-onset obesity, hyperinsulinemia, increased intracellular triacylglycerol content and reduced β-cell mass in Langerhans islets. Moreover, we have recently reported that AQP7 upregulation in β-cells after bariatric surgery, an effective weight loss surgical procedure, contributes, in part, to the improvement of pancreatic steatosis and insulin secretion through the increase of intracytoplasmic glycerol in obese rats. Human studies remain scarce and controversial, with some rare cases of loss-of function mutations of the *AQP7* gene being associated with the onset of type 2 diabetes. The present Review is focused on the role of aquaporins in the physiology and pathophysiology of the pancreas, highlighting the role of pancreatic AQP7 as a novel player in the control of β-cell function and a potential anti-diabetic-drug.

Keywords: aquaporin, glycerol, pancreas, insulin signaling, obesity, type 2 diabetes, bariatric surgery

INTRODUCTION

The movement of water through the lipid bilayers of cell membranes is essential for homeostasis. Aquaporins (AQPs) are channel-forming integral membrane proteins of the major intrinsic protein (MIP) family that allow the water transport across the cell membranes (King et al., 2004; Soveral et al., 2017; Yang, 2017). The secondary structure of AQPs consists of six transmembrane α-helices and two highly conserved, hydrophobic asparagine-proline-alanine (NPA) consensus motifs (Jung et al., 1994). The three-dimensional structure of AQPs resembles an hourglass with the NPA motifs forming the aperture of a very tight water channel pore of ~2 Å in diameter. In the cellular membranes, AQPs exist as a tetrameric assembly of individually active subunits. Professor Peter Agre was awarded the 2003 Nobel Prize in Chemistry for the discovery and characterization of the first water channel protein AQP1 (Agre, 2009). To date, thirteen aquaporins have been discovered (AQP0-AQP12) in mammalian tissues, which are classified into three subgroups depending on their permeability and structure: orthodox aquaporins, aquaglyceroporins and superaquaporins (Verkman et al., 2014). Orthodox aquaporins (AQP0, 1, 2, 4, 5, 6, and 8) are considered pure water channels, whereas aquaglyceroporins (AQP3, 7, 9, and 10) are permeated by water and other small solutes, such as glycerol or urea (Oliva et al., 2010). Superaquaporins (AQP11 and 12) exhibit very low homology to the other groups of AQPs due to their unique asparagine-proline-cysteine (NPC) motifs (Soveral et al., 2017) and their subcellular localization on the membrane of intracellular organelles instead of the plasma membrane (Ishibashi, 2006; Calvanese et al., 2013).

The human *AQP7* gene, mapped to chromosome 9p13.3, was cloned from the adipose tissue in 1997 (originally named AQPap) (Ishibashi et al., 1997, 1998). The glycerol channel AQP7 plays a crucial role in the control of triacylglycerols (TG) accumulation and glucose homeostasis with *Aqp7*-KO mice exhibiting adult-onset obesity, impaired insulin secretion and insulin resistance (Maeda et al., 2004; Hara-Chikuma et al., 2005; Hibuse et al., 2005; Matsumura et al., 2007). AQP7 is markedly increased during adipocyte differentiation, because the *AQP7* gene promoter contains putative response elements for peroxisome proliferator-activated receptor α and γ (PPARα and PPARγ), the master transcription factor of adipogenesis (Kishida et al., 2001; Walker et al., 2007; Méndez-Giménez et al., 2015). In this sense, the administration of the PPARγ agonists rosiglitazone or pioglitazone, which are insulin-sensitizing drugs, to rodents has been shown to upregulate AQP7 expression in the adipose tissue (Kishida et al., 2001; Lee et al., 2005; Rodríguez et al., 2015b). Although AQP7 was considered the unique glycerol channel in human adipose tissue, AQP3, AQP5, AQP9, AQP10, and AQP11 also represent novel pathways for glycerol transport in human adipocytes (Frühbeck and Gómez-Ambrosi, 2001; Rodríguez et al., 2011b; Laforenza et al., 2013; Madeira et al., 2014b, 2015). In the basal state, perilipin-1 binds to AQP7 in the lipid droplets, thereby preventing localization of AQP7 to the plasma membrane where it can exert glycerol efflux activity (Hansen et al., 2016). In circumstances of negative energy balance, such as fasting or exercise, TG are hydrolyzed to glycerol and free fatty acids (FFA) by adipose triglyceride lipase (ATGL) as well as hormone-sensitive lipase (HSL) enzymes (Frühbeck et al., 2014; Méndez-Giménez, 2017). Both FFA and glycerol are released into the bloodstream and can be used as energy substrates in peripheral tissues. Several lipolytic stimuli, such as catecholamines, leptin, atrial natriuretic peptide, uroguanylin and guanylin, regulate the expression and translocation of aquaglyceroporins from the cytosolic fraction (AQP3) or the lipid droplets (AQP7) to the plasma membrane facilitating glycerol release from adipocytes (Kishida et al., 2000; Walker et al., 2007; Rodríguez et al., 2011b, 2015b, 2016). By contrast, lipogenic stimuli, such ghrelin and dexamethasone, downregulate the expression of AQP7 in adipocytes, which results in an increase in intracellular glycerol (Fasshauer et al., 2003; Rodríguez et al., 2009), a metabolite that induces changes in the conformation and enzymatic activity of glycerol kinase (GK), favoring the conversion of glycerol to glycerol-3-phosphate (Yeh et al., 2004). The consequent increase in glycerol-3-phosphate concentrations induces TG biosynthesis, leading to a progressive adipocyte hypertrophy (Hara-Chikuma et al., 2005). Noteworthy, the gene expression of the main lipogenic enzymes are downregulated in visceral adipose tissue of obese subjects (Ortega et al., 2010).

Circulating glycerol constitutes an important energy substrate during fasting with the liver being responsible for about 70–90% of whole-body glycerol metabolism (Reshef et al., 2003). AQP9 constitutes the main route for hepatocyte glycerol uptake (Jelen et al., 2011; Calamita et al., 2012), although the human liver also expresses the aquaglyceroporins AQP3, AQP7, and AQP10 (Rodríguez et al., 2014). AQP9 is mainly localized in the sinusoidal plasma membrane that faces the portal vein (Elkjaer et al., 2000; Nicchia et al., 2001; Gena et al., 2013; Rodríguez et al., 2014). In hepatocytes, glycerol is phosphorylated to glycerol-3-phosphate by GK, and glycerol-3-phosphate constitutes a precursor for hepatic gluconeogenesis as well as for the *de novo* TG synthesis (Rodríguez et al., 2014). The proportion of glycerol used for hepatic gluconeogenesis or lipogenesis mainly depends on the nutritional state (Kuriyama et al., 2002; Calamita et al., 2012), but a sexual dimorphism has been also observed in hepatocyte glycerol utilization (Nicchia et al., 2001; Lebeck et al., 2015; Rodríguez et al., 2015a). The close coordination between adipose and hepatic aquaglyceroporins is required for the control of whole-body glucose homeostasis as well as lipid accumulation in both rodents (Kuriyama et al., 2002; Rodríguez et al., 2015b) and humans (Catalán et al., 2008; Miranda et al., 2009; Rodríguez et al., 2011b).

The existence of several AQPs has been identified in the pancreas (**Table 1**), an exocrine and endocrine organ of the digestive system that plays an essential role in the onset of insulin resistance and type 2 diabetes (Delporte, 2014). Exocrine and endocrine cells account for 90 and 10%, respectively, of

Abbreviations: AQP, aquaporin; ATGL, adipose triglyceride lipase; DHAP, dihydroxyacetone phosphate; GK, glycerol kinase; GLP-1, glucagon-like peptide 1; GPD, glycerol-3-phosphate dehydrogenase; FFA, free fatty acids; HSL, hormone-sensitive lipase; NAFLD, non-alcoholic fatty liver disease; PPAR, peroxisome proliferator-activated receptor; TG, triacylglycerols.

TABLE 1 | Tissue distribution and biological function of pancreatic aquaporins.

Type	Exocrine/endocrine pancreas	Cellular location	Biological function	References
AQP0	Not detected (mice, rats and humans)	–	–	Isokpehi et al., 2009
AQP1	Exocrine pancreas (rat and humans)	Acinar cells, intercalated ducts and capillaries	Pancreatic fluid secretion	Koyama et al., 1997; Hurley et al., 2001; Ko et al., 2002; Burghardt et al., 2003
AQP2	Not detected (rats and humans)	–	–	Hurley et al., 2001; Isokpehi et al., 2009
AQP3	Exocrine pancreas (humans)	Acinar and collecting duct cells	Marker of tumor aggressiveness in pancreatic ductal adenocarcinomas	Ishibashi et al., 1995; Burghardt et al., 2003; Direito et al., 2017
AQP4	Negligible expression (rat and humans)	–	–	Koyama et al., 1997; Hurley et al., 2001; Burghardt et al., 2003
AQP5	Exocrine pancreas (humans)	Intercalated and intralobular ductal cells	Pancreatic fluid secretion and marker of tumor differentiation in pancreatic ductal adenocarcinomas	Burghardt et al., 2003; Direito et al., 2017
AQP6	Not detected (mice, rats and humans)	–	–	Isokpehi et al., 2009
AQP7	Endocrine pancreas (mice and rats)	β- and δ-cells	Control of insulin synthesis and secretion, triacylglycerol accumulation and proliferation of β-cells	Matsumura et al., 2007; Best et al., 2009; Méndez-Giménez et al., 2017
AQP8	Exocrine pancreas (rat and humans)	Acinar cells	Pancreatic fluid secretion	Koyama et al., 1997; Calamita et al., 2001; Hurley et al., 2001; Burghardt et al., 2003
AQP9	Not detected (rats and humans)	–	–	Isokpehi et al., 2009
AQP10	Not detected (humans)	–	–	Hatakeyama et al., 2001; Méndez-Giménez et al., 2017
AQP11	Negligible expression (humans)	–	–	Isokpehi et al., 2009
AQP12	Exocrine and endocrine pancreas (rats)	Acinar cells and β-cells	Maturation and exocytosis of zymogen granules, marker of pancreatic damage in acute pancreatitis and pancreatic steatosis	Itoh et al., 2005; Ohta et al., 2009; Méndez-Giménez et al., 2017

AQP, aquaporin.

the total pancreatic cells. Exocrine cells comprise acinar cells, which synthesize and secrete digestive enzymes, and ductal cells that release most of the pancreatic juice. Endocrine cells are organized into small clusters of cells termed islets of Langerhans, which are composed by five cell subtypes, α-cells (20% of the total cells producing glucagon), β-cells (∼70% producing insulin), δ-cells (10% producing somatostatin), polypeptide cells (5% producing PP) and ε-cells (<1% producing ghrelin). In the present review, we have focused on the role of AQPs in the physiology and pathophysiology of the pancreas, highlighting the role of pancreatic AQP7, which has emerged as a novel player in the control of β-cell function (Matsumura et al., 2007; Best et al., 2009; Louchami et al., 2012; Méndez-Giménez et al., 2017).

AQUAPORINS IN THE EXOCRINE PANCREAS: REGULATION OF PANCREATIC FLUID SECRETION AND MARKERS OF PANCREATIC DAMAGE

The exocrine pancreas secretes daily a large volume of HCO_3^--rich fluid containing digestive enzymes to neutralize gastric acid that enters into the duodenum and to digest dietary nutrients (Hurley et al., 2001). The epithelial cells lining the ductal system and, to a lesser extent, acinar cells of the exocrine pancreas generate near-isotonic fluids, a mechanism that requires a high transepithelial water permeability (Hurley et al., 2001; Ko et al., 2002; Burghardt et al., 2003). Several AQPs, including AQP1, AQP5, AQP8, and AQP12, contribute to the high water permeability of apical and basolateral membranes of both acinar and ductal cells of the exocrine pancreas (**Table 1**). However, it is tempting to speculate that the existence of other unidentified water channels in the exocrine pancreas, since $HgCl_2$, a non-selective AQP blocker, reduces total water permeability by as much as 90% in isolated rat acinar cells (Hurley et al., 2001) and 78% in isolated rat interlobular ducts (Ko et al., 2002). In the human pancreas, AQP8 is exclusively expressed in the apical membrane of pancreatic acinar cells, whereas AQP1 and AQP5 are abundantly expressed in the apical and basolateral membranes of the epithelial cells of intercalated ducts, which is probably the main site of pancreatic fluid secretion (Burghardt et al., 2003; **Figure 1**). In this sense, pancreatic fluid secretion starts with the secretion of a small volume of isotonic-like fluid rich in NaCl from acinar cells with AQP8 allowing water efflux to the lumen. Subsequently, intercalated ducts, secrete Na^+, $HCO3^-$, and Cl^- with AQP1 and AQP5 allowing water movement from ductal cells to the ductal lumen (Delporte, 2014). The digestive enzymes within the pancreatic juice are synthesized in acinar cells and are stored in secretory vesicles termed zymogen granules in the apical pole of the cell. Interestingly, AQP12 is expressed in the pancreatic acinar cells with an intracellular localization in the rough endoplasmic

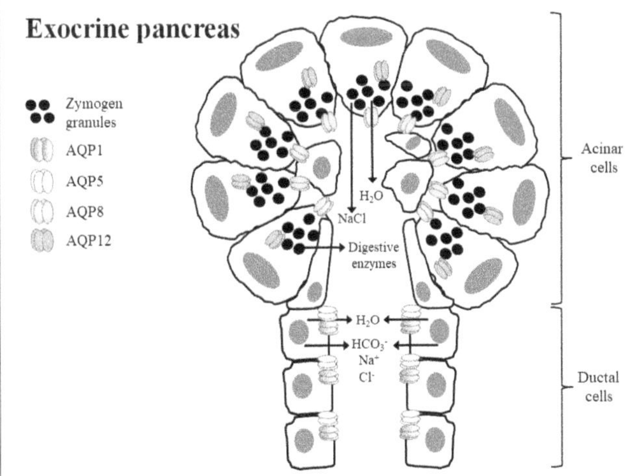

FIGURE 1 | Role of aquaporins in isotonic fluid secretion and zymogen granule exocytosis in the exocrine pancreas. The primary function of pancreatic acinar cells is to synthesize and secrete digestive enzymes, which are stored in zymogen granules in the apical poles. AQP12, which is located in the cytoplasm, contributes to the proper formation, maturation and exocytosis of zymogen granules, a process dependent on water transport across the membranes. Acinar cells also secrete a small volume of a NaCl-enriched isotonic fluid. The water efflux from acinar cells to the lumen is mainly mediated by AQP8. Ductal cells secrete Na^+, Cl^-, $HCO3^-$ as well as large amounts of water via AQP1 and AQP5 in order to form the final isotonic pancreatic fluid.

reticulum and the membranes of zymogen granules near the rough endoplasmic reticulum (Itoh et al., 2005; **Figure 1**). AQP12 not only participates in the secretion of pancreatic isotonic fluid, but it is also involved in the proper maturation and exocytosis of the zymogen granules in murine pancreatic acinar cells (Itoh et al., 2005; Ohta et al., 2009). There is evidence of expression of AQP12 in the human pancreas (Isokpehi et al., 2009), and its tissue distribution and function warrants further investigation.

The pancreatic exocrine function is severely impaired during pancreatitis, the inflammation of the pancreas, which is divided in acute and chronic types (Delporte, 2014; Ravi Kanth and Nageshwar Reddy, 2014). The clinical symptoms of acute pancreatitis include upper abdominal pain, nausea, vomiting and increased serum levels of the digestive enzymes amylase and lipase. Chronic pancreatitis is characterized by recurrent abdominal pain, damage of the pancreatic parenchyma with inflammation and fibrosis, ductal dilation, necrosis and finally a progressive loss of exocrine (maldigestion) and endocrine (diabetes mellitus) functions. Changes in both AQP1 and AQP12 have been observed during the onset of acute and chronic pancreatitis, reflecting their potential as markers of pancreatic damage. AQP1 is overexpressed in the pancreatic ducts of patients with autoimmune pancreatitis, which showed chronic pancreatitis characterized by a severely impaired secretion of digestive enzymes from acinar cells as well as pancreatic fluid and HCO_3^- secretion from ducts (Ko et al., 2009; Koyama et al., 2010). The upregulation of AQP1 might constitute a compensatory mechanism to overcome the slowed fluid movement across the pancreatic endothelia and ducts, which alter the convective flow of pancreatic digestive enzymes through the pancreatic duct. On the other hand, AQP12 deficiency increases the susceptibility of caerulein, a cholecystokinin-8 analog inducing acute pancreatitis (Ohta et al., 2009). Accordingly, AQP12-KO mice show more numerous and larger exocytic vacuoles in acinar cells, an important cellular hallmark of early pancreatitis, than control mice.

Likewise, a deregulation of AQPs has been also detected in other pathophysiological conditions of the pancreas, such as obesity-associated pancreatic steatosis (Méndez-Giménez et al., 2017) or pancreatic ductal adenocarcinoma (Direito et al., 2017). AQP12 is upregulated in the pancreas of obese rats with the increased pancreatic *Aqp12* mRNA levels being positively associated with markers of insulin resistance and ectopic lipid overload (Méndez-Giménez et al., 2017). A strong immunoreactivity for AQP3 and AQP5 is observed in the ductal cells of patients with pancreatic ductal adenocarcinomas that is associated to tumor aggressiveness and tumor differentiation, respectively (Direito et al., 2017).

AQUAPORIN-7 IN THE ENDOCRINE PANCREAS: CONTROL OF INSULIN RELEASE, TRIACYLGLYCEROL ACCUMULATION AND β-CELL PROLIFERATION

Circulating glucose is the most relevant regulator of proinsulin synthesis and insulin secretion in pancreatic β-cells (Muoio and Newgard, 2008). However, glycerol constitutes another metabolite involved in nutrient-induced insulin release through the activation of the glycerol-phosphate shuttle, a metabolic pathway that replenishes cytosolic NAD^+ levels necessary to maintain glycolysis, which in turn provides pyruvate for anaplerosis (Skelly et al., 2001). AQP7 has been identified in pancreatic β-cells of murine and rat endocrine pancreas (**Figure 2**), but not in the acini or the ducts of the exocrine pancreas, as well as in the rat pancreatic BRIN-BD11 and RIN-m5F β-cell lines (Matsumura et al., 2007; Best et al., 2009; Delporte et al., 2009; Méndez-Giménez et al., 2017). AQP7 transports urea and glycerol in β-cells, resulting in a similar β-cell swelling, activation of the volume-regulated anion channel and insulin secretion (Best et al., 2009). Nonetheless, glycerol triggers a more marked and sustained effect on membrane potential (Best et al., 2009). Extracellular glycerol is transported into β-cells through AQP7, transformed into glycerol-3-phosphate by the activation of the GK enzyme activity and entered into the glycerol-3-phosphate shuttle (Rodríguez et al., 2011a; **Figure 3**). In this metabolic process, glycerol-3-phosphate is converted into dihydroxyacetone phosphate (DHAP) in a reaction catalyzed by the inner membrane-bound mitochondrial glycerol-3-phosphate dehydrogenase (GPD) that reduces FAD^+ to $FADH_2$ that enters in the mitochondrial oxidative phosphorylation process to generate ATP (Skelly et al., 2001; Matsumura et al., 2007; Rodríguez et al., 2011a; Méndez-Giménez, 2017). The subsequent increase in the cytosolic ATP/ADP ratio induces the closure of ATP-sensitive K^+ channels, depolarization of the plasma

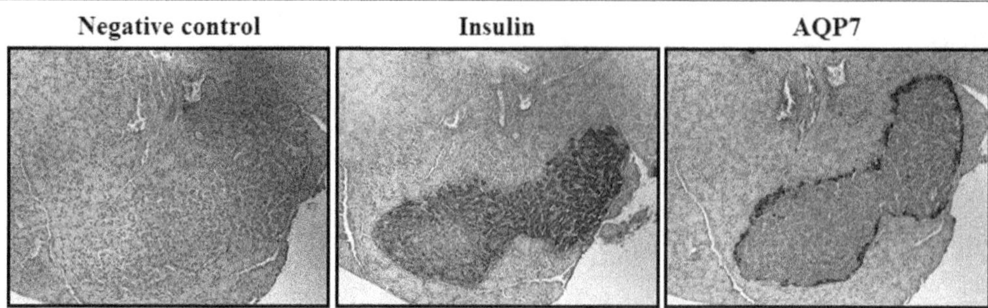

FIGURE 2 | AQP7 distribution in β-cells of Langerhans islets. Immunohistochemistry showing the location of insulin and AQP7 in Langerhans islets in serial sections of rat pancreas using specific primary antibodies (magnification 100x). Negative control was obtained in the absence of primary antibody. The detailed methodology is described in the following reference (Méndez-Giménez et al., 2017).

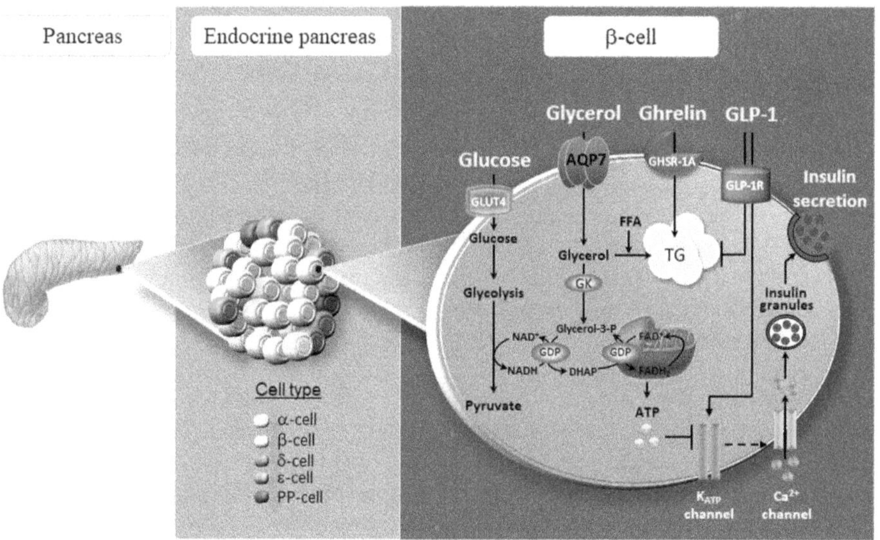

FIGURE 3 | Role of AQP7 in insulin secretion and triacylglycerol accumulation in β-cells of the endocrine pancreas. AQP7 facilitates glycerol influx to β-cells. The increase in intracellular glycerol and the consequent activation of glycerol kinase (GK) activity, in turn, stimulate the pro-insulin mRNA and insulin secretion, probably through their participation in the glycolysis and glycerol-phosphate shuttle activities in the β-cell. Glycerol can be also used as a substrate for *de novo* synthesis of TG. Both ghrelin and glucagon-like peptide 1 (GLP-1) down-regulate AQP7 expression in β-cells. The subsequent increase in intracellular glycerol might be used for the biosynthesis of triacylglycerols (TG) induced by ghrelin as well as for insulin synthesis and secretion triggered by GLP-1. GDP, glycerol-3-phosphate dehydrogenase; GLUT4, glucose transporter 4; PP, pancreatic polypeptide.

membrane, activation of voltage-dependent Ca^{2+} channels followed by a rapid influx of Ca^{2+} that triggers insulin exocytosis. *Aqp7*-KO mice show increased β-cell glycerol content and GK activity, which result in higher basal and glucose-induced insulin secretion (Matsumura et al., 2007; Louchami et al., 2012). Interestingly, AQP7 deficiency is associated with reduced β-cell mass caused by a decrease in β-cell proliferation, but it is also related to increased insulin-1 and insulin-2 transcript levels indicating a more efficient insulin biosynthesis and secretion (Matsumura et al., 2007).

Short-term exposure of β-cells to FFA increases glucose-stimulated insulin secretion, but chronic exposure to high FFA levels promotes β-cell hypertrophy and insulin hypersecretion, ultimately causing β-cell dysfunction and death through lipoapoptosis (El-Assaad et al., 2003; Méndez-Giménez et al., 2017). β-cells require a continuous sense fuel load, particularly glucose, and they cannot protect themselves by blocking glucose uptake to avoid excess nutrient load and their capacity to store fuel excess in the form of TG is limited (Mugabo et al., 2017). Excess-fuel detoxification pathways comprise glycerol and FFA formation and release to the extracellular milieu and the diversion of glucose carbons to TG and cholesterol esters in β-cells. In this regard, AQP7 plays an important role in the modulation of intraislet glycerol concentration and TG synthesis (**Figure 3**; Matsumura et al., 2007; Louchami et al., 2012; Méndez-Giménez et al., 2017). AQP7 deficiency in mice causes an increased intracellular glycerol and the GK activity resulting in an increase in TG concentration in the Langerhans islets (Hibuse et al., 2005; Matsumura et al., 2007).

OBESITY IS ASSOCIATED WITH DEREGULATION OF AQUAGLYCEROPORINS IN THE ADIPOSE TISSUE, LIVER AND PANCREAS

AQP7-KO mice display a clear phenotype of adult-onset obesity and hyperinsulinemia (Maeda et al., 2004; Hibuse et al., 2005; Matsumura et al., 2007), but the impact of AQP7 loss-of-function homozygous mutations in human obesity and diabetes remains controversial. In a study conducted in 160 adult Japanese subjects, those individuals carrying homozygous missense mutations (R12C, V59L, and G264V) and silent mutations (A103A and G250G) in the *AQP7* gene neither exhibit obesity nor diabetes (Kondo et al., 2002). Nonetheless, Kondo and colleagues found that the unique case homozygous for G264V mutation in the *AQP7* gene exhibited an impaired exercise-induced increase in plasma glycerol in spite of the increased plasma noradrenaline (Kondo et al., 2002), confirming the role of AQP7 in adipocyte lipolysis. Hyperglyceroluria and platelet secretion defect have been also attributed to the G264V variant of *AQP7* gene in three children homozygous for this non-functional mutation (Goubau et al., 2013). In another cohort of 178 Caucasian subjects, one single case of a subject homozygous for the G264V mutation exhibited glycerol levels below the 10th percentile, overweight and type 2 diabetes (Ceperuelo-Mallafré et al., 2007). Moreover, a study performed in 977 Caucasian individuals detected a single-nucleotide polymorphism (A593G) in the human *AQP7* gene promoter that was related to decreased AQP7 expression in the adipose tissue as well as with type 2 diabetes (Prudente et al., 2007). Further studies are required to analyze the real impact of *AQP7* gene variants in the onset of obesity and type 2 diabetes. Nonetheless, growing evidence support the strong metabolic impact of the regulation of AQP7 expression in the onset of obesity and its associated comorbidities (Frühbeck, 2005; Frühbeck et al., 2006; Méndez-Giménez et al., 2014). Human obesity is associated with a deregulation in the expression of aquaglyceroporins in adipose tissue (Marrades et al., 2006; Ceperuelo-Mallafré et al., 2007; Prudente et al., 2007; Catalán et al., 2008; Rodríguez et al., 2011b) and liver (Catalán et al., 2008; Miranda et al., 2009; Rodríguez et al., 2014). Visceral adipose tissue of obese patients shows an upregulation of AQP3 and AQP7, which might be related to the increased lipolytic rate in this fat depot (Catalán et al., 2008; Rodríguez et al., 2011b). In contrast, AQP7 is downregulated in the subcutaneous adipose tissue leading to the promotion of an intracellular glycerol accumulation and a progressive adipocyte hypertrophy (Rodríguez et al., 2011b). Moreover, our group found a reduction of glycerol permeability and AQP9 expression in the liver of obese patients with non-alcoholic fatty liver disease (NAFLD) in parallel to the degree of hepatic steatosis, being further aggravated in insulin-resistant patients (Rodríguez et al., 2014). The downregulation of AQP9 seems to be a compensatory mechanism whereby the liver counteracts further TG accumulation within its parenchyma as well as reduces hepatic gluconeogenesis in obese patients with NAFLD.

Obesity is commonly associated with insulin resistance and type 2 diabetes. Under normal conditions, the pancreatic islet β-cells increase insulin secretion sufficiently to overcome the reduced efficiency of insulin action, thereby maintaining normal glucose tolerance. In order to maintain an appropriate long-term glycemic control in insulin-resistant states, the number of pancreatic islet β-cells or β-cell mass, is expanded (de Koning et al., 2008; Méndez-Giménez, 2017). The β-cell dysfunction is characterized by a decreased insulin gene expression, blunted glucose-stimulated insulin secretion as well as increased β-cell apoptosis rates (Wajchenberg, 2007). Obesity-associated insulin resistance has been attributed to ectopic lipid overload, with lipotoxicity being a major contributor of β-cell dysfunction (Lee et al., 2010; van Raalte et al., 2010; Ou et al., 2013). Since glycerol also constitutes an important metabolite for insulin exocytosis and TG synthesis in β-cells, we analyzed the impact of obesity and weight loss achieved by bariatric surgery on pancreatic AQP7 in a recent study (Méndez-Giménez et al., 2017). As expected hyperinsulinemic and insulin-resistant obese rats exhibited adaptive changes in β-cell mass as well as pancreatic steatosis. Bariatric surgery improved β-cell dysfunction in obese rats, as evidenced by reduced pancreatic β-cell apoptosis, steatosis and insulin secretion. Interestingly, both weight gain and weight loss achieved by bariatric surgery were associated with increased pancreatic AQP7 mRNA and protein levels (Méndez-Giménez et al., 2017). AQP7 upregulation in the pancreas might constitute an adaptive response of β-cells to increase glycerol uptake and the subsequent insulin synthesis and secretion, which seems nevertheless inefficient to reduce the hyperglycemia in the obese state, but not after bariatric surgery. Further studies are needed to validate the potential role of AQP7 in β-cell function in the human pancreas.

ROLE OF AQP7 IN GHRELIN- AND GLP-1-INDUCED IMPROVEMENT OF PANCREATIC β-CELL FUNCTION AFTER BARIATRIC SURGERY

Bariatric surgery significantly improves insulin sensitivity within days after this procedure, which implicates mechanisms independent of weight loss that involve the modulation of intrinsic gut hormones via the gastro-entero-insular axis (Frühbeck, 2015; Méndez-Giménez, 2017). The incretin hormone glucagon-like peptide-1 (GLP-1) is among the most widely studied modulators of β-cell function, with the incretin effect accounting for 70% of the insulin secretion after an oral glucose tolerance test (Hussain et al., 2016). At the endocrine pancreas, GLP-1 binds its receptor GLP-1R and suppresses glucagon secretion from α-cells and potentiates insulin secretion from β-cells in a glucose-dependent manner. On the other hand, ghrelin represents a survival factor promoting cell survival *in vitro* in HIT-T15 pancreatic β-cells (Granata et al., 2006) and *in vivo* in streptozotocin-induced diabetic mice (Bando et al., 2013). Interestingly, we found that acylated and desacyl ghrelin induced intracellular lipid accumulation in RIN-m5F β-cells (Méndez-Giménez et al., 2017), which is in agreement with the lipogenic effect of ghrelin isoforms in other metabolic tissues, including adipose tissue and liver (Rodríguez et al., 2009; Porteiro et al., 2013; Ezquerro et al., 2016). We confirmed the water (*Pf*) and glycerol (*Pgly*) permeability of the rat RIN-m5F β-cells (Méndez-Giménez et al., 2017), which exhibited permeability values within the range of the *Pf* and *Pgly* measured in mature murine 3T3-L1 adipocytes with endogenous AQP7 expression (Madeira et al., 2013). To gain further insight into the molecular mechanisms triggering the improvement of β-cell function, the role of ghrelin and GLP-1 in the expression of pancreatic AQP7 was studied (**Figure 3**). Acylated and desacyl ghrelin constitute negative regulators of AQP7 in adipocytes and this downregulation contributes, in part, to the lipid accumulation in fat cells (Rodríguez et al., 2009). Accordingly, acylated and desacyl ghrelin diminished the AQP7 expression in parallel to an increased TG content in RIN-m5F β-cells (Méndez-Giménez et al., 2017). Interestingly, GLP-1 showed a tendency toward a downregulation of AQP7 in RIN-m5F β-cells with the AQP7 protein expression being negatively associated with insulin release (Méndez-Giménez et al., 2017). Thus, it seems plausible that the reduction of AQP7 induced by ghrelin and GLP-1 might result in intracellular glycerol accumulation, which can be used for the biosynthesis of TG as well as for insulin synthesis and secretion in β-cells (**Figure 3**).

CONCLUSIONS

Although there is compelling evidence from murine and human studies that AQP7 might constitute an effective anti-diabetic drug target (Rodríguez et al., 2011a; Méndez-Giménez et al., 2014; da Silva and Soveral, 2017), the discovery and development of pharmacological AQP modulators has been slow, in part because current efforts to identify inhibitors are hampered by challenges in screening assays and in targeting the compact, pore-containing AQP molecule (Verkman et al., 2014).

Several heavy metals, such as mercury chloride ($HgCl_2$), silver sulfide (AgS) or gold(III) compound [Au(phen)Cl_2]Cl (phen=1,10-phenatroline) (Auphen) constitute AQP7 inhibitors (Preston et al., 1993; Delporte et al., 2009; Madeira et al., 2014a). Hg^{2+} ions bind specifically the mercury-sensitive cysteine located just in front of the second NPA box of several AQPs (Preston et al., 1993). This covalent modification of cysteine residues either induces the blockage or conformational change of the AQP pore causing the inhibition of water permeability. Silver ($AgNO_3$ or AgS) or gold ($HAuCl_4$ or Auphen) compounds interact with sulfhydryl groups of proteins, such as the thiolates of cysteine residues in the vicinity of conserved NPA motifs and thus effectively inhibit water and glycerol permeability to a higher extent than $HgCl_2$ (Niemietz and Tyerman, 2002; Martins et al., 2012). However, the AQP inhibitors $HgCl_2$ or AgS cause major irreversible cytotoxic effects in β-cells (Best et al., 2009). In this context, the design of novel small-molecule modulators of AQP7 expression/function may have clinical applications in the therapy of type 2 diabetes. The use of well-designed experimental strategies is of utmost importance for aquaporin drug discovery. The most frequently used biophysical and biological approaches to detect AQP activity and/or function include: (i) cell models with AQP gene overexpression or silencing for functional analysis; (ii) water and/or glycerol permeability assays by using techniques based on volume-dependent optical properties, such as stopped-flow light-scattering spectrophotometry, or osmotic swelling assays; and (iii) computational methods for the analysis of the target of novel candidate molecules in the three-dimensional AQP structure models (for extensive review of these methods, please refer to; Madeira et al., 2016).

From a clinical point of view, the possibility of regulating the pancreatic AQP7 function, by the upregulation of AQP expression or possibly by gene transfer in rare cases of loss-of-function mutations of the *AQP7* gene, may also be beneficial in obesity, insulin resistance and type 2 diabetes. Nonetheless, additional data related to novel mutations, single nucleotide polymorphisms, epigenetic and transcription changes and protein stability are needed to better establish a firm mechanistic basis for the contribution of AQP7 in the etiopathogenesis of these metabolic diseases.

AUTHOR CONTRIBUTIONS

AR: Conception and design of research; LM-G, GF, and AR: Prepared figures; LM-G, GF, and AR: Drafted the manuscript; LM-G, SE, IdS, GS, GF, and AR: Edited and revised manuscript; LM-G, SE, IdS, GS, GF, and AR: Approved final version of manuscript.

ACKNOWLEDGMENTS

This work was supported by Fondo de Investigación Sanitaria-FEDER (FIS PI16/00221 and PI16/01217) from the Instituto de Salud Carlos III, and the Department of Health of the Gobierno de Navarra (61/2014). CIBEROBN is an initiative of the Instituto de Salud Carlos III, Spain. SE was recipient of a predoctoral grant from the Spanish Ministerio de Educación, Cultura y Deporte (FPU15/02599) and IdS received a PhD fellowship (PD/BD/113634/2015) from Fundação para a Ciência e a Tecnologia, Portugal.

REFERENCES

Agre, P. (2009). The 2009 Lindau Nobel Laureate Meeting: Peter Agre, Chemistry 2003. *J. Vis. Exp.* 34:1565. doi: 10.3791/1565

Bando, M., Iwakura, H., Ariyasu, H., Koyama, H., Hosoda, K., Adachi, S., et al. (2013). Overexpression of intraislet ghrelin enhances β-cell proliferation after streptozotocin-induced β-cell injury in mice. *Am. J. Physiol. Endocrinol. Metab.* 305, E140–E148. doi: 10.1152/ajpendo.00112.2013

Best, L., Brown, P. D., Yates, A. P., Perret, J., Virreira, M., Beauwens, R., et al. (2009). Contrasting effects of glycerol and urea transport on rat pancreatic ?-cell function. *Cell. Physiol. Biochem.* 23, 255–264. doi: 10.1159/000218172

Burghardt, B., Elkaer, M. L., Kwon, T. H., Rácz, G. Z., Varga, G., Steward, M. C., et al. (2003). Distribution of aquaporin water channels AQP1 and AQP5 in the ductal system of the human pancreas. *Gut* 52, 1008–1016. doi: 10.1136/gut.52.7.1008

Calamita, G., Gena, P., Ferri, D., Rosito, A., Rojek, A., Nielsen, S., et al. (2012). Biophysical assessment of aquaporin-9 as principal facilitative pathway in mouse liver import of glucogenetic glycerol. *Biol. Cell* 104, 342–351. doi: 10.1111/boc.201100061

Calamita, G., Mazzone, A., Bizzoca, A., Cavalier, A., Cassano, G., Thomas, D., et al. (2001). Expression and immunolocalization of the aquaporin-8 water channel in rat gastrointestinal tract. *Eur. J. Cell Biol.* 80, 711–719. doi: 10.1078/0171-9335-00210

Calvanese, L., Pellegrini-Calace, M., and Oliva, R. (2013). *In silico* study of human aquaporin AQP11 and AQP12 channels. *Protein Sci.* 22, 455–466. doi: 10.1002/pro.2227

Catalán, V., Gómez-Ambrosi, J., Pastor, C., Rotellar, F., Silva, C., Rodríguez, A., et al. (2008). Influence of morbid obesity and insulin resistance on gene expression levels of AQP7 in visceral adipose tissue and AQP9 in liver. *Obes. Surg.* 18, 695–701. doi: 10.1007/s11695-008-9453-7

Ceperuelo-Mallafré, V., Miranda, M., Chacón, M. R., Vilarrasa, N., Megia, A., Gutiérrez, C., et al. (2007). Adipose tissue expression of the glycerol channel aquaporin-7 gene is altered in severe obesity but not in type 2 diabetes. *J. Clin. Endocrinol. Metab.* 92, 3640–3645. doi: 10.1210/jc.2007-0531

da Silva, I. V., and Soveral, G. (2017). Aquaporins in obesity. *Adv. Exp. Med. Biol.* 969, 227–238. doi: 10.1007/978-94-024-1057-0_15

de Koning, E. J., Bonner-Weir, S., and Rabelink, T. J. (2008). Preservation of beta-cell function by targeting beta-cell mass. *Trends Pharmacol. Sci.* 29, 218–227. doi: 10.1016/j.tips.2008.02.001

Delporte, C. (2014). Aquaporins in salivary glands and pancreas. *Biochim. Biophys. Acta* 1840, 1524–1532. doi: 10.1016/j.bbagen.2013.08.007

Delporte, C., Virreira, M., Crutzen, R., Louchami, K., Sener, A., Malaisse, W. J., et al. (2009). Functional role of aquaglyceroporin 7 expression in the pancreatic β-cell line BRIN-BD11. *J. Cell. Physiol.* 221, 424–429. doi: 10.1002/jcp.21872

Direito, I., Paulino, J., Vigia, E., Brito, M. A., and Soveral, G. (2017). Differential expression of aquaporin-3 and aquaporin-5 in pancreatic ductal adenocarcinoma. *J. Surg. Oncol.* 115, 980–996. doi: 10.1002/jso.24605

El-Assaad, W., Buteau, J., Peyot, M. L., Nolan, C., Roduit, R., Hardy, S., et al. (2003). Saturated fatty acids synergize with elevated glucose to cause pancreatic β-cell death. *Endocrinology* 144, 4154–4163. doi: 10.1210/en.2003-0410

Elkjaer, M., Vajda, Z., Nejsum, L. N., Kwon, T., Jensen, U. B., Amiry-Moghaddam, M., et al. (2000). Immunolocalization of AQP9 in liver, epididymis, testis, spleen, and brain. *Biochem. Biophys. Res. Commun.* 276, 1118–1128. doi: 10.1006/bbrc.2000.3505

Ezquerro, S., Méndez-Giménez, L., Becerril, S., Moncada, R., Valentí, V., Catalán, V., et al. (2016). Acylated and desacyl ghrelin are associated with hepatic lipogenesis, b-oxidation and autophagy: role in NAFLD amelioration after sleeve gastrectomy in obese rats. *Sci. Rep.* 6:39942. doi: 10.1038/srep39942

Fasshauer, M., Klein, J., Lossner, U., Klier, M., Kralisch, S., and Paschke, R. (2003). Suppression of aquaporin adipose gene expression by isoproterenol, TNF?, and dexamethasone. *Horm. Metab. Res.* 35, 222–227. doi: 10.1055/s-2003-39478

Frühbeck, G. (2005). Obesity: aquaporin enters the picture. *Nature* 438, 436–437. doi: 10.1038/438436b

Frühbeck, G. (2015). Bariatric and metabolic surgery: a shift in eligibility and success criteria. *Nat. Rev. Endocrinol.* 11, 465–477. doi: 10.1038/nrendo.2015.84

Frühbeck, G., Catalán, V., Gómez-Ambrosi, J., and Rodríguez, A. (2006). Aquaporin-7 and glycerol permeability as novel obesity drug-target pathways. *Trends Pharmacol. Sci.* 27, 345–347. doi: 10.1016/j.tips.2006.05.002

Frühbeck, G., and Gómez-Ambrosi, J. (2001). Rationale for the existence of additional adipostatic hormones. *FASEB J.* 15, 1996–2006. doi: 10.1096/fj.00-0829hyp

Frühbeck, G., Méndez-Giménez, L., Fernández-Formoso, J. A., Fernández, S., and Rodríguez, A. (2014). Regulation of adipocyte lipolysis. *Nutr. Res. Rev.* 27, 63–93. doi: 10.1017/S095442241400002X

Gena, P., Mastrodonato, M., Portincasa, P., Fanelli, E., Mentino, D., Rodríguez, A., et al. (2013). Liver glycerol permeability and aquaporin-9 are dysregulated in a murine model of non-alcoholic fatty liver disease. *PLoS ONE* 8:e78139. doi: 10.1371/journal.pone.0078139

Goubau, C., Jaeken, J., Levtchenko, E. N., Thys, C., Di Michele, M., Martens, G. A., et al. (2013). Homozygosity for aquaporin 7 G264V in three unrelated children with hyperglyceroluria and a mild platelet secretion defect. *Genet. Med.* 15, 55–63. doi: 10.1038/gim.2012.90

Granata, R., Settanni, F., Trovato, L., Destefanis, S., Gallo, D., Martinetti, M., et al. (2006). Unacylated as well as acylated ghrelin promotes cell survival and inhibit apoptosis in HIT-T15 pancreatic β-cells. *J. Endocrinol. Invest.* 29, RC19–RC22. doi: 10.1007/BF03347367

Hansen, J. S., Krintel, C., Hernebring, M., Haataja, T. J., de Marè, S., Wasserstrom, S., et al. (2016). Perilipin 1 binds to aquaporin 7 in human adipocytes and controls its mobility via protein kinase A mediated phosphorylation. *Metabolism* 65, 1731–1742. doi: 10.1016/j.metabol.2016.09.004

Hara-Chikuma, M., Sohara, E., Rai, T., Ikawa, M., Okabe, M., Sasaki, S., et al. (2005). Progressive adipocyte hypertrophy in aquaporin-7-deficient mice: adipocyte glycerol permeability as a novel regulator of fat accumulation. *J. Biol. Chem.* 280, 15493–15496. doi: 10.1074/jbc.C500028200

Hatakeyama, S., Yoshida, Y., Tani, T., Koyama, Y., Nihei, K., Ohshiro, K., et al. (2001). Cloning of a new aquaporin (AQP10) abundantly expressed in duodenum and jejunum. *Biochem. Biophys. Res. Commun.* 287, 814–819. doi: 10.1006/bbrc.2001.5661

Hibuse, T., Maeda, N., Funahashi, T., Yamamoto, K., Nagasawa, A., Mizunoya, W., et al. (2005). Aquaporin 7 deficiency is associated with development of obesity through activation of adipose glycerol kinase. *Proc. Natl. Acad. Sci. U.S.A.* 102, 10993–10998. doi: 10.1073/pnas.0503291102

Hurley, P. T., Ferguson, C. J., Kwon, T. H., Andersen, M. L., Norman, A. G., Steward, M. C., et al. (2001). Expression and immunolocalization of aquaporin water channels in rat exocrine pancreas. *Am. J. Physiol. Gastrointest. Liver Physiol.* 280, G701–G709. doi: 10.1152/ajpgi.2001.280.4.G701

Hussain, M. A., Akalestou, E., and Song, W. J. (2016). Inter-organ communication and regulation of β-cell function. *Diabetologia* 59, 659–667. doi: 10.1007/s00125-015-3862-7

Ishibashi, K. (2006). Aquaporin subfamily with unusual NPA boxes. *Biochim. Biophys. Acta* 1758, 989–993. doi: 10.1016/j.bbamem.2006.02.024

Ishibashi, K., Kuwahara, M., Gu, Y., Kageyama, Y., Tohsaka, A., Suzuki, F., et al. (1997). Cloning and functional expression of a new water channel abundantly expressed in the testis permeable to water, glycerol, and urea. *J. Biol. Chem.* 272, 20782–20786. doi: 10.1074/jbc.272.33.20782

Ishibashi, K., Sasaki, S., Saito, F., Ikeuchi, T., and Marumo, F. (1995). Structure and chromosomal localization of a human water channel (AQP3) gene. *Genomics* 27, 352–354. doi: 10.1006/geno.1995.1055

Ishibashi, K., Yamauchi, K., Kageyama, Y., Saito-Ohara, F., Ikeuchi, T., Marumo, F., et al. (1998). Molecular characterization of human Aquaporin-7 gene and its chromosomal mapping. *Biochim. Biophys. Acta* 1399, 62–66. doi: 10.1016/S0167-4781(98)00094-3

Isokpehi, R. D., Rajnarayanan, R. V., Jeffries, C. D., Oyeleye, T. O., and Cohly, H. H. (2009). Integrative sequence and tissue expression profiling of chicken and mammalian aquaporins. *BMC Genom.* 10(Suppl. 2):S7. doi: 10.1186/1471-2164-10-s2-s7

Itoh, T., Rai, T., Kuwahara, M., Ko, S. B., Uchida, S., Sasaki, S., et al. (2005). Identification of a novel aquaporin, AQP12, expressed in pancreatic acinar cells. *Biochem. Biophys. Res. Commun.* 330, 832–838. doi: 10.1016/j.bbrc.2005.03.046

Jelen, S., Wacker, S., Aponte-Santamaría, C., Skott, M., Rojek, A., Johanson, U., et al. (2011). Aquaporin-9 protein is the primary route of hepatocyte glycerol uptake for glycerol gluconeogenesis in mice. *J. Biol. Chem.* 286, 44319–44325. doi: 10.1074/jbc.M111.297002

Jung, J. S., Preston, G. M., Smith, B. L., Guggino, W. B., and Agre, P. (1994). Molecular structure of the water channel through aquaporin CHIP. The hourglass model. *J. Biol. Chem.* 269, 14648–14654.

King, L. S., Kozono, D., and Agre, P. (2004). From structure to disease: the evolving tale of aquaporin biology. *Nat. Rev. Mol. Cell Biol.* 5, 687–698. doi: 10.1038/nrm1469

Kishida, K., Kuriyama, H., Funahashi, T., Shimomura, I., Kihara, S., Ouchi, N., et al. (2000). Aquaporin adipose, a putative glycerol channel in adipocytes. *J. Biol. Chem.* 275, 20896–20902. doi: 10.1074/jbc.M001119200

Kishida, K., Shimomura, I., Nishizawa, H., Maeda, N., Kuriyama, H., Kondo, H., et al. (2001). Enhancement of the aquaporin adipose gene expression by a peroxisome proliferator-activated receptor γ. *J. Biol. Chem.* 276, 48572–48579. doi: 10.1074/jbc.M108213200

Ko, S. B., Mizuno, N., Yatabe, Y., Yoshikawa, T., Ishiguro, H., Yamamoto, A., et al. (2009). Aquaporin 1 water channel is overexpressed in the plasma membranes of pancreatic ducts in patients with autoimmune pancreatitis. *J. Med. Invest.* 56(Suppl.), 318–321. doi: 10.2152/jmi.56.318

Ko, S. B., Naruse, S., Kitagawa, M., Ishiguro, H., Furuya, S., Mizuno, N., et al. (2002). Aquaporins in rat pancreatic interlobular ducts. *Am. J. Physiol. Gastrointest Liver Physiol.* 282, G324–G331. doi: 10.1152/ajpgi.00198.2001

Kondo, H., Shimomura, I., Kishida, K., Kuriyama, H., Makino, Y., Nishizawa, H., et al. (2002). Human aquaporin adipose (AQPap) gene. Genomic structure, promoter analysis and functional mutation. *Eur. J. Biochem.* 269, 1814–1826. doi: 10.1046/j.1432-1033.2002.02821.x

Koyama, K. I., Yasuhara, D., Nakahara, T., Harada, T., Uehara, M., Ushikai, M., et al. (2010). Changes in acyl ghrelin, des-acyl ghrelin, and ratio of acyl ghrelin to total ghrelin with short-term refeeding in female inpatients with restricting-type anorexia nervosa. *Horm. Metab. Res.* 42, 595–598. doi: 10.1055/s-0030-1252017

Koyama, Y., Yamamoto, T., Kondo, D., Funaki, H., Yaoita, E., Kawasaki, K., et al. (1997). Molecular cloning of a new aquaporin from rat pancreas and liver. *J. Biol. Chem.* 272, 30329–30333. doi: 10.1074/jbc.272.48.30329

Kuriyama, H., Shimomura, I., Kishida, K., Kondo, H., Furuyama, N., Nishizawa, H., et al. (2002). Coordinated regulation of fat-specific and liver-specific glycerol channels, aquaporin adipose and aquaporin 9. *Diabetes* 51, 2915–2921. doi: 10.2337/diabetes.51.10.2915

Laforenza, U., Scaffino, M. F., and Gastaldi, G. (2013). Aquaporin-10 represents an alternative pathway for glycerol efflux from human adipocytes. *PLoS ONE* 8:e54474. doi: 10.1371/journal.pone.0054474

Lebeck, J., Cheema, M. U., Skowronski, M. T., Nielsen, S., and Praetorius, J. (2015). Hepatic AQP9 expression in male rats is reduced in response to PPARalpha agonist treatment. *Am. J. Physiol. Gastrointest. Liver Physiol.* 308, G198–G205. doi: 10.1152/ajpgi.00407.2013

Lee, D. H., Park, D. B., Lee, Y. K., An, C. S., Oh, Y. S., Kang, J. S., et al. (2005). The effects of thiazolidinedione treatment on the regulations of aquaglyceroporins and glycerol kinase in OLETF rats. *Metab. Clin. Exp.* 54, 1282–1289. doi: 10.1016/j.metabol.2005.04.015

Lee, Y., Lingvay, I., Szczepaniak, L. S., Ravazzola, M., Orci, L., and Unger, R. H. (2010). Pancreatic steatosis: harbinger of type 2 diabetes in obese rodents. *Int. J. Obes.* 34, 396–400. doi: 10.1038/ijo.2009.245

Louchami, K., Best, L., Brown, P., Virreira, M., Hupkens, E., Perret, J., et al. (2012). A new role for aquaporin 7 in insulin secretion. *Cell. Physiol. Biochem.* 29, 65–74. doi: 10.1159/000337588

Madeira, A., Camps, M., Zorzano, A., Moura, T. F., and Soveral, G. (2013). Biophysical assessment of human aquaporin-7 as a water and glycerol channel in 3T3-L1 adipocytes. *PLoS ONE* 8:e83442. doi: 10.1371/journal.pone.0083442

Madeira, A., de Almeida, A., de Graaf, C., Camps, M., Zorzano, A., Moura, T. F., et al. (2014a). A gold coordination compound as a chemical probe to unravel aquaporin-7 function. *Chembiochem* 15, 1487–1494. doi: 10.1002/cbic.201402103

Madeira, A., Fernández-Veledo, S., Camps, M., Zorzano, A., Moura, T. F., Ceperuelo-Mallafré, V., et al. (2014b). Human aquaporin-11 is a water and glycerol channel and localizes in the vicinity of lipid droplets in human adipocytes. *Obesity* 22, 2010–2017. doi: 10.1002/oby.20792

Madeira, A., Mósca, A. F., Moura, T. F., and Soveral, G. (2015). Aquaporin-5 is expressed in adipocytes with implications in adipose differentiation. *IUBMB Life* 67, 54–60. doi: 10.1002/iub.1345

Madeira, A., Moura, T. F., and Soveral, G. (2016). Detecting aquaporin function and regulation. *Front. Chem.* 4:3. doi: 10.3389/fchem.2016.00003

Maeda, N., Funahashi, T., Hibuse, T., Nagasawa, A., Kishida, K., Kuriyama, H., et al. (2004). Adaptation to fasting by glycerol transport through aquaporin 7 in adipose tissue. *Proc. Natl. Acad. Sci. U.S.A.* 101, 17801–17806. doi: 10.1073/pnas.0406230101

Marrades, M. P., Milagro, F. I., Martínez, J. A., and Moreno-Aliaga, M. J. (2006). Differential expression of aquaporin 7 in adipose tissue of lean and obese high fat consumers. *Biochem. Biophys. Res. Commun.* 339, 785–789. doi: 10.1016/j.bbrc.2005.11.080

Martins, A. P., Marrone, A., Ciancetta, A., Galán Cobo, A., Echevarría, M., Moura, T. F., et al. (2012). Targeting aquaporin function: potent inhibition of aquaglyceroporin-3 by a gold-based compound. *PLoS ONE* 7:e37435. doi: 10.1371/journal.pone.0037435

Matsumura, K., Chang, B. H., Fujimiya, M., Chen, W., Kulkarni, R. N., Eguchi, Y., et al. (2007). Aquaporin 7 is a β-cell protein and regulator of intraislet glycerol content and glycerol kinase activity, β-cell mass, and insulin production and secretion. *Mol. Cell. Biol.* 27, 6026–6037. doi: 10.1128/MCB.00384-07

Méndez-Giménez, L. (2017). *Role of Aquaporins in the Improvement of Adiposity and Non-alcoholic Fatty Liver Disease after Bariatric Surgery.* Ph.D. thesis, G. Frühbeck, and A. Rodríguez (directors). University of Navarra, Pamplona, Spain.

Méndez-Giménez, L., Becerril, S., Camões, S. P., da Silva, I. V., Rodrigues, C., Moncada, R., et al. (2017). Role of aquaporin-7 in ghrelin- and GLP-1-induced improvement of pancreatic β-cell function after sleeve gastrectomy in obese rats. *Int. J. Obes.* 41, 1394–1402. doi: 10.1038/ijo.2017.135

Méndez-Giménez, L., Becerril, S., Moncada, R., Valentí, V., Ramírez, B., Lancha, A., et al. (2015). Sleeve gastrectomy reduces hepatic steatosis by improving the coordinated regulation of aquaglyceroporins in adipose tissue and liver in obese rats. *Obes. Surg.* 25, 1723–1734. doi: 10.1007/s11695-015-1612-z

Méndez-Giménez, L., Rodríguez, A., Balaguer, I., and Frühbeck, G. (2014). Role of aquaglyceroporins and caveolins in energy and metabolic homeostasis. *Mol. Cell. Endocrinol.* 397, 78–92. doi: 10.1016/j.mce.2014.06.017

Miranda, M., Ceperuelo-Mallafré, V., Lecube, A., Hernández, C., Chacón, M. R., Fort, J. M., et al. (2009). Gene expression of paired abdominal adipose AQP7 and liver AQP9 in patients with morbid obesity: relationship with glucose abnormalities. *Metab. Clin. Exp.* 58, 1762–1768. doi: 10.1016/j.metabol.2009.06.004

Mugabo, Y., Zhao, S., Lamontagne, J., Al-Mass, A., Peyot, M. L., Corkey, B. E., et al. (2017). Metabolic fate of glucose and candidate signaling and excess-fuel detoxification pathways in pancreatic β-cells. *J. Biol. Chem.* 292, 7407–7422. doi: 10.1074/jbc.M116.763060

Muoio, D. M., and Newgard, C. B. (2008). Mechanisms of disease: molecular and metabolic mechanisms of insulin resistance and β-cell failure in type 2 diabetes. *Nat. Rev. Mol. Cell Biol.* 9, 193–205. doi: 10.1038/nrm2327

Nicchia, G. P., Frigeri, A., Nico, B., Ribatti, D., and Svelto, M. (2001). Tissue distribution and membrane localization of aquaporin-9 water channel: evidence for sex-linked differences in liver. *J. Histochem. Cytochem.* 49, 1547–1556. doi: 10.1177/002215540104901208

Niemietz, C. M., and Tyerman, S. D. (2002). New potent inhibitors of aquaporins: silver and gold compounds inhibit aquaporins of plant and human origin. *FEBS Lett.* 531, 443–447. doi: 10.1016/S0014-5793(02)03581-0

Ohta, E., Itoh, T., Nemoto, T., Kumagai, J., Ko, S. B., Ishibashi, K., et al. (2009). Pancreas-specific aquaporin 12 null mice showed increased susceptibility to caerulein-induced acute pancreatitis. *Am. J. Physiol. Cell Physiol.* 297, C1368–C1378. doi: 10.1152/ajpcell.00117.2009

Oliva, R., Calamita, G., Thornton, J. M., and Pellegrini-Calace, M. (2010). Electrostatics of aquaporin and aquaglyceroporin channels correlates with their transport selectivity. *Proc. Natl. Acad. Sci. U.S.A.* 107, 4135–4140. doi: 10.1073/pnas.0910632107

Ortega, F. J., Mayas, D., Moreno-Navarrete, J. M., Catalán, V., Gómez-Ambrosi, J., Esteve, E., et al. (2010). The gene expression of the main lipogenic enzymes is downregulated in visceral adipose tissue of obese subjects. *Obesity* 18, 13–20. doi: 10.1038/oby.2009.202

Ou, H. Y., Wang, C. Y., Yang, Y. C., Chen, M. F., and Chang, C. J. (2013). The association between nonalcoholic fatty pancreas disease and diabetes. *PLoS ONE* 8:e62561. doi: 10.1371/journal.pone.0062561

Porteiro, B., Díaz-Ruíz, A., Martínez, G., Senra, A., Vidal, A., Serrano, M., et al. (2013). Ghrelin requires p53 to stimulate lipid storage in fat and liver. *Endocrinology* 154, 3671–3679. doi: 10.1210/en.2013-1176

Preston, G. M., Jung, J. S., Guggino, W. B., and Agre, P. (1993). The mercury-sensitive residue at cysteine 189 in the CHIP28 water channel. *J. Biol. Chem.* 268, 17–20.

Prudente, S., Flex, E., Morini, E., Turchi, F., Capponi, D., De Cosmo, S., et al. (2007). A functional variant of the adipocyte glycerol channel aquaporin 7 gene is associated with obesity and related metabolic abnormalities. *Diabetes* 56, 1468–1474. doi: 10.2337/db06-1389

Ravi Kanth, V., and Nageshwar Reddy, D. (2014). Genetics of acute and chronic pancreatitis: an update. *World J. Gastrointest Pathophysiol.* 5, 427–437. doi: 10.4291/wjgp.v5.i4.427

Reshef, L., Olswang, Y., Cassuto, H., Blum, B., Croniger, C. M., Kalhan, S. C., et al. (2003). Glyceroneogenesis and the triglyceride/fatty acid cycle. *J. Biol. Chem.* 278, 30413–30416. doi: 10.1074/jbc.R300017200

Rodríguez, A., Catalán, V., Gómez-Ambrosi, J., and Frühbeck, G. (2011a). Aquaglyceroporins serve as metabolic gateways in adiposity and insulin resistance control. *Cell Cycle* 10, 1548–1556. doi: 10.4161/cc.10.10.15672

Rodríguez, A., Catalán, V., Gómez-Ambrosi, J., García-Navarro, S., Rotellar, F., Valentí, V., et al. (2011b). Insulin- and leptin-mediated control of aquaglyceroporins in human adipocytes and hepatocytes is mediated via the PI3K/Akt/mTOR signaling cascade. *J. Clin. Endocrinol. Metab.* 96, E586–E597. doi: 10.1210/jc.2010-1408.

Rodríguez, A., Gena, P., Méndez-Giménez, L., Rosito, A., Valentí, V., Rotellar, F., et al. (2014). Reduced hepatic aquaporin-9 and glycerol permeability are related to insulin resistance in non-alcoholic fatty liver disease. *Int. J. Obes.* 38, 1213–1220. doi: 10.1038/ijo.2013.234

Rodríguez, A., Gómez-Ambrosi, J., Catalán, V., Ezquerro, S., Méndez-Giménez, L., Becerril, S., et al. (2016). Guanylin and uroguanylin stimulate lipolysis in human visceral adipocytes. *Int. J. Obes.* 40, 1405–1415. doi: 10.1038/ijo.2016.66

Rodríguez, A., Gómez-Ambrosi, J., Catalán, V., Gil, M. J., Becerril, S., Sáinz, N., et al. (2009). Acylated and desacyl ghrelin stimulate lipid accumulation in human visceral adipocytes. *Int. J. Obes.* 33, 541–552. doi: 10.1038/ijo.2009.40

Rodríguez, A., Marinelli, R. A., Tesse, A., Frühbeck, G., and Calamita, G. (2015a). Sexual dimorphism of adipose and hepatic aquaglyceroporins in health and metabolic disorders. *Front. Endocrinol.* 6:171. doi: 10.3389/fendo.2015.00171

Rodríguez, A., Moreno, N. R., Balaguer, I., Méndez-Giménez, L., Becerril, S., Catalán, V., et al. (2015b). Leptin administration restores the altered adipose and hepatic expression of aquaglyceroporins improving the non-alcoholic fatty liver of ob/ob mice. *Sci. Rep.* 5:12067. doi: 10.1038/srep12067.

Skelly, R. H., Wicksteed, B., Antinozzi, P. A., and Rhodes, C. J. (2001). Glycerol-stimulated proinsulin biosynthesis in isolated pancreatic rat islets via adenoviral-induced expression of glycerol kinase is mediated via mitochondrial metabolism. *Diabetes* 50, 1791–1798. doi: 10.2337/diabetes.50.8.1791

Soveral, G., Nielsen, S., and Casini, A. (2017). *Aquaporins in Health and Disease: New Molecular Targets for Drug Discovery.* Boca Raton, FL: CRC Press.

van Raalte, D. H., van der Zijl, N. J., and Diamant, M. (2010). Pancreatic steatosis in humans: cause or marker of lipotoxicity? *Curr. Opin. Clin. Nutr. Metab. Care* 13, 478–485. doi: 10.1097/MCO.0b013e32833aa1ef

Verkman, A. S., Anderson, M. O., and Papadopoulos, M. C. (2014). Aquaporins: important but elusive drug targets. *Nat. Rev. Drug Discov.* 13, 259–277. doi: 10.1038/nrd4226

Wajchenberg, B. L. (2007). β-cell failure in diabetes and preservation by clinical treatment. *Endocr. Rev.* 28, 187–218. doi: 10.1210/10.1210/er.2006-0038

Walker, C. G., Holness, M. J., Gibbons, G. F., and Sugden, M. C. (2007). Fasting-induced increases in aquaporin 7 and adipose triglyceride lipase mRNA expression in adipose tissue are attenuated by peroxisome proliferator-activated receptor alpha deficiency. *Int. J. Obes.* 31, 1165–1171. doi: 10.1038/sj.ijo.0803555

Yang, B. (2017). *Aquaporins. Advances in Experimental Medicine and Biology Book Series 969*, Dordrecht: Springer.

Yeh, J. I., Charrier, V., Paulo, J., Hou, L., Darbon, E., Claiborne, A., et al. (2004). Structures of enterococcal glycerol kinase in the absence and presence of glycerol: correlation of conformation to substrate binding and a mechanism of activation by phosphorylation. *Biochemistry* 43, 362–373. doi: 10.1021/bi034258o

8

Nutritional Stress Induced by Amino Acid Starvation Results in Changes for Slc38 Transporters in Immortalized Hypothalamic Neuronal Cells and Primary Cortex Cells

Sofie V. Hellsten, Rekha Tripathi, Mikaela M. Ceder and Robert Fredriksson*

Molecular Neuropharmacology, Department of Pharmaceutical Biosciences, Uppsala University, Uppsala, Sweden

***Correspondence:**
Rekha Tripathi
rekha.tripathi@farmbio.uu.se

Amino acid sensing and signaling is vital for cells, and both gene expression and protein levels of amino acid transporters are regulated in response to amino acid availability. Here, the aim was to study the regulation of all members of the SLC38 amino acid transporter family, *Slc38a1-11*, in mouse brain cells following amino acid starvation. We reanalyzed microarray data for the immortalized hypothalamic cell line N25/2 subjected to complete amino acid starvation for 1, 2, 3, 5, or 16 h, focusing specifically on the SLC38 family. All 11 *Slc38* genes were expressed in the cell line, and *Slc38a1*, *Slc38a2,* and *Slc38a7* were significantly upregulated at 5 h and most strongly at 16 h. Here, protein level changes were measured for SLC38A7 and the orphan family member SLC38A11 which has not been studied under different amino acid starvation condition at protein level. At 5 h, no significant alteration on protein level for either SLC38A7 or SLC38A11 could be detected. In addition, primary embryonic cortex cells were deprived of nine amino acids, the most common amino acids transported by the SLC38 family members, for 3 h, 7 h or 12 h, and the gene expression was measured using qPCR. *Slc38a1*, *Slc38a2*, *Slc38a5*, *Slc38a6*, *Slc38a9,* and *Slc38a10* were upregulated, while *Slc38a3* and *Slc38a7* were downregulated. *Slc38a8* was upregulated at 5 h and downregulated at 12 h. In conclusion, several members from the SLC38 family are regulated depending on amino acid levels and are likely to be involved in amino acid sensing and signaling in brain.

Keywords: SLC38 transporters, amino acid starvation, gene expression, protein expression, glutamine transporters

INTRODUCTION

Amino acid sensing and signaling is important for cells to control metabolism and protein synthesis, as well as catabolism and autophagy (Hyde et al., 2003; Kilberg et al., 2005). The amino acid sensing machinery is mainly mediated via the mechanistic target of rapamycin complex 1 (mTORC1) and the amino acid response (AAR) pathway (Gallinetti et al., 2013; Efeyan et al., 2015). These pathways are activated depending on amino acid availability and when the cells have plenty of amino acids, the mTORC1 pathway is activated to maintain protein synthesis and cellular growth (Laplante and Sabatini, 2012). The RAG kinase complex (Rag A/B and Rag C/D) are activated and translocate mTORC1 to the lysosomes where it binds the Ragulator complex. The pathway is fully activated when the lysosomal GDP bound protein Rheb becomes GTP bound in response to growth factors and encounters the mTORC1 complex (Jewell et al., 2013). Contrary, when the cells have scarce levels of amino acids the AAR pathway is activated, leading to reduced protein synthesis (Efeyan et al., 2015). The GCN2 kinases senses the limitation by binding to uncharged tRNAs (Deval et al., 2009) and phosphorylates the eukaryotic initiation factor 2α (eiF2α) which strongly inhibits the cap dependent translation (Harding et al., 2000; Zhang et al., 2002). The activating transcription factor 4 (ATF4) is upregulated by repressed translation (Averous et al., 2004) and bind elements termed amino acid response elements (AAREs) or nutrient sensing response elements (NSREs) in other genes. These elements are short nucleotide sequences and genes holding these are hence transcriptionally upregulated (Barbosa-Tessmann et al., 2000; Fafournoux et al., 2000; Bruhat et al., 2002).

Amino acids are important regulators of gene expression (Fafournoux et al., 2000) and numerous amino acid transporters are transcriptionally regulated in response to amino acid levels. These transporters are suggested to function as tranceptors, as they can both function as transporters as well as amino acid sensors (Hundal and Taylor, 2009). Several amino acid transporters from the Solute carrier (SLC) superfamily are transcriptionally altered depending on amino acid levels (Taylor, 2014). The SLCs are the largest group of transporters in human and comprises over 400 members divided into 65 families (Hediger et al., 2013)[1]. The members in each SLC family share at least 20 % protein sequence identity with another family member, and therefore also functional characteristics (Hediger et al., 2004). The SLCs are membrane-bound uniporters, symporters, or antiporters, with a diverse substrate profile and transport, among others, amino acids, sugars, fatty acids, vitamins, hormones, ions, and drugs (Hediger et al., 2013). One of the amino acid transporter families is the SLC38 family; the sodium coupled neutral amino acid transporter (SNAT) family, which holds 11 members, encoded by the genes *Slc38a1-11* (Sundberg et al., 2008). All members are functionally characterized (Bröer, 2014; Rebsamen et al., 2015; Hellsten et al., 2017b) except for SLC38A6 and SLC38A11, but SLC38A6 is histologically characterized in mouse brain (Bagchi et al., 2014). These transporters translocate small neutral amino acids, mostly glutamine, alanine, and asparagine (Bröer, 2014). Members from this family are shown to be involved in amino acid sensing and signaling, and SLC38A2 was upregulated on both gene and protein levels after amino acid starvation in BeWo cells (Novak et al., 2006). In the *Slc38a2* gene an AARE is identified in the first intron (Palii et al., 2006). Moreover, SLC38A9 is located to lysosomes and it is a component of the Ragulator-Rag complex responsible for amino acid sensing and activation of the mTORC1 (Jung et al., 2015; Rebsamen et al., 2015; Wang et al., 2015). SLC38A1 was recently found to be regulated in an amino acid responsive way (Bröer et al., 2016). In brain, several of the family members are proposed to participate in the glutamate/GABA-glutamine cycle which occurs between neurons and astrocytes (Bröer, 2014; Scalise et al., 2016).

[1]http://slc.bioparadigms.org/

In this study the aim was to study the transcriptional regulation of the SLC38 family members in a mouse neuronal cell-line following amino acid starvation, to identify which transporters could be involved in amino acid sensing and signaling in brain. Data from expression microarrays of the N25/2 cell-line exposed to complete amino acid starvation from a previous study (Hellsten et al., 2017c)was reanalyzed specifically for the SLC38 family. We also investigate regulatory changes at the protein level of SLC38A7 using western blot, since this member was transcriptionally upregulated in the hypothalamic cell line and has not previously been studied. In addition, changes at the protein level were also studied for SLC38A11using western blot which was chosen because this is the only family member that is still orphan. In addition, primary embryonic cortex cells were deprived of nine amino acids, glycine, L-alanine, L-asparagine, L-glutamine, L-histidine, L-isoleucine, L-leucine, L-serine, and L-valine, the most common amino acids transported by the SLC38 members and the gene expression changes were measured for the entire family using qPCR.

MATERIALS AND METHODS

Heat Map Analysis

Genesis version 1.7.6 was used to generate both heat maps. The microarray and analysis of data was performed in Hellsten et al. (2017c) and the array data can be accessed from the NCBI-GEO database with accession number GSE61402. The heat map displaying the gene expression changes measured with microarray for the *Slc38* genes in the immortalized hypothalamic cell line N25/2 was obtained by using the difference in log2 gene expression scores between the starved and control cells. *Slc38a1*, *Slc38a9*, and *Slc3810* had two probes each on the DNA chip and the expression score from both probes were used in the heat map analysis. The heat map presenting the gene expression changes measured with qPCR after partial amino acid starvation in primary cortex cells was generated by using the difference between the normalized mean values of expression in starved and control cells.

Culturing and Complete Amino Acid Starvation of the Immortalized Hypothalamic Cell Line N25/2

The starvation experiment was performed in Hellsten et al. (2017c). Briefly, the mouse immortalized embryonic hypothalamic cell line N25/2, (mHypoE-N25/2, CEDARLANE, Canada) was cultured in Dulbecco's modified Eagles medium (DMEM) supplemented with 10% Fetal Bovine Serum (FBS), 1% Penicillin-Streptomycin and 1% Fungizone® Antimycotic at 37°C in 5% CO_2, 95% air. Cells were grown in Nunclon surface dishes 150 × 20 mm (Thermo Scientific, USA) to 70–90% confluency before starvation experiment. Medium for the experiment was prepared using Earle's balanced salt solution (EBSS) supplemented with 1 mM Sodium Pyruvate 100 mM, 4X MEM Vitamin Solution. The control medium was as well supplemented with 0.4 mM glycine, 0.4 mM L-arginine, 0.2 mM L-cystine, 4.0 mM L-glutamine, 0.2 mM L-histidine, 0.8 mM L-isoleucine, 0.8 mM L-leucine, 0.8 mM L-lysine, 0.2 mM L-methionine, 0.4 mM L-phenylalanine, 0.4 mM L-serine, 0.8 mM L-threonine, 0.08 mM L-tryptophan, 0.4 mM L-tyrosine and 0.8 mM L-valine (Sigma-Aldrich, USA). The complete DMEM medium was replaced with starvation EBSS medium or control EBSS medium. The cells were incubated in the different media for 1, 2, 3, 5, or 16 h before RNA was extracted using RNeasy Midi Kit (Qiagen, Germany), following the manufacturers protocol. The samples from 1, 2, 3, and 16 h were run in singlets in each treatment group (starved and control), while the samples from 5 h were run in quadruplicates. Protein was extracted from three replicates in each treatment group from 5 h using the Allprep® DNA/RNA/Protein Mini kit (Qiagen, Germany) following manufacturers protocol. The protein concentration was measured using the Protein Quantification kit-Rapid (Sigma-Aldrich, USA) in FALCON® 96 well Clear Microtest Plate (Corning, USA) in FLUOstar Omega (BMG LABTECH, Germany) with the Omega MARS software.

Western Blot Analysis of Protein Expression in the Hypothalamic Cell Line N25/2

Ten microliters (~9–11 μg) of protein samples were diluted in 15 μl of sample buffer [95% 2 × Lammeli's sample buffer (Bio-Rad, USA), 5% 2-mercaptoethanol (Sigma-Aldrich, USA)] was added and the samples were incubated at 95°C for 5 min. Twenty-five microliters of samples were loaded in wells together with 15 μl Page ruler™ Prestained Protein ladder, 10–180 kDa (Thermo Fisher Scientific, USA). Electrophoresis was performed at 250 V for approximately 25 min with gel Mini-protean TGX Precast Gels 4–15%, 10 well comb, 50 μl/well (Bio-Rad, USA) with running buffer (0.025 M Trizma base, 0.192 M Glycine, 0.1% SDS). Proteins were transferred to a 0.2 μm PVDF membrane using the Trans-Blot® Turbo™ Mini PVDF Transfer Packs (Bio-Rad, USA) in the Trans-Blot® Turbo™ Transfer System for 7 min (Bio-Rad, USA). The membrane was incubated in blocking buffer [5% Blotting grade blocker Non-fat dry Milk (Bio-Rad, USA) in TTBS (0.15 M NaCl, 0.01 M Trizma base, 0.05% Tween-20, pH = 8.0)] for 1 h, before incubation in the custom made polyclonal anti-SLC38A7 (produced in rabbit) (Innovagen, Sweden) (NH_2-CVMSKEPDGASGSPW-CONH2), which was used in Hägglund et al. (2011) diluted 1:200 or the custom made polyclonal anti-SLC38A11 (produced in rabbit) (Innovagen, Sweden) (MSYQQPQLSGPLQRC) diluted 1:100 with β-actin (produced in mouse) (Sigma-Aldrich, USA) diluted 1:1000 in blocking buffer overnight at 4°C. The membrane was washed 3 × 10 min in TTBS before 1 h incubation in goat-anti-rabbit horseradish peroxidase antibody (Invitrogen, USA) diluted 1:5000 in blocking buffer. The membrane was washed 4 × 10 min in TTBS and the blot was developed using Clarity Western ECL Substrate and visualized using a CCD camera (Bio-Rad, USA). For SLC38A7 the membrane was washed 6 × 10min in TTBS after development and the membrane was incubated in β-actin diluted 1:1000 in blocking buffer overnight and the membrane was treated as stated above. With the exception that the membrane was incubated in goat-anti-mouse horseradish peroxidase antibody (Invitrogen, USA) diluted 1:10000 for 1 h. For SLC38A11 the membrane was washed in TTBS 6 × 10 min after development and incubated in goat-anti-mouse horseradish peroxidase antibody (Invitrogen, USA) diluted 1:10000 in blocking buffer followed by development as stated above.

Calculations of Normalized Protein Expression

The western blots were quantified using ImageJ software and the protein expression was normalized against β-actin. GraphPad Prism 5 (Graph Pad software, USA) was used to generate graphs and for statistical calculations. Unpaired *t*-test were performed with significance levels (*≤0.05, **≤0.01, ***≤0.001).

Ethical Statement

Experiments including mice were approved by local ethical committee in Uppsala (Uppsala Djurförsöksetiska Nämnd, Uppsala district court) (Permit Number C67/13), following the guidelines of European Communities Council Directive (2010/63). C57Bl6/J mice (Taconic M&B, Denmark) were used and the mice had free access to water and standard R3 chow (Lantmännen, Sweden). The mice were housed in a temperature, light/dark, and humidity controlled room. Mice were mated in the animal facility and pregnancies were confirmed by the mucus plug.

Preparation and Partial Amino Acid Starvation of Primary Embryonic Cortex Cells

The preparation and starvation of primary cells were performed as described in Perland et al. (2017). Briefly, a pregnant female mouse was euthanized by cervical dislocation at embryonic day e14.5. Cortices were dissected from the embryos and placed in ice cold PBS (137.0 mM NaCl, 2.7 mM KCl, 8.1 mM Na_2HPO_4) supplemented with 10.0 mM glucose (all from Sigma-Aldrich, USA). The tissues were chemically dissociated using a DNase/Papain solution prior mechanical dissociation. Single cells were filtered through a 70 μm nylon cell strainer (BD Stockholm, Sweden) before plated at a density of 7.5×10^4-1.5×10^5 cells per well in PLL coated 6 well plates (Invitrogen, USA) using plating media. Following cell adhering, the plating media was replaced with growth media supplemented with B27 (Gibco®, Life technologies, USA). 75% of the medium was changed every third day and the cells grew for 10 days before starvation experiment. The control medium was prepared using EBSS (Gibco®, Life technologies, USA) supplemented with 2.0 mM GlutaMAX™ and the amino acids glycine, L-alanine, L-arginine, L-asparagine, L-cysteine, L-histidine, L-isoleucine, L-leucine, L-lysine, L-methionine, L-phenylalanine, L-proline, L-serine, L-threonine, L-tryptophan, L-tyrosine, and L-valine (Sigma-Aldrich, USA) was added in the same concentrations as in the Neurobasal® A medium. The starved medium was prepared using EBSS supplemented with L-arginine, L-cysteine,

L-lysine, L-methionine, L-phenylalanine, L-proline, L-threonine, L-tryptophan, and L-tyrosine (Sigma-Aldrich, USA) in the same concentrations as in the Neurobasal® A medium. Both the control and starvation medium was supplemented with 1.0 mM Sodium-Pyruvate, 1% Penicillin-Streptomycin, 2% B-27® (50X), 4X MEM Vitamin Solution (100X) (Gibco®, Life technologies, USA) and 10.9 mM HEPES (1 M) buffer solution (Gibco®, Life technologies, USA). Hence, the starved cells were deprived of glycine, L-alanine, L-asparagine, L-glutamine, L-histidine, L-isoleucine, L-leucine, L-serine and L-valine, which are among the most common amino acids transported by the SLC38 family and their precursors. The experiment was run in triplicates in each treatment group (starved vs. control cells) and the cells were treated in the limited amino acid medium or the complete amino acid medium for 3, 7, or 12 h before RNA was extracted using RNeasy Midi Kit (Qiagen, Germany), following the manufacturers protocol. cDNA synthesis was performed using the High-Capacity RNA-to-cDNA kit (Invitrogen, USA) according to the manufacturers protocol and the cDNA from the triplicates in each treatment group were pooled. The cDNA concentrations were measured using a ND-spectrophotometer (NanoDrop Technologies, USA).

qPCR Analysis of Gene Expression in Primary Embryonic Cortex Cells

The cDNA samples were analyzed using qPCR on MyiQ thermal cycler (Bio-Rad Laboratories, Sweden). Primers were designed using Beacon Designer v.8 (Premier Biosoft, USA) and the primers used are listed in **Table 1**. Housekeeping genes used for normalization were mouse *mβ-Actin*, *mGlycerylaldehyde 3-phosphate dehydrogenase* and *mHistone 3a*. Sixty nanograms cDNA per qPCR reaction was combined with 0.05 μl of each primer (100 pmol/μl), 3.6 μl 10X DreamTaq buffer (Thermo Fischer Scientific), 0.2 μl of 25 mM dNTP mix (Thermo Fischer Scientific), 1μl DMSO, 0.5 μl SYBR Green (Invitrogen) and 0.08 μl of Dream Taq (5U/μl, Thermo Fisher scientific). The volume was adjusted to 20 μl with water. The amplification was performed as follow; initial denaturation, 95.0°C for 30s, 45 cycles of: 95.0°C for 10s, 55.8–60.0°C for 30s and 72.0°C for 30s. Cycling was followed by melt curve performance for 81 cycles, starting at 55.0°C, with steps of 0.5°C and 10s intervals. All qPCRs were run in triplicates and water was used as a negative control.

Data Analysis and Normalized Expression Calculations

The MyIQ software (Bio-Rad Laboratories, Sweden) was used to obtain the qPCR cycle threshold (Ct) -values and melt curve data. The melting curves were compared to the negative control to verify that only one product was amplified. The triplicates for the raw Ct-values were compared and excluded if the difference was greater than 0.5. For *Slc38a4* and *Slc38a11*, no Ct outliers could be removed due to high Ct values (Ct > 35). The efficiency for each primer pair was determined using LinRegPCR v7.5 and the average qPCR primer efficiency and standard deviation were calculated after significant outliers were removed using Grubbs outlier test (GraphPad Software, USA). The delta Ct-method was used to transform the Ct-values into relative quantities with standard deviations for each treatment time. Geometric means of all housekeeping genes were calculated and the normalized mRNA levels were calculated by dividing the relative Ct-values of the sample by the geometric mean of the housekeeping genes relative Ct-values. Unpaired *t*-tests (*≤0.05, **≤0.01, ***≤0.001) were performed using GraphPad Prism 5 (GraphPad Software, USA) between the control cells and the starved cells.

TABLE 1 | Primers used for qPCR.

Primer	Forward/Reverse
Slc38a1	F:tga cga gag tca cgc aga gat g, R:gag cag tat gag aac aag cga agc
Slc38a2	F:tct act cgc tgg ttc ttc, R:aat aaa ctt gtc act tcc ctt
Slc38a3	F:act ctt gtc ttc ttc cct ctc ctc, R:gcc tcc ctt ctc cca gca g
Slc38a4	F:tct cac tct aca cca aca cta agg, R:act cta tac tgg caa ccg tca ttc
Slc38a5	F:tgg agg tgt ctg gtc tct aat aa, R:ggc agt gag gca act cta agg
Slc38a6	F:gga aga aca cca cag acc aga atc, R:tgc tct ctt gcc tct tgc tct c
Slc38a7	F:att gtt gtt ctc cca tcc atc cc, R:act gtg aaa ggc agc act tgg
Slc38a8	F:cgt ggt gac tcg gga cag, R:ta caa gcc agg gac act aag g
Slc38a9	F:ttg aaa gcg agg gaa atg atg gtc, R:atg gga atg agg gtc act gag aag
Slc38a10	F:tgg tga agg ctc cga aga aag g, R:act tgg ctt ggg tct gaa ctg g
Slc38a11	F:act ttc aat tcg gaa cct, R:cat cag tgc taa tct tgt g
mβ-Actin (mActb)	F:cct tct tgg gta tgg aat cct gtg, R:cag cac tgt gtt ggc ata gag g
mGlycerylaldehyde 3-phosphate dehydrogenase (mGAPDH)	F:gcc ttc cgt gtt cct acc, R:gcc tgc ttc acc acc ttc
mHistone3a (mH3a)	F:cct tgt ggg tct gtt tga, R:cag ttg gat gtc ctt ggg

RESULTS

Microarray Analysis of Gene Expression in the Immortalized Hypothalamic Cell Line N25/2

The immortalized hypothalamic cell line N25/2 was completely starved of amino acids and the gene expression was analyzed using microarray in Hellsten et al. (2017c). All 11 genes encoding members of the SLC38 family were expressed in the cell line (expression score > 5.0). *Slc38a1*, *Slc38a9*, and *Slc38a10* had two probes each on the microarray and the results were comparable between the probes. The regulation of the *Slc38* genes is presented in the heat map (**Figure 1**). The red color represents upregulation and green color represents downregulation of gene expression. In

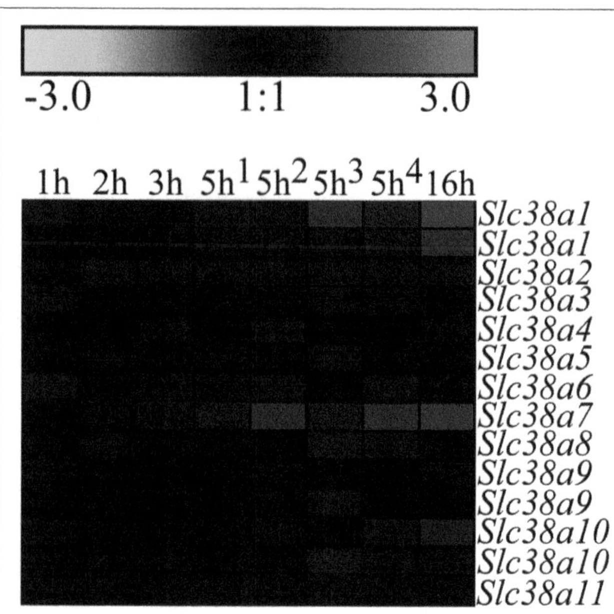

FIGURE 1 | Heat map analysis of the gene expression changes for *Slc38a1-11* after complete amino acid starvation performed on the immortalized hypothalamic cell line N25/2. A heat map of the gene expression changes measured with microarray between starved cells and controls at 1, 2, 3, 5, or 16 h. The color scale represents the log2 difference between starved and control cells. Green color represents downregulation and red color represent upregulation of gene expression. Note that *Slc38a1*, *Slc38a9*, and *Slc3810* had two probes each on the gene chip and the expression scores from both probes are presented in the heat map.

Table 2, all differences in log2 expression scores and the adjusted *P*-value at 5 h of starvation, and in addition the system, substrates and location in brain for all family members are presented. *Slc38a1*, *Slc38a2*, and *Slc38a7* were significantly upregulated at 5 h (i.e., adj. *P*-value < 0.01) of amino acid starvation, and strongly upregulated at 16 h of starvation. *Slc38a3*, *Slc38a4*, *Slc38a5*, *Slc38a6*, *Slc38a8*, *Slc38a9*, *Slc38a10*, and *Slc38a11* were not significantly changed at 5 h in the array.

Protein Expression of SLC38A7 And SLC38A11 in the Immortalized Hypothalamic Cell Line N25/2

We chose to study SLC38A7 and SLC38A11 on protein level. This, because SLC38A7 was transcriptionally upregulated in the hypothalamic cell line and this transporter has not previously been studied on protein level. While the other two SLC38 family members (*Slc38a1* and *Slc38a2*) found to be transcriptionally upregulated in the N25/2 hypothalamic cells have previously been studied in several studies and therefore we found it most interesting to investigate the regulation of SLC38A7. In addition, SLC38A11 is currently the only family member that has not been either studied histologically or functionally so therefore we found it interested to study this transporter on protein level in the hypothalamic cells. The protein expression of SLC38A7 was analyzed using western blot and a band was detected with approximate size of 62 kDa in all samples except first replicate of starved cells (**Figure 2A**). β-actin was used for normalization and the blot is displayed in **Figure 2B**. SLC38A7 was upregulated in the second sample while downregulated in the third sample of starved cells compared with the controls. In the first starved sample, SLC38A7 was not detected, however β-actin was detected. The normalized protein levels for SLC38A7 were calculated in each replicate (1, 2 and 3) in each treatment group (**Figure 2C**). The expression of SLC38A7 was combined in the starved cells and control cells (mean value normalized protein expression ± SD) and overall the protein expression of SLC38A7 was not significantly changed ($p = 0.6886$; **Figure 2D**). The protein expression of the orphan family member SLC38A11 was analyzed using western blot and in the blot a band with approximate size of 46 kDa was detected (**Figure 3A**). The predicted size of SLC38A11 in mouse is 49.6 kDA (453 amino acids, NP_796048) and hence the blot indicates specific binding of the anti-SLC38A11 antibody. β-actin was used to normalize the protein expression and was detected in all replicates in each treatment group (**Figure 3B**). SLC38A11 was downregulated after starvation in the first and second sample, while upregulated in the third sample (**Figure 3C**). The expression of SLC38A11 was combined in the starved cells and control cells (mean value normalized protein expression ± SD) and these results indicate that the protein expression of SLC38A11 was unchanged ($p = 0.4108$; **Figure 3D**).

qPCR Analysis of Gene Expression in the Primary Embryonic Cortex Cells

Primary cortex cells were partly deprived of the most common amino acids transported by the SLC38 family, as well as their precursors, for 3, 7, and 12 h. Subsequently, the gene expression was measured with qPCR for *Slc38a1-11* (**Figure 4A**). All genes were detected in the primary cells, however *Slc38a4* and *Slc38a11* had low mRNA expression (i.e., CT>35) and these results should hence be considered with caution. *Slc38a1* was upregulated at 12 h ($p = 0.0495$). *Slc38a2* expression was increased at all three deprivation timepoints 3 h ($p = 0.0012$), 7 h ($p = 0.0026$), and 12 h ($p = 0.0026$). *Slc38a3* was downregulated at 12 h (p=0.0158), *Slc38a4* expression was unchanged at all three timepoints and *Slc38a5* expression was increased at 7 h ($p = 0.0159$) and 12 h ($p = 0.0304$). *Slc38a6* expression was upregulated at 3 h ($p = 0.0079$) and 7 h ($p = 0.0057$). *Slc38a7* expression was decreased at 7 h ($p = 0.0054$) and*Slc38a8* was upregulated at 3 h ($p = 0.0059$) of deprivation but downregulated at 12 h ($p = 0.0323$). *Slc38a9* was upregulated early at 3 h ($p = 0.0165$) while *Slc38a10* was upregulated late at 12 h ($p = 0.0201$). *Slc38a11* expression was increased at 3 h ($p = 0.0295$) and decreased at 12 h ($p = 0.0455$). The heat map (**Figure 4B**) summarizes the gene expression changes measured with qPCR for each *Slc38* gene.

DISCUSSION

Amino acid sensing and signaling are crucial for cells to control basic functions and transporters involved in these processes often act as amino acid sensors (Efeyan et al., 2015). In many cancer cells, amino acid transporters are upregulated to enable

TABLE 2 | Summary of the microarray data and the SLC38 transporters.

Gene	1 h	2 h	3 h	5 h[1]	5 h[2]	5 h[3]	5 h[4]	Adj. *P*-value (5 h)	16 h	System A/N	Substrates	Main location in brain
Slc38a1	−0.25	−0.08	−0.02	0.72	0.64	1.17	1.00	0.00009461	1.52	A	Gln, Ala, Asn, Cys, His, Ser	GABAergic neurons (Solbu et al., 2010)
	0.07	0.02	0.14	0.55	0.59	0.56	0.83	0.00010526	1.22			
Slc38a2	0.23	0.68	0.63	0.64	0.64	0.63	0.68	0.00001176	0.78	A	Ala, Asn, Cys, Gln, Gly, His, Met, Pro, Ser	Glutamatergic neurons (González-González et al., 2005)
Slc38a3	−0.28	−0.02	0.014	0.06	0.20	−0.20	−0.13	0.93754260	−0.01	N	Gln, His, Ala, Asn	Astrocytes (Boulland et al., 2003)
Slc38a4	−0.02	0.07	−0.20	−0.07	−0.29	−0.05	0.11	0.73438555	−0.21	A	Ala, Asn, Cys, Gly, Ser, Thr	?
Slc38a5	0.07	−0.13	0.15	0.26	0.06	−0.23	−0.04	0.96736096	−0.04	N	Gln, Asn, His, Ser	Astrocytes (Cubelos et al., 2005)
Slc38a6	−0.36	−0.10	−0.24	−0.21	−0.32	0.06	−0.29	0.12927331	−0.15	?	?	Glutamatergic neurons (Bagchi et al., 2014)
Slc38a7	0.17	0.34	0.72	0.86	1.17	0.91	1.25	0.00002241	1.38	N (Hägglund et al., 2011)	Gln, His, Ser, Ala, Asn	GABAergic and glutamatergic neurons (Hägglund et al., 2011)
Slc38a8	0.00	−0.21	0.26	0.10	0.08	−0.45	−0.31	0.49605581	−0.10	A (Hägglund et al., 2015)	Gln, Arg, Ala, Asp, Leu, His, Asn, Pro, Glu	GABAergic and glutamatergic neurons (Hägglund et al., 2015)
Slc38a9	−0.13	0.18	0.01	−0.01	0.33	0.22	0.09	0.26471418	0.37	?	Arg, Gln, His, Pro, Lys, Glu, Leu	GABAergic and glutamatergic neurons (Hellsten et al., 2017a)
	0.07	0.17	0.09	0.03	−0.09	−0.36	0.17	0.68362400	0.10	?		
Slc38a10	−0.15	−0.09	−0.08	−0.08	−0.17	−0.06	−0.36	0.16057397	−0.62	A (Hellsten et al., 2017b)	Gln, Glu, Ala, D-Asp, Ser (Hellsten et al., 2017b)	Neurons and astrocytes (Hellsten et al., 2017b)
	0.02	0.02	0.12	0.09	−0.04	−0.38	−0.22	0.30033341	−0.21			
Slc38a11	0.21	0.04	0.18	0.18	0.04	−0.10	0.17	0.65258319	−0.07	?	?	?

Difference in log2 expression scores between the starved and control cells from the microarray analysis is presented (1–16 h), as well as the system, substrates and astrocytic/GABAergic/glutamatergic-neuronal location in brain for the transporters. Information about system classification and substrate profile were obtained from SLC tables (http://www.bioparadigms.org/slc/intro.htm) otherwise stated, (? Not known).

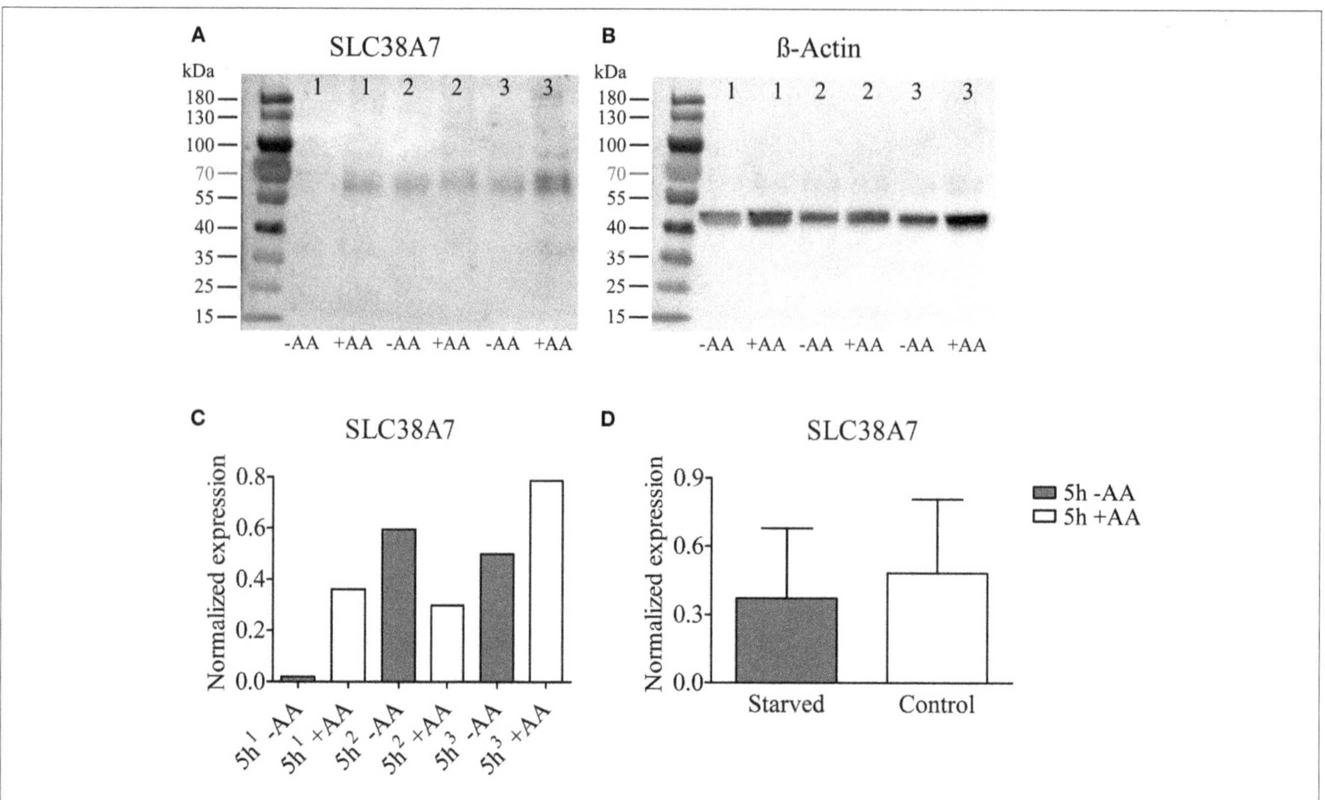

FIGURE 2 | Western blot analysis of SLC38A7 protein expression in the immortalized hypothalamic cell line N25/2 after complete starvation at 5 h. **(A)** The blot (developed for 18.4 s) displays the protein expression of SLC38A7 in three replicates (1, 2, 3) from each treatment group. The predicted size of the mouse SLC38A7 protein is 49.9 kDA (463 amino acids, NP_766346) and a band with approximately size of 62 kDa was detected. **(B)** The blot (developed for 3.1 s) displays the protein expression of β-actin in each sample which was used for normalization of protein expression in each sample. **(C)** The graph illustrates the normalized protein expression of SLC38A7 in the starved cells compared with the amino acid treated controls for each replicate. **(D)** The graph represents the normalized protein expression of all replicates in each group (mean value of protein expression ± SD). An unpaired *t*-test was performed between the protein expression in starved cells and controls. No difference ($p = 0.6886$) was detected on protein level for SLC38A7.

rapid cell growth and are therefore potential drug targets e.g. as SLC1A5, SLC6A15, SLC7A5, and SLC7A11 (Bhutia et al., 2015). Here, complete and partial amino acid starvation of cells was performed to study the regulation of the amino acid transporters in the SLC38 family in mouse brain cells. The hypothalamic cell line N25/2 was used to measure changes in expression levels on gene and protein levels during complete amino acid starvation, and primary cortex cells, comprising both neurons and astrocytes, were partly deprived of amino acids to study gene expression changes. A murine hypothalamic cell line and primary cells from different brain regions were used in this study to obtain a more comprehensive understanding of the regulation. *Slc38a2* was upregulated in the hypothalamic cell line and at all three timepoints in the primary cortex cells. *Slc38a2* is known to be transcriptionally induced by amino acid starvation (Gaccioli et al., 2006) and this gene holds an AARE (Palii et al., 2006). SLC38A2 follows adaptive regulation in response to amino acid stress by GCN pathway (Taylor, 2014). Along with this *Slc38a9* is also known as an arginine sensor and regulate the mTORC1 pathway. Moreover, *Slc38a1* was also transcriptionally induced in both cell types, however only late in the primary cortex cells, and SLC38A1 expression was recently found to be regulated by amino acid starvation (Bröer et al., 2016). SLC38A1 and SLC38A2 are mostly expressed on neurons in brain and the main function of these proteins are suggested to be uptake of glutamine in GABAergic respectively glutamatergic neurons (Bak et al., 2006). In cancer cells, SLC38A1 and SLC38A2 are involved in providing glutamine for glutaminolysis (Bröer et al., 2016). Both *Slc38a1* (Mackenzie et al., 2003) and *Slc38a2* (Yao et al., 2000) encode system A transporters, which system *Slc38a8* (Hägglund et al., 2015) also is classified to. *Slc38a8* was also initially upregulated in the primary cortex cells. Among transporters classified to system N, *Slc38a7* (Hägglund et al., 2011) showed increased expression in the hypothalamic cell line while reduced in the cortex cells. The dissimilarity in regulation pattern could be due to different starvation times and the fact that the hypothalamic cells are completely starved while the cortex cells are partly deprived of amino acids, also the cultures are inherently different, because the primary cultures are embryonic and mixed cultures of neurons and glia cells, while the N25/2 cultures are only neurons. The gene expression of the functionally orphan protein SLC38A6 was upregulated in the primary cortex cells. In a previous study, this transporter was shown to be expressed specifically on glutamatergic neurons (Bagchi et al., 2014). Assuming SLC38A6

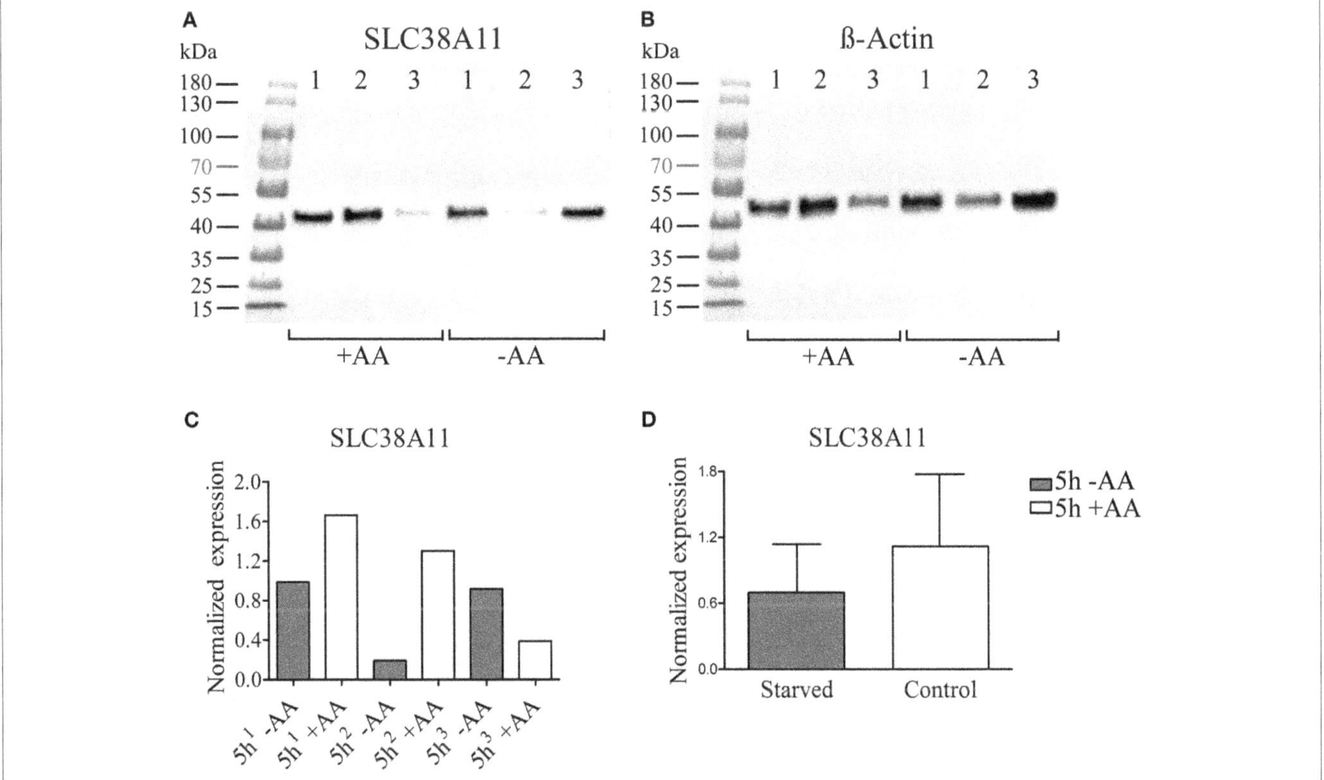

FIGURE 3 | Western blot analysis of SLC38A11 protein expression in the immortalized hypothalamic cell line N25/2 after complete starvation at 5 h. **(A)** The blot (developed for 2.0 s) show the protein expression of SLC38A11 in three replicates (1, 2, 3) in each treatment group. The predicted size of the mouse SLC38A11 protein is 49.6 kDA (453 amino acids, NP_796048) and a band with approximate size of 46 kDA was detected. **(B)** The blot (developed for 2.0 s) visualizes the protein expression of β-actin which was used to normalize the protein expression in each sample. **(C)** The graph displays the normalized protein expression of SLC38A11 in the starved cells compared with the amino acid treated controls for each sample. **(D)** The graph represents the normalized protein expression of all replicates in each treatment group (mean value of protein expression ± SD). An unpaired *t*-test was performed between the protein expression in starved cells and controls. No difference ($p = 0.4108$) of protein expression for SLC38A11 was measured.

is a transporter for glutamine as speculated in Bagchi et al. (2014), its role could be in importing glutamine into the presynapes of glutamatergic neurons, where it will be used as substrate for glutamine synthesis. If so, it makes sense that SLC38A6 is upregulated in response to lack of glutamine in the starved state, so neurons can maintain glutamine levels in the pre-synapse. SLC38A7 (Hägglund et al., 2011) and SLC38A8 (Hägglund et al., 2015) are suggested to facilitate uptake of glutamine in neurons and the expression levels of these transcripts were altered in the cortex cells. An interesting point of view is that it is possible that *Slc38* genes encodes proteins with similar localization and function, are regulated differently; as one protein could have housekeeping functions while the other protein is responding to stress. For example, SLC38A3 and SLC38A5 have similar expression and function in brain, and these genes had altered gene expression in opposite direction. These proteins are also closely phylogenetically related (Hägglund et al., 2015). This theory can also be applied to SLC38A7 and SLC38A8 which also are phylogenetically closely related and co-expressed on most neurons (Hägglund et al., 2015) and initially regulated in the opposite direction after partial amino acid starvation, and in the hypothalamic cell line *Slc38a7* was transcriptionally induced while *Slc38a8* was not. In a previous study, SLC38A7 co-localized with lysosomes in HeLa cells and was found to mediate flux of glutamine and asparagine and hence crucial for growth of cancer cells (Verdon et al., 2017). SLC38A9 is located on lysosomes and is a component of the amino acid sensing Ragulator-Rag complex responsible for activation of mTORC1 (Jung et al., 2015; Rebsamen et al., 2015; Wang et al., 2015) and in mouse brain SLC38A9 immunostaining is detected in both GABAergic and glutamatergic neurons (Hellsten et al., 2017a). Expression of *Slc38a9* was not altered by complete amino acid starvation in hypothalamic cells but initially upregulated in the primary cortex cells. In a previous study where mice were food deprived for 24 h before euthanasia, *Slc38a9* was upregulated in cortex while unaffected in hypothalamus in brain (Hellsten et al., 2017a). A hallmark of the SLC38 family is adaptive regulation with modulator of nutrient stress, and these transporters are translocated within the cell, e.g., to and from the plasma membrane depending on different stimulus such as amino acid levels (Bröer and Gether, 2012; Bröer, 2014). Studying gene expression levels is a good approach to pinpoint which genes are responding to alterations in amino acid levels, but to understand how the regulation of gene expression affects

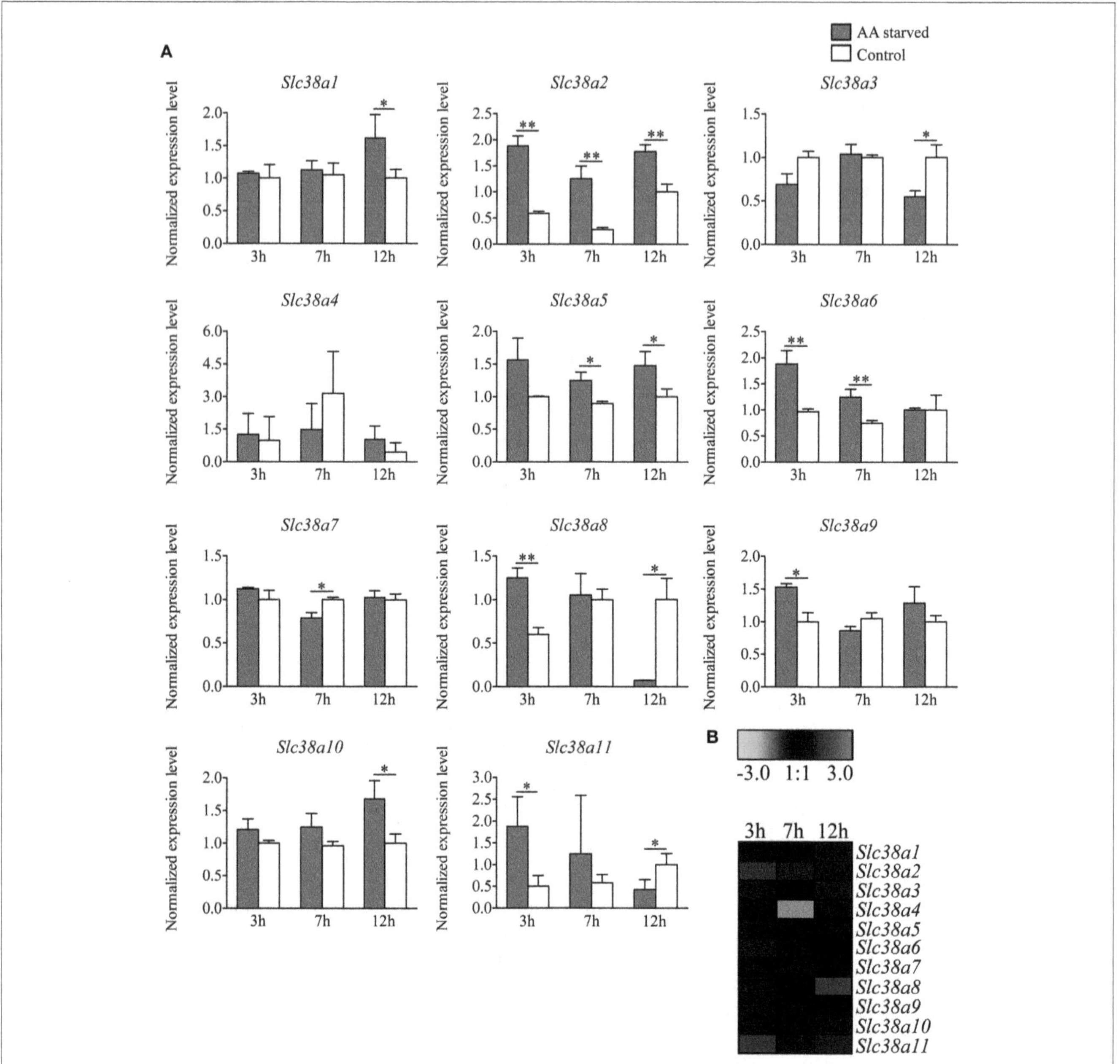

FIGURE 4 | Gene expression analysis of *Slc38a1-11* in primary cortex cells at 3h, 7h and 12h treatment. **(A)** Gene expression data from the primary cortex cells using qPCR for *Slc38a1-11*. The gene expression levels were normalized against *mβ-Actin*, *mGlycerylaldehyde 3-phosphate dehydrogenase,* and *mHistone 3a* and the normalized expression level ± SD ($n = 3$) is presented for each gene. Dark gray bars represent amino acid starved cells and white bars represent amino acid treated controls. Unpaired t-tests were used between starved cells and controls (*≤0.05, **≤0.01) to analyze alteration in gene expression. The x-axis represents time of treatment in hours and the y-axis represents the normalized mRNA expression levels. **(B)** Heat map analysis summarizing the gene expression alterations measured with qPCR for *Slc38a1-11*. The color scale represents the difference between the mean value of normalized expression in starved and control cells. Green color represents downregulation and red color represent upregulation of gene expression.

the cellular function, alterations on protein levels are crucial to study. The system A transporters SLC38A1 (Bröer et al., 2016) and SLC38A2 (Novak et al., 2006) are known to be upregulated on protein level in response to amino acid starvation. Apart from SLC38A1 and SLC38A2 the only other transporter that had significantly changed expression at 5 h was *Slc38a7*. We investigated if these changes could also be detected on protein level and found that the protein expression of SLC38A7 was unchanged at 5 h in the hypothalamic cell line. We have however verified that *Slc38a7* was upregulated in the hypothalamic cell line at 5 h at the mRNA level using qPCR in Hellsten et al. (2017c).This is likely a result of the fact that changes in protein levels occurs later than on mRNA level and has not yet manifested itself at the timepoint we are measuring changes at the protein level. We also investigated changes in protein levels of SLC38A11, the last orphan member of the SLC38 family. The gene expression of *Slc38a11* was measured in a previous study and was overall low in the rat brain (Sundberg et al., 2008), and both in the hypothalamic cell line and the cortex cells the mRNA levels were low. However, SLC38A11 protein levels could easily be detected in the hypothalamic cell line, but no effect on mRNA and protein levels were detected.

Neurons have low ability for *de-novo* synthesis of glutamine and other amino acids compared to other cells and is therefore dependent on import of these compounds provided either by astrocytes or glia cells or from import into the brain via the blood brain barrier (Bixel et al., 2001; Lieth et al., 2001; Schousboe, 2018). Therefore, plasma membrane expressed transporters on neuronal cells are crucial for maintaining homeostasis of amino acids and this transport needs to be tightly controlled. The main way, as far as currently understood, of regulating transport mediated by SLCs is for the cells to change number of transporters by, in the short term, alter surface expression and over longer timespans regulate number of transporters at the transcription and protein synthesis levels. Nerve cells have five or possibly six transporters from the SLC38 family which could possibly contribute in importing glutamine into neurons (Schiöth et al., 2013; Bröer, 2014). The data presented in this paper shows that in a neuronal cell-line, SLC38A1, SLC38A2, and SLC38A7 are regulated in response to amino acid starvation. In the nervous system, SLC38A1 and SLC38A2 are found on certain neuronal populations while SLC38A7, together with SLC38A8, are ubiquitously expressed on most neurons (Hägglund et al., 2011). This suggests that glutamine import into neurons by the SLC38 family could be dependent on SLC38A8, which is ubiquitously expressed on neurons, as housekeeping transporter and SLC38A7 together with one of or both SLC38A1 and SLC38A2 for the regulated transport. Expression of SLC38A6 is not regulated in the N25/2 cells and this transporter is found only on excitatory neurons (Bagchi et al., 2014) suggesting a role specifically for importing glutamine for the glutamine/glutamate/GABA cycle. However, our data from primary cultures, which are mixed cultures of different neuronal subtypes and non-neuronal cells such as astrocytes and glia cells, which is closer to a true representation of the *in vivo* situation, suggests that the situation is much more complex *in vivo* because here we show that all SLC38 members except for Slc38a4 can be regulated in response to amino acid starvation. Interestingly, some are being upregulated and others downregulated in response to amino acid starvation. In the *in vivo* situation, the SLC38 family of transporters is most likely regulated differently on different cell-types to maintain glutamine homeostasis as close as possible for the brain in total.

CONCLUSION

In conclusion, three (*Slc38a1, Slc38a2,* and *Slc38a7*) of eleven members from the SLC38 family, have increased transcription following 5 h of complete amino acid starvation in the hypothalamic cell line N25/2. However, no regulation of SLC38A7 could be measured on protein level at 5 h. Following partial amino acid starvation of primary embryonic mouse cortex cells genes encoding all 11 SLC38 family members except *Slc38a4* were altered. Genes encoding both system A and N transporters were transcriptionally regulated upon changes in amino acid levels. Several of the SLC38 family members are possibly involved in amino acid sensing and signaling in brain.

AUTHOR CONTRIBUTIONS

SH wrote and drafted manuscript, planned and performed starvation experiments, microarray data analysis, generation of heat maps, qPCR and qPCR analysis, statistics, protein sample preparations and western blot; RT protein sample preparations, western blot, analysis of western blots and revised the draft paper; MC cDNA synthesis, qPCR and qPCR analysis; RF drafted manuscript, planned experiments. All authors have read and approved of the manuscript and helped with interpretation of results.

FUNDING

This study was supported by the Swedish Research Council, The Novo Nordisk foundation, Åhlens foundation, Engkvist Foundation, Gunvor and Josef Anérs foundation and Magnus Bergvalls foundation.

ACKNOWLEDGMENTS

Thanks to Emelie Perland and Emilia Lekholm for assistance with preparations of primary cells.

REFERENCES

Averous, J., Bruhat, A., Jousse, C., Carraro, V., Thiel, G., and Fafournoux, P. (2004). Induction of CHOP expression by amino acid limitation requires both ATF4 expression and ATF2 phosphorylation. *J. Biol. Chem.* 279, 5288–5297.doi: 10.1074/jbc.M311862200

Bagchi, S., Baomar, H. A., Al-Walai, S., Al-Sadi, S., and Fredriksson, R. (2014). Histological analysis of SLC38A6 (SNAT6) expression in mouse brain shows selective expression in excitatory neurons with high expression in the synapses. *PLoS ONE* 9:e95438. doi: 10.1371/journal.pone.0095438

Bak, L. K., Schousboe, A., and Waagepetersen, H. S. (2006). The glutamate/GABA-glutamine cycle: aspects of transport, neurotransmitter homeostasis and ammonia transfer. *J. Neurochem.* 98, 641–653. doi: 10.1111/j.1471-4159.2006.03913.x

Barbosa-Tessmann, I. P., Chen, C., Zhong, C., Siu, F., Schuster, S. M., Nick, H. S., et al. (2000). Activation of the human asparagine synthetase gene by the amino acid response and the endoplasmic reticulum stress response pathways occurs by common genomic elements. *J. Biol. Chem.* 275, 26976–26985. doi: 10.1074/jbc.M000004200

Bhutia, Y. D., Babu, E., Ramachandran, S., and Ganapathy, V. (2015). Amino acid transporters in cancer and their relevance to "glutamine addiction": novel targets for the design of a new class of anticancer drugs. *Cancer Res.* 75, 1782–1788. doi: 10.1158/0008-5472.CAN-14-3745

Bixel, M. G., Yoshiharu, S., Susan, M. H., and Bernd, H. (2001). Distribution of key enzymes of branched-chain amino acid metabolism in glial and neuronal cells in culture. *J. Histochem. Cytochem.* 49, 407–418. doi: 10.1177/002215540104900314

Boulland, J. L., Rafiki, A., Levy, L. M., Storm-Mathisen, J., and Chaudhry, F. A. (2003). Highly differential expression of SN1, a bidirectional glutamine transporter, in astroglia and endothelium in the developing rat brain. *Glia* 41, 260–275. doi: 10.1002/glia.10188

Bröer, A., Rahimi, F., and Broer, S. (2016). Deletion of amino acid transporter ASCT2 (SLC1A5) reveals an essential role for transporters SNAT1 (SLC38A1) and SNAT2 (SLC38A2) to sustain glutaminolysis in cancer cells. *J. Biol. Chem.* 291, 13194–13205. doi: 10.1074/jbc.M115.700534

Bröer, S. (2014). The SLC38 family of sodium-amino acid co-transporters. *Pflugers Arch.* 466, 155–172. doi: 10.1007/s00424-013-1393-y

Bröer, S., and Gether, U. (2012). The solute carrier 6 family of transporters. *Br. J. Pharmacol.* 167, 256–278. doi: 10.1111/j.1476-5381.2012.01975.x

Bruhat, A., Averous, J., Carraro, V., Zhong, C., Reimold, A. M., Kilberg, M. S., et al. (2002). Differences in the molecular mechanisms involved in the transcriptional activation of the CHOP and asparagine synthetase genes in response to amino acid deprivation or activation of the unfolded protein response. *J. Biol. Chem.* 277, 48107–48114. doi: 10.1074/jbc.M206149200

Cubelos, B., Gonzalez-Gonzalez, I. M., Gimenez, C., and Zafra, F. (2005). Amino acid transporter SNAT5 localizes to glial cells in the rat brain. *Glia* 49, 230–244. doi: 10.1002/glia.20106

Deval, C., Chaveroux, C., Maurin, A. C., Cherasse, Y., Parry, L., Carraro, V., et al. (2009). Amino acid limitation regulates the expression of genes involved in several specific biological processes through GCN2-dependent and GCN2-independent pathways. *FEBS J.* 276, 707–718. doi: 10.1111/j.1742-4658.2008.06818.x

Efeyan, A., Comb, W. C., and Sabatini, D. M. (2015). Nutrient-sensing mechanisms and pathways. *Nature* 517, 302–310. doi: 10.1038/nature14190

Fafournoux, P., Bruhat, A., and Jousse, C. (2000). Amino acid regulation of gene expression. *Biochem. J.* 351, 1–12. doi: 10.1042/bj3510001

Gaccioli, F., Huang, C. C., Wang, C., Bevilacqua, E., Franchi-Gazzola, R., Gazzola, G. C., et al. (2006). Amino acid starvation induces the SNAT2 neutral amino acid transporter by a mechanism that involves eukaryotic initiation factor 2α phosphorylation and cap-independent translation. *J. Biol. Chem.* 281, 17929–17940. doi: 10.1074/jbc.M600341200

Gallinetti, J., Harputlugil, E., and Mitchell, J. R. (2013). Amino acid sensing in dietary-restriction-mediated longevity: roles of signal-transducing kinases GCN2 and TOR. *Biochem. J.* 449, 1–10. doi: 10.1042/BJ20121098

González-González, I. M., Cubelos, B., Gimenez, C., and Zafra, F. (2005). Immunohistochemical localization of the amino acid transporter SNAT2 in the rat brain. *Neuroscience* 130, 61–73. doi: 10.1016/j.neuroscience.2004.09.023

Hägglund, M. G., Hellsten, S. V., Bagchi, S., Philippot, G., Lofqvist, E., Nilsson, V. C., et al. (2015). Transport of L-glutamine, L-alanine, L-arginine and L-histidine by the neuron-specific Slc38a8 (SNAT8) in CNS. *J. Mol. Biol.* 427, 1495–1512. doi: 10.1016/j.jmb.2014.10.016

Hägglund, M. G., Sreedharan, S., Nilsson, V. C., Shaik, J. H., Almkvist, I. M., Backlin, S., et al. (2011). Identification of SLC38A7 (SNAT7) protein as a glutamine transporter expressed in neurons. *J. Biol. Chem.* 286, 20500–20511. doi: 10.1074/jbc.M110.162404

Harding, H. P., Novoa, I., Zhang, Y., Zeng, H., Wek, R., Schapira, M., et al. (2000). Regulated translation initiation controls stress-induced gene expression in mammalian cells. *Mol. Cell* 6, 1099–1108. doi: 10.1016/S1097-2765(00)00108-8

Hediger, M. A., Clemencon, B., Burrier, R. E., and Bruford, E. A. (2013). The ABCs of membrane transporters in health and disease (SLC series): introduction. *Mol. Aspects Med.* 34, 95–107. doi: 10.1016/j.mam.2012.12.009

Hediger, M. A., Romero, M. F., Peng, J. B., Rolfs, A., Takanaga, H., and Bruford, E. A. (2004). The ABCs of solute carriers: physiological, pathological and therapeutic implications of human membrane transport proteinsIntroduction. *Pflugers Arch.* 447, 465–468. doi: 10.1007/s00424-003-1192-y

Hellsten, S. V., Eriksson, M. M., Lekholm, E., Arapi, V., Perland, E., and Fredriksson, R. (2017a). The gene expression of the neuronal protein, SLC38A9, changes in mouse brain after *in vivo* starvation and high-fat diet. *PLoS ONE* 12:e0172917. doi: 10.1371/journal.pone.0172917

Hellsten, S. V., Hagglund, M. G., Eriksson, M. M., and Fredriksson, R. (2017b). The neuronal and astrocytic protein SLC38A10 transports glutamine, glutamate, and aspartate, suggesting a role in neurotransmission. *FEBS Open Biol.* 7, 730–746. doi: 10.1002/2211-5463.12219

Hellsten, S. V., Lekholm, E., Ahmad, T., and Fredriksson, R. (2017c). The gene expression of numerous SLC transporters is altered in the immortalized hypothalamic cell line N25/2 following amino acid starvation. *FEBS Open Biol.* 7, 249–264. doi: 10.1002/2211-5463.12181

Hundal, H. S., and Taylor, P. M. (2009). Amino acid transceptors: gate keepers of nutrient exchange and regulators of nutrient signaling. *Am. J. Physiol. Endocrinol. Metab.* 296, E603–E613. doi: 10.1152/ajpendo.91002.2008

Hyde, R., Taylor, P. M., and Hundal, H. S. (2003). Amino acid transporters: roles in amino acid sensing and signalling in animal cells. *Biochem. J.* 373, 1–18. doi: 10.1042/bj20030405

Jewell, J. L., Russell, R. C., and Guan, K. L. (2013). Amino acid signalling upstream of mTOR. *Nat. Rev. Mol. Cell. Biol.* 14, 133–139. doi: 10.1038/nrm3522

Jung, J., Genau, H. M., and Behrends, C. (2015). Amino acid-dependent mTORC1 regulation by the lysosomal membrane protein SLC38A9. *Mol. Cell. Biol.* 35, 2479–2494. doi: 10.1128/MCB.00125-15

Kilberg, M. S., Pan, Y. X., Chen, H., and Leung-Pineda, V. (2005). Nutritional control of gene expression: how mammalian cells respond to amino acid limitation. *Annu. Rev. Nutr.* 25, 59–85. doi: 10.1146/annurev.nutr.24.012003.132145

Laplante, M., and Sabatini, D. M. (2012). mTOR signaling in growth control and disease. *Cell* 149, 274–293. doi: 10.1016/j.cell.2012.03.017

Lieth, E., LaNoue, K. F., Berkich, D. A., Xu, B., Ratz, M., Taylor, C., et al. (2001). Nitrogen shuttling between neurons and glial cells during glutamate synthesis. *J. Neurochem.* 76, 1712–1723. doi: 10.1046/j.1471-4159.2001.00156.x

Mackenzie, B., Schafer, M. K., Erickson, J. D., Hediger, M. A., Weihe, E., and Varoqui, H. (2003). Functional properties and cellular distribution of the system A glutamine transporter SNAT1 support specialized roles in central neurons. *J. Biol. Chem.* 278, 23720–23730. doi: 10.1074/jbc.M212718200

Novak, D., Quiggle, F., and Haafiz, A. (2006). Impact of forskolin and amino acid depletion upon system a activity and SNAT expression in BeWo cells. *Biochimie* 88, 39–44. doi: 10.1016/j.biochi.2005.07.002

Palii, S. S., Thiaville, M. M., Pan, Y. X., Zhong, C., and Kilberg, M. S. (2006). Characterization of the amino acid response element within the human sodium-coupled neutral amino acid transporter 2 (SNAT2) system a transporter gene. *Biochem. J.* 395, 517–527. doi: 10.1042/BJ20051867

Perland, E., Hellsten, S. V., Lekholm, E., Eriksson, M. M., Arapi, V., and Fredriksson, R. (2017). The novel membrane-bound proteins MFSD1 and MFSD3 are putative SLC transporters affected by altered nutrient intake. *J. Mol. Neurosci.* 61, 199–214. doi: 10.1007/s12031-016-0867-8

Rebsamen, M., Pochini, L., Stasyk, T., de Araujo, M. E., Galluccio, M., Kandasamy, R. K., et al. (2015). SLC38A9 is a component of the lysosomal amino acid sensing machinery that controls mTORC1. *Nature* 519, 477–481. doi: 10.1038/nature14107

Scalise, M., Pochini, L., Galluccio, M., and Indiveri, C. (2016). Glutamine transport. from energy supply to sensing and beyond. *Biochim. Biophys. Acta* 1857, 1147–1157. doi: 10.1016/j.bbabio.2016.03.006

Schiöth, H. B., Roshanbin, S., Hagglund, M. G., and Fredriksson, R. (2013). Evolutionary origin of amino acid transporter families SLC32, SLC36 and SLC38 and physiological, pathological and therapeutic aspects. *Mol. Aspects Med.* 34, 571–585. doi: 10.1016/j.mam.2012.07.012

Schousboe, A. (2018). Metabolic signaling in the brain and the role of astrocytes in control of glutamate and GABA neurotransmission. *Neurosci. Lett.* doi: 10.1016/j.neulet.2018.01.038. [Epub ahead of print].

Solbu, T. T., Bjorkmo, M., Berghuis, P., Harkany, T., and Chaudhry, F. A. (2010). SAT1, a glutamine transporter, is preferentially expressed in GABAergic neurons. *Front. Neuroanat.* 4:1. doi: 10.3389/neuro.05.001.2010

Sundberg, B. E., Waag, E., Jacobsson, J. A., Stephansson, O., Rumaks, J., Svirskis, S., et al. (2008). The evolutionary history and tissue mapping of amino acid transporters belonging to solute carrier families SLC32, SLC36, and SLC38. *J. Mol. Neurosci.* 35, 179–193. doi: 10.1007/s12031-008-9046-x

Taylor, P. M. (2014). Role of amino acid transporters in amino acid sensing. *Am. J. Clin. Nutr.* 99, 223S–230S. doi: 10.3945/ajcn.113.070086

Verdon, Q., Boonen, M., Ribes, C., Jadot, M., Gasnier, B., and Sagne, C. (2017). SNAT7 is the primary lysosomal glutamine exporter required for extracellular protein-dependent growth of cancer cells. *Proc. Natl. Acad. Sci. U.S.A.* 114, E3602–E3611. doi: 10.1073/pnas.1617066114

Wang, S., Tsun, Z. Y., Wolfson, R. L., Shen, K., Wyant, G. A., Plovanich, M. E., et al. (2015). Metabolism. lysosomal amino acid transporter SLC38A9 signals arginine sufficiency to mTORC1. *Science* 347, 188–194. doi: 10.1126/science.1257132

Yao, D., Mackenzie, B., Ming, H., Varoqui, H., Zhu, H., Hediger, M. A., et al. (2000). A novel system A isoform mediating Na+/neutral amino acid cotransport. *J. Biol. Chem.* 275, 22790–22797. doi: 10.1074/jbc.M002965200

Zhang, P., McGrath, B. C., Reinert, J., Olsen, D. S., Lei, L., Gill, S., et al. (2002). The GCN2 eIF2α kinase is required for adaptation to amino acid deprivation in mice. *Mol. Cell. Biol.* 22, 6681–6688. doi: 10.1128/MCB.22.19.6681-6688.2002

9

The Physiopathological Role of the Exchangers Belonging to the SLC37 Family

Anna Rita Cappello†, Rosita Curcio†, Rosamaria Lappano, Marcello Maggiolini and Vincenza Dolce*

Department of Pharmacy, Health and Nutritional Sciences, University of Calabria, Rende, Italy

***Correspondence:**
Marcello Maggiolini
marcellomaggiolini@yahoo.it;
marcello.maggiolini@unical.it

†These authors have contributed equally to this work.

The human *SLC37* gene family includes four proteins SLC37A1-4, localized in the endoplasmic reticulum (ER) membrane. They have been grouped into the SLC37 family due to their sequence homology to the bacterial organophosphate/phosphate (Pi) antiporter. SLC37A1-3 are the less characterized isoforms. SLC37A1 and SLC37A2 are Pi-linked glucose-6-phosphate (G6P) antiporters, catalyzing both homologous (Pi/Pi) and heterologous (G6P/Pi) exchanges, whereas SLC37A3 transport properties remain to be clarified. Furthermore, SLC37A1 is highly homologous to the bacterial glycerol 3-phosphate permeases, so it is supposed to transport also glycerol-3-phosphate. The physiological role of SLC37A1-3 is yet to be further investigated. SLC37A1 seems to be required for lipid biosynthesis in cancer cell lines, *SLC37A2* has been proposed as a vitamin D and a phospho-progesterone receptor target gene, while mutations in the *SLC37A3* gene appear to be associated with congenital hyperinsulinism of infancy. SLC37A4, also known as glucose-6-phosphate translocase (G6PT), transports G6P from the cytoplasm into the ER lumen, working in complex with either glucose-6-phosphatase-α (G6Pase-α) or G6Pase-β to hydrolyze intraluminal G6P to Pi and glucose. G6PT and G6Pase-β are ubiquitously expressed, whereas G6Pase-α is specifically expressed in the liver, kidney and intestine. G6PT/G6Pase-α complex activity regulates fasting blood glucose levels, whereas G6PT/G6Pase-β is required for neutrophil functions. G6PT deficiency is responsible for glycogen storage disease type Ib (GSD-Ib), an autosomal recessive disorder associated with both defective metabolic and myeloid phenotypes. Several kinds of mutations have been identified in the *SLC37A4* gene, affecting G6PT function. An increased autoimmunity risk for GSD-Ib patients has also been reported, moreover, SLC37A4 seems to be involved in autophagy.

Keywords: SLC37A1-4, endoplasmic reticulum, glucose-6-phosphate translocase, G6PT deficiency, glycogen storage disease type Ib

INTRODUCTION

The SLC37 family belongs to the largest human solute-carrier (SLC) superfamily, comprising more than 52 gene families, and over 400 membrane-bound proteins catalyzing the transport of metabolites across biological membranes (He et al., 2009; Perland and Fredriksson, 2017).

So far, four isoforms have been identified, named SLC37A1-4 (Bartoloni and Antonarakis, 2004; Chou and Mansfield, 2014). They are transmembrane proteins located in the endoplasmic reticulum (ER) membrane (Pan et al., 2011), and have been grouped into the SLC37 family due to their sequence homology to the bacterial organophosphate/phosphate (Pi) antiporter (Pao et al., 1998). Moreover, in the membrane transporter classification system included in the transport classification database, SLC37 carriers are reported to belong to the OPA family, classified as 2.A.1.4 (http://www.tcdb.org/). SLC37A1-4 translocases are also called sugar-phosphate exchangers SPX1-4 (Bartoloni et al., 2000; Takahashi et al., 2000; Bartoloni and Antonarakis, 2004), and are predicted to consist of 10–12 transmembrane domains (Chou and Mansfield, 2014).

SLC37A1, SLC37A2, and SLC37A4 are Pi-linked glucose-6-phosphate (G6P) antiporters, catalyzing both homologous (Pi/Pi) and heterologous (G6P/Pi) exchanges, and are inhibited to a very different extend by cholorogenic acid, while SLC37A3 transport activity is yet to be determinated (Chen et al., 2008; Pan et al., 2011).

SLC37A1, SLC37A2, and SLC37A3 are the less characterized SLC37 family members (Chou and Mansfield, 2014). SLC37A1 gene appears to be involved in breast (Iacopetta et al., 2010) and colorectal (Kikuchi et al., 2018) cancers. *SLC37A2* has been recently proposed as a vitamin D (Wilfinger et al., 2014; Saksa et al., 2015) and a phospho-progesterone receptor (Knutson et al., 2017) target gene. Moreover, in obese murine models its expression seems to be related to chronic inflammation that supports metabolic syndrome (Kim et al., 2007). In dairy cattle, a *SLC37A2* mutation appears to be responsible for increased female infertility due to embryonic death (Fritz et al., 2013; Reinartz and Dist, 2016). The *SLC37A3* gene has been possibly related to congenital hyperinsulinemia (Proverbio et al., 2013). Furthermore, this gene seems to be involved in epigenetic modifications, because its methylation level depends on fasting glucose blood levels, at least after a significant weight loss (Benton et al., 2015). SLC37A4, also known as glucose-6-phosphate translocase (G6PT), is the more extensively studied isoform, and is a member of the multicomponent glucose-6-phosphatase system (G6Pase-system). In the liver and kidney, the activity of this complex is required to maintain blood glucose homeostasis (Bartoloni and Antonarakis, 2004). Additionally, it supports neutrophil and macrophage functions (Chou and Mansfield, 2014).

In the past, G6Pase-system was believed to consist of a glucose-6-phosphatase, with its active site facing the ER lumen, and three translocases (known as T1-3). In detail, T1 mediated G6P import through the ER membrane, whereas T2 and T3 catalyzed Pi and glucose efflux from the ER cavity, respectively (Gerin et al., 2001). Moreover, the presence of a regulatory 21 kDa hepatic microsomal glucose-6-phosphatase stabilizing protein (SP) was also hypothesized (Burchell et al., 1985). The existence of T2, T3, and SP has never been proven.

Based on recent scientific literature, T1 corresponds to G6PT, and it works in complex with either glucose-6-phosphatase-α (G6Pase-α, also called G6PC1) or glucose-6-phosphatase-β (G6Pase-β, known as G6PC3; Chou et al., 2002).

G6Pase-α is specifically expressed in the liver, kidney, and intestine, and it hydrolyzes intraluminal G6P to Pi and glucose, then this sugar exits the cell and enters the bloodstream to maintain interprandial blood glucose homeostasis (Chou and Mansfield, 2014).

G6PT deficiency is responsible for glycogen storage disease type Ib (GSD-Ib, OMIM232220), whereas G6Pase-α impairment causes GSD type Ia (GSD-Ia, OMIM232200) (Chou et al., 2010a,b). Both disorders prevent the final steps of gluconeogenesis and glycogenolysis; as a result, endogenous glucose production is severely compromised creating metabolic impairment, consisting of fasting hypoglycemia, hyperlipidemia, hyperuricemia, lactic acidemia, growth retardation, and amassing of glycogen and fat in the liver and kidneys, causing hepatomegaly and nephromegaly, respectively (Chou et al., 2002, 2010b).

In neutrophils, G6PT is functionally coupled to the ubiquitous G6Pase-β, in order to support neutrophil and macrophage functions (Chou et al., 2010a,b; Jun et al., 2010). G6Pase-β deficiency results in severe congenital neutropenia (Boztug et al., 2009). This condition has been considered as a glycogen storage disease I related syndrome (GSD-Irs, OMIM 612541).

Unlike GSD-Ia, both GSD-Irs (Cheung et al., 2007; Jun et al., 2010; McDermott et al., 2010) and GSD-Ib (Kim et al., 2008; Jun et al., 2014) can cause neutropenia and myeloid dysfunction.

In this review, we focus on the physiopathological role of the SLC37A family members, in particular on the best characterized G6PT, highlighting its role in autophagy, an increased autoimmunity risk for GSD-Ib patients, as well as new promising therapeutic strategies for GSD-Ib.

SLC37A1 FAMILY MEMBER

The human SLC37A1 protein, also knows as SPX1, is encoded by the *SLC37A1* gene (NM_018964), mapped to chromosome 21q22.3, and containing 19 coding exons and 7 untranslated exons. Alternative splicing origins different transcripts, although the predicted protein sequence is identical, consisting of 533 amino acids, with a calculated molecular weight of 58 kDa (Bartoloni et al., 2000). This latter contains a mitochondrial cleavage site, as well as both N- and C-terminal ER signals for the ER retention (Bartoloni et al., 2000). This protein displays 59, 35, and 22% sequence identity with the human SLC37A2, SLC37A3 and SLC37A4 proteins, respectively (Chou et al., 2013), and it is 86% identical to its mouse homolog (Bartoloni and Antonarakis,

Abbreviations: AMPK, 5′ AMP-activated protein kinase; ATG, autophagy-related gene; CBA, chicken β-actin; CRC, colorectal cancer; WAT, white adipose tissue; CHI, congenital hyperinsulinism of infancy; Tconvs, conventional T cells; FOXP3, forkhead box P3; G6Pase-α, promoter/enhancer GPE; G6Pase-system, glucose-6-phosphatase system; G6PT, glucose-6-phosphate translocase; GSD-I, glycogen storage disease type I; G-CSF, granulocyte colony-stimulating factor; HIF-1α, hypoxia-inducible transcriptional factor-1α; IBD, inflammatory bowel disease; mTORC1, mammalian target of rapamycin complex 1; miGT, minimal G6PT promoter/enhancer; OPA, organophosphate/phosphate antiporter; PPAR-γ, peroxisome proliferator-activated receptor-γ; phospho-Ser294 PR, phospho-Ser294 progesterone receptor; CMV, cytomegalovirus; rAAV, recombinant adeno-associated virus; Tregs, regulatory T cells; RUNX2, runt-related transcription factor 2; SLC, solute-carrier; SP, stabilizing protein; SPX, sugar-phosphate exchangers; TCR, T cell receptor; ULK1, unc-51 like autophagy activating kinase 1; VDR, vitamin D receptor.

2004). SLC37A1 and SLC37A2 isoforms are the most related, while all the remaining pairwise sequence comparisons between the other SLC37 family members show lower sequence identity; hence, it is feasible that they might have had an independent evolution.

The human SLC37A1 protein shares 30 and 71% sequence identity to bacterial GlpT and *Mus musculus* SLC37A2, respectively (Takahashi et al., 2000); suggesting that mammalian SLC37A1 could be able to transport glycerol-3-phosphate (G3P), probably catalyzing an heterologous G3P/Pi exchange; therefore its gene was also called G3PP (Bartoloni et al., 2000).

A G3P transport activity has never been demonstrated, althought SLC37A1 association with glycolipid metabolism has been suggested (Bartoloni and Antonarakis, 2004; Dolce et al., 2011). The hypothetical role of SLC37A1 as a G3P exchanger has been postulated in cancer cells (Iacopetta et al., 2010). In details, in estrogen receptor (ESR) negative SkBr3 breast cancer cells (Lappano et al., 2017), as well as in ESR positive endometrial Ishikawa tumor cells, the expression of the SLC37A1 transcript was proven to be upregulated by the epidermal growth factor (EGF), through the EGF receptor/mitogen-activated protein kinase/Fos transduction pathway. Notably, in the same work the SLC37A1 protein localization in the ER was also demonstrated, supporting the hypothesis that this protein could import G3P into the ER lumen to sustain phospholipid biosynthesis, required to promote cancer progression (Iacopetta et al., 2010).

The functional role of SLC37A1 was also investigated in other human diseases. Analyses led in patients affected by glycerol kinase deficiency-like syndrome, with glyceroluria but lacking mutations in the human glycerol kinase gene, found only non-pathogenetic sequence variants in the human *SLC37A1* gene, excluding its implication in this defect (Bartoloni et al., 2000).

Furthermore, this gene critically maps to autosomal recessive nonsyndromic deafness locus (DFNB10), on chromosome 21q22.3, but its involvement in the pathogenesis of this disease was also excluded by mutational analysis (Bartoloni et al., 2000).

More recently, *SLC37A1* upregulation (at the mRNA and protein levels) was found in patients with colorectal cancer (CRC), and it was associated with positive venous invasion, liver metastasis, and poor patient outcomes (Kikuchi et al., 2018). Moreover, in a colon cancer cell line, LS180, *SLC37A1* upregulation was positively correlated to Sialyl Lewis A and Sialyl Lewis X levels. These carbohydrate antigens are ligands for the adhesion molecule E selectin, and are responsible for the adhesion of cancer cells to the endothelium during metastasis, which is a typical process of cancer progression (Bartella et al., 2016; Iacopetta et al., 2017). Their positive modulation suggests that *SLC37A1* might play a key role in the hematogenous metastasis of CRC, even if the underlying mechanisms remain unclear (Kikuchi et al., 2018).

Currently, it is proven that SLC37A1 can catalyze both heterologous G6P/Pi and homologous Pi/Pi exchanges, but it is poorly sensitive to chlorogenic acid and is not functionally coupled to G6Pases. On this basis, it is unlikely that it is involved in blood glucose homeostasis (Pan et al., 2011), so its physiological role remains to be clarified.

SLC37A1 mRNA is ubiquitously expressed, although mainly in adult kidney, spleen, liver, small intestine, bone marrow, as well as in fetal liver, brain, and spleen (Bartoloni et al., 2000). In the main gluconeogenetic organs, liver, and kidney, the relative SLC37A1 transcript levels are rather low with respect to the SLC37A4 levels, since they represent <2%, whereas in the intestine and pancreas they constitute 60 and 69%, respectively, of those observed for SLC37A4 (Pan et al., 2011). In macrophages, the SLC37A1 transcript level is 43% of that found for SLC37A4, while in neutrophils, it is markedly (about 280 %) higher, suggesting that SLC37A1 might have a key role in such cells (Chou and Mansfield, 2014).

SLC37A2 FAMILY MEMBER

SLC37A2, also knows as SPX2, was firstly identified in a work, conducted on mice and aimed to detect cAMP inducible genes playing a role in promoting cholesterol efflux from the macrophage cell line RAW264 via apoE and apoA1 (Takahashi et al., 2000). Two murine transcripts were identified, originated by the use of alternative polyadenylation sites. Both transcripts are highly expressed in bone marrow derived macrophages, and encode a 510 amino-acid protein with a predicted molecular weight of 55 kDa (Takahashi et al., 2000).

A further study showed that *SLC37A2* is abundantly expressed in murine macrophages, spleen and thymus, as well as in white adipose tissue (WAT) of genetically obese mouse models, since WAT is subject to considerable macrophage infiltrations, and this promotes obesity-associated chronic inflammation underlying metabolic syndrome and other comorbidities of obesity (Kim et al., 2007). The murine SLC37A2 protein undergoes post-translational modifications by N-linked glycosylation, and it migrates as a heterogeneous species of 50–75 kDa (Kim et al., 2007).

The human SLC37A2 protein is encoded by the *SLC37A2* gene (NM_198277), mapped to chromosome 11q24.2 and consisting of 18 coding exons. Alternative splicing originates four different transcripts. Only the longest isoform has been characterized (Pan et al., 2011). The corresponding human SLC37A2 transcript is expressed in murine liver, kidney, intestine, and pancreas, however the related expression levels are <4.5% of those found for SLC37A4 (Pan et al., 2011). Noticeably, the SLC37A2 transcript levels increase 46-fold during differentiation of human monocytic leukemia cells (THP-1) to macrophages (Kim et al., 2007).

The human SLC37A2 protein consists of 505 amino acids and displays 59, 36, and 23% sequence identity with the human SLC37A1, SLC37A3, and SLC37A4 proteins, respectively (Chou et al., 2013). Moreover, it is 90% identical to its mouse homolog (Bartoloni and Antonarakis, 2004). Like the murine protein, also the human protein is post-translationally modified by N-linked glycosylation.

The SLC37A2 protein is able to catalyze both G6P/Pi and Pi/Pi exchanges (Pan et al., 2011). Similarly to SLC37A1, the SLC37A2 transport activity is poorly sensitive to chlorogenic acid and the protein is not functionally coupled to G6Pases, as well as it seems not to be involved in blood glucose homeostasis (Pan et al., 2011). Hence, the functional role of SLC37A2 is yet to be understood. Recently, *SLC37A2* has been found as a vitamin D target gene (Wilfinger et al., 2014; Saksa et al., 2015). Vitamin D_3 may affect gene regulation via the binding of its metabolite, 1α,25-dihydroxyvitamin D_3 (1,25$(OH)_2D_3$), to the transcription factor vitamin D receptor (VDR). In monocytic and macrophage-like cells, the human *SLC37A2* gene contains a conserved VDR-binding site allowing such modulation, although only in monocytic cells *SLC37A2* is an early responding target gene, potentially useful as a biomarker of vitamin D_3 status in the hematopoietic system (Wilfinger et al., 2014). In addition, in human peripheral blood mononuclear cells, changes in the expression of the *SLC37A2* gene, together with those of other primary vitamin D target genes, are systematically associated with the alteration in the circulating form of vitamin D_3. Remarkably, during vitamin D_3 supplementation in pre-diabetic subjects those features allow a distinction into high and low responder patients (Saksa et al., 2015).

Remarkably, in dairy cattle a deleterious homozygous mutation (g.28879810C>T) was detected in an aborted fetus. This mutation was predicted to introduce a premature stop codon, strongly impairing protein structure, and it was believed to be responsible for embryonic lethality (Reinartz and Dist, 2016). The same mutation, leading to embryonic lethal defects with increased female infertility was also detected in another study (Fritz et al., 2013).

Considering that the *SLC37A2* gene carries a VDR binding site, and that vitamin D_3 may be involved in many biological pathways, such as calcium and phosphate homeostasis, cell growth, intracellular metabolism, as well as innate and adaptive immunity, embryonic death could depend on a deficit in such processes (Reinartz and Dist, 2016).

Recently, human *SLC37A2* has also been proposed as a phospho-Ser294 progesterone receptor (phospho-Ser294 PR) target gene (Knutson et al., 2017). PR Ser294 phosphorylation is a common event in breast cancer progression, and its activity is significantly associated with invasive lobular carcinoma. The runt-related transcription factor 2 (RUNX2) is an osteoblast differentiation transcription factor expressed in developing breast epithelial cells; it appears to be required in the regulation of phospho-Ser294 PR target genes. In this regard, human *SLC37A2* represents a good candidate as target gene, because it is expressed in monocytes, as well as in breast and cervical tissues, and it was found to contain multiple RUNX2 binding motifs immediately upstream and within the gene; moreover, its expression is proven to be upregulated by progestin in multiple cell line models (Knutson et al., 2017).

SLC37A3 FAMILY MEMBER

The human SLC37A3 protein, also knows as SPX3, is the less characterized SLC37 family member. It is encoded by the *SLC37A3* gene (NM_207113), mapped to chromosome 7q34 and containing 17 coding exons. Alternative splicing originates three different transcripts (Bartoloni and Antonarakis, 2004).

One isoform, consisting of 494 amino acids, displays 35, 36, and 22% sequence identity with the human SLC37A1, SLC37A2, and SLC37A4 proteins, respectively (Chou et al., 2013), and it is 90% identical to its mouse and rat homologs (Bartoloni and Antonarakis, 2004). Even though SLC37A3 is an ER-associated protein, it fails to show an uptake activity (Pan et al., 2011), hence its functional properties remain to be clarified. Remarkably, the SLC37A3 transcript is extremely expressed in murine neutrophils, pancreas, and, to a lesser extent, in the liver, kidney, intestine, and macrophages (Pan et al., 2011; Chou et al., 2013), suggesting a possible functional role in the immune system and pancreas (Chou and Mansfield, 2014). In this latter regard, the human *SLC37A3* gene could contribute to the pathogenesis of congenital hyperinsulinism of infancy (CHI). In detail, a mutation in this gene was found in one patient with CHI in which the molecular basis of the disease remained unknown, highligting that it could be responsible for the dysregulation of insulin secretion (Proverbio et al., 2013), even if the biological role of SLC37A3 in pancreatic insulin secretion has never been clarified.

More recently, epigenetic mechanisms were demonstrated to modify the human *SLC37A3* gene, since a robust correlation between change in fasting glucose and DNA methylation level within the human *SLC37A3* gene was found in subcutaneous adipose, after gastric bypass followed by a significant weight loss (Benton et al., 2015). This could suggest a possible involvement of SLC37A3 in obesity-related metabolic dysfunction.

SLC37A4 FAMILY MEMBER

SLC37A4 is the best functionally characterized SLC37 family member (Chen et al., 2000, 2002, 2008). The human protein is encoded by a single copy gene, *SLC37A4* (NM_001467, OMIM 602671), mapped to chromosome 11q23 (Annabi et al., 1998), containing nine coding exons (Marcolongo et al., 1998; Gerin et al., 1999; Hiraiwa et al., 1999), and firstly isolated from a human bladder tumor cDNA library (Gerin et al., 1997).

This protein displays 20, 25, and 26% sequence identity with bacterial protein UhpT, GlpT, and UhpC, respectively (Gerin et al., 1997). UhpT and GlpT are OPAs (Maloney and Wilson, 1996), while UhpC is a putative G6P receptor controlling UhpT expression (Island et al., 1992).

SLC37A4 protein is scarcely related to the other SLC37 family members, as it shares 22% amino acid sequence homology with both SLC37A1 and SLC37A3, and it is 23% homologous to SLC37A2 (Chou et al., 2013). The human SLC37A4 protein is highly conserved in other species. Murine and rat homologous proteins share 98% sequence homology, as well as 95 and 93% sequence homology to the human protein, respectively (Lin et al., 1998). Two human tissue-specific splicing isoforms have been identified, because alternative splicing of exon 7 leads to the expression of two transcripts, G6PT and variant G6PT (vG6PT), differing by the inclusion of a 66-bp exon 7 sequence in vG6PT, and encoding proteins of 429 and 451 amino acids, respectively (Gerin et al., 1997; Hiraiwa et al., 1999; Lin et al., 2000). Human vG6PT contains 22 additional amino acids, and it is active in microsomal G6P transport; it has been detected in the brain, heart and skeletal muscle (Lin et al., 2000). G6PT mRNA is ubiquitously expressed, although at the highest levels in the liver, kidney, intestine (Lin et al., 1998; Pan et al., 2011), and in haematopoietic progenitor cells (Ihara et al., 2000). The physiological implications of those different expression patterns remain unclear. In this regard, inclusion of exon 7 sequence might increase vG6PT sensitivity for degradation, since in mouse models the turnover rate of vG6PT seems to be increased during myogenesis of muscle cells (Shieh et al., 2007). Both G6PT and vG6PT appear to be similarly active in G6P transport (Lin et al., 2000), although the majority of studies used G6PT.

Human G6PT is a hydrophobic protein whose transmembrane topology has been long debated. Hydropathy profile analysis predicted either 10 (Hoffman and Stoffel, 1993) or 12 transmembrane domains (Gerin et al., 1997). Protease protection and glycosylation scanning assays suggested a 10-transmembrane domains model, with both N- and C-termini protruding on the cytoplasmic side of the ER membrane (Pan et al., 1999). Conversely, homology modeling proposed a model containing 12 transmembrane α-helices (Almqvist et al., 2004). More recently, glycosylation scanning and protease sensitivity studies have indicated that the 10-domains model is more probable (Pan et al., 2009).

G6PT biological function is to translocate G6P from the cytoplasm into the ER lumen, where it is hydrolyzed to glucose and Pi either by G6Pase-α (Lei et al., 1996; Chou et al., 2010a,b) or by G6Pase-β (Shieh et al., 2003; Chou et al., 2010a,b).

In the past, only one G6Pase isoform was known, expressed exclusively in the liver, kidney and intestine (Lin et al., 1998). In 2003, a second isoform, ubiquitously expressed, was discovered and called G6Pase-β (Shieh et al., 2003). Consequently, the original isoform was renamed G6Pase-α. Both proteins are transmembrane phosphohydrolases essential for the last step of gluconeogenesis. They have similar topology (Pan et al., 1998; Shieh et al., 2003) and mechanism of action as regards G6P hydrolysis (Ghosh et al., 2002, 2004); their active sites are located inside the ER lumen, hence both enzymes require to be coupled with a functional G6PT to hydrolyze intraluminal G6P. On the other hand, G6Pase activity is required in turn for an efficient G6P transport (Lei et al., 1996).

Since G6PT is ubiquitous, tissue expression profiles of G6Pase-α or G6Pase-β, and the resulting G6PT/G6Pase complexes, reflect the different GSD-Ia, -Ib or -Irs phenotypes.

On this basis, when the G6PT/G6Pase-α complex is present in the main gluconeogenic organs (liver, kidney, and intestine), G6Pase-α mutations cause a defective glucose production with impaired blood glucose homeostasis between meals, that is the first biochemical hallmark of GSD-Ia (Chou et al., 2010a,b).

In neutrophils and macrophages, the G6PT/G6Pase-β complex preserves energy homeostasis and functionality, hence G6Pase-β mutations are responsible for GSD-Irs, an autosomal recessive disorder characterized by neutropenia and neutrophil dysfunction (Chou et al., 2010a,b), often associated with congenital cardiac and uro-genital anomalies (Boztug et al., 2009).

On the other hand, G6PT mutations underlie GSD-Ib, which implies either impaired metabolism as in GSD-Ia, or neutropenia and neutrophil dysfunction as in GSD-Irs (Chou et al., 2010a,b), even if in neutrophils and macrophages G6PT expression levels are rather low (Chou et al., 2013).

PHYSIOPATHOLOGICAL ROLE OF SLC37A4

SLC37A4, known as G6PT or SPX4, is able to catalize both homologous Pi/Pi and heterologous G6P/Pi exchanges between the ER lumen and the cytoplasm (Chen et al., 2008). Early studies led on intact liver microsomes showed that the high specificity of G6PT for G6P is responsible for substrate specificity of the G6PT/G6Pase-α complex, since G6Pase-α is less specific for G6P (Arion et al., 1972, 1975).

G6PT transport activity is specifically and strongly inhibited by chlorogenic acid (Arion et al., 1997, 1998; Hemmerle et al., 1997; Hiraiwa et al., 1999; Chen et al., 2008), acting as a reversible, competitive inhibitor. Also some chlorogenic acid derivatives, S3483 (Arion et al., 1998; Leuzzi et al., 2003), and S4048 (Herling et al., 1999), competitively inhibit G6PT, even more potently than chlorogenic acid. They have been used in studies concerning metabolic impairment in GSD-1 animal models (Bandsma et al., 2001; Grefhorst et al., 2010).

Several studies have established that G6P uptake activity needs not only an active G6PT, but also a functional G6Pase (Lei et al., 1996; Shieh et al., 2003; Chen et al., 2008; Pan et al., 2011). In this regard, hepatic microsomes isolated from G6Pase-α-deficient (GSD-Ia) mice, maintaining a functional G6PT, showed decreased G6P uptake activity, when compared to wild type hepatic microsomes (Lei et al., 1996). Accordingly, in a GSD-Ia mouse model, G6P transport activity could be restored by gene therapy supporting G6Pase-α function (Zingone et al., 2000). On this basis, functional coupling between G6PT and G6Pase-α became evident. A first explanation was suggested considering that G6PT provided the enzyme's substrate by importing cytoplasmic G6P into the ER lumen. Secondly, the physical interaction between G6Pase-α and G6PT, probably mediated by allosteric mechanisms, could support transport activity. This functional coupling was verified achieving functional cell-based activity assays for recombinant G6PT proteins, in order to measure G6P transport activity (Hiraiwa et al., 1999; Chen et al., 2000, 2002, 2008; Pan et al., 2011). According to these studies, it was demonstrated that microsomes expressing a functional G6Pase-α, but lacking an active G6PT (G6Pase-α+/+/G6PT -/-) showed little or no G6P uptake activity. In the same way, microsomes expressing an active G6PT but having a defective G6Pase-α (G6Pase-α -/- /G6PT+/+) exhibited poor G6P uptake rates, and microsomes expressing functional G6Pase-α and G6PT (G6Pase-α+/+/G6PT+/+) had strikingly increased G6P uptake rates (Chou and Mansfield, 2014). Furthermore, using a reconstitution procedure into proteoliposomes (Della Rocca et al., 2015; Curcio et al., 2016) preloaded with Pi, G6PT was proven to be an antiporter able to efficiently exchange G6P/Pi, without needing for a G6Pase-α coexpression (Chen et al.,

2008). Those evidences suggested that G6Pase-α coexpression might increase intraluminal Pi concentration, in order to create a driving Pi gradient, useful for supporting G6PT antiporter activity. Cell-based assays and functional reconstitution into proteoliposomes were also successfully employed to characterize 23 SLC37A4 mutations identified in GSD-Ib patients (Chen et al., 2008).

SLC37A4 AND AUTOPHAGY

Recently, SLC37A4 was identified as a key activator of autophagy pathway, able to negatively regulate mammalian target of rapamycin complex 1 (mTORC1) activity (Ahn et al., 2015). Autophagy is activated under nutrient deficiency to preserve cell homeostasis, and its deficit is associated with several human diseases (Jiang and Mizushima, 2014). Amino acids deprivation induces autophagy by inhibiting mTORC1 (Sancak et al., 2010), conversely, mTORC1 inhibits autophagy by phosphorylating unc-51 like autophagy activating kinase 1 (ULK1) (Jung et al., 2009) and autophagy/beclin-1 regulator 1, in order to ubiquitinate ULK1 for degradation (Nazio et al., 2013). Autophagy can also be triggered by ER stresses (Kouroku et al., 2007) or hypoxia (Bellot et al., 2009). On the other hand, prolonged ER stress leads to the inhibition of autophagy flux (Lee H. et al., 2012). Among the several autophagy-related genes (ATGs), ULK1 plays a key role, since it encodes a serine/threonine kinase essential for the initiation step of autophagy, because it forms complexes that are mainly controlled by mTORC 1 (Ganley et al., 2009) and 5′ AMP-activated protein kinase (AMPK) (Kim et al., 2011).

Among the ATGs encoded proteins, ATG9 is a membrane polypeptide depending on ULK1 activity, that regulates autophagosomes biogenesis by delivering them membrane source derived from the *trans* Golgi network (Young et al., 2006). SLC37A4 seems to promote the initiation step of autophagy acting upstream of mTORC1. In detail, SLC37A4 overexpression increases the interaction between N-terminal Venus-tagged ULK1 (ULK1-VN) and C-terminal Venus-tagged ATG9 (ATG9-VC), improving autophagic flux independent of G6PT transport activity (Ahn et al., 2015).

Previous studies demonstrated that G6PT-mTORC1 signaling is essential in promoting autophagy in hepatic cell lines, in addition, mTORC1 failure is often related to metabolic diseases, including type 2 diabetes and cancer (Zoncu et al., 2011). In this regard, it was proposed that this translocase could affect mTORC1 function through calcium mobilization (Chen et al., 2003). Furthermore, it was also suggested that G6PT could modulate mTORC1 through AMPK, which in turn is an energy sensor activated in response to augmented cellular AMP, ADP or calcium levels (Mihaylova and Shaw, 2011). Since AMPK can regulate autophagy through either direct ULK1 phosphorylation or mTORC1 inhibition (Hawley et al., 2005), disruption of calcium mobilization due to SLC37A4 dysfunction might influence both AMPK and mTORC1, leading to autophagy inhibition (Ahn et al., 2015).

SLC37A4 DEFECT LEADS TO GSD-Ib

SLC37A4 is the G6PT shared by the G6PT/G6Pase-α or -β complexes and responsible for GSD-Ib (Chou et al., 2002, 2010b; Chou and Mansfield, 2014).

Early studies based on the activity of the G6PT/G6Pase-α complex suggested the existence of five GSD-I subtypes, referred to as Ia (affecting the G6Pase catalytic subunit), Ib (affecting G6PT), IaSP, Ic, and Id, believed to arise from T2, T3, and SP deficiency, respectively (Lei et al., 1995; Matern et al., 2002). Furthermore, G6Pase-β deficit was responsible for the onset of GSD-Irs (Boztug et al., 2009).

In the past, partial kinetic analysis demonstrated a deficit of Pi export from the microsomal lumen, suggesting the existence of a third form of GSD-I, called GSD-Ic (OMIM 232240), caused by the involvement of a third gene postulated in the pathogenesis of the disease (Nordlie et al., 1983). Subsequently, genotyping studies found out detrimental mutations in the human SLC37A4 gene (Veiga-da-Cunha et al., 1998; Galli et al., 1999; Janecke et al., 2000), therefore it was confirmed that either GSD-Ib or -Ic were caused by mutations occurring in the same gene (Veiga-da-Cunha et al., 1999). Additional defects, reported in patients, affected either microsomal glucose translocation (Lei et al., 1995), or SP, a hypothetical 21-kD protein, able to stabilize the G6Pase catalytic unit *in vitro* (Burchell et al., 1985). These conditions were initially classified as GSD-Id and GSD-IaSP (Burchell and Waddell, 1990), respectively. A patient diagnosed with GSD-IaSP was found to be homozygous for a *G6Pase* mutation, so GSD-IaSP was reclassified as GSD-Ia (Lei et al., 1995). In the same way, the diagnosis of GSD-Id was withdrawn, because this disorder was caused by a single mutation found in the human *SLC37A4* gene (Veiga-da-Cunha et al., 1999, 2000). As a result, GSD-Ib was implicated in all the reported cases of non-GSD-Ia (Chou et al., 2010b).

G6PT deficiency causes GSD-Ib, an autosomal recessively inherited disease, involving ~20% of all GSD-I patients (Chou et al., 2002, 2010b). This disorder is not limited to any racial or ethnic group, although the prevalence of some mutations is higher in whites and Japanese ethnicity (Chou et al., 2010b).

Up to date, 110 separate mutations have been identified in the *SLC37A4* gene of GSD-Ib and non-GSD-Ia studied patients, including 61 missense/nonsense 1 regulatory and 17 splicing mutations, 29 small insertion/deletions, and 2 gross deletions (http://www.hgmd.cf.ac.uk/ac/gene.php?gene=SLC37A4). They were distributed throughout the gene. The missense mutation c.443C>T (A148V) seems to be restricted to Korean population, since it has not been reported in other ethnic groups (Rihwa et al., 2017). Several residues critical for G6PT function reside in the consensus sequence shared by the SLC37 family members (**Figure 1**), as well as by other OPA family members (Chou and Mansfield, 2014). In the topological model proposed for G6PT according to glycosylation scanning and protease sensitivity studies (Pan et al., 2009), many mutations are located in the first ER luminal loop (**Figure 2**). Here, a conserved arginine (R28), corresponding to R46 in UhpT and essential for activity (Lloyd and Kadner, 1990), is believed to constitute part of the substrate binding site and is required for G6P transport

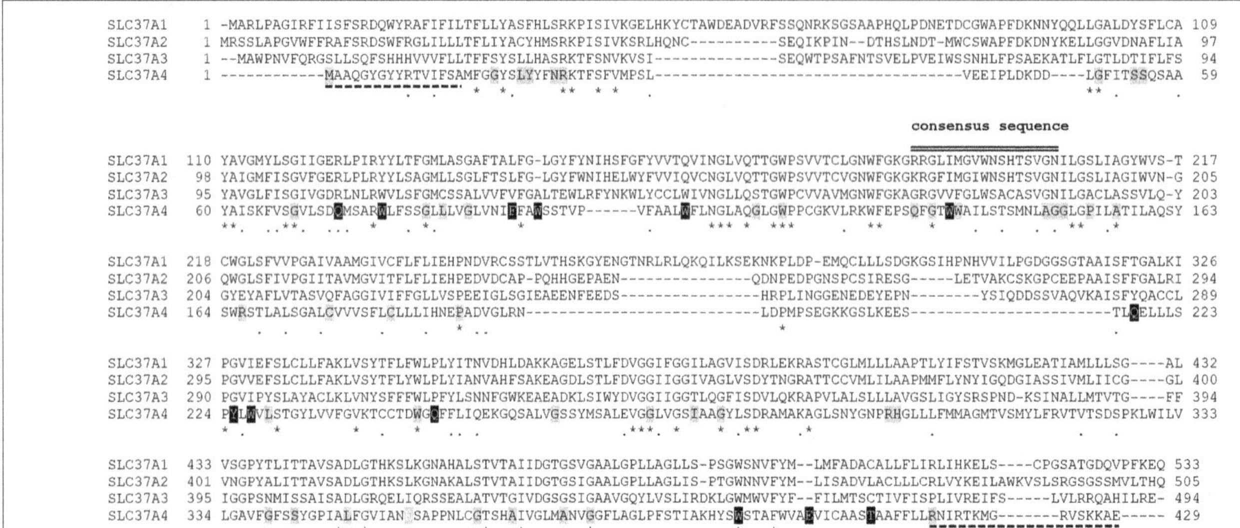

FIGURE 1 | Alignment of the amino acid sequences of human SLC37A1, SLC37A2, SLC37A3, and SLC37A4 showing the location of nonsense and missense mutations identified in GSD-Ib patients. The aligned amino acid sequences are GENBANK accession numbers NP_061837.3 (SLC37A1), NP_938018.1 (SLC37A2), AAH46567.1 (SLC37A3), and CAG33014.1 (SLC37A4). Sequence conservation is indicated by an asterisk for identical residues, a dot for conserved substitutions, and a gap for non-conserved residues. The organo-phosphate/Pi antiporter family consensus sequence, ProSite PDOC00726, shared by the SLC37 family members is indicated by black double lines. Dashed black lines show lacking residues at the N- or C- terminal end in mutants MIV and R415X, respectively. Nonsense and missense mutations are highlighted in black or gray, respectively. Alignment has been performed by ClustalW.

(Pan et al., 2009). Furthermore, N-terminal residues and helix 1 play a key role in transport activity, because the N-terminal mutation called MIV, lacking the N-terminal domain (residues1-7) and the first part of helix 1 (residues 8-16), abolishes transport function (Chen et al., 2002), but it does not interfere with G6PT stability (Chou and Mansfield, 2014). Conversely, the C-terminal domain deeply affects protein stability, since the nonsense mutation R415X, eliminating the whole cytoplasmic tail, causes a more rapid G6PT degradation with respect to the wild-type (Chen et al., 2000). Moreover, integrity of helix 10 is structurally important, because nonsense mutations E401X and T408X reduce G6PT expression and affect its folding (Chou and Mansfield, 2014).

SLC37A4 DEFECT: BIOCHEMICAL FEATURES AND CLINICAL PHENOTYPES

GSD-Ib-related symptoms are associated with both defective metabolic and myeloid phenotypes (Chou et al., 2010a,b). GSD-Ib metabolic phenotype is shared with GSD-Ia. Interprandial blood glucose homeostasis is controlled by the liver, the principal gluconeogenic organ, and to a lesser extent, by the kidney and intestine. Between meals, G6P produced in these organs during gluconeogenesis and glycogenolysis is imported into the ER lumen by G6PT, where it is hydrolyzed by G6Pase-α to produce glucose, then exported back into the bloodstream (**Figure 3A**; Chen, 2001; Chou et al., 2002). Since G6PT, as well as G6Pase-α, are abundantly expressed in gluconeogenic organs, when G6PT is defective the G6PT/G6Pase-α complex activity is defective. As a result of an inadequate glucose production, patients suffer from fasting hypoglycemia. At the same time, G6P cytoplasmic elevation leads to an abnormal storage of glycogen, which causes progressive nephromegaly and hepatomegaly (favoring a protruding abdomen), along with hyperlipidaemia, hyperuricemia, and lactic acidemia, besides, hepatomegaly is worsened by liver fat accumulation (Chen, 2001; Chou et al., 2002; **Figure 3B**). In GSD-Ib patients, short stature, xanthomas, and diarrhea have also been reported; additionally, fasting hypoglycemia may cause seizure. Signs and symptoms of the disorder generally develop during the childhood, around the age of 3 or 4 months, when babies start to sleep through the night, not eating as frequently as newborns. Affected children have a typical aspect with puffy cheeks and doll-like facies (Bartram et al., 1981). Untreated GSD-Ib is childhood lethal (Chou and Mansfield, 2011). Long-term complications include growth retardation, delayed puberty, osteoporosis, pancreatitis, gout, pulmonary hypertension, polycystic ovaries, and increased risk of hepatocellula adenoma (Chou et al., 2002, 2010b; Rake et al., 2002).

GSD-Ib myeloid phenotype is shared with GSD-Irs. A faulty G6PT/G6Pase-β complex activity causes neutrophil dysfunction and congenital neutropenia, therefore either GSD-Ib or GSD-Irs patients suffered from recurrent infections.

In neutrophils, glucose imported into the cytoplasm via GLUT1 is metabolized by hexokinase to G6P, which in turn enters the ER lumen through G6PT, where it can accumulate until it is hydrolyzed to glucose by G6Pase-β and transported back into the cytoplasm. Intracytoplasmic G6P/glucose ratio is affected by several pathways, such as glycolysis, pentose phosphate pathway, and recycling of G6P/glucose between the ER lumen and the cytoplasm (Jun et al., 2010; **Figure 4A**).

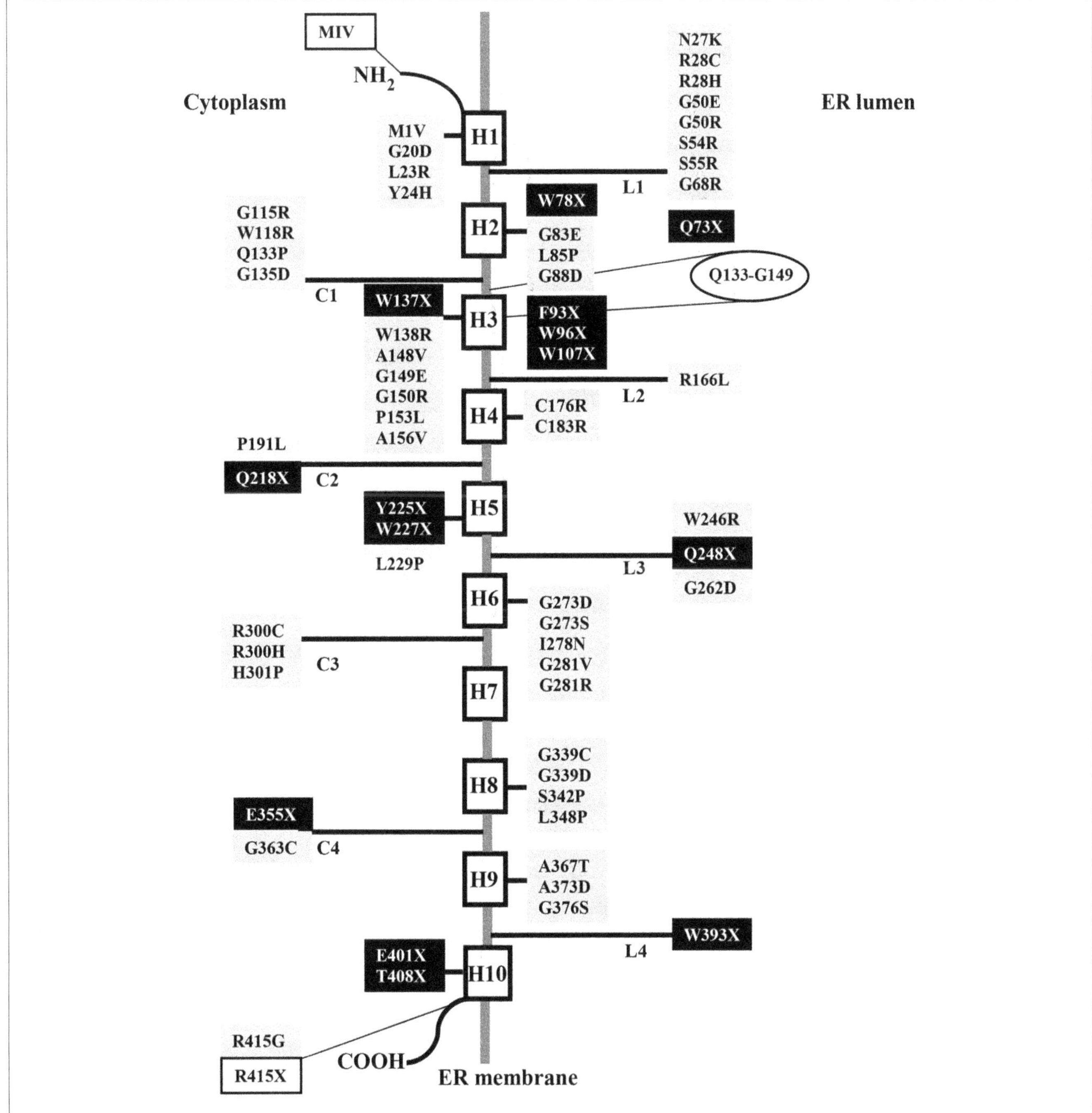

FIGURE 2 | Schematic topological model of human G6PT displaying nonsense and missense mutations identified in GSD-Ib patients. Nonsense and missense mutations are highlighted in black or gray, respectively. The extension of the consensus sequence is reported in an ellipse. White boxes represent mutations that eliminate the N- or C- terminal domain.

The G6PT/G6Pase-β complex plays a key role in the third pathway, because glucose recycling decreases cytoplasmic G6P/glucose ratio, so regulating the previously mentioned cytoplasmic pathways for G6P metabolism. As a consequence, G6PT impairment arises a lack of glucose recycling that can cause impaired neutrophil, macrophage, and monocytes functionality, as well as energy homeostasis, leading to reduced intracellular levels of G6P, lactate, ATP and NADPH (McCawley et al., 1993; Jun et al., 2010). A defective G6PT can also cause reduced neutrophil respiratory burst, chemotaxis, calcium mobilization and phagocytic activities (**Figure 4B**; Kilpatrick et al., 1990; Chou et al., 2010a; Jun et al., 2014).

Furthermore, in G6PT-deficient neutrophils, reduced respiratory burst was associated with an impaired activation of NADPH oxidase, a multicomponent enzyme promoting

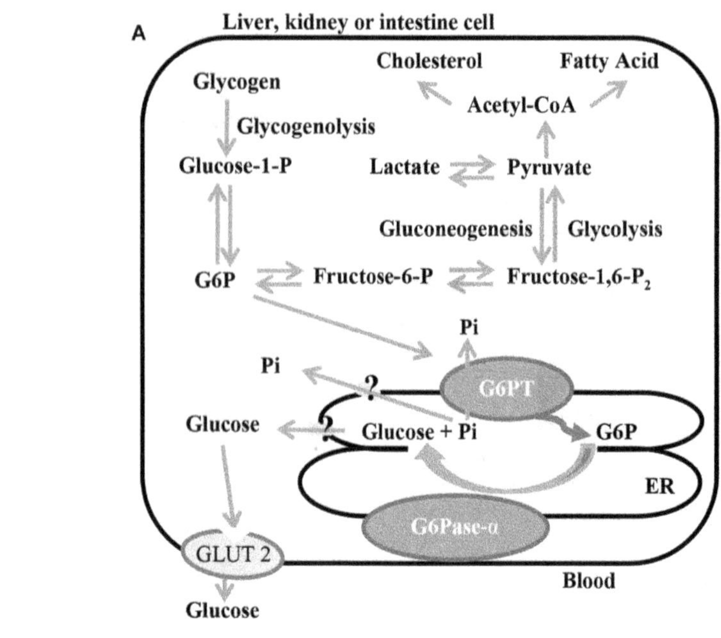

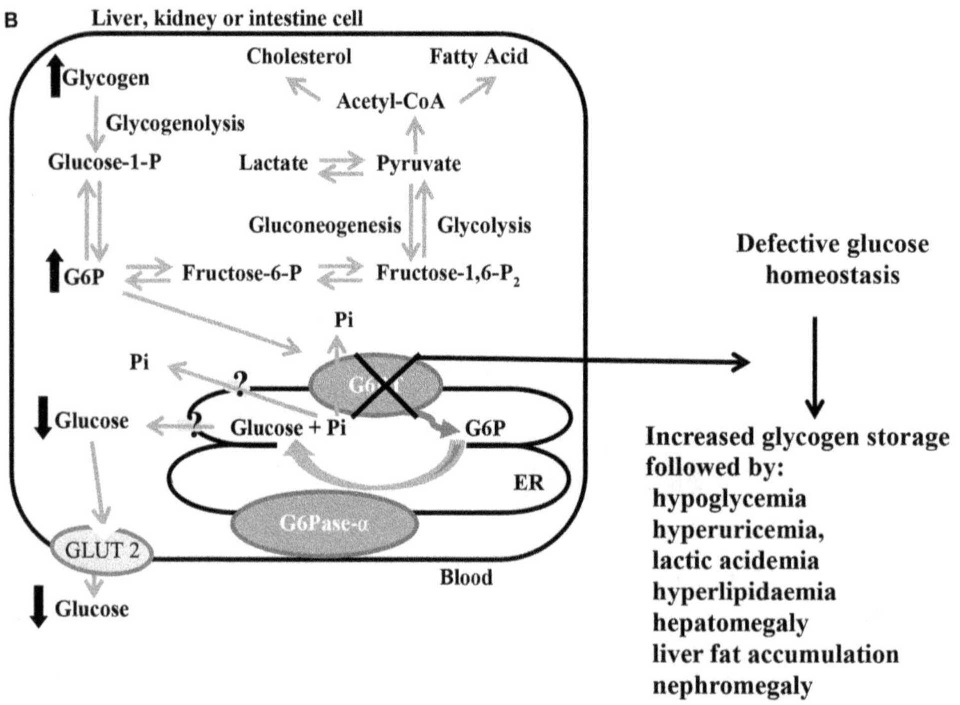

FIGURE 3 | Primary metabolic pathways of G6P in the liver, kidney, and intestine, in normal **(A)** and defective G6PT **(B)** cells. Schematic cell harboring an extended endoplasmic reticulum (ER). G6Pase-α and G6PT are embedded in the ER membrane; the glucose transporter GLUT2 is embedded in the plasma membrane. Black arrows indicate metabolic changes due to defective SLC37A4. G6P, glucose-6-phosphate; G6Pase-α, glucose-6-phosphatase-α; G6PT, glucose-6-phosphate translocase; GLUT2, glucose transporter 2; P, phosphate; Pi, inorganic phosphate.

the production of reactive oxygen species (Jun et al., 2014). Neutrophil metabolism is dependent on anaerobic glycolysis for ATP production. Under hypoxia the protein levels of the hypoxia-inducible transcriptional factor-1α (HIF-1α) increase (Bárdos and Ashcroft, 2005), and neutrophils display defective respiratory burst activity (McGovern et al., 2011). HIF-1α is

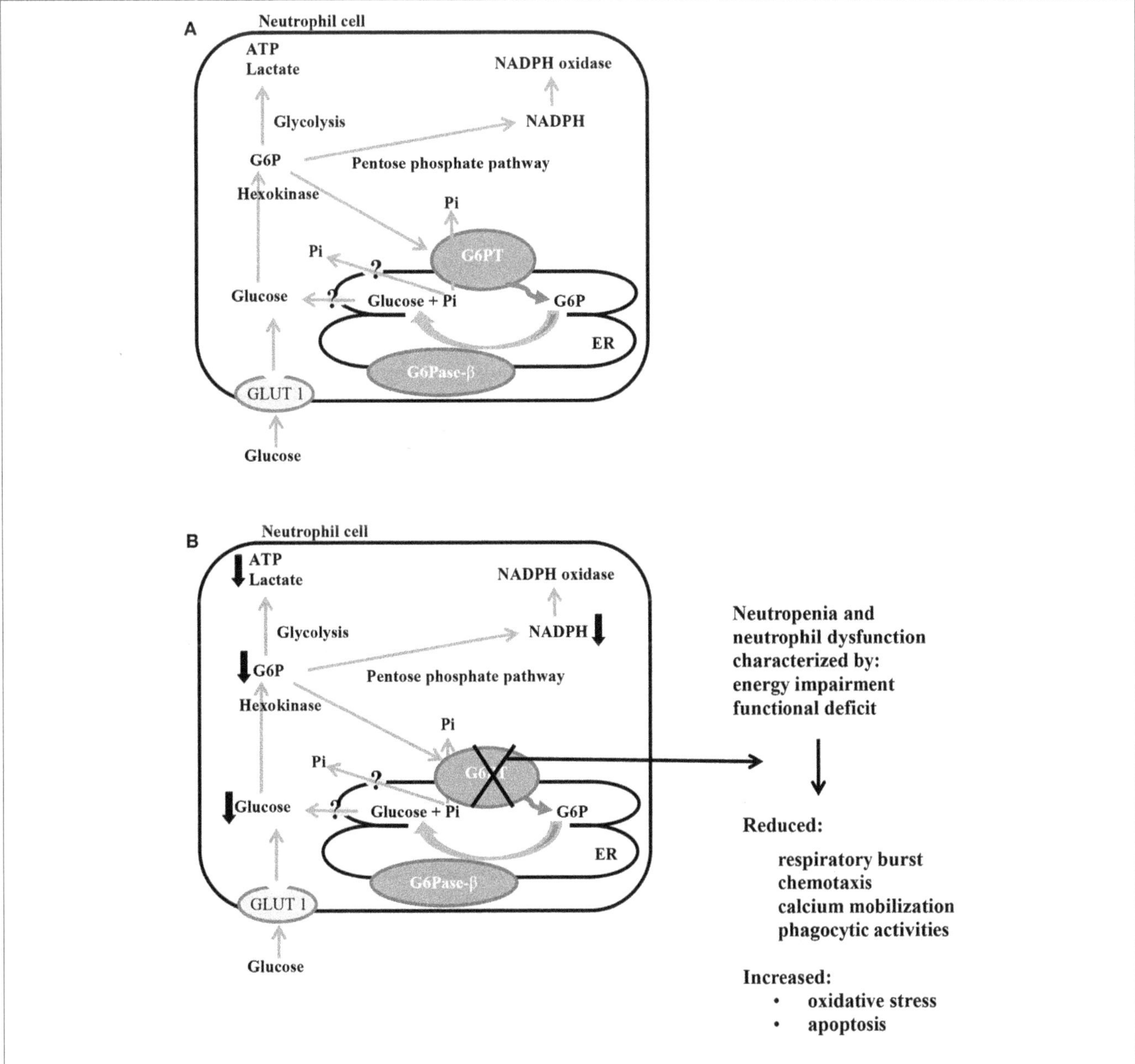

FIGURE 4 | Main metabolic pathways of G6P in normal **(A)** and defective G6PT **(B)** neutrophils. Schematic cell showing an extended endoplasmic reticulum (ER) and the three major pathways (glycolysis, pentose phosphate pathway, and ER cycling) in which G6P is involved. G6Pase-β and G6PT are embedded in the ER membrane; GLUT 1 is embedded in the plasma membrane. Black arrows indicate metabolic changes due to defective SLC37A4.: G6P, glucose-6-phosphate; G6Pase-β, glucose-6-phosphatase-β; G6PT, glucose-6-phosphate translocase; GLUT 1, glucose transporter 1; P, phosphate; Pi, inorganic phosphate; ATP, adenosine triphosphate; NADPH, nicotinamide adenine dinucleotide phosphate.

also an upstream activator of peroxisome proliferator-activated receptor-γ (PPAR-γ) (Krishnan et al., 2009), a nuclear receptor involved in the regulation of lipid and glucose metabolism, influencing inflammation and many other diseases (Kvandova et al., 2016). It was observed that in neutrophils PPAR-γ is constitutively expressed, and its activation leads to chemotaxis inhibition (Reddy et al., 2008). On this basis, it was supposed that the activation of the HIF-1α/PPAR-γ pathway in neutrophils of GSD-Ib patients could trigger neutrophil dysfunction, impairing chemotaxis and calcium mobilization activities (Jun et al., 2014).

GSD-Ib patients may also experience oral symptoms, consisting of dental caries, periodontal diseases, gingivitis, delayed dental maturation and eruption, oral bleeding diathesis and ulcers (Mortellaro et al., 2005). Remarkably, not all GSD-Ib patients manifest neutropenia or frequent infections (Kure et al., 2000; Melis et al., 2005; Angaroni et al., 2006; Martens et al., 2006). In this regard, in a multicentre study investigating the genotype/phenotype correlation on a cohort of 25 GSD-Ib patients, no correlation was found between individual mutations and the presence of neutropenia, bacterial infections or systemic complications. This evidence might suggest the existence of unknown factors able to influence immune phenotype, such as polymorphisms, proteins or genes, capable of modulating neutrophil differentiation, maturation, and apoptosis (Melis et al., 2005). Considering that neutrophils of GSD-Ib patients exhibited enhanced apoptosis, a causal relationship between apoptosis and neutropenia was hypothesized (Kuijpers et al., 2003; Jun et al., 2014). This theory was supported by further studies conducted on animal models, demonstrating that either neutrophils from *G6Pase-β* $^{-/-}$ mice or those from *G6PT* $^{-/-}$ mice exhibited enhanced ER stress and apoptosis (Cheung et al., 2007; Kim et al., 2008). So, neutrophil ER stress, higher oxidative stress and apoptosis might be underlying causes of neutropenia in GSD-Ib (Jun et al., 2010). In addition, neutrophil apoptosis in both *G6Pase-β* $^{-/-}$ (Jun et al., 2011) and *G6PT* $^{-/-}$ (Kim et al., 2008) mice was mediated by the intrinsic apoptosis pathway. In GSD-Ib, a maturation arrest seems not to be responsible for neutrophil dysfunction (Jun et al., 2014). Since neutrophils, as well as macrophages, have to import glucose from the blood by the glucose transporters (Pessin and Bell, 1992), these cells critically depend on the G6PT/G6Pase-β complex activity, especially when the need for glucose rises (Jun et al., 2014). This might provide a rationale for neutropenia caused by enhanced neutrophil ER stress, oxidative stress and apoptosis, when G6PT and/or G6Pase-β are defective (Kuijpers et al., 2003; Kim et al., 2008; Jun et al., 2010, 2014).

AUTOIMMUNITY RISK OF SLC37A4 DEFECT

A strong association was found between GSD-Ib and inflammatory bowel disease (IBD), because many GSD-Ib patients with chronic gastrointestinal inflammation were diagnosed with IBD, which was clinically indistinguishable from idiopathic Crohn disease, assuming the involvement of an impaired mucosal innate immunity in the pathogenesis of IBD (Dieckgraefe et al., 2002). The association between neutropenia and IBD was supported by Visser et al., in a retrospective European study, showing that up to 77% of patients with GSD-Ib presented also neutropenia, as well as many GSD-Ib patients suffering from perioral or perianal infections (Visser et al., 2000).

In patients with GSD-Ib an increased risk for Crohn-like disease was reported (Melis et al., 2003), along with a severe deficit of hypothalamus-pituitary-thyroid axis, causing an increased prevalence of thyroid autoimmunity and hypothyroidism (Melis et al., 2007). In one patient, the occurrence of myasthenia gravis was also described (Melis et al., 2008). These observations paved the way to the hypothesis that GSD-Ib patients, but not those affected by GSD-Ia, were at increased risk for autoimmune disorders. The different risk degree between GSD-Ia and GSD-Ib patients might be related to the presence of neutropenia and neutrophil dysfunction only in GSD-Ib (Melis et al., 2007). Some studies have also suggested an association between lymphopenia and autoimmunity (Merayo-Chalico et al., 2016). Chronic lymphopenia might promote autoimmunity inducing the homeostatic expansion of T cell, which represents a normal compensatory reaction during lymphopenic conditions (King et al., 2004).

Recent studies have highlighted the molecular mechanisms underlying the increased frequency of autoimmunity disorders shown in GSD-Ib patients (Melis et al., 2017).

Regulatory T cells (Tregs) are a subset of CD4+ T cells involved in maintaining tolerance to self-antigens, and they play a critical role in human autoimmune diseases, because their imbalance seems to be responsible for the failure of local regulatory mechanisms (Dejaco et al., 2006). Those cells mediate their suppressive function by acting directly on conventional T cells (Tconvs) and antigen-presenting cells, such as dendritic cells (Rueda et al., 2016). Tregs express the transcription factor forkhead box P3 (FOXP3), which is very important for Tregs development and function, since defects in the FOXP3 gene cause a human lethal autoimmune disease (Bennett et al., 2001).

Treg responses can be modulated by several metabolic pathways (Buck et al., 2015), particularly by glycolysis, able to affect human Treg induction and function (De Rosa et al., 2015). In this regard, a defective engagement of glycolysis upon suboptimal T cell receptor (TCR) stimulation of conventional T cells (Tconvs) has been observed in several human autoimmune diseases, and it has been associated with a decreased suppressive function of Tregs (De Rosa et al., 2015).

In GSD-Ib, a defective G6PT causes a decreased capacity to mobilize glucose, leading to diminished glucose utilization. Consequently, a reduced engagement of glycolysis in T cells occurs upon suboptimal TCR stimulation; additionally, qualitative and quantitative alterations of peripheral regulatory T cells (pTregs) have been observed, along with impaired FOXP3 expression by Tconvs during low TCR activation (Melis et al., 2017).

THERAPEUTIC APPROACHES FOR SLC37A4 DEFECT

Clinical therapies consist of dietary treatment, granulocyte colony-stimulating factor (G-CSF) therapy and transplantations.

Since recurrent hypoglycemia is responsible for lactic acidosis, hyperuricemia and hypertriglyceridemia, the primary goal of nutritional therapy is to achieve a stable normoglycemia. In addition, dietary treatment aims to reduce metabolic impairment, delaying some of the long-term GSD-Ib consequences. Unfortunately, elevated triglycerides and cholesterol blood levels may persist regardless of diet, along with their consequences (Cappello et al., 2016); moreover, even if nutritional therapy can improve long-term outcomes for many patients, several long-term complications remain. Recommended diet composition is 60–70% calories from carbohydrates, 10–15% from proteins and the remaining from fats (Goldberg and Slonim, 1993). Small frequent feedings rich in complex carbohydrates (particularly those higher in fiber) have to be regularly ingested over 24 h to achieve a good metabolic control (Wolfsdorf and Weinstein, 2003; Kishnani et al., 2014). GSD-Ib, as well as GSD-Ia patients, can use the same nutritional therapy to avoid hypoglycemia, especially nighttime (Chou et al., 2010b).

Cornstarch therapy in GSD-I is used since the early 1980s (Chen et al., 1984). Raw uncooked cornstarch is a slowly digested carbohydrate, which allows a slow release of glucose able to prolong the length of euglycemia between meals (Sidbury et al., 1986).

Glucose requirement normally decreases with age, so adults have a longer fasting tolerance with respect to children. Traditionally, in children older than 3 years, as well as in adults, normoglycemia during nighttime is maintained by the ingestion at bedtime of uncooked corn starch (Wolfsdorf and Crigler, 1997; Weinstein and Wolfsdorf, 2002; Shah and O'Dell, 2013) or of modified forms of corn starch (Bhattacharya et al., 2007; Correia et al., 2008). In children <3 years continuous tube feeding is usually needed (Greene et al., 1976), because the level of pancreatic amylase able to hydrolyze raw starch is low before 3 years of age (Chou et al., 2010b). A recent controlled crossover study enrolling adult GSD-Ia and GSD-Ib patients, highlighted that nighttime glucose control can be achieved also by the ingestion of a cooked pasta meal at bedtime, allowing a more palatable alternative to corn starch use (Hochuli et al., 2015).

G-CSF administration promotes the production of granulocytes (Mehta et al., 2015), increasing neutrophile numbers and reducing the frequency and severity of infections in GSD-Ib patients, but it can not improve neutrophile dysfunction (Visser et al., 2002). G-CSF also appears to increase neutrophil survival (Jun et al., 2011). In this regard, studies led *in vivo*, on murine *G6Pase-β*-deficient models, highlighted that G-CSF therapy was able to normalize neutrophil energy homeostasis and to improve functionality, as supported by improved neutrophil glucose uptake and increased G6P, ATP, and lactate intracellular concentrations (Jun et al., 2011).

A recent study has evidenced a partial improvement of neutrophil respiratory burst activity in a GSD-Ib patient by oral administration of galactose, even though the role of galactose in sugar metabolism of GSD-Ib neutrophils remains to be clarified (Letkemann et al., 2017).

Neutropenia associated with IBD can be treated by using a combination of G-CSF and 5-aminosalicylic acid (Visser et al., 2002; Koeberl et al., 2009; Chou et al., 2010b; Shah and O'Dell, 2013).

In some GSD-Ib patients, metabolic abnormalities can be corrected by liver or combined liver/kidney transplantation, since such operations have improved metabolic control, restoring normal fasting tolerance (Boers et al., 2014). Patients with impending renal failure are suggested to consider combined liver/kidney transplantation (Labrune, 2002). In GSD-Ib patients, myeloid dysfunctions can be treated by bone marrow transplantation, which appears to be a promising approach, even if it requires further validation (Pierre et al., 2008). According to the guidelines from the European study on GSD-I, liver transplantation is suggested in GSD-I patients with unresectable hepatocellular adenomas unresponsive to nutritional therapy, mainly if adenomas are associated with serious compression or hemorrhage, or in the case of enhanced risk of transformation into hepatocellular carcinomas (Rake et al., 2002). Although liver transplantation improves metabolic impairment (Reddy et al., 2009), its usefulness on renal disease and neutropenia or neutrophil dysfunction is yet to be settled.

GENE THERAPY FOR SLC37A4 DEFECT

Gene therapy represents a promising strategy to correct metabolic abnormalities in all GSD-I patients (Chou and Mansfield, 2011), although currently it seems not to compensate for myeloid and renal dysfunction in GSD-Ib patients (Kwon et al., 2017).

Several gene transfer vectors, including recombinant adeno-associated virus (rAAV) vectors, have been developed and tested, either on GSD-Ia or on GSD-Ib animal models (Chou et al., 2015; Kwon et al., 2017).

G6PT knockout (*G6PT*$^{-/-}$) mice are excellent *G6PT*-deficient murine models, since they exhibit all the metabolic and myeloid dysfunctions typical of human GSD-Ib (Chen et al., 2003). Some studies led on those mice showed that recombinant adenovirus-mediated *G6PT* gene transfer was able to deliver the transgene to the liver and bone marrow, improving metabolic and myeloid defects; however, this therapy was short-lived, owing to the fast loss of vector-mediated gene expression (Yiu et al., 2007).

Further studies led on such mice showed that a human *G6PT* expressing recombinant AAV serotypes 2/8 vector (rAAV8) directed by a hybrid chicken β-actin (CBA) promoter and a cytomegalovirus (CMV) enhancer, was able to deliver the transgene primarily to the liver, thus normalizing metabolic abnormalities. Nevertheless, two of the five treated mice survived for 51–72 weeks, developed multiple hepatocellular adenomas, and one experienced cancer transformation (Yiu et al., 2009). So, this therapeutic approach, while allowing normoglicemia, could not prevent long term complications of hepatocellular adenoma.

A further work, on *G6Pase-α*-deficient murine models (manifesting all the symptoms of human GSD-Ia), was led in order to compare two different gene transfer methods. In one case, murine *G6Pase-α* gene transfer *in vivo* was mediated by recombinant AAV serotypes 2/1 (rAAV1) or rAAV8 vectors, and expression was directed by hybrid CBA promoter/CMV enhancer. In the other case, a rAAV8 vector expressing human G6Pase-α directed by its promoter/enhancer (GPE) was employed (Yiu et al., 2010).

This work highlighted that the gluconeogenic tissue-specific human GPE was more effective in directing persistent *in vivo* hepatic transgene expression with respect to the CBA promoter/CMV enhancer, because human GPE utilization triggered a lesser humoral immune response, allowing complete normalization of hepatic G6Pase-α deficiency

(Yiu et al., 2010). In addition, in murine GSD-Ia models, the use of a *G6Pase-α*-expressing rAAV vector under the GPE control was able to correct metabolic defects with no hepatocellular adenoma development (Lee Y. M. et al., 2012).

On this basis, recently two different liver directed gene therapy approaches were tested on $G6PT^{-/-}$ mice, using rAAV-GPE-*G6PT* and rAAV-miGT-*G6PT*, this latter consisted of a human *G6PT* expressing rAAV directed by human minimal *G6PT* promoter/enhancer (miGT) (Hiraiwa and Chou, 2001; Kwon et al., 2017).

Both vectors could deliver the *hG6PT* transgene to the liver, correcting metabolic anomalies, but rAAV-GPE-*G6PT* vector directed by the *hG6Pase-α* promoter/enhancer had greater efficacy. A full restoration of normal G6PT activity was not necessary to obtain significant therapeutic benefits, since a restoration of 3-62% seemed to confer protection against age-related obesity and insulin resistance, while restoration <6% exposed to hepatic cancer risk (Kwon et al., 2017).

AUTHOR CONTRIBUTIONS

AC, RC and RL conducted literary review, wrote the article and prepared publication-ready figures, MM and VD designed and edited the article.

ACKNOWLEDGMENTS

This work was supported by Associazione Italiana per la Ricerca sul Cancro (MM grant no. 16719/2015).

REFERENCES

Ahn, H. H., Oh, Y., Lee, H., Lee, W., Chang, J. W., Pyo, H. K., et al. (2015). Identification of glucose-6-phosphate transporter as a key regulator functioning at the autophagy initiation step. *FEBS Lett.* 589, 2100–2109. doi: 10.1016/j.febslet.2015.05.018

Almqvist, J., Huang, Y., Hovmöller, S., and Wang, D. N. (2004). Homology modeling of the human microsomal glucose 6-phosphate transporter explains the mutations that cause the glycogen storage disease type Ib. *Biochemistry* 43, 9289–9297. doi: 10.1021/bi049334h

Angaroni, C. J., Labrune, P., Petit, F., Sastre, D., Capra, A. E., Dodelson de Kremer, R., et al. (2006). Glycogen storage disease type Ib without neutropenia generated by a novel splice-site mutation in the glucose-6-phosphate translocase gene. *Mol. Genet. Metab.* 88, 96–99. doi: 10.1016/j.ymgme.2005.12.011

Annabi, B., Hiraiwa, H., Mansfield, B. C., Lei, K. J., Ubagai, T., Polymeropoulos, M. H., et al. (1998). The gene for glycogen storage disease type 1b maps to chromosome 11q23. *Am. J. Hum. Genet.* 62, 400–405. doi: 10.1086/301727

Arion, W. J., Canfield, W. K., Ramos, F. C., Schindler, P. W., Burger, H. J., Hemmerle, H., et al. (1997). Chlorogenic acid and hydroxynitrobenzaldehyde: new inhibitors of hepatic glucose 6-phosphatase. *Arch. Biochem. Biophys.* 339, 315–322. doi: 10.1006/abbi.1996.9874

Arion, W. J., Canfield, W. K., Ramos, F. C., Su, M. L., Burger, H. J., Hemmerle, H., et al. (1998). Chlorogenic acid analogue S 3483: a potent competitive inhibitor of the hepatic and renal glucose-6-phosphatase systems. *Arch. Biochem. Biophys.* 351, 279–285. doi: 10.1006/abbi.1997.0563

Arion, W. J., Wallin, B. K., Carlson, P. W., and Lange, A. J. (1972). The specificity of glucose 6-phosphatase of intact liver microsomes. *J. Biol. Chem.* 247, 2558–2565.

Arion, W. J., Wallin, B. K., Lange, A. J., and Ballas, L. M. (1975). On the involvement of a glucose 6-phosphate transport system in the function of microsomal glucose 6-phosphatase. *Mol. Cell. Biochem.* 6, 75–83. doi: 10.1007/BF01732001

Bandsma, R. H., Wiegman, C. H., Herling, A. W., Burger, H. J., ter Harmsel, A., Meijer, A. J., et al. (2001). Acute inhibition of glucose-6-phosphate translocator activity leads to increased de novo lipogenesis and development of hepatic steatosis without affecting VLDL production in rats. *Diabetes* 50, 2591–2597. doi: 10.2337/diabetes.50.11.2591

Bárdos, J. I., and Ashcroft, M. (2005). Negative and positive regulation of HIF-1: a complex network. *Biochim. Biophys. Acta* 1755, 107–120. doi: 10.1016/j.bbcan.2005.05.001

Bartella, V., De Francesco, E. M., Perri, M. G., Curcio, R., Dolce, V., Maggiolini, M., et al. (2016). The G protein estrogen receptor (GPER) is regulated by endothelin-1 mediated signaling in cancer cells. *Cell. Signal.* 28, 61–71. doi: 10.1016/j.cellsig.2015.11.010

Bartoloni, L., and Antonarakis, S. E. (2004). The human sugar-phosphate/phosphate exchanger family SLC37. *Pflugers Arch.* 447, 780–783. doi: 10.1007/s00424-003-1105-0

Bartoloni, L., Wattenhofer, M., Kudoh, J., Berry, A., Shibuya, K., Kawasaki, K., et al. (2000). Cloning and characterization of a putative human glycerol 3-phosphate permease gene (SLC37A1 or G3PP) on 21q22.3: mutation analysis in two candidate phenotypes, DFNB10 and a glycerol kinase deficiency. *Genomics* 70, 190–200. doi: 10.1006/geno.2000.6395

Bartram, C. R., Przyrembel, H., Wendelz, U., Bremer, H. J., Schaub, J., and Haas, J. R. (1981). Glyeogenosis type I b complicated by severe granuloeytopenia resembling inherited Neutropenia. *Eur. J. Pediatr.* 137, 81–84. doi: 10.1007/BF00441175

Bellot, G., Garcia-Medina, R., Gounon, P., Chiche, J., Roux, D., Pouysségur, J., et al. (2009). Hypoxia-induced autophagy is mediated through hypoxia-inducible factor induction of BNIP3 and BNIP3L via their BH3 domains. *Mol. Cell. Biol.* 29, 2570–2581. doi: 10.1128/MCB.00166-09

Bennett, C. L., Christie, J., Ramsdell, F., Brunkow, M. E., Ferguson, P. J., Whitesell, L., et al. (2001). The immune dysregulation, polyendocrinopathy, enteropathy, X-linked syndrome (IPEX) is caused by mutations of FOXP3. *Nat. Genet.* 27, 20–21. doi: 10.1038/83713

Benton, M. C., Johnstone, A., Eccles, D., Harmon, B., Hayes, M. T., and Lea, R. A. (2015). An analysis of DNA methylation in human adipose tissue reveals differential modification of obesity genes before and after gastric bypass and weight loss. *Genome Biol.* 16:8. doi: 10.1186/s13059-014-0569-x

Bhattacharya, K., Orton, R. C., Qi, X., Mundy, H., Morley, D. W., Champion, M. P., et al. (2007). A novel starch for the treatment of glycogen storage diseases. *J. Inherit. Metab. Dis.* 30, 350–357. doi: 10.1007/s10545-007-0479-0

Boers, S. J., Visser, G., Smit, P. G., and Fuchs, S. A. (2014). Liver transplantation in glycogen storage disease type I. *Orphanet J. Rare Dis.* 9:47. doi: 10.1186/1750-1172-9-47

Boztug, K., Appaswamy, G., Ashikov, A., Schäffer, A. A., Salzer, U., Diestelhorst, J., et al. (2009). A syndrome with congenital neutropenia and mutations in G6PC3. *N. Engl. J. Med.* 360, 32–43. doi: 10.1056/NEJMoa0805051

Buck, M. D., O'Sullivan, D., and Pearce, E. L. (2015). T cell metabolism drives immunity. *J. Exp. Med.* 212, 1345–1360. doi: 10.1084/jem.20151159

Burchell, A., and Waddell, I. D. (1990). Diagnosis of a novel glycogen storage disease: type 1aSP. *J. Inherit. Metab. Dis.* 13, 247–249. doi: 10.1007/BF01799362

Burchell, A., Burchell, B., Monaco, M., Walls, H. E., and Arion, W. J. (1985). Stabilization of glucose-6-phosphatase activity by a 21000-dalton hepatic microsomal protein. *Biochem. J.* 230, 489–495. doi: 10.1042/bj2300489

Cappello, A. R., Dolce, V., Iacopetta, D., Martello, M., Fiorillo, M., Curcio, R., et al. (2016). Bergamot (Citrus bergamia Risso) flavonoids and their potential benefits in human hyperlipidemia and atherosclerosis: an overview. *Mini Rev. Med. Chem.* 16, 619–629. doi: 10.2174/1389557515666150709110222

Chen, L. Y., Lin, B., Pan, C. J., Hiraiwa, H., and Chou, J. Y. (2000). Structural requirements for the stability and microsomal transport activity of the human glucose-6-phosphate transporter. *J. Biol. Chem.* 275, 34280–34286. doi: 10.1074/jbc.M006439200

Chen, L. Y., Pan, C. J., Shieh, J. J., and Chou, J. Y. (2002). Structure-function analysis of the glucose-6-phosphate transporter deficient in glycogen storage disease type Ib. *Hum. Mol. Genet.* 11, 3199–3207. doi: 10.1093/hmg/11.25.3199

Chen, L. Y., Shieh, J. J., Lin, B., Pan, C. J., Gao, J. L., Murphy, P. M., et al. (2003). Impaired glucose homeostasis, neutrophil trafficking and function in mice lacking the glucose-6-phosphate transporter. *Hum. Mol. Genet.* 12, 2547–2558. doi: 10.1093/hmg/ddg263

Chen, S. Y., Pan, C. J., Nandigama, K., Mansfield, B. C., Ambudkar, S. V., and Chou, J. Y. (2008). The glucose-6-phosphate transporter is a phosphate-linked antiporter deficient in glycogen storage disease type Ib and Ic. *FASEB J.* 22, 2206–2213. doi: 10.1096/fj.07-104851

Chen, Y. T. (2001). "Glycogen storage diseases," in *The Metabolic and Molecular Bases of Inherited Disease, 8th Edn*, eds C. R. Scriver, A. L. Beaudet, W. S. Sly, and D. Valle (New York, NY: McGraw-Hill), 1521–1551.

Chen, Y. T., Cornblath, M., and Sidbury, J. B. (1984). Cornstarch therapy in type I glycogen-storage disease. *N. Engl. J. Med.* 310, 171–175. doi: 10.1056/NEJM198401193100306

Cheung, Y. Y., Kim, S. Y., Yiu, W. H., Pan, C. J., Jun, H. S., Ruef, R. A., et al. (2007). Impaired neutrophil activity and increased susceptibility to bacterial infection in mice lacking glucose-6-phosphatase-beta. *J. Clin. Invest.* 117, 784–793. doi: 10.1172/JCI30443

Chou, J. Y., and Mansfield, B. C. (2011). Recombinant AAV-directed gene therapy for type I glycogen storage diseases. *Expert Opin. Biol. Ther.* 11, 1011–1024. doi: 10.1517/14712598.2011.578067

Chou, J. Y., and Mansfield, B. C. (2014). The SLC37 family of sugar-phosphate/phosphate exchangers. *Curr. Top. Membr.* 73, 357–382. doi: 10.1016/B978-0-12-800223-0.00010-4

Chou, J. Y., Jun, H. S., and Mansfield, B. C. (2010a). Neutropenia in type Ib glycogen storage disease. *Curr. Opin. Hematol.* 17, 36–42. doi: 10.1097/MOH.0b013e328331df85

Chou, J. Y., Jun, H. S., and Mansfield, B. C. (2010b). Glycogen storage disease type I and G6Pase-b deficiency: etiology and therapy. *Nat. Rev. Endocrinol.* 6, 676–688. doi: 10.1038/nrendo.2010.189

Chou, J. Y., Sik Jun, H., and Mansfield, B. C. (2013). The SLC37 family of phosphate-linked sugar phosphate antiporters. *Mol. Aspects Med.* 34, 601–611. doi: 10.1016/j.mam.2012.05.010

Chou, J. Y., Jun, H. S., and Mansfield, B. C. (2015). Type I glycogen storage diseases: disorders of the glucose-6-phosphatase/glucose-6-phosphate transporter complexes. *J. Inherit. Metab. Dis.* 38, 511–519. doi: 10.1007/s10545-014-9772-x

Chou, J. Y., Matern, D., Mansfield, B. C., and Chen, Y. T. (2002). Type I glycogen storage diseases: disorders of the glucose-6-phosphatase complex. *Curr. Mol. Med.* 2, 121–143. doi: 10.2174/1566524024605798

Correia, C. E., Bhattacharya, K., Lee, P. J., Shuster, J. J., Theriaque, D. W., Shankar, M. N., et al. (2008). Use of modified cornstarch therapy to extend fasting in glycogen storage disease types Ia and Ib. *Am. J. Clin. Nutr.* 88, 1272–1276. doi: 10.3945/ajcn.2008.26352

Curcio, R., Muto, L., Pierri, C. L., Montalto, A., Lauria, G., Onofrio, A., et al. (2016). New insights about the structural rearrangements required for substrate translocation in the bovine mitochondrial oxoglutarate carrier. *Biochim. Biophys. Acta* 1864, 1473–1480. doi: 10.1016/j.bbapap.2016.07.009

De Rosa, V., Galgani, M., Porcellini, A., Colamatteo, A., Santopaolo, M., Zuchegna, C., et al. (2015). Glycolysis controls the induction of human regulatory T cells by modulating the expression of FOXP3 exon 2 splicing variants. *Nat. Immunol.* 16, 1174–1184. doi: 10.1038/ni.3269

Dejaco, C., Duftner, C., Grubeck-Loebenstein, B., and Schirmer, M. (2006). Imbalance of regulatory T cells in human autoimmune diseases. *Immunology* 117, 289–300. doi: 10.1111/j.1365-2567.2005.02317.x

Della Rocca, B. M., Miniero, D. V., Tasco, G., Dolce, V., Falconi, M., Ludovico, A., et al. (2015). Substrate-induced conformational changes of the mitochondrial oxoglutarate carrier: a spectroscopic and molecular modelling study. *Mol. Membr. Biol.* 22, 443–452. doi: 10.1080/09687860500269335

Dieckgraefe, B. K., Korzenik, J. R., Husain, A., and Dieruf, L. (2002). Association of glycogen storage disease 1b and Crohn disease: results of a North American survey. *Eur. J. Pediatr.* 161, S88–S92. doi: 10.1007/BF02680002

Dolce, V., Cappello, A. R., Lappano, R., and Maggiolini, M. (2011). Glycerophospholipid synthesis as a novel drug target against cancer. *Curr. Mol. Pharmacol.* 4, 167–175. doi: 10.2174/1874467211104030167

Fritz, S., Capitan, A., Djari, A., Rodriguez, S. C., Barbat, A., Baur, A., et al. (2013). Detection of haplotypes associated with prenatal death in dairy cattle and identification of deleterious mutations in GART, SHBG and SLC37A2. *PLoS ONE* 8:e65550. doi: 10.1371/journal.pone.0065550

Galli, L., Orrico, A., Marcolongo, P., Fulceri, R., Burchell, A., Melis, D., et al. (1999). Mutations in the glucose-6-phosphate transporter (G6PT) gene in patients with glycogen storage diseases type 1b and 1c. *FEBS Lett.* 459, 255–258.

Ganley, I. G., Lam du, H., Wang, J., Ding, X., Chen, S., and Jiang, X. (2009). ULK1.ATG13.FIP200 complex mediates mTOR signaling and is essential for autophagy. *J. Biol. Chem.* 284, 12297–12305. doi: 10.1074/jbc.M900573200

Gerin, I., Noel, G., and Van Schaftingen, E. (2001). Novel arguments in favor of the substrate-transport model of glucose-6-phosphatase. *Diabetes* 50, 1531–1538. doi: 10.2337/diabetes.50.7.1531

Gerin, I., Veiga-da-Cunha, M., Achouri, Y., Collet, J. F., and Van Schaftingen, E. (1997). Sequence of a putative glucose-6-phosphate translocase, mutated in glycogen storage disease type 1b. *FEBS Lett.* 419, 235–238. doi: 10.1016/S0014-5793(97)01463-4

Gerin, I., Veiga-da-Cunha, M., Noël, G., and Van Schaftingen, E. (1999). Structure of the gene mutated in glycogen storage disease type Ib. *Gene* 227, 189–195. doi: 10.1016/S0378-1119(98)00614-3

Ghosh, A., Shieh, J. J., Pan, C. J., and Chou, J. Y. (2004). Histidine 167 is the phosphate acceptor in glucose-6-phosphatase-beta forming a phosphohistidine enzyme intermediate during catalysis. *J. Biol. Chem.* 279, 12479–12483. doi: 10.1074/jbc.M313271200

Ghosh, A., Shieh, J. J., Pan, C. J., Sun, M. S., and Chou, J. Y. (2002). The catalytic center of glucose-6-phosphatase. HIS176 is the nucleophile forming the phosphohistidine-enzyme intermediate during catalysis. *J. Biol. Chem.* 277, 32837–32842. doi: 10.1074/jbc.M201853200

Goldberg, T., and Slonim, A. E. (1993). Nutrition therapy for hepatic glycogen storage diseases. *J. Am. Diet. Assoc.* 93, 1423–1430. doi: 10.1016/0002-8223(93)92246-T

Greene, H. L., Slonim, A. E., O'Neill, J. A. Jr., and Burr, I. M. (1976). Continuous nocturnal intragastric feeding for management of type 1 glycogen-storage disease. *N. Engl. J. Med.* 294, 423–425. doi: 10.1056/NEJM197602192940805

Grefhorst, A., Schreurs, M., Oosterveer, M. H., Cortés, V. A., Havinga, R., Herling, A. W., et al. (2010). Carbohydrate response-element-binding protein (ChREBP) and not the liver X receptor α (LXRα) mediates elevated hepatic lipogenic gene expression in a mouse model of glycogen storage disease type 1. *Biochem. J.* 432, 249–254. doi: 10.1042/BJ20101225

Hawley, S. A., Pan, D. A., Mustard, K. J., Ross, L., Bain, J., Edelman, A. M., et al. (2005). Calmodulin-dependent protein kinase kinase beta is an alternative upstream kinase for AMP-activated protein kinase. *Cell Metab.* 2, 9–19. doi: 10.1016/j.cmet.2005.05.009

He, L., Vasiliou, K., and Nebert, D. W. (2009). Analysis and update of the human solute carrier (SLC) gene superfamily. *Hum. Genomics* 3, 195–206. doi: 10.1186/1479-7364-3-2-195

Hemmerle, H., Burger, H. J., Below, P., Schubert, G., Rippel, R., Schindler, P. W., et al. (1997). Chlorogenic acid and synthetic chlorogenic acid derivatives: novel inhibitors of hepatic glucose-6-phosphate translocase. *J. Med. Chem.* 40, 137–145. doi: 10.1021/jm9607360

Herling, A. W., Burger, H., Schubert, G., Hemmerle, H., Schaefer, H., and Kramer, W. (1999). Alterations of carbohydrate and lipid intermediary metabolism during inhibition of glucose-6-phosphatase in rats. *Eur. J. Pharmacol.* 386, 75–82. doi: 10.1016/S0014-2999(99)00748-7

Hiraiwa, H., and Chou, J. Y. (2001). Glucocorticoids activate transcription of the gene for glucose-6-phosphate transporter, deficient in glycogen storage disease type 1b. *DNA Cell Biol.* 20, 447–453. doi: 10.1089/104454901316976073

Hiraiwa, H., Pan, C. J., Lin, B., Moses, S. W., and Chou, J. Y. (1999). Inactivation of the glucose-6-phosphate transporter causes glycogen storage disease type 1b. *J. Biol. Chem.* 274, 5532–5536. doi: 10.1074/jbc.274.9.5532

Hochuli, M., Christ, E., Meienberg, F., Lehmann, R., Krützfeldt, J., and Baumgartner, M. R. (2015). Alternative nighttime nutrition regimens in glycogen storage disease type I: a controlled crossover study. *J. Inherit. Metab. Dis.* 38, 1093–1098. doi: 10.1007/s10545-015-9864-2

Hoffman, K., and Stoffel, W. (1993). TMbase—A database of membrane spanning protein segments. *Biol. Chem.* 347, 166–170.

Iacopetta, D., Carocci, A., Sinicropi, M. S., Catalano, A., Lentini, G., Ceramella, J., et al. (2017). Old drug scaffold, new activity: Thalidomide-correlated compounds exert different effects on breast cancer cell growth and progression. *Chem. Med. Chem.* 12, 381–389. doi: 10.1002/cmdc.201600629

Iacopetta, D., Lappano, R., Cappello, A. R., Madeo, M., De Francesco, E. M., Santoro, A., et al. (2010). SLC37A1 gene expression is up-regulated by epidermal growth factor in breast cancer cells. *Breast Cancer Res. Treat.* 122, 755–764. doi: 10.1007/s10549-009-0620-x

Ihara, K., Nomura, A., Hikino, S., Takada, H., and Hara, T. (2000). Quantitative analysis of glucose-6-phosphate translocase gene expression in various human tissues and haematopoietic progenitor cells. *J. Inherit. Metab. Dis.* 23, 583–592. doi: 10.1023/A:1005677912539

Island, M. D., Wei, B. Y., and Kadner, R. J. (1992). Structure and function of the uhp genes for the sugar phosphate transport system in *Escherichia coli* and *Salmonella typhimurium*. *J. Bacteriol.* 174, 2754–2762. doi: 10.1128/jb.174.9.2754-2762.1992

Janecke, A. R., Linder, M., Erdel, M., Mayatepek, E., Möslinger, D., Podskarbi, T., et al. (2000). Mutation analysis in glycogen storage disease type 1 non-a. *Hum. Genet.* 107, 285–289. doi: 10.1007/s004390000371

Jiang, P., and Mizushima, N. (2014). Autophagy and human diseases. *Cell Res.* 24, 69–79. doi: 10.1038/cr.2013.161

Jun, H. S., Lee, Y. M., McDermott, D. H., DeRavin, S. S., Murphy, P. M., Mansfield, B. C., et al. (2010). Lack of glucose recycling between endoplasmic reticulum and cytoplasm underlies cellular dysfunction in glucose-6-phosphatase-beta-deficient neutrophils in a congenital neutropenia syndrome. *Blood* 116, 2783–2792. doi: 10.1182/blood-2009-12-258491

Jun, H. S., Lee, Y. M., Song, K. D., Mansfield, B. C., and Chou, J. Y. (2011). G-CSF improves murine G6PC3-deficient neutrophil function by modulating apoptosis and energy homeostasis. *Blood* 117, 3881–3892. doi: 10.1182/blood-2010-08-302059

Jun, H. S., Weinstein, D. A., Lee, Y. M., Mansfield, B. C., and Chou, J. Y. (2014). Molecular mechanisms of neutrophil dysfunction in glycogen storage disease type Ib. *Blood* 123, 2843–2853. doi: 10.1182/blood-2013-05-5 02435

Jung, C. H., Jun, C. B., Ro, S. H., Kim, Y. M., Otto, N. M., Cao, J., et al. (2009). ULK-Atg13-FIP200 complexes mediate mTOR signaling to the autophagy machinery. *Mol. Biol. Cell* 20, 1992–2003. doi: 10.1091/mbc.E08-12-1249

Kikuchi, D., Saito, M., Saito, K., Watanabe, Y., Matsumoto, Y., Kanke, Y., et al. (2018). Upregulated solute carrier family 37 member 1 in colorectal cancer is associated with poor patient outcome and metastasis. *Oncol. Lett.* 15, 2065–2072. doi: 10.3892/ol.2017.7559

Kilpatrick, L., Garty, B. Z., Lundquist, K. F., Hunter, K., Stanley, C. A., Baker, L., et al. (1990). Impaired metabolic function and signaling defects in phagocytic cells in glycogen storage disease type 1b. *J. Clin. Invest.* 86, 196–202. doi: 10.1172/JCI114684

Kim, J. Y., Tillison, K., Zhou, S., Wu, Y., and Smas, C. M. (2007). The major facilitator superfamily member Slc37a2 is a novel macrophage-specific gene selectively expressed in obese white adipose tissue. *Am. J. Physiol. Endoc. M.* 293, E110–E120. doi: 10.1152/ajpendo.00404.2006

Kim, J., Kundu, M., Viollet, B., and Guan, K. L. (2011). AMPK and mTOR regulate autophagy through direct phosphorylation of Ulk1. *Nat. Cell Biol.* 13, 132–141. doi: 10.1038/ncb2152

Kim, S. Y., Jun, H. S., Mead, P. A., Mansfield, B. C., and Chou, J. Y. (2008). Neutrophil stress and apoptosis underlie myeloid dysfunction in glycogen storage disease type Ib. *Blood* 111, 5704–5711. doi: 10.1182/blood-2007-12-129114

King, C., Ilic, A., Koelsch, K., and Sarvetnick, N. (2004). Homeostatic expansion of T cells during immune insufficiency generates autoimmunity. *Cell* 117, 265–277. doi: 10.1016/S0092-8674(04)00335-6

Kishnani, P. S., Austin, S. L., Abdenur, J. E., Arn, P., Bali, D. S., Boney, A., et al. (2014). Diagnosis and management of glycogen storage disease type I: a practice guideline of the American College of Medical Genetics and Genomics. *Genet. Med.* 16:e1. doi: 10.1038/gim.2014.128

Knutson, T. P., Truong, T. H., Ma, S., Brady, N. J., Sullivan, M. E., Raj, G., et al. (2017). Posttranslationally modified progesterone receptors direct ligand-specific expression of breast cancer stem cell-associated gene programs. *J. Hematol. Oncol.* 10:89. doi: 10.1186/s13045-017-0462-7

Koeberl, D. D., Kishnani, P. S., Bali, D., and Chen, Y. T. (2009). Emerging therapies for glycogen storage disease type I. *Trends Endocrinol. Metab.* 20, 252–258. doi: 10.1016/j.tem.2009.02.003

Kouroku, Y., Fujita, E., Tanida, I., Ueno, T., Isoai, A., Kumagai, H., et al. (2007). ER stress (PERK/eIF2alpha phosphorylation) mediates the polyglutamine-induced LC3 conversion, an essential step for autophagy formation. *Cell Death Differ.* 14, 230–239. doi: 10.1038/sj.cdd.4401984

Krishnan, J., Suter, M., Windak, R., Krebs, T., Felley, A., Montessuit, C., et al. (2009). Activation of a HIF1α-PPARgamma axis underlies the integration of glycolytic and lipid anabolic pathways in pathologic cardiac hypertrophy. *Cell Metab.* 9, 512–524. doi: 10.1016/j.cmet.2009.05.005

Kuijpers, T. W., Maianski, N. A., Tool, A. T., Smit, G. P., Rake, J. P., Roos, D., et al. (2003). Apoptotic neutrophils in the circulation of patients with glycogen storage disease type 1b (GSD1b). *Blood* 101, 5021–5024. doi: 10.1182/blood-2002-10-3128

Kure, S., Hou, D. C., Suzuki, Y., Yamagishi, A., Hiratsuka, M., Fukuda, T., et al. (2000). Glycogen storage disease type Ib without neutropenia. *J. Pediatr.* 137, 253–256. doi: 10.1067/mpd.2000.107472

Kvandova, M., Majzúnová, M., and Dovinová, I. (2016). The role of PPARgamma in cardiovascular diseases. *Physiol. Res.* 65(Suppl. 3), S343–S363.

Kwon, J. H., Lee, Y. M., Cho, J. H., Kim, G. Y., Anduaga, J., Starost, M. F., et al. (2017). Liver-directed gene therapy for murine glycogen storage disease type Ib. *Hum. Mol. Genet.* 26, 4395–4405. doi: 10.1093/hmg/ddx325

Labrune, P. (2002). Glycogen storage disease type I: indications for liver and/or kidney transplantation. *Eur. J. Pediatr.* 161(Suppl. 1), S53–S55. doi: 10.1007/BF02679995

Lappano, R., Sebastiani, A., Cirillo, F., Rigiracciolo, D. C., Galli, G. R., Curcio, R., et al. (2017). The lauric acid-activated signaling prompts apoptosis in cancer cells. *Cell Death Discov.* 3:17063. doi: 10.1038/cddiscovery.2017.63.eCollection 2017

Lee, H., Noh, J. Y., Oh, Y., Kim, Y., Chang, J. W., Chung, C. W., et al. (2012). IRE1 plays an essential role in ER stress-mediated aggregation of mutant huntingtin via the inhibition of autophagy flux. *Hum. Mol. Genet.* 21, 101–114. doi: 10.1093/hmg/ddr445

Lee, Y. M., Jun, H. S., Pan, C. J., Lin, S. R., Wilson, L. H., Mansfield, B. C., et al. (2012). Prevention of hepatocellular adenoma and correction of metabolic abnormalities in murine glycogen storage disease type Ia by gene therapy. *Hepatology* 56, 1719–1729. doi: 10.1002/hep.25717

Lei, K. J., Chen, H., Pan, C. J., Ward, J. M., Mosinger, B., Lee, E. J., et al. (1996). Glucose-6-phosphatase dependent substrate transport in the glycogen storage disease type 1a mouse. *Nat. Genet.* 13, 203–209. doi: 10.1038/ ng0696-203

Lei, K. J., Shelly, L. L., Lin, B., Sidbury, J. B., Chen, Y. T., Nordlie, R. C., et al. (1995). Mutations in the glucose-6-phosphatase gene are associated with glycogen storage disease types 1a and 1aSP but not 1b and 1c. *J. Clin. Invest.* 95, 234–240. doi: 10.1172/JCI117645

Letkemann, R., Wittkowski, H., Antonopoulos, A., Podskabi, T., Haslamc, S. M., Föll, D., et al. (2017). Partial correction of neutrophil dysfunction by oral galactose therapy in glycogen storage disease type Ib. *Int. Immunopharmacol.* 44, 216–225. doi: 10.1016/j.intimp.2017.01.020

Leuzzi, R., Bánhegyi, G., Kardon, T., Marcolongo, P., Capecchi, P. L., Burger, H. J., et al. (2003). Inhibition of microsomal glucose-6-phosphate transport in human neutrophils results in apoptosis: a potential explanation for neutrophil dysfunction in glycogen storage disease type 1b. *Blood* 101, 2381–2887. doi: 10.1182/blood-2002-08-2576

Lin, B., Annabi, B., Hiraiwa, H., Pan, C. J., and Chou, J. Y. (1998). Cloning and characterization of cDNAs encoding a candidate glycogen storage disease type 1b protein in rodents. *J. Biol. Chem.* 273, 31656–31670. doi: 10.1074/jbc.273.48.31656

Lin, B., Pan, C. J., and Chou, J. Y. (2000). Human variant glucose-6-phosphate transporter is active in microsomal transport. *Hum. Genet.* 107, 526–552. doi: 10.1007/s004390000404

Lloyd, A. D., and Kadner, R. J. (1990). Topology of the *Escherichia coli* UhpT sugar-phosphate transporter analyzed by using TnphoA fusions. *J. Bacteriol.* 172, 1688–1693. doi: 10.1128/jb.172.4.1688-1693.1990

Maloney, P.C., and Wilson, T. H. (1996) *Escherichia coli and Salmonella: Cellular and Molecular Biology*. Washington, DC: ASM Press. 1130–1148.

Marcolongo, P., Barone, V., Priori, G., Pirola, B., Giglio, S., Biasucci, G., et al. (1998). Structure and mutation analysis of the glycogen storage disease type 1b gene. *FEBS Lett.* 436, 247–250. doi: 10.1016/S0014-5793(98) 01129-6

Martens, D. H., Kuijpers, T. W., Maianski, N. A., Rake, J. P., Smit, G. P., and Visser, G. (2006). A patient with common glycogen storage disease type Ib mutations without neutropenia or neutrophil dysfunction. *J. Inherit. Metab. Dis.* 29, 224–225. doi: 10.1007/s10545-006-0146-x

Matern, D., Seydewitz, H. H., Bali, D., Lang, C., and Chen, Y. T. (2002). Glycogen storage disease type I: diagnosis and phenotype/genotype correlation. *Eur. J. Pediatr.* 161, S10–S19. doi: 10.1007/s00431-002-0998-5

McCawley, L. J., Korchak, H. M., Cutilli, J. R., Stanley, C. A., Baker, L., Douglas, S. D., et al. (1993). Interferon-gamma corrects the respiratory burst defect *in vitro* in monocyte-derived macrophages from glycogen storage disease type 1b patients. *Pediatr. Res.* 34, 265–269. doi: 10.1203/00006450-199309000-00005

McDermott, D. H., De Ravin, S. S., Jun, H. S., Liu, Q., Priel, D. A., Noel, P., et al. (2010). Severe congenital neutropenia resulting from G6PC3 deficiency with increased neutrophil CXCR4 expression and myelokathexis. *Blood* 116, 2793–2802. doi: 10.1182/blood-2010-01-265942

McGovern, N. N., Cowburn, A. S., Porter, L., Walmsley, S. R., Summers, C., Thompson, A. A. R., et al. (2011). Hypoxia selectively inhibits respiratory burst activity and killing of *Staphylococcus aureus* in human neutrophils. *J. Immunol.* 186, 453–463. doi: 10.4049/jimmunol.1002213

Mehta, H. M., Malandra, M., and Corey, S. J. (2015). G-CSF and GM-CSF in Neutropenia. *J. Immunol.* 195, 1341–1349. doi: 10.4049/jimmunol.1500861

Melis, D., Balivo, R., Della Casa, R., Romano, A., Taurisano, R., Capaldo, B., et al. (2008). Myasthenia gravis in a patient affected by glycogen storage disease type Ib: a further manifestation of an increased risk for autoimmune disorders? *J. Inherit. Metab. Dis.* 31 (Suppl. 2), S227–S231. doi: 10.1007/s10545-008-0810-4

Melis, D., Carbone, F., Minopoli, G., La Rocca, C., Perna, F., De Rosa, V., et al. (2017). Cutting edge: increased autoimmunity risk in glycogen storage disease type 1b is associated with a reduced engagement of glycolysis in T Cells and an impaired regulatory T cell function. *J. Immunol.* 198, 3803–3808. doi: 10.4049/jimmunol.1601946

Melis, D., Fulceri, R., Parenti, G., Marcolongo, P., Gatti, R., Parini, R., et al. (2005). Genotype/phenotype correlation in glycogen storage disease type 1b: a multicentre study and review of the literature. *Eur. J. Pediatr.* 164, 501–508. doi: 10.1007/s00431-005-1657-4

Melis, D., Parenti, G., Della Casa, R., Sibilio, M., Berni Canani, R., Terrin, G., et al. (2003). Crohn's-like ileo-colitis in patients affected by glycogen storage disease Ib: two years_ follow-up of patients with a wide spectrum of gastrointestinal signs. *Acta Paediatr.* 92, 1415–1421. doi: 10.1111/j.1651-2227.2003.tb00825.x

Melis, D., Pivonello, R., Parenti, G., Della Casa, R., Salerno, M., Lombardi, G., et al. (2007). Increased prevalance of thyroid autoimmunity and hypothyroidism in patients with glycogen storage disease type 1. *J. Pediatr.* 150, 300–305. doi: 10.1016/j.jpeds.2006.11.056

Merayo-Chalico, J., Rajme-Lopez, S., Barrera-Vargas, A., Alcocer-Varela, J., Diaz-Zamudio, M., and Gomez-Martìn, D. (2016). Lymphopenia and autoimmunity: a double-edged sword. *Hum. Immunol.* 77, 921–929. doi: 10.1016/j.humimm.2016.06.016

Mihaylova, M. M., and Shaw, R. J. (2011). The AMPK signalling pathway coordinates cell growth, autophagy and metabolism. *Nat. Cell Biol.* 13, 1016–1023. doi: 10.1038/ncb2329

Mortellaro, C., Garagiola, U., Carbone, V., Cerutti, F., Marci, V., and Bonda, P. L. (2005). Unusual oral manifestations and evolution in glycogen storage disease type Ib. *J. Craniofac. Surg.*16, 45–52. doi: 10.1097/00001665-200501000-00010

Nazio, F., Strappazzon, F., Antonioli, M., Bielli, P., Cianfanelli, V., Bordi, M., et al. (2013). MTOR inhibits autophagy by controlling ULK1 ubiquitylation, self-association and function through AMBRA1 and TRAF6. *Nat. Cell Biol.* 15, 406–416. doi: 10.1038/ncb2708

Nordlie, R. C., Sukalski, K. A., Munoz, J. M., and Baldwin, J. J. (1983). Type 1c, a novel glycogenosis. *J. Biol. Chem.* 258, 9739–9744.

Pan, C. J., Chen, S. Y., Jun, H. S., Lin, S. R., Mansfield, B. C., and Chou, J. Y. (2011). SLC37A1 and SLC37A2 are phosphate-linked, glucose-6-phosphate antiporters. *PLoS ONE* 6:e23157. doi: 10.1371/journal.pone.0023157

Pan, C. J., Chen, S. Y., Lee, S., and Chou, J. Y. (2009). Structure-function study of glucose-6-phosphate transporter, an eukaryotic antiporter deficient in glycogen storage disease type Ib. *Mol. Genet. Metab.* 96, 32–37. doi: 10.1016/j.ymgme.2008.10.005

Pan, C. J., Lei, K. J., Annabi, B., Hemrika, W., and Chou, J. Y. (1998). Transmembrane topology of glucose-6-phosphatase. *J. Biol. Chem.* 273, 6144–6148. doi: 10.1074/jbc.273.11.6144

Pan, C. J., Lin, B., and Chou, J. Y. (1999). Transmembrane topology of human glucose-6-phosphate transporter. *J. Biol. Chem.* 274, 13865–13869. doi: 10.1074/jbc.274.20.13865

Pao, S. S., Paulsen, I. T., and Saier, M. H. Jr. (1998). Major facilitator superfamily. *Microbiol. Mol. Biol. Rev.* 62, 1–34.

Perland, E., and Fredriksson, R. (2017). Classification systems of secondary active transporters.*Trends Pharmacol. Sci.* 38, 305–315. doi: 10.1016/j.tips.2016.11.008

Pessin, J. E., and Bell, G. I. (1992). Mammalian facilitative glucose transporter family: structure and molecular regulation. *Annu. Rev. Physiol.* 54, 911–930. doi: 10.1146/annurev.ph.54.030192.004403

Pierre, G., Chakupurakal, G., McKiernan, P., Hendriksz, C., Lawson, S., and Chakrapani, A. (2008). Bone marrow transplantation in glycogen storage disease type 1b. *J. Pediatr.* 152, 286–288. doi: 10.1016/j.jpeds.2007.09.031

Proverbio, M. C., Mangano, E., Gessi, A., Bordoni, R., Spinelli, R., Asselta, R., et al. (2013). Whole genome SNP genotyping and exome sequencing reveal novel genetic variants and putative causative genes in congenital hyperinsulinism. *PLoS ONE* 8:e68740. doi: 10.1371/journal.pone.0068740

Rake, J. P., Visser, G., Labrune, P., Leonard, J. V., Ullrich, K., and Smit, G. P. (2002). Glycogen storage disease type I: diagnosis, management, clinical course and outcome. Results of the European Study on Glycogen Storage Disease Type I (ESGSDI). *Eur. J. Pediatr.* 161, S20–S34. doi: 10.1007/BF02679990

Reddy, R. C., Narala, V. R., Keshamouni, V. G., Milam, J. E., Newstead, M. W., and Standiford, T. J. (2008). Sepsis-induced inhibition of neutrophil chemotaxis is mediated by activation of peroxisome proliferator-activated receptor-{gamma}. *Blood* 112, 4250–4258. doi: 10.1182/blood-2007-12-128967

Reddy, S. K., Austin, S. L., Spencer-Manzon, M., Koeberl, D. D., Clary, B. M., Desai, D. M., et al. (2009). Liver transplantation for glycogen storage disease type Ia. *J. Hepatol.* 51, 483–490. doi: 10.1016/j.jhep.2009.05.026

Reinartz, S., and Dist, O. (2016). Validation of deleterious mutations in vorderwald cattle. *PLoS ONE* 11:e0160013. doi: 10.1371/journal.pone.0160013

Rihwa, C., Hyung-Doo, P., Jung Min, K., Jeongho, L., Dong Hwan, L., Suk Jin, H., et al. (2017). Novel SLC37A4 mutations in korean patients with glycogen storage disease Ib. *Ann. Lab. Med.* 37, 261–266. doi: 10.3343/alm.2017.37.3.261

Rueda, C. M., Jackson, C. M., and Chougnet, C. A. (2016). Regulatory T-Cell-mediated suppression of conventional T-Cells and dendritic cells by different cAMP intracellular pathways. *Front. Immunol.* 7:216. doi: 10.3389/fimmu.2016.00216

Saksa, N., Neme, A., Ryynänen, J., Uusitupa, M., de Mello, V. D., Voutilainen, S., et al. (2015). Dissecting high from lowresponders in a vitamin D3 intervention study. *J. Steroid Biochem. Mol. Biol.* 148, 275–282. doi: 10.1016/j.jsbmb.2014.11.012

Sancak, Y., Bar-Peled, L., Zoncu, R., Markhard, A. L., Nada, S., and Sabatini, D. M. (2010). Regulator-Rag complex targets mTORC1 to the lysosomal surface and is necessary for its activation by amino acids. *Cell* 141, 290–303. doi: 10.1016/j.cell.2010.02.024

Shah, K. K., and O'Dell, S. D. (2013). Effect of dietary interventions in the maintenance of normoglycaemia in glycogen storage disease type 1a: a systematic review and meta-analysis. *J. Hum. Nutr. Diet.* 26, 329–339. doi: 10.1111/jhn.12030

Shieh, J. J., Chen, C. T., and Huang, W. R. (2007). The variant glucose-6-phosphate transporter decreases protein stability and requires MyoD-dependent alternative splicing during myogenesis of muscle cells. *FASEB J.* 21:A243.

Shieh, J. J., Pan, C. J., Mansfield, B. C., and Chou, J. Y. (2003). Glucose-6-phosphate hydrolase, widely expressed outside the liver, can explain age-dependent resolution of hypoglycemia in glycogen storage disease type Ia. *J. Biol. Chem.* 278, 47098–47103. doi: 10.1074/jbc.M309472200

Sidbury, J. B., Chen, Y. T., and Roe, C. R. (1986). The role of raw starches in the treatment of type I glycogenosis. *Arch. Intern. Med.* 146:370–373. doi: 10.1001/archinte.1986.00360140200029

Takahashi, Y., Miyata, M., Zheng, P., Imazato, T., Horwitz, A., and Smith, J. D. (2000). Identification of cAMP analogue inducible genes in RAW264 macrophages. *Biochim. Biophys. Acta* 1492, 385–394. doi: 10.1016/S0167-4781(00)00133-0

Veiga-da-Cunha, M., Gerin, I., and Van Schaftingen, E. (2000). How many forms of glycogen storage disease type I? *Eur. J. Pediatr.* 159, 314–318. doi: 10.1007/s004310051279

Veiga-da-Cunha, M., Gerin, I., Chen, Y.-T., de Barsy, T., de Lonlay, P., Dionisi-Vici, C., et al. (1998). A gene on chromosome 11q23 coding for a putative glucose-6-phosphate translocase is mutated in glycogenstorage disease types Ib and Ic. *Am. J. Hum. Genet.* 63, 976–983. doi: 10.1086/302068

Veiga-da-Cunha, M., Gerin, I., Chen, Y. T., Lee, P. J., Leonard, J. V., Maire, I., et al. (1999). The putative glucose 6-phosphate translocase gene is mutated in essentially all cases of glycogen storage disease type I non-a. *Eur. J. Hum. Genet.* 7, 717–723. doi: 10.1038/sj.ejhg.5200366

Visser, G., Rake, J. P., Fernandes, J., Labrune, P., Leonard, J. V., Moses, S., et al. (2000). Neutropenia, neutrophil dysfunction, and inflammatory bowel disease in glycogen storage disease type Ib: results of the European Study on Glycogen storage disease type I. *J. Pediatr.* 137, 187–191. doi: 10.1067/mpd.2000.105232

Visser, G., Rake, J. P., Labrune, P., Leonard, J. V., Moses, S., Ullrich, K., et al. (2002). Granulocyte colony-stimulating factor in glycogen storage disease type 1b. results of the European Study on Glycogen Storage Disease Type 1. *Eur. J. Pediatr.* 161, S83–S87. doi: 10.1007/BF02680001

Weinstein, D. A., and Wolfsdorf, J. I. (2002). Effect of continuous glucose therapywith uncooked cornstarch on the long-term clinical course of type 1a glycogen storage disease. *Eur. J. Pediatr.* 161(Suppl. 1), S35–S39. doi: 10.1007/BF02679991

Wilfinger, J., Seuter, S., Tuomainen, T. P., Virtanen, J. K., Voutilainen, S., Nurmi, T., et al. (2014). Primary vitamin D receptor target genes as biomarkers for the vitamin D3 status in the hematopoietic system. *J. Nutr. Biochem.* 25, 875–884. doi: 10.1016/j.jnutbio.2014.04.002

Wolfsdorf, J. I., and Crigler, J. F. Jr. (1997). Cornstarch regimens for nocturnal treatment of young adults with type I glycogen storage disease. *Am. J. Clin. Nutr.* 65, 1507–1511 doi: 10.1093/ajcn/65.5.1507

Wolfsdorf, J. I., and Weinstein, D. A. (2003). Glycogen storage diseases. *Rev. Endocr. Metab. Disord.* 4, 95–102. doi: 10.1023/A:1021831621210

Yiu, W. H., Lee, Y. M., Peng, W. T., Pan, C. J., Mead, P. A., Mansfield, B. C., et al. (2010). Complete normalization of hepatic G6PC deficiency in murine glycogen storage disease type Ia using gene therapy. *Mol. Ther.* 18, 1076–1084. doi: 10.1038/mt.2010.64

Yiu, W. H., Pan, C. J., Allamarvdasht, A., Kim, S. Y., and Chou, J. Y. (2007). Glucose-6-phosphate transporter gene therapy corrects metabolic and myeloid abnormalities in glycogen storage disease type Ib mice. *Gene Ther.*14, 219–226. doi: 10.1038/sj.gt.3302869

Yiu, W. H., Pan, C. J., Mead, P. A., Starost, M. F., Mansfield, B. C., and Chou, J. Y. (2009). Normoglycemia alone is insufficient to prevent long term complications of hepatocellular adenoma in glycogen storage disease type Ib mice. *J. Hepatol.* 51, 909–917. doi: 10.1016/j.jhep.2008.11.026

Young, A. R., Chan, E. Y., Hu, X. W., Kochl, R., Crawshaw, S. G., High, S., et al. (2006). Starvation and ULK1-dependent cycling of mammalian Atg9 between the TGN and endosomes. *J. Cell Sci.* 119, 3888–3900. doi: 10.1242/jcs.03172

Zingone, A., Hiraiwa, H., Pan, C.-J., Lin, B., Chen, H., Ward, J. M., et al. (2000). Correction of glycogen storage disease type 1a in a mouse model by gene therapy. *J. Biol. Chem.* 275, 828–832. doi: 10.1074/jbc.275.2.828

Zoncu, R., Efeyan, A., and Sabatini, D. M. (2011). MTOR: from growth signal integration to cancer, diabetes and ageing. *Nat. Rev. Mol. Cell Biol.* 12, 21–35. doi: 10.1038/nrm3025

10

The Sodium Sialic Acid Symporter from *Staphylococcus aureus* has Altered Substrate Specificity

Rachel A. North[1,2,3†], Weixiao Y. Wahlgren[3,4†], Daniela M. Remus[1,2], Mariafrancesca Scalise[5], Sarah A. Kessans[1,2], Elin Dunevall[3], Elin Claesson[3], Tatiana P. Soares da Costa[6], Matthew A. Perugini[6], S. Ramaswamy[7], Jane R. Allison[2,8,9], Cesare Indiveri[5], Rosmarie Friemann[3,4] and Renwick C. J. Dobson[1,10*]*

***Correspondence:**
Rosmarie Friemann
rosmarie.friemann@gu.se
Renwick C. J. Dobson
renwick.dobson@canterbury.ac.nz

† These authors have contributed equally to this work.

[1] School of Biological Sciences, University of Canterbury, Christchurch, New Zealand, [2] Biomolecular Interaction Centre, University of Canterbury, Christchurch, New Zealand, [3] Department of Chemistry and Molecular Biology, University of Gothenburg, Gothenburg, Sweden, [4] Centre for Antibiotic Resistance Research, University of Gothenburg, Gothenburg, Sweden, [5] Unit of Biochemistry and Molecular Biotechnology, Department DiBEST (Biologia, Ecologia, Scienze della Terra), University of Calabria, Arcavacata di Rende, Italy, [6] Department of Biochemistry and Genetics, La Trobe Institute for Molecular Science, La Trobe University, Melbourne, VIC, Australia, [7] The Institute for Stem Cell Biology and Regenerative Medicine, Bangalore, India, [8] Centre for Theoretical Chemistry and Physics, Institute of Natural and Mathematical Sciences, Massey University, Auckland, New Zealand, [9] Maurice Wilkins Centre for Molecular Biodiscovery, University of Auckland, Auckland, New Zealand, [10] Department of Biochemistry and Molecular Biology, Bio21 Molecular Science and Biotechnology Institute, University of Melbourne, Parkville, VIC, Australia

Mammalian cell surfaces are decorated with complex glycoconjugates that terminate with negatively charged sialic acids. Commensal and pathogenic bacteria can use host-derived sialic acids for a competitive advantage, but require a functional sialic acid transporter to import the sugar into the cell. This work investigates the sodium sialic acid symporter (SiaT) from *Staphylococcus aureus* (*Sa*SiaT). We demonstrate that *Sa*SiaT rescues an *Escherichia coli* strain lacking its endogenous sialic acid transporter when grown on the sialic acids *N*-acetylneuraminic acid (Neu5Ac) or *N*-glycolylneuraminic acid (Neu5Gc). We then develop an expression, purification and detergent solubilization system for *Sa*SiaT and demonstrate that the protein is largely monodisperse in solution with a stable monomeric oligomeric state. Binding studies reveal that *Sa*SiaT has a higher affinity for Neu5Gc over Neu5Ac, which was unexpected and is not seen in another SiaT homolog. We develop a homology model and use comparative sequence analyses to identify substitutions in the substrate-binding site of *Sa*SiaT that may explain the altered specificity. *Sa*SiaT is shown to be electrogenic, and transport is dependent upon more than one Na^+ ion for every sialic acid molecule. A functional sialic acid transporter is essential for the uptake and utilization of sialic acid in a range of pathogenic bacteria, and developing new inhibitors that target these transporters is a valid mechanism for inhibiting bacterial growth. By demonstrating a route to functional recombinant *Sa*SiaT, and developing the *in vivo* and *in vitro* assay systems, our work underpins the design of inhibitors to this transporter.

Keywords: antibiotic resistance, sialic acids, SiaT, sodium solute symporter, *Staphylococcus aureus*

INTRODUCTION

Mammalian cell surfaces are decorated with complex glycoconjugates, such as glycoproteins and glycolipids. Found at the terminal non-reducing positions of these cell-surface glycoconjugates are negatively charged sialic acids, which mediate a diverse array of cellular interactions, recognition and adhesion.

Sialic acids comprise a large family of nine-carbon acidic monosaccharides, the most common of which is *N*-acetylneuraminic acid (Neu5Ac). While Neu5Ac is ubiquitously synthesized, the closely related sialic acid, *N*-glycolylneuraminic acid (Neu5Gc) is not. Although Neu5Ac and Neu5Gc sialic acids are widely expressed on mammalian tissues, human cells do not synthesize Neu5Gc. This is because humans have an inactivating mutation in the gene encoding CMP-*N*-acetylneuraminic acid hydroxylase, the rate-limiting enzyme for the generation of Neu5Gc in the cells of other mammals (Varki, 2001).

Mammalian commensal and pathogenic bacteria that colonize sialic acid rich tissues, such as the respiratory or gastrointestinal tract, have evolved mechanisms to use host-derived sialic acids for a competitive advantage; this suggests a link between sialic acid uptake/utilization and survival *in vivo* (Almagro-Moreno and Boyd, 2009). Some bacteria, such as *Haemophilus influenzae* (Vimr et al., 2000; Bouchet et al., 2003), and *Neisseria meningitides* (Vimr et al., 2004) incorporate sialic acid into their cell surface macromolecules to trick the host's innate immune response. Others, such as *Escherichia coli* (Vimr and Troy, 1985; Chang et al., 2004), *Staphylococcus aureus* (Olson et al., 2013), and *Vibrio vulnificus* (Jeong et al., 2009) use a suite of enzymes (North et al., 2013, 2014a,b, 2016) to degrade sialic acids as a source of carbon, nitrogen and energy. Notably, *H. influenzae* also metabolizes sialic acids in this way, and must make a metabolic decision between cell surface sialylation and sialic acid degradation (Vimr et al., 2000).

Bacteria that import sialic acids have evolved multiple mechanisms of transport across the cytoplasmic membrane. To date, four unique transporter families have been recognized, including those from the ATP binding cassette (ABC) (Post et al., 2005), tripartite ATP-independent periplasmic (TRAP) (Allen et al., 2005), major facilitator superfamily (MFS) (Vimr and Troy, 1985), and sodium solute symporter (SSS) (Severi et al., 2010; Wahlgren et al., 2018) transporter families (North et al., 2017). Whilst most bacteria possess only one type of sialic acid transporter, there are a few exceptions that are predicted to express two family types (Severi et al., 2010). It is not understood why these organisms produce more than one type of sialic acid transporter, but it is possible that they import sialic acid derivatives that are known in biological contexts.

Developing novel inhibitors that target bacterial sialic acid transporters may be a valid mechanism for inhibiting bacterial growth—several lines of evidence support this. It has been shown that a dedicated and functional sialic acid membrane transporter is required for the uptake of sialic acids (Vimr and Troy, 1985; Severi et al., 2005, 2010). Moreover, *in vivo* mouse studies demonstrate that sialic acid uptake and utilization is essential for colonization and persistence in a range of pathogenic bacteria (Chang et al., 2004; Almagro-Moreno and Boyd, 2009; Jeong et al., 2009; Pezzicoli et al., 2012). Knocking out the respective sialic acid transporter genes in *Salmonella enterica serovar* Typhirium and *Clostridium difficile* impairs outgrowth during post-antibiotic expansion (Ng et al., 2013), and *E. coli* during intestinal inflammation (Huang et al., 2015). Humans readily synthesize the Neu5Ac type of sialic acid and have dedicated membrane transporters to deploy it onto their surface. These share little homology to the bacterial transporters (North et al., 2017) so inhibitors to the bacterial transporters may not be toxic.

Recently, we determined the high-resolution outward-facing, and open, substrate-bound structure of the SiaT sialic acid transporter from *Proteus mirabilis* (*Pm*SiaT) (Wahlgren et al., 2018). SiaT transporters belong to the SSS family. *Pm*SiaT adopts the LeuT-fold with Neu5Ac bound near the center of the protein, and two Na^+ ions for transport.

This work investigates the SiaT sodium sialic acid symporter from *S. aureus* (*Sa*SiaT). We demonstrate that *Sa*SiaT can be purified and stably occupies a monomeric oligomeric state. We characterize the functionality of *Sa*SiaT with two different sialic acids, and the kinetics of sialic acid membrane transport.

MATERIALS AND METHODS

Molecular Biology Techniques

The *S. aureus* (strain RF122*) siaT* (Accession AJ938182.1) gene was codon optimized for *E. coli* (GeneArt, ThermoFischer Scientific; Supplementary Figure 1). For purification of recombinant protein and functional studies, *siaT* was amplified by PCR using *Sa_siaT*-F1 and *Sa_siaT*-R1 oligonucleotides (Supplementary Table 1) and cloned into the pWarf(-) (Hsieh et al., 2010) vector using the In-Fusion HD Cloning Kit (Clontech). The pWarf(-) vector carries a C-terminal human rhinovirus 3C protease (HRV3C) cleavage site followed by a green fluorescence protein (GFP)-tag and an 8 × histidine (His)-tag. The amplified fragment was cloned into pWarf(-) digested with the BamHI (3′) and XhoI (5′) restriction enzymes to generate pWarf(-)*Sa_siaT* with kanamycin resistance. This was transformed into Stellar™ Competent Cells (Clontech), purified using the DNA-Spin™ Plasmid DNA Purification Kit (iNtRon Biotechnology), and verified by DNA sequencing (Eurofins).

For bacterial growth experiments, *siaT* was amplified by PCR using *Sa_siaT*-F2 and *Sa_siaT*-R2 oligonucleotides (Supplementary Table 1) and cloned into the low-copy vector pJ422-01 also using the In-Fusion HD Cloning Kit. The amplified fragment was cloned into pJ422-01 digested with the EcoR1 (3′) and Nde1 (5′) restriction enzymes to generate pJ422-01*Sa_siaT* with Zeocin™ resistance. This was transformed into Stellar™ Competent Cells (Clontech), purified using the DNA-Spin™ Plasmid DNA Purification Kit (iNtRon Biotechnology), and verified by DNA sequencing (Genetic Analysis Service, University of Otago). The pJ422-01*Sa_siaT* plasmid was subsequently transformed into the *E. coli* JW3193 Δ*nanT* strain

[NBRP (NIG, Japan): *E. coli*] (Baba et al., 2006) generating the complementation strain *E. coli* JW3193 Δ*nanT-siaT*.

Protein Production and Purification

The pWarf(-)*Sa_siaT* plasmid was transformed into *E. coli* Lemo21(DE3) and grown in terrific broth media supplemented with kanamycin (50 μg/mL), chloramphenicol (34 μg/mL), L-rhamnose (100 μM), and induced with 0.4 mM isopropyl β-D-1-thiogalactopyranoside (IPTG) at 26°C overnight, with shaking at 180 rpm. For isothermal titration calorimetry and proteoliposome measurements, the protein was expressed in PASM-5052 auto-induction media (Lee et al., 2014). Cells were solubilized in phosphate-buffered saline (PBS), supplemented with cOmplete™ EDTA free protease inhibitor tablets (Roche), lysozyme (0.5 mg/mL), DNaseI (5 μg/mL), $MgCl_2$ (2 mM) and lysed by sonication using a Hielscher UP200S Ultrasonic Processor at 70% amplitude in cycles of 0.5 s on, 0.5 s off, for 30 min. Cell debris was pelleted by centrifugation at 24,000 g, for 25 min, at 4°C and the cell membranes were collected by ultracentrifugation at 230,000 g, for 2 h, at 4°C and stored at −80°C until further use. Cell membranes were solubilized in 2% (w/v) n-dodecyl-ß-D-maltoside (DDM) for 2 h at 4°C and unsolublized material was removed by ultracentrifugation at 150,000 g. The protein was first purified using immobilized metal affinity chromatography; the supernatant was loaded onto a 5 mL HisTrap HP column (GE Healthcare) equilibrated with Buffer A (70 mM Tris-HCl, pH 8.0, 150 mM NaCl, 20 mM imidazole, 6% glycerol, 5 mM β-mercaptoethanol, and 0.0174% (w/v) DDM). The column was washed with Buffer A, followed by a 10% wash with Buffer B (Buffer A with 500 mM imidazole) and protein was eluted using 50% Buffer B. Protein was concentrated and simultaneously exchanged into Buffer C (50 mM Tris-HCl, pH 8.0, 150 mM NaCl, 0.0174% (w/v) DDM). For analytical ultracentrifugation experiments, Buffer C contained 0.174% DDM. The GFP-tag was cleaved with HRV3C protease in a 1:12.5 mass ratio (HRV3C:*Sa*SiaT) at 4°C for 18 h. Size exclusion chromatography was performed as a final purification step using a HiLoad 16/60 Superdex 200 column in Buffer C. Protein concentration was determined using a NanoDrop 1000 spectrophotometer at 280 nm, using an extinction coefficient of 75,750 $M^{-1}cm^{-1}$, and a molecular weight of 56.7 kDa following HRV3C cleavage of the GFP-tag.

Analytical Ultracentrifugation

Sedimentation velocity experiments were performed in a Beckman Coulter Model XL-I analytical ultracentrifuge equipped with UV/Vis scanning optics. Reference buffer solution (50 mM Tris-HCl, 150 mM NaCl, pH 8.0) and sample solutions (including reference buffer solution with 0.174% DDM, and *Sa*SiaT at four concentrations: 0.6, 0.4, 0.2, and 0.1 mg mL^{-1}) were loaded into 12 mm double-sector cells with standard Epon 2-channel centerpieces and quartz windows. Cells were mounted in an eight hole An-50 Ti rotor and centrifuged at 50,000 rpm at 12°C. Interference and absorbance measurements at a wavelength of 280 nm were recorded over a radial position range of 5.8 to 7.3 cm within the cell, with measurements taken at sediment boundary intervals of 0.003 cm. The partial specific volume of *Sa*SiaT was calculated using SEDNTERP (Laue et al., 1992) and buffer density and buffer viscosity were experimentally measured with an Anton Paar DMA4100M density meter and Anton Paar Lovis 2000 ME microviscometer, respectively. The van Holde-Weischet and 2DSA-Monte Carlo analyses were performed using UltraScan III (Demeler and van Holde, 2004; Brookes and Demeler, 2007; Demeler and Brookes, 2007; Demeler, 2010).

Bacterial Growth Experiment

E. coli strains JW3193 Δ*nanT*, JW3193 Δ*nanT_siaT*, *and E. coli* BW25113, which served as a wild type control, were grown (37°C, 250 rpm) overnight in low salt Luria-Bertani (LB) media. For Δ*nanT_siaT*, the LB media was supplemented with Zeocin™ (25 μg/mL). Overnight cultures were diluted to an OD_{600} of 0.05 and further grown (37°C, 250 rpm) in low salt LB media supplemented with 1 mM IPTG until they reached mid-logarithmic phase (OD_{600} of 0.35). Bacterial cultures were harvested by centrifugation (6,000 rpm, 10 min, 4°C), washed three times in M9 minimal media and diluted to an OD_{600} of 0.5. Cultures (20 μL) were added to a Costar Flat Bottom 96 well plate with lid containing M9 minimal media (180 μL) supplemented with Zeocin™ (25 μg/mL), IPTG (1 mM), thiamin hydrochloride (7 μM) and either *N*-acetylneuraminic acid (Neu5Ac, 4 mg/mL, 12.9 mM), *N*-glycolylneuraminic acid (Neu5Gc, 4 mg/mL, 12.3 mM) or glucose (0.4%) as the sole carbon source. In addition, bacterial growth was monitored in M9 minimal media without any carbon source. Growth at 37°C, with shaking at 250 rpm, was recorded at 600 nm every 10 min using the FLUOstar Omega microplate reader (BMG labtech). Growth curves represent the mean of four measurements ± standard error of the mean, or three measurements ± standard error of the mean for the control experiments.

Microscale Thermophoresis

The binding affinities for two sialic acids and purified *Sa*SiaT were determined using microscale thermophoresis. Experiments were performed on a Monolith NT.LabelFree instrument (NanoTemper Technologies) (Wienken et al., 2010; Soares da Costa et al., 2016; Stifter et al., 2018). Purified *Sa*SiaT was diluted to 2 μM in PBS buffer supplemented with 0.0174% (w/v) DDM, and incubated with Neu5Ac (from 0.3 μM to 10 mM), and Neu5Gc (0.08 μM to 2.5 mM), for 5 min prior to taking measurements. The samples were loaded into Monolith NT Standard Treated Capillaries (NanoTemper Technologies). Microscale thermophoresis measurements were carried out at 25°C using 20% LED power, and 20% microscale thermophoresis infrared laser power. The dissociation constants (K_d) were determined using the mass action equation *via* the NT Analysis software version 1.5.41 (NanoTemper Technologies), using the signal from Thermophoresis + T-jump for triplicate experiments.

Isothermal Calorimetry

Purified *Sa*SiaT was concentrated to a final concentration of 170–240 μM using membrane ultrafiltration with a molecular weight cutoff of 50 kDa. The flow through was used to dilute 100 mM stock solutions of sialic acid to concentrations of 2.5–4 mM for Neu5Ac and 2–2.4 mM for Neu5Gc. Protein sample (206 μL) was loaded into the sample cell, and 70 μL of the respective sialic acid was loaded into the injection syringe. The system was equilibrated to 25°C with a stirring speed of 750 rpm. Titration curves were initiated by a 1 μL injection followed by 4 μL injections every 180 s. Background corrections were obtained by injection of sialic acids into buffer and buffer into protein with the same parameters. Biological triplicate experiments were analyzed using ORIGIN 7 with the first injection excluded. The curves were fitted into a single-site binding isotherm and K_d values were determined. Measurements were made using a Micro-200 Isothermal titration calorimeter or a PEAQ Isothermal titration calorimeter (MicroCal, Malvern).

Sequence Alignment and Homology Modeling of SiaT in an Outward-Facing Open Conformation

Multiple protein sequence alignment was performed between *Sa*SiaT and additional SiaT from various bacterial species, as described elsewhere (Wahlgren et al., 2018). This was used to compare conservation of the Neu5Ac binding site between organisms. A second multiple protein sequence alignment was performed between SiaT from 19 strains of *S. aureus*, to compare conservation of the Neu5Ac binding site between different isolates. These include *S. aureus* RF122, *S. aureus* ED133, *S. aureus* NR153, *S. aureus* XQ, *S. aureus* 93b_S9, *S. aureus* CFSAN007883, *S. aureus* HZW450, *S. aureus* MS4, *S. aureus* SA268, *S. aureus* SA40, *S. aureus* SA957, *S. aureus* M013, *S. aureus* FDA209P, *S. aureus* FDAARGOS_43, *S. aureus* NRS271, *S. aureus* MW2, *S. aureus* NRS143, *S. aureus* USA400-0051, *S. aureus* EDCC5464. Alignments were generated using *ClustalW* (Larkin et al., 2007).

The outward-facing open conformation of *Sa*SiaT was modeled on the outward-facing open structure of SiaT from *P. mirabilis* (*Pm*SiaT). These transporters share ~41% sequence identity. To build a homology model, an alignment between the two protein sequences was first generated using a global sequence alignment with *EMBOSS stretcher* (Myers and Miller, 1988). *MEDELLER* (Kelm et al., 2010) was used to create the model of *Sa*SiaT in the outward-facing open conformation using *Pm*SiaT (pdb entry 5nv9) as a template structure. Next, GROMACS 5.1.2 (Abraham et al., 2015) was used for energy minimization of the *Sa*SiaT homology model, using the GROMOS 54A7 force field. The resulting structure was superimposed onto the *Pm*SiaT structure with Neu5Ac bound using a Structural Alignment of Multiple Proteins (STAMP) structure-based sequence alignment in VMD MultiSeq. The structure was manually edited using COOT (without further energy minimization) to remove a clash between the sidechain of Tyr79 and the Neu5Ac. The sidechain was rotated to overlay with that of the corresponding residue (Phe78) in the template *Pm*SiaT structure. Other residues in the substrate binding site of the homology model were rotated to better represent the conformations found in the substrate bound *Pm*SiaT template.

Proteoliposome Assays

Purified *Sa*SiaT was reconstituted into proteoliposomes using a protocol previously optimized for *Pm*SiaT, with some modifications (Wahlgren et al., 2018). Briefly, 5 μg of protein was mixed with 120 μL 10% $C_{12}E_8$, 100 μL of 10% egg yolk phospholipids (w/v, sonicated as previously described to form liposomes, Scalise et al., 2014). Next, 20 mM of K^+-gluconate buffered by 20 mM Tris-HCl, pH 7.0 was added to create a final volume of 700 μL. The mixture was incubated with 0.5 g Amberlite XAD-4 resin under rotatory stirring (1,200 rev/min) at 25°C for 40 min (Scalise et al., 2015). After reconstitution, 600 μL of proteoliposomes were loaded onto a Sephadex G-75 column (0.7 cm diameter × 15 cm height) pre-equilibrated with 20 mM Tris-HCl, pH 7.0, 40 mM sucrose to balance internal osmolarity. To generate a K^+ diffusion potential, valinomycin (0.75 μg/mg phospholipid) prepared in ethanol was added to the proteoliposomes following Sephadex G-75 column chromatography, as previously described (Scalise et al., 2014; Wahlgren et al., 2018). As a control, ethanol was added to proteoliposomes, which did not exert any effect on the transport activity. After 10 s of incubation with valinomycin/ethanol, transport was started by adding 50 μM [^{3}H]-Neu5Ac to the proteoliposomes in the presence of 25 mM NaCl. The initial rate of transport was measured by stopping the reaction after 5 min, i.e., within the initial linear range of [^{3}H]-Neu5Ac uptake into the proteoliposomes. Transport was terminated once [^{3}H]-Neu5Ac was removed by loading each proteoliposome sample (100 μL) on a Sephadex G-75 column (0.6 cm diameter × 8 cm height). Proteoliposomes were eluted with 1 mL 50 mM NaCl and collected in 4 mL of scintillation mixture, vortexed and counted. Radioactivity uptake in liposome controls (without incorporated protein) was negligible with respect to transport data. Uptake data were fitted in a first-order rate equation for time course plots, and kinetic data were fitted with a Michaelis-Menten or Hill equations. Non-linear fitting analysis was performed by Grafit software (version 5.0.13). To measure the specific activity of *Sa*SiaT, the amount of protein was estimated by NanoDrop. All measurements are presented as means ± SD from three independent experiments.

RESULTS AND DISCUSSION

Expression of *Sa*SiaT Rescues an *E. Coli* Strain That Lacks its Endogenous Sialic Acid Transporter

To demonstrate sialic acid transport by *Sa*SiaT, we first showed that *Sa*SiaT rescues the growth of an *E. coli* strain lacking the endogenous NanT sialic acid transporter (Δ*nanT*) when grown on Neu5Ac or Neu5Gc (**Figure 1**). The Neu5Ac and Neu5Gc differ by the addition of a hydroxyl at the C11 methyl of the *N*-acetyl group in Neu5Gc (**Figure 1A**). While *E. coli* JW3193 Δ*nanT* grows in M9 minimal media supplemented with glucose (**Table 1**), it is not able to utilize Neu5Ac or Neu5Gc as the sole carbon source (**Figure 1B**, data in green). After complementation of *E. coli* JW3193 Δ*nanT* with pJ422-01*Sa_siaT* (to produce *E. coli* JW3193

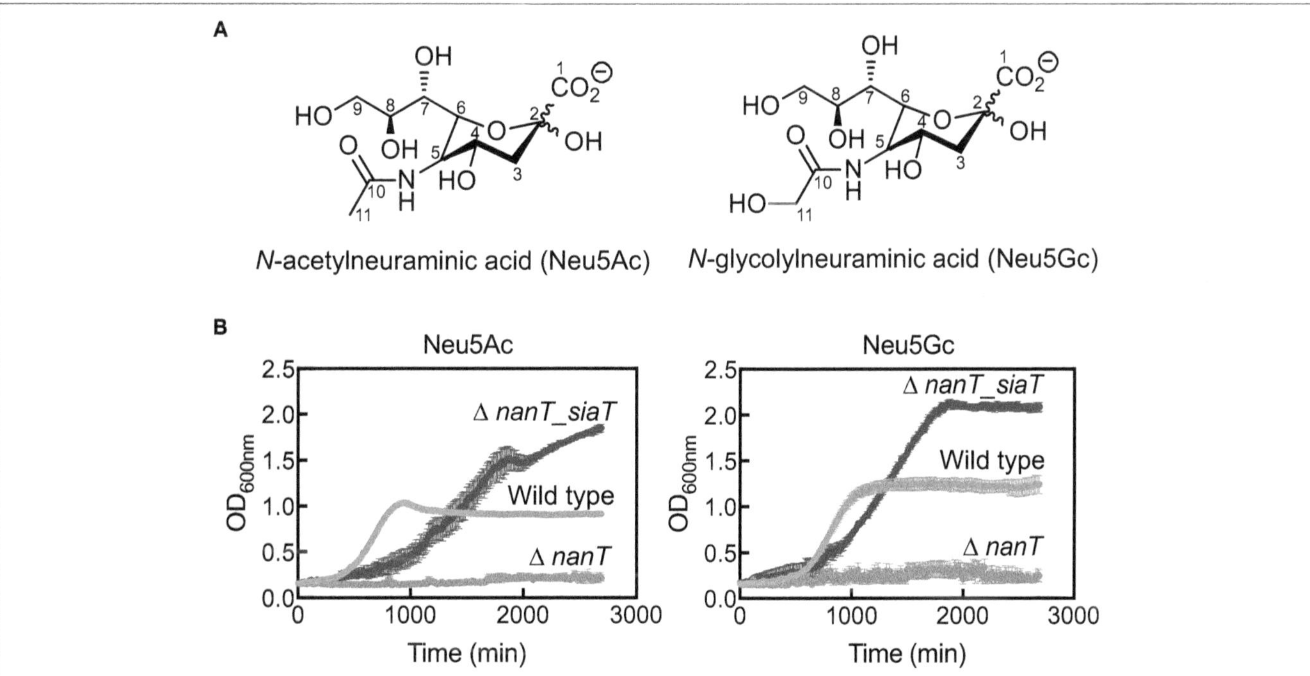

FIGURE 1 | Bacterial growth experiments demonstrate *Sa*SiaT function. **(A)** The chemical structures of Neu5Ac and Neu5Gc. **(B)** Growth of *E. coli* wild type (orange), Δ*nanT* (green), and its complemented derivative Δ*nant_siaT* (blue) on Neu5Ac and Neu5Gc. While Δ*nanT* is unable to utilize Neu5Ac and Neu5Gc, *Sa*SiaT is able to rescue the growth of Δ*nanT* on both Neu5Ac and Neu5Gc sialic acids as the sole carbon source.

TABLE 1 | Growth rates of the *E. coli* wild type, Δ*nanT* and Δ*nanT_siaT* in M9 minimal media containing different carbon sources.

Strain	Neu5Ac	Neu5Gc	Glucose	No carbon source
Wild type	3.56 (0.04) × 10^{-3}	3.3 (0.1) × 10^{-3}	5.5 (0.2) × 10^{-3}	–
Δ*nanT*	–	–	4.3 (0.5) × 10^{-3}	–
Δ*nanT_siaT*	1.3 (0.3) × 10^{-3}	1.9 (0.05) × 10^{-3}	3.86 (0.05) × 10^{-3}	–

Values represent the growth rate/min. A dash (–) indicates no growth. Values in brackets represent the standard error of measurement, where n = 4.

Δ*nanT_siaT*), the ability to grow on both sialic acids is restored (**Figure 1B**, data in blue). Notably, the growth rate of Δ*nanT_siaT* is faster when grown in M9 minimal media containing Neu5Gc as the sole carbon source, as opposed to Neu5Ac (**Table 1**). This could reflect more efficient transport of Neu5Gc, due to a higher affinity for Neu5Gc compared to Neu5Ac.

Curiously, *E. coli* Δ*nanT_siaT* reached higher final optical density compared to wild type *E. coli* BW25113 (**Figure 1B**, data in blue compared to data in orange). This was unexpected, perhaps suggesting that the native *E. coli* NanT may be regulated in some way, thereby limiting sialic acid uptake. *E. coli* Δ*nanT_siaT* exhibits an extended lag-phase compared to wild type *E. coli* BW25113. Since SiaT expression was pre-induced with IPTG (see section Materials and Methods), it is likely that the growth lag is due to an increased metabolic burden caused by the overexpression of SiaT itself. This also explains the reduced growth rates of Δ*nanT_siaT* compared to the wild type (**Table 1**).

In short, we demonstrate that the *Sa*SiaT is functional *in vivo* and observe a preference for Neu5Gc in terms of maximum growth rate.

Recombinant *Sa*SiaT Is Stably Purified as a Single Species

*Sa*SiaT was successfully overexpressed, solubilized, and purified to homogeneity in buffer containing DDM detergent. The profile from size exclusion chromatography (**Figure 2A**) shows a dominant peak at ~55 mL, with a shoulder to the left that is consistent with a small amount of a larger component, possibly an aggregate. Analytical ultracentrifugation studies at protein concentrations ranging from 0.1 to 0.6 mg/mL were used to assess the stability and oligomeric state of purified recombinant *Sa*SiaT prior to functional studies. Analyses of absorbance data from analytical ultracentrifugation experiments, using van Holde-Weischet sedimentation coefficient distributions (**Figure 2B**), reveal a largely monodisperse solution with a major component at ~8 S. However, as evidenced by the shift of the distribution

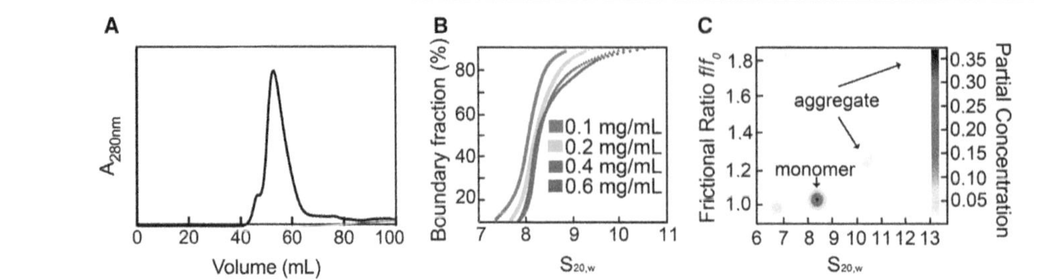

FIGURE 2 | Recombinant *Sa*SiaT can be stably purified and occupies a predominantly single oligomeric state. **(A)** Size-exclusion chromatography trace of *Sa*SiaT at its final purification step. To the left of a main dominant peak there is a small shoulder, which may represent aggregate. **(B)** van Holde-Weischet sedimentation coefficient distributions show a dominant component at ~8 S. **(C)** 2DSA-Monte Carlo analysis of sedimentation velocity data of *Sa*SiaT at 0.6 mg/mL, as implemented by UltraScan III, shows a main peak comprising 70% of the signal.

to the right, the van Holde-Weischet analysis also suggests that some protein may be aggregated. 2DSA-Monte Carlo analysis (**Figure 2C**) determines a major component at 8.2 S with a frictional ratio of 1.05, which is consistent with a molecular weight of 160 kDa (assuming a mass averaged v-bar of 0.76 for the detergent:protein complex). This is consistent with a *Sa*SiaT monomer surrounded by ~200 DDM molecules. This monomeric species represents ~70% of the total sample. The 2DSA-Monte Carlo analysis also shows a series of larger components ranging from 10.5 to 13.0 S with an increasing frictional ratio, that represent a small amount of aggregate. Overall, our studies demonstrate that *Sa*SiaT can be stably expressed and purified using the detergent DDM. Furthermore, when solubilized in DDM, it is largely a monomer that associates with ~200 DDM molecules in solution.

Binding Studies Demonstrate That *Sa*SiaT Has an Altered Specificity

Given the increased growth rate observed when grown on Neu5Gc compared to Neu5Ac, the binding affinity of Neu5Ac and Neu5Gc to recombinant *Sa*SiaT was determined using microscale thermophoresis (**Figure 3A**) and isothermal titration calorimetry (**Figure 3B**). By microscale thermophoresis, *Sa*SiaT has a considerably higher affinity for the Neu5Gc sialic acid (K_d = 39 ± 4 μM) compared to the Neu5Ac sialic acid (K_d = 113 ± 6 μM). Consistent with this, isothermal titration calorimetry experiments confirmed that *Sa*SiaT has a higher affinity for Neu5Gc (K_d = 18 ± 2 μM) than Neu5Ac (K_d = 106 ± 2 μM). Interestingly, *Pm*SiaT is the opposite, and displays a more similar, but higher binding affinity for Neu5Ac (K_d^{Neu5Ac} = 58 ± 1 μM) compared to Neu5Gc (K_d^{Neu5Gc} = 85 ± 2 μM) using microscale thermophoresis (Wahlgren et al., 2018). Thus, *Sa*SiaT reveals different substrate specificity compared to *Pm*SiaT.

Three Substitutions in the Active Site of *Sa*SiaT may Explain Altered Substrate Specificity

To reconcile at the molecular level the observed difference in substrate specificity, and ultimately, the difference between *Sa*SiaT and *Pm*SiaT, amino acid sequence analyses and homology modeling were used to examine the differences in the active site.

The Neu5Ac binding site, as determined in *Pm*SiaT (pdb entry 5nv9), is conserved among SiaT transporters from a number of bacterial species (**Figure 4A**) (Wahlgren et al., 2018). When comparing the sequences between *Sa*SiaT and *Pm*SiaT, there are three substitutions in *Sa*SiaT (*Pm*SiaT-Gln82 to *Sa*SiaT-Asn83, *Pm*SiaT-Phe78 to *Sa*SiaT-Tyr79, and *Pm*SiaT-Phe243 to *Sa*SiaT-Asn244, **Figure 4A**) that we predict are involved in substrate binding. These residues are highly conserved among *S. aureus* isolates (Supplementary Figure 2); they are, therefore, not specific to any particular isolate of *S. aureus*.

To map these substitutions within the putative active site, a homology model of *Sa*SiaT was built based upon the outward-facing open structure of *Pm*SiaT (pdb entry 5nv9) (**Figure 4B**). Superposition of the *Sa*SiaT homology model with *Pm*SiaT (r.m.s.d. = 0.172 Å for 364 α-carbon atoms) demonstrates that the *Pm*SiaT-Gln82 to *Sa*SiaT-Asn83, *Pm*SiaT-Phe243 to *Sa*SiaT-Asn244, and *Pm*SiaT-Phe78 to *Sa*SiaT-Tyr79 substitutions in *Sa*SiaT may be responsible for the altered substrate specificity observed in the binding experiments, since they are close to the C11 methyl group of the *N*-acetyl moiety of Neu5Ac (**Figure 4B**), which is hydroxylated in Neu5Gc.

In the *Pm*SiaT crystal structure, the side chain of Gln82 (*Sa*SiaT-Asn83) is in a position to form two hydrogen bonds with the hydroxyl group at C9 and the hydroxyl group at C7 of the Neu5Ac glycerol tail (**Figure 4C**) (Wahlgren et al., 2018). In *Sa*SiaT, the side chain of the Asn83 substitution is shorter than a Gln, which creates more space in the substrate-binding cavity. *Sa*SiaT-Asn83 may be in a position to bond the additional C11 hydroxyl of Neu5Gc (**Figure 4C**), but only if the C11 hydroxyl points toward the glycerol tail. Like *Pm*SiaT-Gln82, *Sa*SiaT-Asn83 is still in position to hydrogen bond the hydroxyl group at C9 of the glycerol tail, albeit with a longer hydrogen bond length.

The C10 carbonyl of the *N*-acetyl moiety in Neu5Ac is coordinated by the amide from the side chain of Gln82 through a water molecule, while the methyl group of the *N*-acetyl moiety of Neu5Ac is facing toward a hydrophobic patch formed by Phe78 and Phe243 (**Figure 4C**) (Wahlgren et al., 2018). In *Sa*SiaT, Tyr79, and Asn244 replace the equivalent positions of

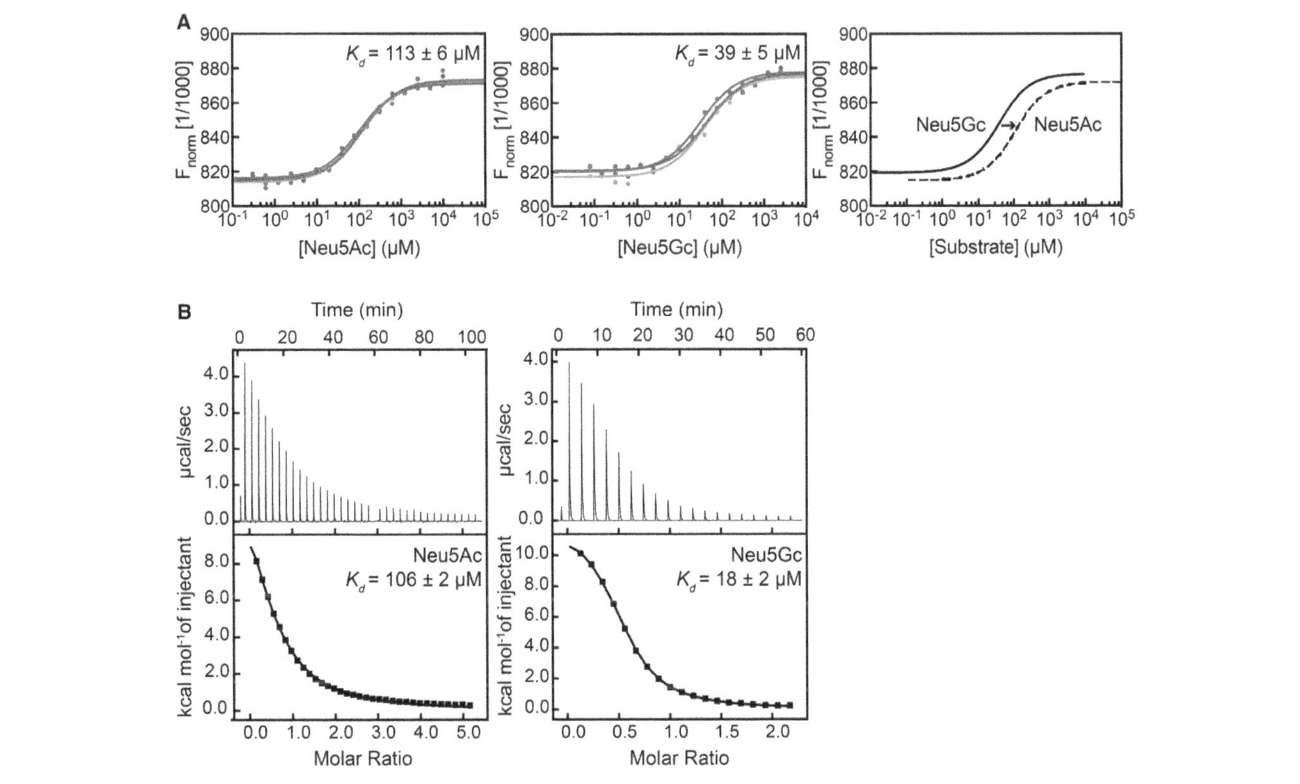

FIGURE 3 | Orthogonal binding experiments demonstrate substrate ambiguity. **(A)** Microscale thermophoresis binding assay to measure the affinity of *Sa*SiaT for Neu5Ac and Neu5Gc sialic acids. Raw data are shown with the fit for three independent experiments with Neu5Ac (left) and Neu5Gc (middle). The K_d values are reported as the mean ± uncertainty in the mean of the fit using the signal from Thermophoresis + T-jump, from triplicate experiments, where $n = 1$ (we define n as the number of different recombinant protein preparations, which we view as equivalent to biological replicates). The K_d and associated error of each fit is given in Supplementary Table 2. The shift in K_d between both sialic acids is shown (right). *Sa*SiaT has a tighter affinity for Neu5Gc than Neu5Ac. **(B)** Representative isothermal titration calorimetry raw data (top panel) and binding isotherm (bottom panel) of one isothermal titration calorimetry experiment obtained by successive titration of Neu5Ac (left) or Neu5Gc (right) with purified *Sa*SiaT. The fit of a single binding site is shown in the bottom panels (black line). K_d values are reported as the mean ± SEM of the fit from three experiments using different protein preparations ($n = 3$).

*Pm*SiaT-Phe78 and *Pm*SiaT-Phe243 (**Figure 4B**). *Sa*SiaT-Asn244 could facilitate a new interaction with the additional C11 hydroxyl group of Neu5Gc, and the side chain hydroxyl group of *Sa*SiaT-Tyr79 could create a more hydrophilic environment in the vicinity, which may be important for Neu5Ac and Neu5Gc discrimination.

There are other examples where the preference for Neu5Gc is mediated by new interactions, *via* hydrogen bonds, with the extra hydroxyl group present in Neu5Gc. A similar preference for Neu5Gc over Neu5Ac has been reported for the subtilase cytotoxin (SubAB) produced by Shiga-toxigenic *E. coli* (Byres et al., 2008), and the porcine rotavirus (Yu et al., 2012), both of which bind to glycans terminating with sialic acids. The crystal structure of SubB-Neu5Gc complex (pdb entry 3dwa) shows that the C11 hydroxyl group of the glycolyl in Neu5Gc forms important hydrogen bonds with the side chain of a Tyr, and the main chain of a Met (Byres et al., 2008). The crystal structure of the porcine rotavirus strain CRW-8 spike protein domain VP8 (pdb entry 3tay) has similar interactions between the glycolyl of Neu5Gc with the side chain of a Thr, and the main chain of a Tyr (Yu et al., 2012). Mutation of these residues results in a significant loss of activity. Similarly, the VP1 capsid protein from human polyomavirus 9 (HPyV9) has a preference for Neu5Gc over Neu5Ac (Khan et al., 2014). However, the VP1 capsid protein from a closely related homolog, monkey-derived simian B-lymphotropic polyomavirus (LPyV), has no such preference (Khan et al., 2014). Again, the preference for Neu5Gc is acquired by specific hydrogen bonds with the glycolyl of Neu5Gc, which LPyV cannot form.

In conclusion, we suggest that the altered specificity of *Sa*SiaT for Neu5Gc over Neu5Ac, compared to *Pm*SiaT, may be afforded by Asn substitutions at the 83 and 244 positions, and a Tyr substitution at position 78, in the substrate-binding site of *Sa*SiaT.

Proteoliposome Assays Delineate the Kinetics of Sialic Acid Membrane Transport

To demonstrate the ability of purified recombinant *Sa*SiaT to not only bind sialic acids, but to also transport them across a lipid membrane, we reconstituted the protein into proteoliposomes using native *E. coli* lipids and measured time dependent

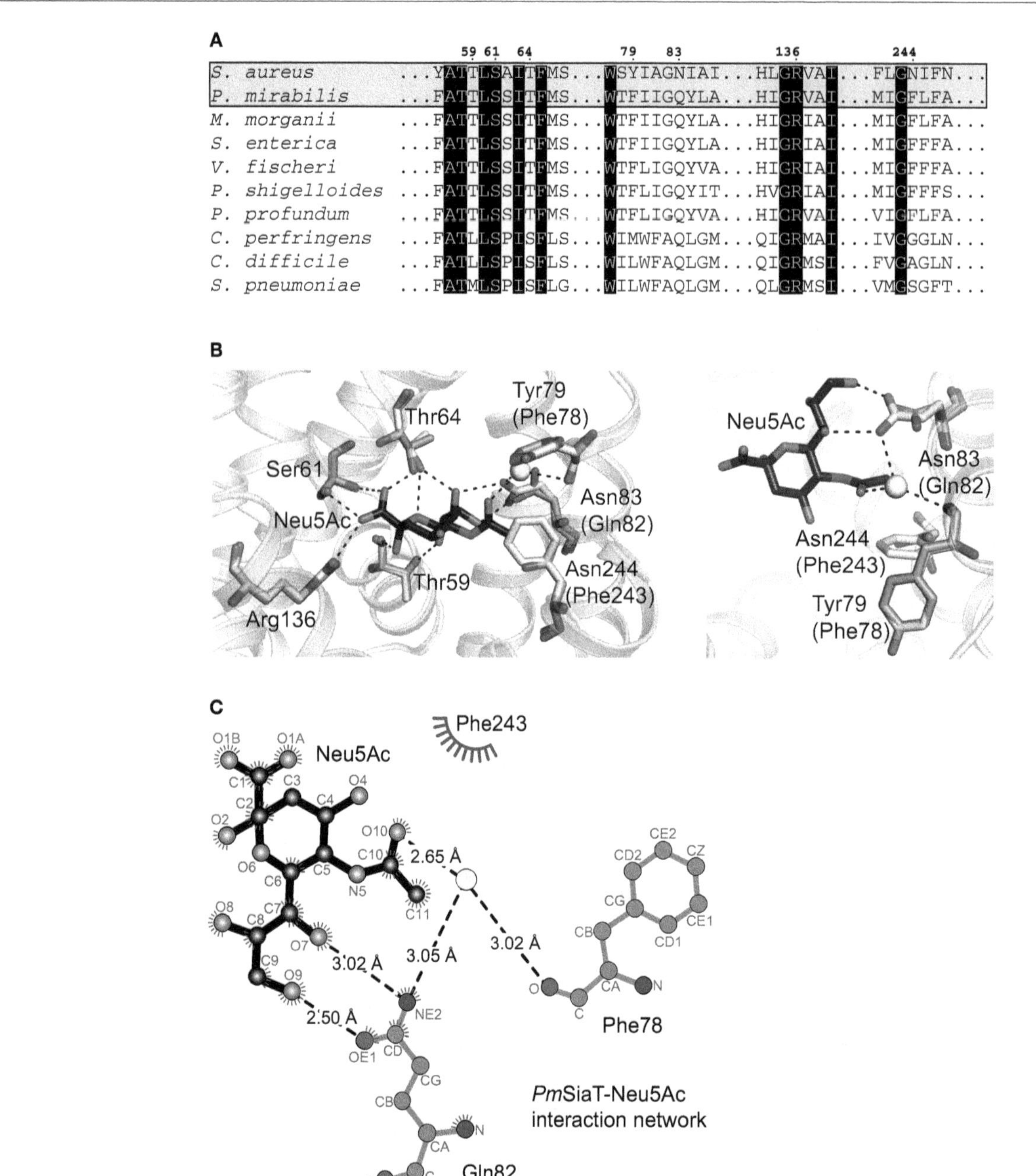

FIGURE 4 | Sequence alignment and homology modeling probe substrate ambiguity. **(A)** Amino acid sequence alignment of *Sa*SiaT with SiaT transporters from eight additional bacterial species (Wahlgren et al., 2018). SiaT transporters from *S. aureus*, *P. mirabilis*, *Morganella morganii*, *S. enterica*, *Vibrio fischeri*, *Plesiomonas shigelloides*, *Photobacterium profundum*, *Clostridium perfringens*, *C. difficile*, and *Streptococcus pneumoniae* are aligned. Important residues in the Neu5Ac binding site in *Pm*SiaT (pdb entry 5nv9) are shown. Residues highlighted with black boxes are highly conserved, and important residues implicated in Neu5Ac binding in *Pm*SiaT are numbered according to *Sa*SiaT. **(B)** Superposition of the *Sa*SiaT homology model (green) and *Pm*SiaT (gray) with Neu5Ac bound (black). Residues are labeled according to *Sa*SiaT, with *Pm*SiaT in parentheses. A water molecule from *Pm*SiaT is shown in yellow. *Pm*SiaT coordinates are from pdb entry 5nv9. Black dashed lines depict hydrogen bonds, or a salt bridge with Arg136. On the right, the binding site has been rotated 90° and the substituted residues are shown. **(C)** The *Pm*SiaT-Neu5Ac interaction network (Wahlgren et al., 2018) with Gln82, Phe78, and Phe243 is represented as a Ligplot$^+$ diagram (Laskowski and Swindells, 2011) using PDB entry 5nv9. Hydrogen bonds (dashed lines), hydrophobic contacts (arcs with spokes), and an interacting water molecule (yellow) are shown.

uptake of [^{3}H]Neu5Ac (**Figure 5A**). The transporter mediated a Na^+-dependent uptake of [^{3}H]Neu5Ac, stimulated by an imposed membrane potential. Similar to *Pm*SiaT (Wahlgren et al., 2018), in the presence of an imposed membrane potential, transport at equilibrium was almost doubled (185 ± 15 nmol/min/mg) compared with transport in the absence of an imposed membrane potential (95 ± 5 nmol/min/mg) (**Figure 5A**). Transport of [^{3}H]Neu5Ac in liposomes without

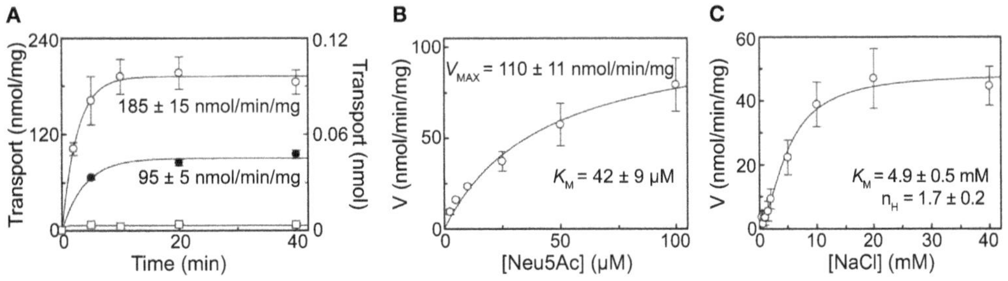

FIGURE 5 | Proteoliposome assays demonstrate the ability to transport sialic acid, which is dependent on Na+. **(A)** Proteoliposome transport was started by adding 50 µM [^{3}H]-Neu5Ac together with 25 mM NaCl to proteoliposomes reconstituted with purified recombinant *Sa*SiaT. In ○, □, valinomycin was added to facilitate K^+ movement prior to transport. In •, ethanol was added instead of valinomycin as a control. On the left Y-axis, specific transport activity is reported. In □, transport was measured in empty liposomes, with transport in empty liposomes reported on the right Y-axis. Transport was stopped at indicated times by passing proteoliposomes through Sephadex-G75 columns. Data were fitted to the first-order rate equation. **(B)** The transport of [^{3}H]-Neu5Ac over a range of concentrations in the presence of 25 mM NaCl was measured in proteoliposomes reconstituted with purified recombinant *Sa*SiaT, with an imposed K^+ diffusion membrane potential, over 5 min. Data were fitted to the Michaelis-Menten equation. **(C)** The transport of 50 µM [^{3}H]-Neu5Ac in the presence of NaCl over a range of concentrations was measured in proteoliposomes reconstituted with purified recombinant *Sa*SiaT, with an imposed K^+ diffusion membrane potential, over 5 min. Data were fitted to the Hill equation. All data are presented as mean ± SD from three independent experiments.

*Sa*SiaT protein was negligible with respect to reconstituted *Sa*SiaT proteoliposomes.

In optimal proteoliposome transport conditions with an imposed membrane potential, [^{3}H]Neu5Ac is transported by *Sa*SiaT with a K_M of 42 ± 9 µM and a V_{max} of 110 ± 11 nmol/min/mg (**Figure 5B**). This is lower (a higher binding affinity) than the measurements made using microscale thermophoresis and isothermal titration calorimetry, which may reflect the altered solubilization of the transporter in lipid, as opposed to detergent. The K_M for [^{3}H]Neu5Ac transport by *Sa*SiaT is almost twice that of *Pm*SiaT (Wahlgren et al., 2018). Consistent with the binding experiments, the molecular basis of this difference is likely that *Sa*SiaT has a lower affinity for Neu5Ac compared to *Pm*SiaT.

The kinetics of Na^+ transport by *Sa*SiaT was measured in proteoliposomes, giving a K_M of 4.9 ± 0.5 mM (**Figure 5C**). As demonstrated by the cooperativity index calculated from the Hill plot, the transport stoichiometry is more than one for Na^+. This is in the same order calculated for *Pm*SiaT, which transport two Na^+ for every Neu5Ac (Wahlgren et al., 2018).

To conclude, proteoliposome experiments demonstrate that the recombinant *Sa*SiaT is functional and able to transport Neu5Ac, that an electrogenic gradient drives transport, that the affinity for Neu5Ac is less than for *Pm*SiaT, and that two Na^+ ions are transported for every sialic acid.

CONCLUSIONS

Overall, we demonstrate that *Sa*SiaT is a functional sialic acid transporter, with a considerably higher binding affinity for Neu5Gc over Neu5Ac. Compared to *Pm*SiaT, in which Neu5Gc and Neu5Ac have similar binding affinities (Wahlgren et al., 2018), *Sa*SiaT has altered substrate specificity. We propose that three residues unique to the *Sa*SiaT substrate-binding site (Tyr79, Asn83, and Asn244) achieve a higher affinity to Neu5Gc. Like SubAB, the porcine rotavirus, and HPyV9, which also have a preference for Neu5Gc over Neu5Ac (Byres et al., 2008; Yu et al., 2012; Khan et al., 2014), specific hydrogen bonds with the C11 hydroxyl of Neu5Gc, and a hydrophilic environment in the vicinity of the Neu5Gc glycolyl chain, afford this specificity (Khan et al., 2014).

Although humans cannot synthesize Neu5Gc, they can acquire it from red meat and milk in the diet (Varki, 2010; Varki et al., 2011). Consequently, metabolic incorporation of Neu5Gc has been identified in the human gut epithelium and kidney vasculature (Tangvoranuntakul et al., 2003; Byres et al., 2008; Banda et al., 2012). Since some bacteria and viruses can discriminate between sialic acid variants (Byres et al., 2008; Yu et al., 2012; Khan et al., 2014; Stencel-Baerenwald et al., 2014), this could, in turn, influence their host or tissue range. It is possible that the ability of *Sa*SiaT to bind Neu5Gc with higher affinity (compared to Neu5Ac) confers an advantage to *S. aureus* in specific niches.

Because a functional sialic acid transporter is essential for the uptake and utilization of sialic acid in a range of pathogenic bacteria, these transporters present a new avenue for drug design. The work presented here underpins the development of inhibitors that target SiaT transporters, and in particular, *S. aureus*.

AUTHOR CONTRIBUTIONS

RF and RD conceived the project. Cloning and expression trials of *Sa*SiaT were carried out by ED and SR. Large-scale expression, membrane preparation, and protein purification were carried out by ED, WW, DR, and RN. Experiments for whole-cell functional analysis were designed by EC, ED, RN, and DR, and carried out by RN and DR. DR analyzed the results. Analytical ultracentrifugation experiments were performed and analyzed by SK. Proteoliposome assays were designed by MS, WW, RD, and CI. MS conducted and analyzed these experiments. Microscale thermophoresis experiments were carried out and analyzed by

RN, TS, and MP. Isothermal titration calorimetry was performed and analyzed by WW. RN, WW, and JA carried out homology modeling and analysis of *Sa*SiaT. RN, WW, DR, MS, SK, CI, JA, RF, and RD wrote the manuscript, while all authors discussed the results and made manuscript revisions.

ACKNOWLEDGMENTS

RD acknowledges the following for funding support, in part: (1) the Marsden Fund Council from Government funding, managed by Royal Society Te Apārangi (contract UOC1506) and (2) the US Army Research Laboratory and US Army Research Office under grant number W911NF-11-1-0481. RF acknowledges the following for funding support: (1) the Swedish Research Council (2011-5790), (2) the Swedish Research Council Formas (2010-1759), (3) the Swedish Governmental Agency for Innovation Systems (VINNOVA) (2013-04655 and 2017-00180), (4) Carl Tryggers Stiftelse för Vetenskaplig Forskning (11:147) and (5) Centre for Antibiotic Resistance Research (CARe) at University of Gothenburg. RN acknowledges EMBO (584-2014). WW acknowledges the Swedish Research Council Formas (221-2013-730), Magnus Bergvalls Stiftelse (2014-00536, 2015-00763, 2016-01606). SR acknowledges the Indo-Swedish grant awarded by the Department of Biotechnology (BT/IN/Sweden/41/SR/2013). JA acknowledges the following for funding support: (1) a Rutherford Discovery Fellowship (15-MAU-001) and (2) the Marsden Fund Council (15-UOA-105). We thank Dr. Mitja Remus-Emsermann (University of Canterbury), for support, guidance, and use of equipment for the bacterial growth assays. We thank Prof. Borries Demeler (University of Texas Health Science Center at San Antonio), for assistance in the analytical ultracentrifugation analysis.

REFERENCES

Abraham, M. J., Murtola, T., Schulz, R., Páll, S., Smith, J. C., Hess, B., et al. (2015). GROMACS: High performance molecular simulations through multi-level parallelism from laptops to supercomputers. *Software X* 1–2, 19–25. doi: 10.1016/j.softx.2015.06.001

Allen, S., Zaleski, A., Johnston, J. W., Gibson, B. W., and Apicella, M. A. (2005). Novel sialic acid transporter of *Haemophilus influenzae*. *Infect. Immun.* 73, 5291–5300. doi: 10.1128/IAI.73.9.5291-5300.2005

Almagro-Moreno, S., and Boyd, E. F. (2009). Insights into the evolution of sialic acid catabolism among bacteria. *BMC Evol. Biol.* 9:118. doi: 10.1186/1471-2148-9-118

Baba, T., Ara, T., Hasegawa, M., Takai, Y., Okumura, Y., Baba, M., et al. (2006). Construction of *Escherichia coli* K-12 in-frame, single-gene knockout mutants: the Keio collection. *Mol. Syst. Biol.* 2:2006.0008. doi: 10.1038/msb4100050

Banda, K., Gregg, C. J., Chow, R., Varki, N. M., and Varki, A. (2012). Metabolism of vertebrate amino sugars with *N*-glycolyl groups: mechanisms underlying gastrointestinal incorporation of the non-human sialic acid xeno-autoantigen *N*-glycolylneuraminic acid. *J. Biol. Chem.* 287, 28852–28864. doi: 10.1074/jbc.M112.364182

Bouchet, V., Hood, D. W., Li, J., Brisson, J.-R., Randle, G. A., Martin, A., et al. (2003). Host-derived sialic acid is incorporated into *Haemophilus influenzae* lipopolysaccharide and is a major virulence factor in experimental otitis media. *PNAS* 100, 8898–8903. doi: 10.1073/pnas.1432026100

Brookes, E. H., and Demeler, B. (2007). "Parsimonious regularization using genetic algorithms applied to the analysis of analytical ultracentrifugation experiments," in *GECCO '07 Proceedings of the 9th annual Conference on Genetic and Evolutionary Computation* (New York, NY).

Byres, E., Paton, A. W., Paton, J. C., Löfling, J. C., Smith, D. F., Wilce, M. C., et al. (2008). Incorporation of a non-human glycan mediates human susceptibility to a bacterial toxin. *Nature* 456, 648–652. doi: 10.1038/nature07428

Chang, D.-E., Smalley, D. J., Tucker, D. L., Leatham, M. P., Norris, W. E., Stevenson, S. J., et al. (2004). Carbon nutrition of *Escherichia coli* in the mouse intestine. *PNAS* 101, 7427–7432. doi: 10.1073/pnas.0307888101

Demeler, B. (2010). Methods for the design and analysis of sedimentation velocity and sedimentation equilibrium experiments with proteins. *Curr. Protoc. Protein. Sci.* Chapter 7, Unit 7.13. doi: 10.1002/0471140864.ps0713s60

Demeler, B., and Brookes, E. (2007). Monte Carlo analysis of sedimentation experiments. *Coll. Polym. Sci.* 286, 129–137. doi: 10.1007/s00396-007-1699-4.

North, R. A., Horne, C. R., Davies, J. S., Remus, D. M., Muscroft-Taylor, A. C., Goyal, P., et al. (2017). "Just a spoonful of sugar": import of sialic acid across bacterial cell membranes. *Biophys. Rev.* 19:425. doi: 10.1007/s12551-017-0343-x

Demeler, B., and van Holde, K. E. (2004). Sedimentation velocity analysis of highly heterogeneous systems. *Anal. Biochem.* 335, 279–288. doi: 10.1016/j.ab.2004.08.039

Hsieh, J. M., Besserer, G. M., Madej, M. G., Bui, H.-Q., Kwon, S., and Abramson, J. (2010). Bridging the gap: a GFP-based strategy for overexpression and purification of membrane proteins with intra and extracellular C-termini. *Protein Sci.* 19, 868–880. doi: 10.1002/pro.365

Huang, Y.-L., Chassard, C., Hausmann, M., von Itzstein M., and Hennet, T. (2015). Sialic acid catabolism drives intestinal inflammation and microbial dysbiosis in mice. *Nat. Commun.* 6:8141. doi: 10.1038/ncomms9141

Jeong, H. G., Oh, M. H., Kim, B. S., Lee, M. Y., Han, H. J., and Choi, S. H. (2009). The capability of catabolic utilization of *N*-acetylneuraminic acid, a sialic acid, is essential for *Vibrio vulnificus* pathogenesis. *Infect. Immun.* 77, 3209–3217. doi: 10.1128/IAI.00109-09

Kelm, S., Shi, J., and Deane, C. M. (2010). MEDELLER: homology-based coordinate generation for membrane proteins. *Bioinformatics* 26, 2833–2840. doi: 10.1093/bioinformatics/btq554

Khan, Z. M., Liu, Y., Neu, U., Gilbert, M., Ehlers, B., Feizi, T., et al. (2014). Crystallographic and glycan microarray analysis of human polyomavirus 9 VP1 identifies *N*-glycolyl neuraminic acid as a receptor candidate. *J. Virol.* 88, 6100–6111. doi: 10.1128/JVI.03455-13

Larkin, M. A., Blackshields, G., Brown, N. P., Chenna, R., McGettigan, P. A., McWilliam, H., et al. (2007). Clustal W and Clustal X version 2.0. *Bioinformatics* 23, 2947–2948. doi: 10.1093/bioinformatics/btm404

Laskowski, R. A., and Swindells, M. B. (2011). LigPlot+: multiple ligand-protein interaction diagrams for drug discovery. *J. Chem. Inf. Model.* 51, 2778–2786. doi: 10.1021/ci200227u

Laue, T. M., Shah, B. D., Ridgeway, T. M., and Pelletier, S. L. (1992). *Analytical Ultracentrifugation in Biochemistry and Polymer Science*. Cambridge: The Royal Society of Chemistry.

Lee, C., Kang, H. J., Hjelm, A., Qureshi, A. A., Nji, E., Choudhury, H., et al. (2014). MemStar: a one-shot *Escherichia coli*-based approach for high-level bacterial membrane protein production. *FEBS Lett.* 588, 3761–3769. doi: 10.1016/j.febslet.2014.08.025

Myers, E. W., and Miller, W. (1988). Optimal alignments in linear space. *Comput. Appl. Biosci.* 4, 11–17.

Ng, K. M., Ferreyra, J. A., Higginbottom, S. K., Lynch, J. B., Kashyap, P. C., Gopinath, S., et al. (2013). Microbiota-liberated host sugars facilitate post-antibiotic expansion of enteric pathogens. *Nature* 502, 96–99. doi: 10.1038/nature12503

Stencel-Baerenwald, J. E., Reiss, K., Reiter, D. M., Stehle, T., and Dermody, T. S. (2014). The sweet spot: defining virus-sialic acid interactions. *Nat. Rev. Microbiol.* 12, 739–749. doi: 10.1038/nrmicro3346

North, R. A., Kessans, S. A., Atkinson, S. C., Suzuki, H., Watson, A. J. A., Burgess, B. R., et al. (2013). Cloning, expression, purification, crystallization and preliminary X-ray diffraction studies of *N*-acetylneuraminate lyase from methicillin-resistant *Staphylococcus aureus*. *Acta Crystallogr. F Struct. Biol. Commun.* 69, 306–312. doi: 10.1107/S1744309113003060

North, R. A., Kessans, S. A., Griffin, M. D. W., Watson, A. J. A., Fairbanks, A. J., and Dobson, R. C. J. (2014a). Cloning, expression, purification, crystallization and preliminary X-ray diffraction analysis of *N*-acetylmannosamine-6-phosphate 2-epimerase from methicillin-resistant *Staphylococcus aureus*. *Acta Crystallogr. F Struct. Biol. Commun.* 70, 650–655. doi: 10.1107/S2053230X14007171

North, R. A., Seizova, S., Stampfli, A., Kessans, S. A., Suzuki, H., Griffin, M. D. W., et al. (2014b). Cloning, expression, purification, crystallization and preliminary X-ray diffraction analysis of *N*-acetylmannosamine kinase from methicillin-resistant *Staphylococcus aureus*. *Acta Crystallogr. F Struct. Biol. Commun.* 70, 643–649. doi: 10.1107/S2053230X14007250

North, R. A., Watson, A. J. A., Pearce, F. G., Muscroft-Taylor, A. C., Friemann, R., Fairbanks, A. J., et al. (2016). Structure and inhibition of *N*-acetylneuraminate lyase from methicillin-resistant *Staphylococcus aureus*. *FEBS Lett.* 590, 4414–4428. doi: 10.1002/1873-3468.12462

Olson, M. E., King, J. M., Yahr, T. L., and Horswill, A. R. (2013). Sialic acid catabolism in *Staphylococcus aureus*. *J. Bact.* 195, 1779–1788. doi: 10.1128/JB.02294-12

Pezzicoli, A., Ruggiero, P., Amerighi, F., Telford, J. L., and Soriani, M. (2012). Exogenous sialic acid transport contributes to group B streptococcus infection of mucosal surfaces. *J. Infect. Dis.* 206, 924–931. doi: 10.1093/infdis/jis451

Post, D. M., Mungur, R., Gibson, B. W., and Munson, R. S. (2005). Identification of a novel sialic acid transporter in *Haemophilus ducreyi*. *Infect. Immun.* 73, 6727–6735. doi: 10.1128/IAI.73.10.6727-6735.2005

Scalise, M., Pochini, L., Panni, S., Pingitore, P., Hedfalk, K., and Indiveri, C. (2014). Transport mechanism and regulatory properties of the human amino acid transporter ASCT2 (SLC1A5). *Amino Acids* 46, 2463–2475. doi: 10.1007/s00726-014-1808-x

Scalise, M., Pochini, L., Pingitore, P., Hedfalk, K., and Indiveri, C. (2015). Cysteine is not a substrate but a specific modulator of human ASCT2 (SLC1A5) transporter. *FEBS Lett.* 589, 3617–3623. doi: 10.1016/j.febslet.2015.10.011

Severi, E., Hosie, A. H., Hawkhead, J. A., and Thomas, G. H. (2010). Characterization of a novel sialic acid transporter of the sodium solute symporter (SSS) family and *in vivo* comparison with known bacterial sialic acid transporters. *FEMS Microbiol. Lett.* 304, 47–54. doi: 10.1111/j.1574-6968.2009.01881.x

Severi, E., Randle, G., Kivlin, P., Whitfield, K., Young, R., Moxon, R., et al. (2005). Sialic acid transport in *Haemophilus influenzae* is essential for lipopolysaccharide sialylation and serum resistance and is dependent on a novel tripartite ATP-independent periplasmic transporter. *Mol. Microbiol.* 58, 1173–1185. doi: 10.1111/j.1365-2958.2005.04901.x

Soares da Costa, T. P., Desbois, S., Dogovski, C., Gorman, M. A., Ketaren, N. E., Paxman, J. J., et al. (2016). Structural determinants defining the allosteric inhibition of an essential antibiotic target. *Structure* 24, 1282–1291. doi: 10.1016/j.str.2016.05.019

Stifter, S. A., Matthews, A. Y., Mangan, N. E., Fung, K. Y., Drew, A., Tate, M. D., et al. (2018). Defining the distinct, intrinsic properties of the novel type I interferon, IFNϵ. *J. Biol. Chem.* 293, 3168–3179. doi: 10.1074/jbc.M117.800755

Tangvoranuntakul, P., Gagneux, P., Diaz, S., Bardor, M., Varki, N., Varki, A., et al. (2003). Human uptake and incorporation of an immunogenic nonhuman dietary sialic acid. *PNAS* 100, 12045–12050. doi: 10.1073/pnas.2131556100

Varki, A. (2001). Loss of *N*-glycolylneuraminic acid in humans: mechanisms, consequences, and implications for hominid evolution. *Am. J. Phys. Anthropol.* (Suppl. 33), 54–69. doi: 10.1002/ajpa.10018

Varki, A. (2010). Uniquely human evolution of sialic acid genetics and biology. *PNAS* 107, 8939–8946. doi: 10.1073/pnas.0914634107

Varki, N. M., Strobert, E., Dick, E. J., Benirschke, K., and Varki, A. (2011). Biomedical differences between human and nonhuman hominids: potential roles for uniquely human aspects of sialic acid biology. *Annu. Rev. Pathol.* 6, 365–393. doi: 10.1146/annurev-pathol-011110-130315

Vimr, E., Lichtensteiger, C., and Steenbergen, S. (2000). Sialic acid metabolism's dual function in *Haemophilus influenzae*. *Mol. Microbiol.* 36, 1113–1123. doi: 10.1046/j.1365-2958.2000.01925.x

Vimr, E. R., Kalivoda, K. A., Deszo, E. L., and Steenbergen, S. M. (2004). Diversity of microbial sialic acid metabolism. *Microbiol. Mol. Biol. Rev.* 68, 132–153. doi: 10.1128/MMBR.68.1.132-153.2004

Vimr, E. R., and Troy, F. A. (1985). Identification of an inducible catabolic system for sialic acids (nan) in *Escherichia coli*. *J. Bact.* 164, 845–853.

Wahlgren, W. Y., Dunevall, E., North, R. A., Paz, A., Scalise, M., Bisignano, P., et al. (2018). Substrate-bound outward-open structure of a Na^+-coupled sialic acid symporter reveals a novel Na^+ site. *Nat. Commun.* 9:1753. doi: 10.1038/s41467-018-04045-7

Wienken, C. J., Baaske, P., Rothbauer, U., Braun, D., and Duhr, S. (2010). Protein-binding assays in biological liquids using microscale thermophoresis. *Nat Commun.* 1:100. doi: 10.1038/ncomms1093

Yu, X., Dang, V. T., Fleming, F. E., von Itzstein M., Coulson, B. S., and Blanchard, H. (2012). Structural basis of rotavirus strain preference toward *N*-acetyl- or *N*-glycolylneuraminic acid-containing receptors. *J. Virol.* 86, 13456–13466. doi: 10.1128/JVI.06975-11

11

Interaction of the New Monofunctional Anticancer Agent Phenanthriplatin with Transporters for Organic Cations

*Anna Hucke [1], Ga Young Park [2], Oliver B. Bauer [3], Georg Beyer [1], Christina Köppen [3], Dorothea Zeeh [1], Christoph A. Wehe [3], Michael Sperling [3,4], Rita Schröter [1], Marta Kantauskaitè [1], Yohannes Hagos [5], Uwe Karst [3], Stephen J. Lippard [2] and Giuliano Ciarimboli [1]**

[1] *Experimental Nephrology, Medical Clinic D, University Hospital, University of Münster, Münster, Germany,* [2] *Department of Chemistry, Massachusetts Institute of Technology, Cambridge, MA, United States,* [3] *Institute of Inorganic and Analytical Chemistry, University of Münster, Münster, Germany,* [4] *European Virtual Institute for Speciation Analysis, Münster, Germany,* [5] *PortaCellTec Biosciences GmbH, Göttingen, Germany*

***Correspondence:**
Giuliano Ciarimboli
gciari@uni-muenster.de

Cancer treatment with platinum compounds is an important achievement of modern chemotherapy. However, despite the beneficial effects, the clinical impact of these agents is hampered by the development of drug resistance as well as dose-limiting side effects. The efficacy but also side effects of platinum complexes can be mediated by uptake through plasma membrane transporters. In the kidneys, plasma membrane transporters are involved in their secretion into the urine. Renal secretion is accomplished by uptake from the blood into the proximal tubules cells, followed by excretion into the urine. The uptake process is mediated mainly by organic cation transporters (OCT), which are expressed in the basolateral domain of the plasma membrane facing the blood. The excretion of platinum into the urine is mediated by exchange with protons via multidrug and toxin extrusion proteins (MATE) expressed in the apical domain of plasma membrane. Recently, the monofunctional, cationic platinum agent phenanthriplatin, which is able to escape common cellular resistance mechanisms, has been synthesized and investigated. In the present study, the interaction of phenanthriplatin with transporters for organic cations has been evaluated. Phenanthriplatin is a high affinity substrate for OCT2, but has a lower apparent affinity for MATEs. The presence of these transporters increased cytotoxicity of phenanthriplatin. Therefore, phenanthriplatin may be especially effective in the treatment of cancers that express OCTs, such as colon cancer cells. However, the interaction of phenanthriplatin with OCTs suggests that its use as chemotherapeutic agent may be complicated by OCT-mediated toxicity. Unlike cisplatin, phenanthriplatin interacts with high specificity with hMATE1 and hMATE2K in addition to hOCT2. This interaction may facilitate its efflux from the cells and thereby decrease overall efficacy and/or toxicity.

Keywords: organic cation transporters, platinum compounds, interaction, toxicity, efficacy, side effects

INTRODUCTION

Cancer is an important cause of death worldwide (Chakraborty et al., 2018). At present, three major therapeutic strategies to treat cancer are used, namely, surgery, radiotherapy, and chemotherapy (Chakraborty et al., 2018). One of the great advances in the treatment of cancer was the introduction of cisplatin as a chemotherapeutic agent (Rosenberg, 1973). Today, platinum derivatives form part of the chemotherapy of almost every second cancer patient (Galanski et al., 2005; Fennell et al., 2016). The currently approved FDA platinum anticancer agents cisplatin, oxaliplatin, and carboplatin have proved efficacious against a wide variety of tumors, with cisplatin treatment considered to be curative for testicular cancer (Einhorn, 2002; Chovanec et al., 2016). Despite their beneficial effects, treatment with these agents is hampered by the development of drug resistance as well as dose-limiting side effects (Rabik and Dolan, 2007; Kuok et al., 2017). To overcome these problems, alternative metal-based anticancer agents are being developed. Current research efforts focus on a variety of non-classical metal anticancer drug candidates (G Quiroga, 2011; Romero-Canelón and Sadler, 2013; Wang and Gao, 2014; Johnstone et al., 2016; Shahsavani et al., 2016), including non-platinum complexes, Pt(IV) constructs, multinuclear constructs, and monofunctional Pt(II) complexes. Monofunctional agents disobey the classical structure-activity relationships (SARs), which stipulate that active platinum complexes should have two labile leaving groups to form bifunctional adducts with DNA targets in the nucleus (Sherman and Lippard, 1987).

Phenanthriplatin, *cis*-$[Pt(NH_3)_2Cl(phenanthridine)]^+$, is a monofunctional anticancer agent having greater efficacy and a complimentary spectrum of cancer cell activity compared to that of the clinically approved platinum agents (Park et al., 2012). These differentiating features suggest the possibility for avoiding drug resistance and dose limiting toxicities. Phenanthriplatin forms highly potent monofunctional adducts on DNA (Kellinger et al., 2013) that are capable of inhibiting both RNA and DNA polymerases. Previous research indicated that phenanthriplatin effectively inhibits the ν, ζ, and κ DNA polymerases, as well as the Klenow fragment (Gregory et al., 2014). Upregulation of Pol η, which performs inefficient but high fidelity translesion synthesis (Gregory et al., 2014), has been demonstrated to play a role in the development of resistance to cisplatin (Hicks et al., 2010). The observation that phenanthriplatin is toxic to both Pol η^+ and Pol η- cells and impervious to other bypass polymerases indicates that phenanthriplatin may escape common cellular resistance mechanisms (Gregory et al., 2014).

In recent years, it has become evident that membrane transporters play an important role not only for resistance to chemotherapeutics, but also for selective uptake of anticancer agents into cancerous cells (Ciarimboli, 2011). Some transporters such as the polyspecific Organic Cation Transporters OCTs (OCT1-3), the Multidrug and Extrusion proteins MATEs (MATE1-2K) and the Copper Transporters 1 and 2 (Ctr1-2) mediate the transport of platinum derivatives through the plasma membrane (Zhang et al., 2006; Lovejoy et al., 2008). Interestingly, OCTs and MATEs share many substrates. Therefore, because of their expression on the basolateral and apical membrane domain, respectively, of secretory epithelial cells, such as those of renal proximal tubules, their concerted action (basolateral uptake by OCTs and apical efflux into the urine by MATEs) mediates the vectorial transport of substrates, resulting in their renal urine excretion (Ciarimboli, 2016). Because transport by MATEs functions as an exchange of substrates with H^+, the slightly acidic pH in the tubular fluid stimulates secretion processes. Indeed, OCTs and MATEs have been implicated in the development of platinum derivatives side effects such as cisplatin nephrotoxicity (Harrach and Ciarimboli, 2015). It is not yet known whether cellular phenanthriplatin uptake is mediated by membrane transporters. We therefore studied its interaction with OCTs and with the efflux transporters hMATEs.

MATERIALS AND METHODS

Cell Culture

Experiments were performed with human embryonic kidney (HEK) 293 cells (CRL-1573; American Type Culture Collection, Rochville, MD), which stably express mOCT1, mOCT2, mOCT3 (Schlatter et al., 2014), hOCT1, hOCT2, hOCT3, (kind gift of Prof. H. Koepsell, University Würzburg), hMATE1 or hMATE2K (Schmidt-Lauber et al., 2012). Some experiments were carried out with mouse embryonic fibroblasts (MEFs) from animals with genetic deletion of Ctr1 ($Ctr1^{-/-}$) or not ($Ctr1^{+/+}$) (Nose et al., 2010), provided by Dr. Yasuhiro Nose, Duke University Medical Center, Durham, USA. HEK 293 cells were grown at 37 °C in 50 mL cell culture flasks (Greiner, Frickenhausen, Germany) in DMEM (Biochrom, Berlin, Germany) containing 3.7 g/L $NaHCO_3$, 1.0 g/L D-glucose, and 2.0 mM L-glutamine (Biochrom), and gassed with 8 % CO_2. Penicillin (100 U/mL), 100 mg/L streptomycin (Biochrom), 10 % fetal calf serum, and, only for OCT transfected cells, 0.8 mg/mL geneticin (PAA Laboratories, Coelbe, Germany) were added to the medium. MATE transfected cells were selected with 0.4–0.5 mg/mL hygromycin B (Invitrogen, San Diego, USA). MEFs were cultured in DMEM supplemented with 20% (v/v) heat-inactivated fetal calf serum, 1 × MEM non-essential amino acids (Biochrom), 100 U/mL penicillin/streptomycin, and 55 μM 2-mercaptoethanol (Öhrvik et al., 2013). The medulloblastoma cell line DAOY was obtained from ATCC-LGC (Promochem, Wesel, Germany). The medulloblastoma cell line UW228 cells was obtained from M. Frühwald (University Children's Hospital Münster, Department of Pediatric Hematology and Oncology, Münster, Germany) with kind permission of J. Silber (Department of Neurological Surgery, University of Washington, Seattle, WA). These cells were cultivated in RPMI 1640 medium (Biochrom, Berlin, Germany) supplemented with 1 mM L-glutamine, 100 U/mL penicillin G, 100 μg/mL streptomycin, and 10% fetal calf serum in 25 cm^2 tissue culture flasks (Greiner Bio One) in a humidified atmosphere of 8% CO_2 at 37°C.

Experiments were performed with cells grown to confluence for 3–8 days from passages 12–80, depending on the cell type used. Culture and functional analyses of these cells were approved by the state government Landesumweltamt Nordrhein-Westfalen, Essen, Germany (no. 521.-M-1.14/00).

Fluorescence Measurements

The interaction of phenanthriplatin with transporters for organic cations (OCT1-3, MATE1, and MATE2K) was investigated by measuring its effects on the uptake of the fluorescent organic cation 4-(4-dimethylamino)styryl-N-methylpyridinium (ASP^+). Microfluorometric measurements of ASP^+ uptake were performed with a fluorescence plate reader (Infinity 200, Tecan, Crailsheim, Germany; excitation at 465 nm, emission at 590 nm) as described previously for cultured HEK 293 cells (Wilde et al., 2009). Before measurements, the culture medium in the wells of the 96 well microtiter plate containing HEK 293 cells was replaced by a HCO_3^--free Ringer-like solution containing (in mM) NaCl 145, K_2HPO_4 1.6, KH_2PO_4 0.4, D-glucose 5, $MgCl_2$ 1, calcium gluconate 1.3, and pH adjusted to 7.4. Fluorescence was measured dynamically at 37°C in each well before and after ASP^+ addition to HCO_3^--free Ringer-like solution, alone or together with increasing phenanthriplatin concentrations, and plotted versus time. ASP^+ (final concentration 1 or 10 μM for experiments with OCTs or MATEs, respectively) was added after the third sampling interval. Emission from the complete area of the well bottom was analyzed four times and averaged for each well. The initial linear fluorescence increase, measured by linear regression within the first 100 s after addition of ASP^+ alone or together with phenanthriplatin, represents specific cellular uptake of ASP^+ across plasma membranes and does not reflect possible toxic effects of phenanthriplatin (Ciarimboli et al., 2005a; Wilde et al., 2009). Background fluorescence was measured for each plate in wells with identical solutions containing no cells and subtracted from each well containing cells. Experiments were performed with cells from one passage of the same day with controls and test replicates in the same plate.

Treatment of Cells and Preparation of Lysates for Inductively Coupled Plasma-Mass Spectrometry (ICP-MS)

The ICP-MS determinations of cellular platinum content were performed via external calibration using an ICP-MS instrument (iCAP Qc, Thermo Fisher Scientific). Briefly, the culture medium of cells grown to confluence was removed and replaced by fresh complete cell culture medium containing 10 or 100 μM phenanthriplatin. In studies with the hOCT2 transporters, 100 μM cimetidine (Cim) was added to the incubation solution for selected wells. In experiments with hMATE1 and hMATE2K cells, 1 mM 1-methyl-4-phenylpyridinium (MPP^+) was added to the incubation solution for selected wells as competitor for the transporter-mediated phenanthriplatin cellular accumulation, since it has a similar affinity for hMATE1 and hMATE2K (4.7 and 3.3 μM, respectively, Astorga et al., 2012). After addition of the platinum containing solutions, the cells were incubated for 10 min. Immediately thereafter, the medium was removed and the cells were washed three times with 2 mL of ice cold phosphate-buffered saline (PBS, Biochrom) to remove all extracellular phenanthriplatin. After the PBS was removed, the cells were lysed with 1 mL distilled water. The plates were then incubated for 7.5 min under a microscope at room temperature to observe swelling and bursting of the cells. To ensure complete lysis, this procedure was followed by additional mechanical stress on the cells for 7.5 min on the plate shaker at 400 rpm. The cell lysates were collected with a cell scraper and transferred to 1.5 mL micro-reaction vessels, which were placed in an ultrasonic bath in ice water to destroy residual cell structures. After vortexing and cooled centrifugation (10 min, 4°C, 16,000 g), the supernatant was transferred to polymethylpentene (PMP) vials for storage at −20°C until platinum and protein analyses were performed. An external calibration using a platinum ICP standard (concentration range 10 ng/L to 2 μg/L) was used for quantification. The acquired platinum concentrations were then normalized to the respective protein concentrations obtained via a Bradford assay.

Bradford Assay for Protein Quantitation

In order to relate Pt quantitation to protein concentration, thereby normalizing for differences in the number of cells, the amount of protein in each sample was analyzed by using the Bradford assay (Bradford, 1976), as previously described (Wehe et al., 2014).

Cytotoxicity Testing

A modified 3-(4,5-dimethylthiazol-2-yl)-2,5-diphenyltetrazolium bromide (MTT) assay (Mosmann, 1983) was used to test the chemosensitivity of cells to phenanthriplatin and, in some experiments, to cisplatin by determining the glycolysis rate via the reduction of the yellow tetrazolium salt MTT to a purple formazan dye, as previously described (Wehe et al., 2014). Briefly, after growing for 24 h in the incubator, cells expressing or not hOCT2, hMATE1, hMATE2 or Ctr1 were treated for 10 min with platinum derivatives. Control cells were incubated with drug-free complete cell culture medium. Afterwards, the medium

TABLE 1 | EC_{50} (μM) values determined for inhibition of ASP^+ uptake by human and murine OCTs in the presence of phenanthriplatin.

	Species	
OCT subtype	**Murine**	**Human**
IC_{50} ($logEC_{50}$ ± SEM) in μM and number of observations (*n*)		
OCT1	17 (−4.77 ± 0.22)	19 (−4.72 ± 0.21)
	n = 6–11	*n* = 6–12
OCT2	2 (−5.64 ± 0.05)	2* (−5.67 ± 0.10)
	n = 6–12	*n* = 6–12
OCT3	3,146* (−2.50 ± 1.07)	21# (−4.67 ± 0.07)
	n = 6–10	*n* = 6–12
MATE1		101§ (−3.99 ± 0.21)
		n = 6–12
MATE2K		57& (−4.24 ± 0.07)
		n = 15–16

The $logIC_{50}$ values ± SEM and the number of observations are also indicated in parenthesis.

**Statistically significant different from the other paralogs (ANOVA); §Statistically significant different from the other paralogs except MATE2K (ANOVA). &Statistically significant different from the other paralogs except OCT1 and MATE1 (ANOVA). The hashtag (#) indicates a statistically significant difference from the murine ortholog (t-test).*

was carefully removed and replaced by 200 μL of fresh complete cell culture medium. After incubation for another 24 h, 10 μL of MTT solution containing 5 mg/mL of the dye were added to each well, and the cells were again incubated for 3 h. The medium was then removed and 100 μL of lysis buffer containing 10% (w/v) sodium dodecyl sulfate and 40% (v/v) dimethylformamide was added to each well. The plates were shaken for 10 min to destroy the cell structure and dissolve the blue formazan dye (Furchert et al., 2007; Wehe et al., 2014). Finally, the absorbance was measured at 590 nm using an automated microtiter plate reader (Infinite M200; Tecan, Männedorf, Switzerland). The percentage of viable cells in the untreated controls was compared to that for the various treatments. Experiments carried out with DAOY and UW228 cells followed a similar protocol except that these cells were incubated for 24 h with phenanthriplatin.

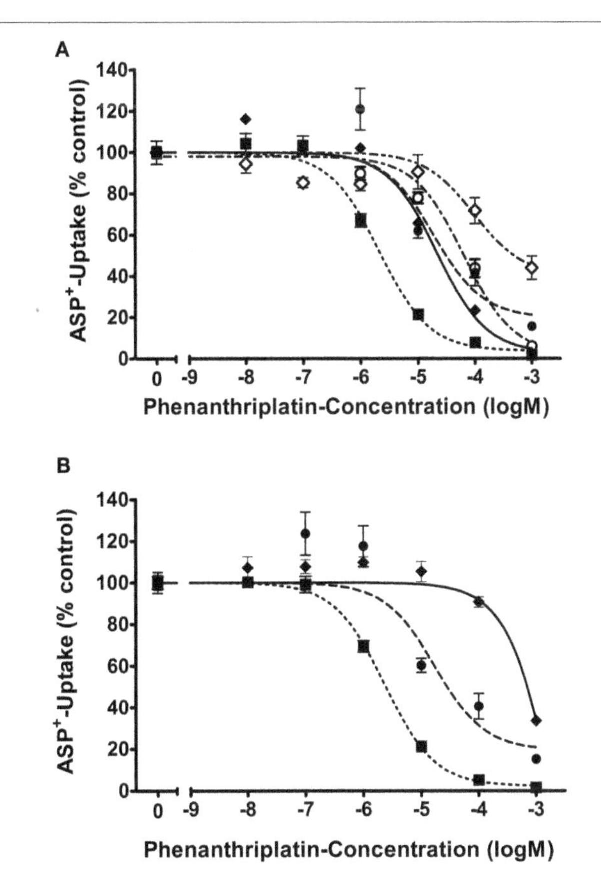

FIGURE 1 | Apparent affinities (IC_{50}) of **(A)** hOCT1 (●; $n = 6$–12), hOCT2 (■; $n = 6$–12), hOCT3 (♦; $n = 6$–12), hMATE2K (O; $n = 15$–16), and hMATE1 (◊; $n = 7$–24) and **(B)** mOCT1 (◊; $n = 6$–11), mOCT2 (●; $n = 6$–12), mOCT3 (■; $n = 6$–10) for phenanthriplatin. Values are means ± SEM expressed as % of ASP^+-uptake in the absence of phenanthriplatin, which was set to 100% (control). The IC_{50} values for the inhibition of initial ASP^+ uptake by phenanthriplatin were 19, 2, 21, 101, and 57 μM for hOCT1, hOCT2, hOCT3, hMATE1, and hMATE2K, respectively. Those for mOCT1, mOCT2, and mOCT3, were 17, 2, and 3,146 μM, respectively.

Western Blotting and SDS-PAGE

For Western blot analysis, DAOY and UW228 cells grown to confluence were solubilized by incubation with PBS containing 1% (w/v) Triton X-100. After 45 min on ice, cell lysates were centrifuged for 1 min at 2,400 g at 4°C. Following this step, the supernatant was diluted in SDS buffer (Roti-Load 1, Roth) with 100 mM dithiothreitol (DTT) and 8% v/v ß-mercaptoethanol and incubated for 5 min at 95°C. The proteins were then separated by SDS-PAGE and transferred to a polyvinylidene fluoride (PVDF) membrane for Western blot analysis. The membranes were blocked with 3% gelatin from cold-water fish skin (Sigma, Munich, Germany). After incubation with the primary antibodies (anti-OCT2 from Alpha Diagnostics, San Antonio, TX, USA at a 1:1,000 dilution and anti-GAPDH from Cell Signaling, Danvers, MA, USA at a 1:2,000 dilution), membranes were incubated with peroxidase-conjugated anti-mouse (DAKO Deutschland, Hamburg, Germany) at a 1:10,000 dilution. Signals were visualized using a Lumi Light detection system (Roche, Mannheim, Germany).

Statistical Analyses

Data are presented as mean values ± SEM, with (n) referring to the number of wells. IC_{50} values defined as the concentration of platinum agent required to inhibit uptake of ASP^+ by 50% and EC_{50} values used to assess cell viability were obtained by sigmoidal concentration-response curve fitting using GraphPad Prism, Version 5.3 (GraphPad Software, San Diego, USA). Unpaired two-sided Student's t-test was employed to prove statistical significance of the effects. For multiple comparisons,

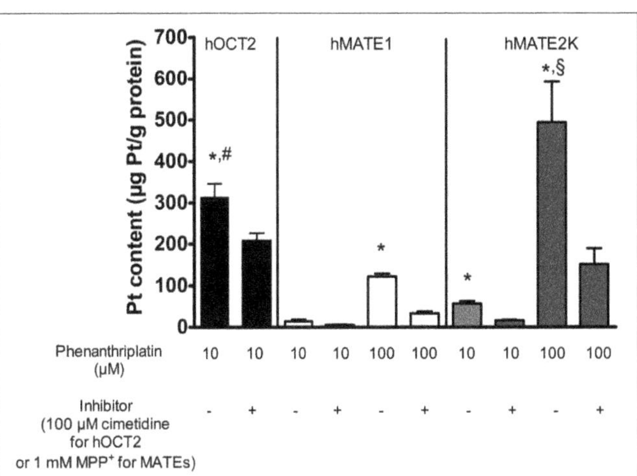

FIGURE 2 | Platinum concentration in lysates from HEK293 cells stably transfected with hOCT2 (black columns), hMATE1 (white columns), or hMATE2K (gray columns) after incubation with phenanthriplatin measured by ICP-MS ($n = 3$–8). The cells were incubated 10 min with 10 μM (hOCT2) or 100 μM (hMATE1 and hMATE2K) phenanthriplatin (Phen) alone or together with 100 μM cimetidine (hOCT2) or 1 mM MPP^+ (hMATE1 and hMATE2K). *indicates a significant difference from all the respective experiments with inhibitor (unpaired t-test); #indicates a significant difference from the other experiments with 10 μM phenanthriplatin alone (ANOVA); §indicates a significant difference from all other experiments in the presence of 100 μM phenanthriplatin (ANOVA).

ANOVA with Bonferroni post-test was used. A *P*-value < 0.05 was considered statistically significant.

Solution and Chemicals

ASP^+ was obtained from Molecular Probes (Leiden, The Netherlands). All standard substances were obtained from Sigma (Munich, Germany) or Merck (Darmstadt, Germany) at highest purity available.

RESULTS

First, the uptake of ASP^+, a known substrate of transporters for organic cations, was investigated in competition with phenanthriplatin. As evident from inspection of **Table 1** and **Figure 1**, similar phenanthriplatin concentrations inhibit ASP^+ uptake to 50% (IC_{50}) for cells overexpressing OCT1 and OCT2 transporters of murine and human origin. The minimum concentration of phenanthriplatin required to inhibit ASP^+ transport by 50% was 2 μM. This value was determined for cells overexpressing both human or mouse OCT2. In contrast, the source of the OCT3 transporter significantly affects the extent of ASP^+ inhibition with phenanthriplatin (3,146 μM for mOCT3 vs. 21 μM for hOCT3).

For what concerns phenanthriplatin interaction with the MATE efflux transporters, a concentration of 101 or 57 μM phenanthriplatin was required to inhibit ASP^+ transport by 50% in cells overexpressing hMATE1 or hMATE2-K, respectively (**Figure 1**).

The cellular accumulation of platinum in HEK 293 cells expressing hOCT2, hMATE1, or hMATE2K was also investigated (**Figure 2**). Platinum concentrations were determined by ICP-MS following 10 min incubation with 10 or 100 μM phenanthriplatin. When incubated with 10 μM phenanthriplatin, HEK293 cells overexpressing hOCT2 showed

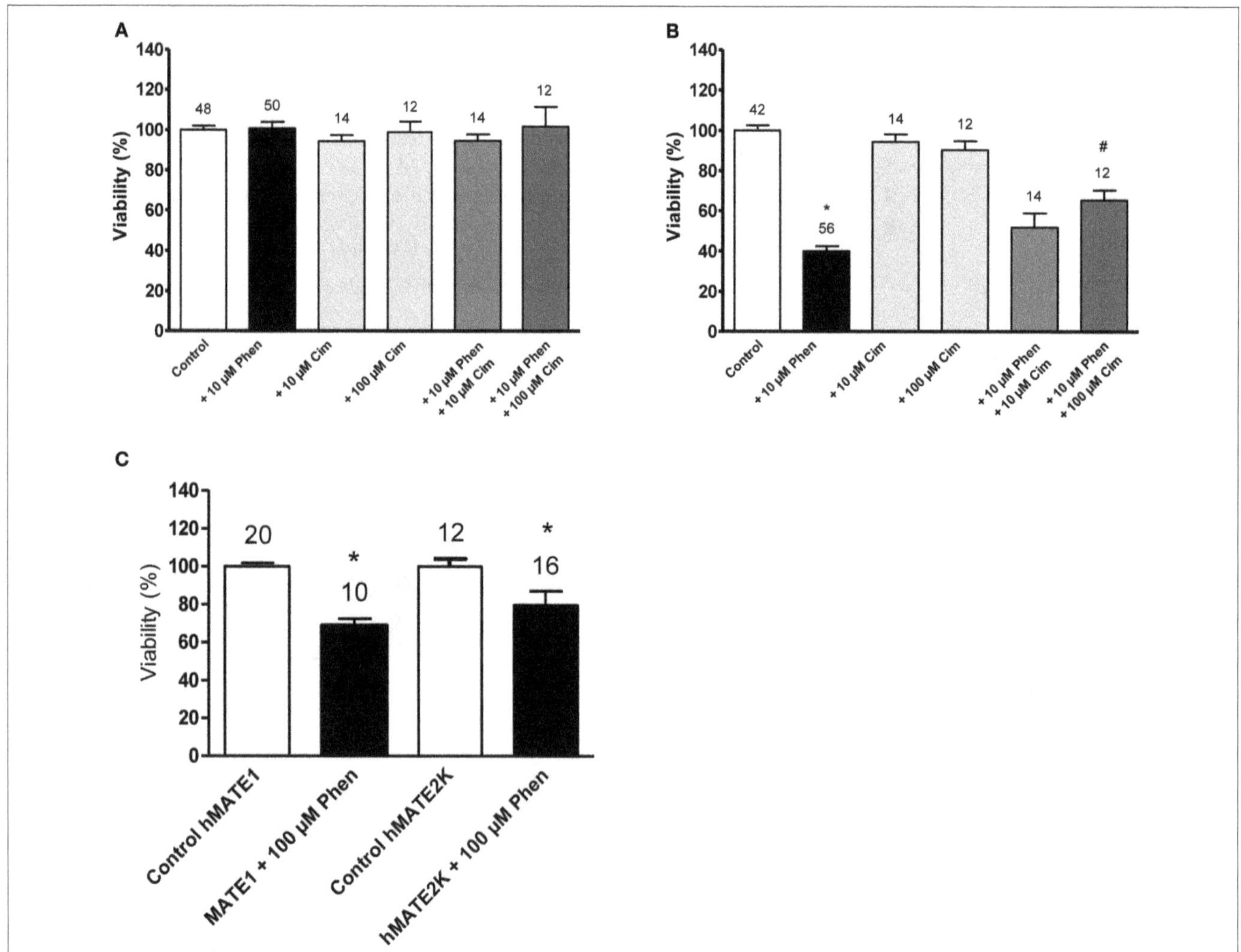

FIGURE 3 | Cell viability (EC_{50}) determined by MTT assay for cells incubated with buffer (control); 10 μM phenanthriplatin (Phen); 10 μM cimetidine (Cim); 100 μM cimetidine; 10 μM phenanthriplatin + 10 μM cimetidine; and 10 μM phenanthriplatin + 100 μM cimetidine, for 10 min. **(A)** HEK 293 WT cells **(B)** HEK 293 hOCT2 cells **(C)** HEK293 hMATE1 and hMATE2K cells. Above the columns is the number of experiments. The asterisk (*) indicates a statistically significant difference compared to the other columns, # a statistically difference compared to all the other columns except than to 10 μM phenanthriplatin + 10 μM cimetidine (ANOVA).

significantly higher phenanthriplatin uptake than HEK293 cells expressing hMATE1 or hMATE2K [340 ± 36 (n = 8), 15 ± 4 (n = 3), and 57 ± 11 (n = 3) μg Pt/g protein, respectively, **Figure 2**]. When phenanthriplatin was co-incubated with 100 μM cimetidine a significant decreased cellular accumulation of platinum in hOCT2 cells was observed (227 ± 19 μg Pt/g protein, n = 8). Incubation of hMATE1 and hMATE2K cells with 100 μM phenanthriplatin resulted in a higher cellular phenanthriplatin accumulation than in experiments using 10 μM phenanthriplatin (122 ± 7 and 494 ± 99 μg Pt/g protein, for hMATE1 and hMATE2K, respectively, both n = 3, **Figure 2**), which was significantly inhibited under co-incubation with 1 mM MPP^+ (33 ± 4 and 151 ± 38 μg Pt/g protein, respectively, both n = 3, **Figure 2**).

These experiments show that both hOCT2 and hMATEs are able to translocate phenanthriplatin across the plasma membrane.

As shown in **Figure 3**, the expression of transporters for organic cations is critical for the cellular toxicity of phenanthriplatin. Cell viability studies show that hOCT2 expression in HEK 293 cells is linked to significant phenanthriplatin toxicity which is reduced upon co-incubation of phenanthriplatin with cimetidine (100 μM), a known substrate for hOCT2 (**Figure 3B**). Cimetidine alone had no significant effect on cell viability. Incubation of cells overexpressing hMATE1 or hMATE2K with 100 μM phenanthriplatin induces significant cell toxicity (**Figure 3C**).

Because the copper transporter 1 (Ctr1) has also been implicated in the cellular uptake of platinum drugs (Holzer et al., 2006), we investigated its possible involvement in phenanthriplatin cellular uptake using MEFs derived from WT ($Ctr1^{+/+}$) and $Ctr1^{-/-}$ mice. We first evaluated whether phenanthriplatin has a toxic effect on MEFs and whether such an effect depends on the expression of Ctr1. **Figure 4** shows that phenanthriplatin is toxic both to $Ctr1^{+/+}$ and $Ctr1^{-/-}$ MEFs. Conversely, cisplatin, a known substrate for Ctr1, (Ishida et al., 2002; Holzer et al., 2004), used as a control, was toxic to $Ctr1^{+/+}$ but not to $Ctr1^{-/-}$ MEFs. Lower phenanthriplatin concentrations (<1 mM) did not change the cell viability in $Ctr1^{+/+}$ and $Ctr1^{-/-}$ MEFs (not shown).

Screening a panel of several tumor cell lines resulted in the identification of two medulloblastoma cell lines, DAOY and UW228, which differed with respect to the expression of mRNA for hOCT2 (Supplementary Figure 2). The differential protein expression of hOCT2 in these two cell lines was determined by Western blot, with DAOY expressing more hOCT2 than UW228 (**Figure 5**). Also other transporters, such as hMATE1, seem to be expressed at lower level in UW228 than DAOY cells (Supplementary Figure 2).

The determination of EC_{50} for phenanthriplatin toxicity measured by MTT assay after 24 h incubation with 10^{-8}–10^{-3} M phenanthriplatin showed that DAOY cells are more sensitive to phenanthriplatin than UW228 cells, EC_{50} = 0.9 vs. 2.8 μM, respectively (**Table 2**). Using these EC_{50} concentrations, we tested whether competition for uptake by hOCT2 by a 10-fold higher cimetidine concentration can protect these cells from phenanthriplatin toxicity. Only DAOY cells could

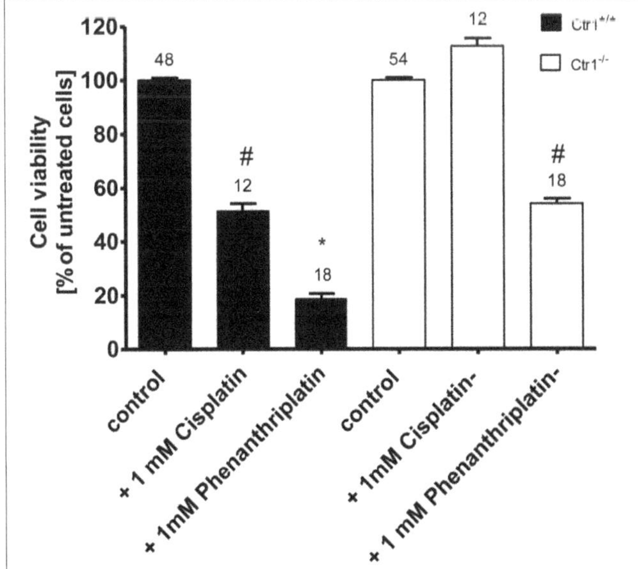

FIGURE 4 | Cell viability of $Ctr1^{+/+}$ and $Ctr1^{-/-}$ MEFs incubated with buffer (control); 1 mM phenanthriplatin or 1 mM cisplatin for 10 min. The number of experiments is listed above each column. The asterisk (*) indicates a statistically significant difference compared to the other columns, # a statistically difference compared to all the other columns except than to 1 mM cisplatin in $Ctr1^{+/+}$ MEFs or to 1 mM phenanthriplatin in $Ctr1^{-/-}$ MEFs (ANOVA).

be efficaciously protected against phenanthriplatin toxicity by cimetidine (**Figure 6**).

DISCUSSION

Transporters for organic cations, when expressed in polarized cells such as hepatocytes and renal proximal tubules cells, mediate the vectorial movement of substances through cells, which under physiological conditions results in the secretion of organic cations into the bile and urine, respectively. hOCT1 and hOCT2 are expressed in the basolateral membrane of hepatocytes and renal proximal tubule cells, respectively, whereas hMATEs are localized on the apical domain of these cells (hMATE2K is only expressed in the kidneys; Harrach and Ciarimboli, 2015). For this reason, hOCT1 and hOCT2 mediate the first step of secretion, that is, the uptake of substrates into the cell, and hMATE1 with hMATE2K are important for the final secretion step that delivers the substrates to the bile and urine. These transporters play an important role in the development of side effects caused by platinum drugs, including cisplatin and oxaliplatin. For example, cisplatin causes significant nephrotoxicity, ototoxicity, and peripheral neurotoxicity, whereas oxaliplatin exerts mainly a toxic effect on peripheral nerves (Rabik and Dolan, 2007; Hucke and Ciarimboli, 2016). Cisplatin is a known substrate of hOCT2 (Ciarimboli et al., 2005b) and hOCT3 (Guttmann et al., 2018), and hOCT2-mediated cisplatin uptake has been implicated in the development of side effects (Ciarimboli et al., 2010; Sprowl

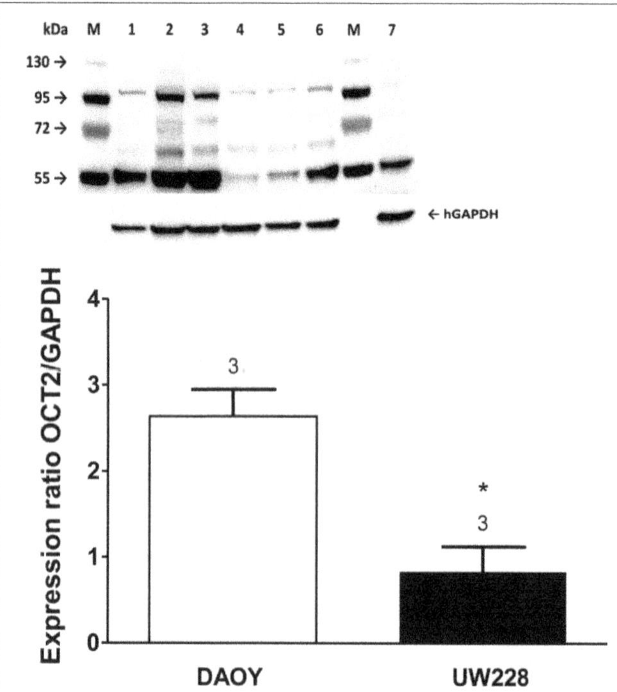

FIGURE 5 | (Upper) Western blot analysis of hOCT2 expression in DAOY and UW228 cells. M is the marker lane. 1, 2, 3 are lysates from three different DAOY passages; 4, 5, and 6 are lysates from three different UW228 passages. Lane 7 contains lysate from hOCT2-HEK cells as a control. The respective bands corresponding to the signal of GAPDH are also shown. **(Lower)** Densitometric analysis of the Western blot, showing the hOCT2 expression in relation to the GAPDH expression. Above the columns is the number of experiments. The asterisk (*) indicates a statistically significant difference compared to the other column (unpaired *t*-test).

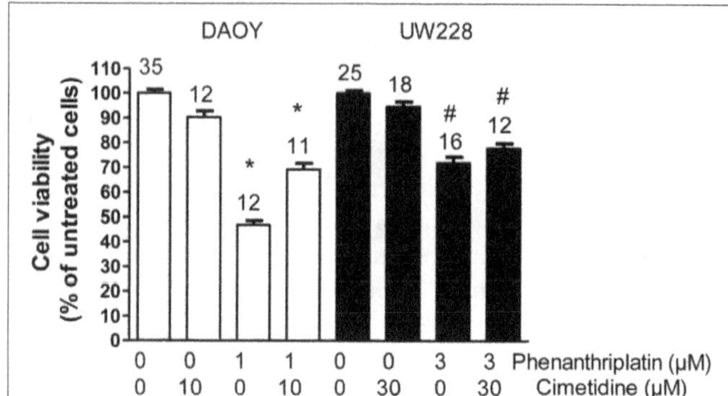

FIGURE 6 | Effects of 24 h incubation of DAOY (empty columns) or UW228 (filled columns) cells with buffer (control) alone and in the presence of 1 or 3 μM phenanthriplatin alone and together with a 10-fold higher concentration of cimetidine on cell viability measured with an MTT-assay. As a further control, experiments performed only in the presence of cimetidine are also shown. Above the columns is the number of experiments. The asterisk (*) indicates a statistically significant difference compared to the other columns, #a statistically difference compared to the control experiments (ANOVA).

TABLE 2 | EC_{50} ($logEC_{50} \pm$ SEM) in μM for viability of DAOY and UW228 cells after 24 h incubation with phenanthriplatin.

DAOY	UW228
IC_{50} ($logEC_{50} \pm$ SEM) in μM	
0.9 (−6.05 ± 0.02)	2.8* (−5.55 ± 0.03)
n = 23–24	*n* = 24

n, number of replicates for tested concentration.
The asterisk (*) denotes a statistical difference from DAOY, unpaired t-test.

et al., 2014; Lanvers-Kaminsky et al., 2015, 2017; Lanvers-Kaminsky and Ciarimboli, 2017). Oxaliplatin is also a known substrate for hOCT2 (Zhang et al., 2006; Yokoo et al., 2007; Yonezawa and Inui, 2011), and uptake by this transporter has been linked to the development of peripheral neurotoxicity (Sprowl et al., 2013). Both cisplatin (see Supplementary Figure 1) and oxaliplatin interact with very low affinity with hMATE1, but only oxaliplatin is a substrate of the kidney-specific hMATE2K and is excreted by this transporter in the urine, explaining the lower nephrotoxicity of oxaliplatin (Yokoo et al., 2007; Estrela et al., 2017).

In the present work, we find that phenanthriplatin is a substrate of hOCT2, hMATE1, and hMATE2K. Co-incubation with specific inhibitors significantly decreased phenanthriplatin accumulation by the transporters. Moreover, expression of these transporters correlated well with phenanthriplatin toxicity.

Phenanthriplatin altered the transport of ASP^+ mediated by hMATE1 and hMATE2K. Compared with the cisplatin inhibition of hMATE1 and hMATE2K (see Supplementary Figure 1), phenanthriplatin is much more able than cisplatin to robustly inhibit the transport of ASP^+ mediated by hMATE1 and hMATE2K (IC_{50} = 101 and 57 μM, respectively). This observation suggests a potential protective action of hMATEs against eventual cellular toxicity.

Comparison of the IC_{50} values for inhibition of ASP^+ transport by human and murine OCTs reveals that OCT1 and OCT2 behave the same in the two species. Conversely, large differences in apparent affinities of hOCT3 and mOCT3 were found. Indeed, different properties for rodent and human orthologues have previously been reported (Schlatter et al., 2014). These results are of great importance for the proper interpretation of translational studies (Schlatter et al., 2014).

The presence of Ctr1 sensitizes MEFs to the toxic effects of cisplatin, as confirmed by experiments with $Ctr1^{-/-}$ MEFs, where no decrease in cell viability after treatment with cisplatin was observed (**Figure 4**). The toxicity of phenanthriplatin was still present in $Ctr1^{-/-}$ MEFs even though at lower level than in $Ctr1^{+/+}$ MEFs. These results suggest that Ctr1 does not have the same importance for phenanthriplatin uptake as it does for cisplatin. Because tumor cells are more sensitive to phenanthriplatin than to cisplatin (Park et al., 2012), we screened the expression of transporters in several tumor cell lines and found that the medulloblastoma cells DAOY and UW228 have different hOCT2 expression, both at the mRNA (not shown) and protein (**Figure 5**) levels. These cells also display a differential sensitivity to phenanthriplatin. The DAOY cells, which express more hOCT2 and hMATE1, show the greatest increase in sensitivity (**Table 2**). Inhibition of phenanthriplatin transport through hOCT2 by cimetidine significantly decreased the toxicity of this compound in DAOY but not in UW228 cells, further supporting a role of hOCT2 in amplifying phenanthriplatin toxicity against tumor cells.

CONCLUSIONS

Here we show that phenanthriplatin interacts with transporters for organic cations and that it is even more effective against tumor cells expressing hOCT2. This observation indicates that phenanthriplatin may be especially effective in the treatment of cancers that express OCTs, such as colon cancer cells. However, the interaction of phenanthriplatin with OCTs suggests that its use as chemotherapeutic agent may be complicated by greater OCT-mediated toxicity. Unlike cisplatin, phenanthriplatin interacts with high specificity with hMATE1 and hMATE2K in addition to hOCT2, which may facilitate its efflux from the cells and thereby decrease overall toxicity.

AUTHOR CONTRIBUTIONS

AH, GYP, OBB, GB, CK, DZ, CAW, MS, RS, MK, YH, and GC performed experiments. AH, GYP, OBB, MS, UK, SJL, and GC planned the study and wrote the manuscript.

ACKNOWLEDGMENTS

This study was supported by the Deutsche Forschungsge meinschaft (grant CI 107/11-1 to GC) and the National Cancer Institute (grant CA034992 to SJL).

REFERENCES

Astorga, B., Ekins, S., Morales, M., and Wright, S. H. (2012). Molecular determinants of ligand selectivity for the human multidrug and toxin extruder proteins MATE1 and MATE2-K. *J. Pharmacol. Exp. Ther.* 341, 743–755. doi: 10.1124/jpet.112.191577

Bradford, M. M. (1976). A rapid and sensitive method for the quantitation of microgram quantities of protein utilizing the principle of protein-dye binding. *Anal. Biochem.* 72, 248–254. doi: 10.1016/0003-2697(76)90527-3

Chakraborty, C., Sharma, A. R., Sharma, G., Sarkar, B. K., and Lee, S. S. (2018). The novel strategies for next-generation cancer treatment: miRNA combined with chemotherapeutic agents for the treatment of cancer. *Oncotarget* 9, 10164–10174. doi: 10.18632/oncotarget.24309

Chovanec, M., Hanna, N., Cary, K. C., Einhorn, L., and Albany, C. (2016). Management of stage I testicular germ cell tumours. *Nat. Rev. Urol.* 13, 663–673. doi: 10.1038/nrurol.2016.164

Ciarimboli, G. (2011). Role of organic cation transporters in drug-induced toxicity. *Expert. Opin. Drug Metab. Toxicol.* 7, 159–174. doi: 10.1517/17425255.2011.547474

Ciarimboli, G. (2016). "Introduction to the cellular transport of organic cations," in *Organic Cation Transporters*, eds G. Ciarimboli, S. Gautron, and E. Schlatter (Heidelberg; New York, NY; Dordrecht; London: Springer), 1–48.

Ciarimboli, G., Deuster, D., Knief, A., Sperling, M., Holtkamp, M., Edemir, B., et al. (2010). Organic cation transporter 2 mediates cisplatin-induced oto- and nephrotoxicity and is a target for protective interventions. *Am. J. Pathol.* 176, 1169–1180. doi: 10.2353/ajpath.2010.090610

Ciarimboli, G., Koepsell, H., Iordanova, M., Gorboulev, V., Dürner, B., Lang, D., et al. (2005a). Individual PKC-phosphorylation sites in organic cation transporter 1 determine substrate selectivity and transport regulation. *J. Am. Soc. Nephrol.* 16, 1562–1570. doi: 10.1681/ASN.2004040256

Ciarimboli, G., Ludwig, T., Lang, D., Pavenstädt, H., Koepsell, H., Piechota, H. J., et al. (2005b). Cisplatin nephrotoxicity is critically mediated via the human organic cation transporter 2. *Am. J. Pathol.* 167, 1477–1484. doi: 10.1016/S0002-9440(10)61234-5

Einhorn, L. H. (2002). Curing metastatic testicular cancer. *Proc. Natl. Acad. Sci. U.S.A.* 99, 4592–4595. doi: 10.1073/pnas.072067999

Estrela, G. R., Wasinski, F., Felizardo, R. J. F., Souza, L. L., Câmara, N. O. S., Bader, M., et al. (2017). MATE-1 modulation by kinin B1 receptor enhances cisplatin efflux from renal cells. *Mol. Cell Biochem.* 428, 101–108. doi: 10.1007/s11010-016-2920-x

Fennell, D. A., Summers, Y., Cadranel, J., Benepal, T., Christoph, D. C., Lal, R., et al. (2016). Cisplatin in the modern era: the backbone of first-line chemotherapy for non-small cell lung cancer. *Cancer Treat. Rev.* 44, 42–50. doi: 10.1016/j.ctrv.2016.01.003

Furchert, S. E., Lanvers-Kaminsky, C., Juürgens, H., Jung, M., Loidl, A., and Frühwald, M. C. (2007). Inhibitors of histone deacetylases as potential therapeutic tools for high-risk embryonal tumors of the nervous system of childhood. *Int. J. Cancer* 120, 1787–1794. doi: 10.1002/ijc.22401

Galanski, M., Jakupec, M. A., and Keppler, B. K. (2005). Update of the preclinical situation of anticancer platinum complexes: novel design strategies and innovative analytical approaches. *Curr. Med. Chem.* 12, 2075–2094. doi: 10.2174/0929867054637626

G Quiroga, A. (2011). Non-classical structures among current platinum complexes with potential as antitumor drugs. *Curr. Top. Med. Chem.* 11, 2613–2622. doi: 10.2174/156802611798040723

Gregory, M. T., Park, G. Y., Johnstone, T. C., Lee, Y. S., Yang, W., and Lippard, S. J. (2014). Structural and mechanistic studies of polymerase eta bypass of phenanthriplatin DNA damage. *Proc. Natl. Acad. Sci. U.S.A.* 111, 9133–9138. doi: 10.1073/pnas.1405739111

Guttmann, S., Chandhok, G., Groba, S. R., Niemietz, C., Sauer, V., Gomes, A., et al. (2018). Organic cation transporter 3 mediates cisplatin and copper cross-resistance in hepatoma cells. *Oncotarget* 9, 743–754. doi: 10.18632/oncotarget.23142

Harrach, S., and Ciarimboli, G. (2015). Role of transporters in the distribution of platinum-based drugs. *Front. Pharmacol.* 6:85. doi: 10.3389/fphar.2015.00085

Hicks, J. K., Chute, C. L., Paulsen, M. T., Ragland, R. L., Howlett, N. G., Guéranger, Q., et al. (2010). Differential roles for DNA polymerases eta, zeta, and REV1 in lesion bypass of intrastrand versus interstrand DNA cross-links. *Mol. Cell Biol.* 30, 1217–1230. doi: 10.1128/MCB.00993-09

Holzer, A. K., Manorek, G. H., and Howell, S. B. (2006). Contribution of the major copper influx transporter CTR1 to the cellular accumulation of cisplatin, carboplatin, and oxaliplatin. *Mol. Pharmacol.* 70, 1390–1394. doi: 10.1124/mol.106.022624

Holzer, A. K., Samimi, G., Katano, K., Naerdemann, W., Lin, X., Safaei, R., et al. (2004). The copper influx transporter human copper transport protein 1 regulates the uptake of cisplatin in human ovarian carcinoma cells. *Mol. Pharmacol.* 66, 817–823. doi: 10.1124/mol.104.001198

Hucke, A., and Ciarimboli, G. (2016). The role of transporters in the toxicity of chemotherapeutic drugs: focus on transporters for organic cations. *J. Clin. Pharmacol.* 56, S157–S172. doi: 10.1002/jcph.706

Ishida, S., Lee, J., Thiele, D. J., and Herskowitz, I. (2002). Uptake of the anticancer drug cisplatin mediated by the copper transporter Ctr1 in yeast and mammals. *Proc. Natl. Acad. Sci. U.S.A.* 99, 14298–14302. doi: 10.1073/pnas.1624 91399

Johnstone, T. C., Suntharalingam, K., and Lippard, S. J. (2016). The next generation of platinum drugs: targeted Pt(II) agents, nanoparticle delivery, and Pt(IV) prodrugs. *Chem. Rev.* 116, 3436–3486. doi: 10.1021/acs.chemrev.5b00597

Kellinger, M. W., Park, G. Y., Chong, J., Lippard, S. J., and Wang, D. (2013). Effect of a monofunctional phenanthriplatin-DNA adduct on RNA polymerase II transcriptional fidelity and translesion synthesis. *J. Am. Chem. Soc.* 135, 13054–13061. doi: 10.1021/ja405475y

Kuok, K. I., Li, S., Wyman, I. W., and Wang, R. (2017). Cucurbit[7]uril: an emerging candidate for pharmaceutical excipients. *Ann. N.Y. Acad. Sci.* 1398, 108–119. doi: 10.1111/nyas.13376

Lanvers-Kaminsky, C., and Ciarimboli, G. (2017). Pharmacogenetics of drug-induced ototoxicity caused by aminoglycosides and cisplatin. *Pharmacogenomics* 18, 1683–1695. doi: 10.2217/pgs-2017-0125

Lanvers-Kaminsky, C., Sprowl, J. A., Malath, I., Deuster, D., Eveslage, M., Schlatter, E., et al. (2015). Human OCT2 variant c.808G>T confers protection effect against cisplatin-induced ototoxicity. *Pharmacogenomics* 16, 323–332. doi: 10.2217/pgs.14.182

Lanvers-Kaminsky, C., Zehnhoff-Dinnesen, A. A., Parfitt, R., and Ciarimboli, G. (2017). Drug-induced ototoxicity: mechanisms, pharmacogenetics, and protective strategies. *Clin. Pharmacol. Ther.* 101, 491–500. doi: 10.1002/cpt.603

Lovejoy, K. S., Todd, R. C., Zhang, S., McCormick, M. S., D'Aquino, J. A., Reardon, J. T., et al. (2008). cis-Diammine(pyridine)chloroplatinum(II), a monofunctional platinum(II) antitumor agent: uptake, structure, function, and prospects. *Proc. Natl. Acad. Sci. U.S.A.* 105, 8902–8907. doi: 10.1073/pnas.0803441105

Mosmann, T. (1983). Rapid colorimetric assay for cellular growth and survival: application to proliferation and cytotoxicity assays. *J. Immunol. Methods* 65, 55–63. doi: 10.1016/0022-1759(83)90303-4

Nose, Y., Wood, L. K., Kim, B. E., Prohaska, J. R., Fry, R. S., Spears, J. W., et al. (2010). Ctr1 is an apical copper transporter in mammalian intestinal epithelial cells *in vivo* that is controlled at the level of protein stability. *J. Biol. Chem.* 285, 32385–32392. doi: 10.1074/jbc.M110.143826

Öhrvik, H. , Nose, Y., Wood, L. K., Kim, B. E., Gleber, S. C., Ralle, M., et al. (2013). Ctr2 regulates biogenesis of a cleaved form of mammalian Ctr1 metal transporter lacking the copper- and cisplatin-binding ecto-domain. *Proc. Natl. Acad. Sci. U.S.A.* 110, E4279–E4288. doi: 10.1073/pnas.1311749110

Park, G. Y., Wilson, J. J., Song, Y., and Lippard, S. J. (2012). Phenanthriplatin, a monofunctional DNA-binding platinum anticancer drug candidate with unusual potency and cellular activity profile. *Proc. Natl. Acad. Sci. U.S.A.* 109, 11987–11992. doi: 10.1073/pnas0.1207670109

Rabik, C. A., and Dolan, M. E. (2007). Molecular mechanisms of resistance and toxicity associated with platinating agents. *Cancer Treat. Rev.* 33, 9–23. doi: 10.1016/j.ctrv.2006.09.006

Romero-Canelón, I., and Sadler, P. J. (2013). Next-generation metal anticancer complexes: multitargeting via redox modulation. *Inorg. Chem.* 52, 12276–12291. doi: 10.1021/ic400835n

Rosenberg, B. (1973). Platinum coordination complexes in cancer chemotherapy. *Naturwissenschaften* 60, 399–406. doi: 10.1007/BF00623551

Schlatter, E., Klassen, P., Massmann, V., Holle, S. K., Guckel, D., Edemir, B., et al. (2014). Mouse organic cation transporter 1 determines properties and regulation of basolateral organic cation transport in renal proximal tubules. *Pflug. Arch.* 466, 1581–1589. doi: 10.1007/s00424-013-1395-9

Schmidt-Lauber, C., Harrach, S., Pap, T., Fischer, M., Victor, M., Heitzmann, M., et al. (2012). Transport mechanisms and their pathology-induced regulation govern tyrosine kinase inhibitor delivery in rheumatoid arthritis. *PLoS ONE* 7:e52247. doi: 10.1371/journal.pone.0052247

Shahsavani, M. B., Ahmadi, S., Aseman, M. D., Nabavizadeh, S. M., Rashidi, M., Asadi, Z., et al. (2016). Anticancer activity assessment of two novel binuclear platinum (II) complexes. *J. Photochem. Photobiol. B* 161, 345–354. doi: 10.1016/j.jphotobiol.2016.05.025

Sherman, S. E., and Lippard, S. J. (1987). Structural aspects of platinum anticancer drug-interactions with Dna. *Chem. Rev.* 87, 1153–1181 doi: 10.1021/cr00081a013

Sprowl, J. A., Ciarimboli, G., Lancaster, C. S., Giovinazzo, H., Gibson, A. A., Du, G., et al. (2013). Oxaliplatin-induced neurotoxicity is dependent on the organic cation transporter OCT2. *Proc. Natl. Acad. Sci. U.S.A.* 110, 11199–11204. doi: 10.1073/pnas.1305321110

Sprowl, J. A., Lancaster, C. S., Pabla, N., Hermann, E., Kosloske, A. M., Gibson, A. A., et al. (2014). Cisplatin-induced renal injury is independently mediated by OCT2 and p53. *Clin. Cancer Res.* 20, 4026–4035. doi: 10.1158/1078-0432.CCR-14-0319

Wang, K., and Gao, E. (2014). Recent advances in multinuclear complexes as potential anticancer and DNA binding agents. *Anticancer Agents Med. Chem.* 14, 147–169. doi: 10.2174/18715206113139990313

Wehe, C. A., Beyer, G., Sperling, M., Ciarimboli, G., and Karst, U. (2014). Assessing the intracellular concentration of platinum in medulloblastoma cell lines after Cisplatin incubation. *J. Trace Elem. Med. Biol.* 28, 166–172. doi: 10.1016/j.jtemb.2014.01.001

Wilde, S., Schlatter, E., Koepsell, H., Edemir, B., Reuter, S., Pavenstädt, H., et al. (2009). Calmodulin-associated post-translational regulation of rat organic cation transporter 2 in the kidney is gender dependent. *Cell Mol. Life Sci.* 66, 1729–1740. doi: 10.1007/s00018-009-9145-z

Yokoo, S., Yonezawa, A., Masuda, S., Fukatsu, A., Katsura, T., and Inui, K. (2007). Differential contribution of organic cation transporters, OCT2 and MATE1, in platinum agent-induced nephrotoxicity. *Biochem. Pharmacol.* 74, 477–487 doi: 10.1016/j.bcp.2007.03.004

Yonezawa, A., and Inui, K. (2011). Organic cation transporter OCT/SLC22A and H(+)/organic cation antiporter MATE/SLC47A are key molecules for nephrotoxicity of platinum agents. *Biochem. Pharmacol.* 81, 563–568. doi: 10.1016/j.bcp.2010.11.016

Zhang, S., Lovejoy, K. S., Shima, J. E., Lagpacan, L. L., Shu, Y., Lapuk, A., et al. (2006). Organic cation transporters are determinants of oxaliplatin cytotoxicity. *Cancer Res.* 66, 8847–8857 doi: 10.1158/0008-5472.CAN-06-0769

12

Targeting Endoplasmic Reticulum and/or Mitochondrial Ca^{2+} Fluxes as Therapeutic Strategy for HCV Infection

*Rosella Scrima [1], Claudia Piccoli [1], Darius Moradpour [2] and Nazzareno Capitanio [1]**

[1] *Department of Clinical and Experimental Medicine, University of Foggia, Foggia, Italy,* [2] *Service of Gastroenterology and Hepatology, Centre Hospitalier Universitaire Vaudois, University of Lausanne, Lausanne, Switzerland*

Correspondence:
Nazzareno Capitanio
nazzareno.capitanio@unifg.it

Chronic hepatitis C is characterized by metabolic disorders and by a microenvironment in the liver dominated by oxidative stress, inflammation and regeneration processes that can in the long term lead to liver cirrhosis and hepatocellular carcinoma. Several lines of evidence suggest that mitochondrial dysfunctions play a central role in these processes. However, how these dysfunctions are induced by the virus and whether they play a role in disease progression and neoplastic transformation remains to be determined. Most *in vitro* studies performed so far have shown that several of the hepatitis C virus (HCV) proteins also localize to mitochondria, but the consequences of these interactions on mitochondrial functions remain contradictory and need to be confirmed in the context of productively replicating virus and physiologically relevant *in vitro* and *in vivo* model systems. In the past decade we have been proposing a temporal sequence of events in the HCV-infected cell whereby the primary alteration is localized at the mitochondria-associated ER membranes and causes release of Ca^{2+} from the ER, followed by uptake into mitochondria. This ensues successive mitochondrial dysfunction leading to the generation of reactive oxygen and nitrogen species and a progressive metabolic adaptive response consisting in decreased oxidative phosphorylation and enhanced aerobic glycolysis and lipogenesis. Here we resume the major results provided by our group in the context of HCV-mediated alterations of the cellular inter-compartmental calcium flux homeostasis and present new evidence suggesting targeting of ER and/or mitochondrial calcium transporters as a novel therapeutic strategy.

Keywords: HCV, mitochondria associated membranes (MAM), calcium channels, viroporin, oxidative phosphorylation, redox signaling

INTRODUCTION

Liver disease related to HCV infection represents a major health burden worldwide (Di Bisceglie, 1998). Recent estimates suggest around 71 million chronically infected individuals, i.e., 1% of the world population (Cf. WHO Global Hepatitis Report 2017 | http://www.who.int/hepatitis/publications/global-hepatitis-report2017/en/). Approximately 80% of acutely infected individuals develop chronic infection which may progress to cirrhosis in 2–20% after 20 years and in 15–30% after 30 years. Once cirrhosis is established, the risk of hepatocellular carcinoma (HCC) development is 1–5% per year (Alter and Seeff, 2000). Great progress has been achieved in the treatment of chronic hepatitis C in recent years. Currently available directly acting antivirals yield sustained virologic response rates >90%, with very well-tolerated and relatively short treatment regimens (Pawlotsky et al., 2015).

HCV is a positive strand RNA virus belonging to the *Flaviviridae* family and *Hepacivirus* genus discovered in 1989 (Choo et al., 1989). It infects hepatocytes, with the main steps of its life cycle involving: binding to membrane receptors and entry into the cell host; uncoating of the genome from the viral capsid; translation of the viral genome at the ER; replication and assembly; as well as release of the virus particles (Moradpour et al., 2007). Notably, HCV replication and virion assembly takes place in a specialized lipid-enriched cellular compartment of the infected host called membranous web (Dubuisson et al., 2002). It is important to remind that HCV is not cytolytic.

MITOCHONDRIAL OXIDATIVE METABOLISM IN HCV INFECTION

The 9.6-kb HCV genome harbors a long open reading frame which is translated into a polyprotein of about 3000 amino acids. This is processed at the level of the ER by cellular and viral proteases to generate 10 proteins. Three of them (structural—core, E1, and E2) contribute to the virus particle, the others (non-structural—p7, NS2, NS3, NS4A, NS4B, NS5A, NS5B) are functional proteins necessary for replication and assembly of the virion (Moradpour and Penin, 2013).

It is amazing how such a limited number of proteins is sufficient to reroute host cell physiology to promote establishment of the infection and viral propagation. An example is given by the capability of HCV to evade innate immunity. This relies in part on the activation of MAVS (mitochondrial antiviral signaling protein) which is anchored on the mitochondrial outer membrane and that after binding of RIG-1 provides a recruiting platform for a number of factors whose activation leads to expression of interferon-β (Seth et al., 2005; West et al., 2011). One of the two viral proteases, the NS3-4A protease, cleaves MAVS, thereby impairing interferon induction (Li et al., 2005; Meylan et al., 2005; Bellecave et al., 2010). The involvement of mitochondria in the viral life cycle is even more pervasive. Indeed, HCV proteins were found to localize at contact sites between the ER and the mitochondrial compartment and move by lateral trafficking to the mitochondrial outer membrane (Mottola et al., 2002; Schwer et al., 2004; Griffin et al., 2005; Kasprzak et al., 2005; Suzuki et al., 2005; Nomura-Takigawa et al., 2006; Rouillé et al., 2006; Ripoli et al., 2010; Horner et al., 2011). The ER-mitochondria contact sites, also known as mitochondria associated membranes (MAMs) (Mannella et al., 1998; Rizzuto et al., 1998), are a well-organized intracellular synapse-like inter-organelle communicating systems whose structural tethering components have been elucidated (Raturi and Simmen, 2013; Giorgi et al., 2015; Giacomello and Pellegrini, 2016). The main proposed function of MAMs is to provide a tightly controlled, localized flux of calcium from the ER store into mitochondria without raising its concentration in the cytosol (Rizzuto and Pozzan, 2006; Krols et al., 2016). Calcium is a recognized physiological modulator of the mitochondrial metabolism, though above a threshold level it becomes cytotoxic (Duchen, 2000).

On this background, we have investigated functional properties of mitochondria in the context of HCV infection. To this aim we used two well-established *in vitro* cell models. One is a tetracycline-regulated system allowing the inducible expression of the entire HCV polyprotein or of defined parts thereof in stably transfected U-2 OS human osteosarcoma cells (Moradpour et al., 1998); in the inducible system only transcription and translation of the viral proteins occurs. The other is an infective system where the virus accomplishes its entire life cycle in the permissive HCC-derived cell line Huh-7.5; to track infected cells GFP was inserted into the HCV genome (Moradpour et al., 2004; Schaller et al., 2007).

The main results of systematic studies carried over the past decade by our group are schematically illustrated in **Figure 1** (Piccoli et al., 2007; Ripoli et al., 2010; Quarato et al., 2012, 2014). It is shown that expression of the HCV proteins both in the inducible system and in Huh 7.5 cells transfected with infectious full-length HCV leads to profound alterations of the mitochondrial functions. These comprise: (i) intra-mitochondrial calcium (mtCa^{2+}) overload; (ii) dissipation of the mitochondrial membrane potential ($\Delta\Psi_m$), which correlates with inhibition of cell respiration and complex I (NADH dehydrogenase) activity; (iii) overproduction of reactive oxygen and nitrogen species (RO/NS). Time-resolved analysis demonstrated that mtCa^{2+} overload was the earliest mitochondria-related alteration following induction of HCV protein expression (Piccoli et al., 2007; Quarato et al., 2012).

INHIBITORS OF THE INTRA-MITOCHONDRIAL CA^{2+} FLUX DAMPEN HCV-MEDIATED MITOCHONDRIAL DYSFUNCTION

The major transporter of Ca^{2+} into mitochondria is the mitochondrial calcium uniporter (MCU) (De Stefani et al., 2011). MCU is part of a complex, comprising also regulatory subunits, mediating a $\Delta\Psi_m$-driven accumulation of calcium ions on the negative site of the inner mitochondrial membrane (Marchi and Pinton, 2014; Granatiero et al., 2017). From the kinetic point of view, MCU is a very low-affinity, high-capacity transporter, meaning that though possessing a relatively high Km for Ca^{2+} its abundance in the inner mitochondrial membranes makes mitochondria an efficient buffering compartment preventing harmful Ca^{2+} rising in the cytosol (Deryabina et al., 2004). The kinetic limitation of MCU is overcome by MAMs, which releasing ER-calcium in its intermembrane space provides a relatively high-concentration Ca^{2+} microdomain (Rizzuto and Pozzan, 2006). The ER possesses a number of calcium releasing channels comprising inositol trisphosphate (IP3) and ryanodine receptors (Patterson et al., 2004; Hamilton, 2005).

Importantly, when cells inducibly expressing the HCV polyprotein were treated with ruthenium red (RR) or Ru360,

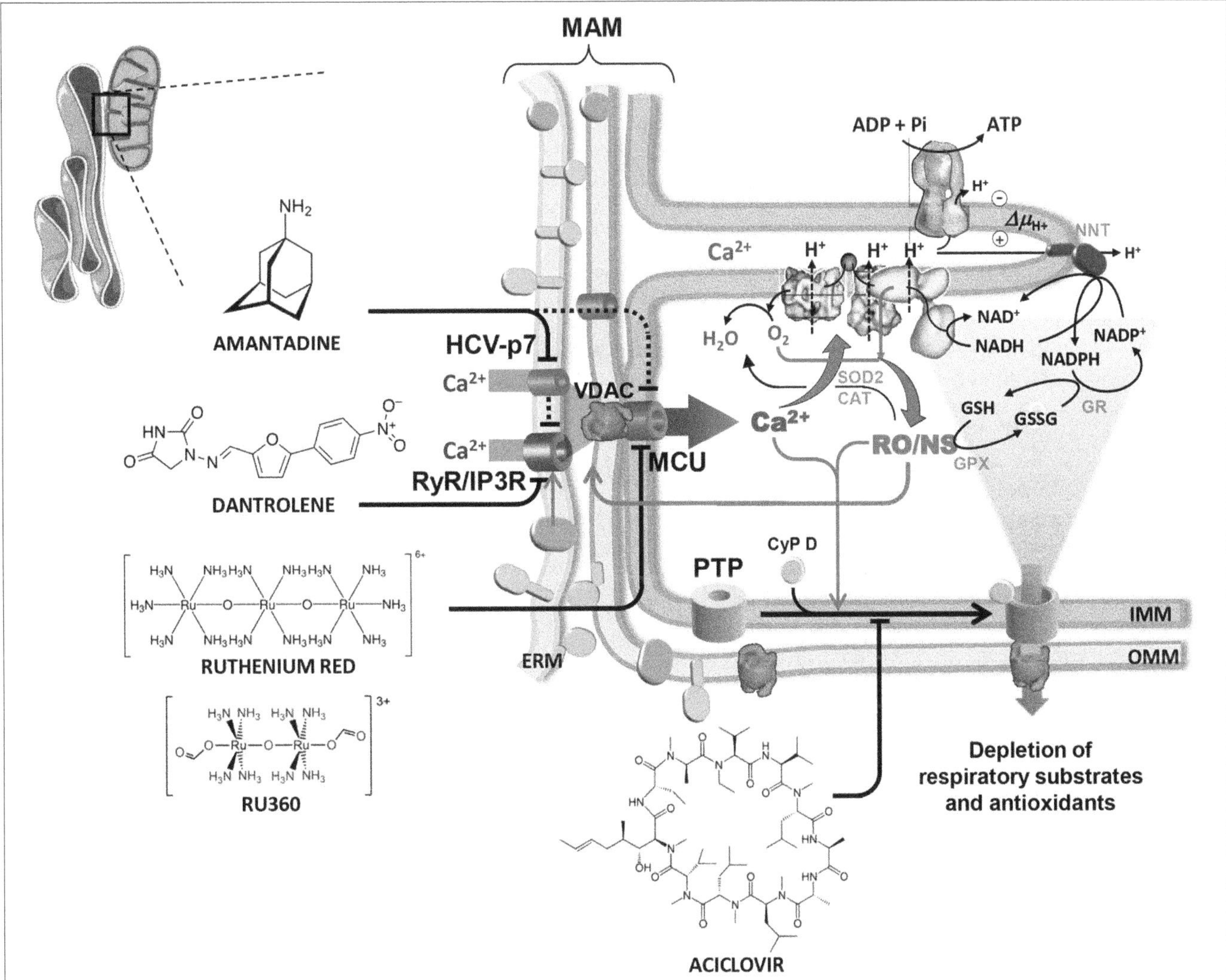

FIGURE 1 | Overview of the alterations in mitochondrial physiology linked to HCV protein expression and of drug-targetable ion channels and translocators. The contact site between endoplasmic reticulum and mitochondria is shown (mitochondrial associated membrane, MAM). HCV proteins are shown in purple on the ER membrane (ERM) and on the outer mitochondrial membrane (OMM) where they are likely transferred from ERM by lateral diffusion. Interaction of HCV proteins with the ERM-located Ca^{2+} transporters (RyR/IP3R) is shown, causing localized increase of the $[Ca^{2+}]$, thereby promoting its uptake within the mitochondria via the voltage-dependent anion channel (VDAC) and the mitochondrial calcium uniporter (MCU) located in the OMM and IMM respectively. The viroporin HCV p7 is also shown to contribute to the mitochondrial Ca^{2+} load. Activation of the ER unfolded protein response (UPR) linked to the stressing accumulation of HCV proteins might also be indirectly involved in the deregulation of the inter-organelle Ca^{2+} fluxes (not shown). The increased intramitochondrial $[Ca^{2+}]$ affects components of the respiratory chain (RC) and activates mitochondrial nitric oxide synthase (not shown, but see text), thereby increasing generation of reactive oxygen and nitrogen species (RO/NS). RC is illustrated within the IMM cristae with complexes I, III, IV (from right to left). The F_oF_1 H^+-ATP synthase is also shown in the upper part of the crista. Electron transfer from NADH to O_2 (forming H_2O) and the chemiosmotic circuitry coupling RC proton pumping to the $\Delta\Psi$-driven ATP synthesis are shown by black arrowed lines. Electron leak from dysfunctional RC leads to ROS formation/accumulation (red arrowed lines) which is mitigated by the concerted action of Mn-superoxidase dismutase 2 (SOD2), catalase (CAT) and glutathione peroxidase (GPX) with glutathione reductase (GR) and nicotinamide nucleotide transhydrogenase (NNT) needed to regenerate reduced glutathione (GSH) at expense of NADPH. The enhanced intramitochondrial levels of Ca^{2+} and RO/NS are shown to activate the permeability transition pore (PTP), illustrated schematically by the cyclophilin D (CyP D)-mediated assembly of OMM and IMM components. Opening of the PTP causes flush out of low molecular weight metabolites comprising $NAD(P)^+/NAD(P)H$ and GSH/GSSG. This leads to further impairment of the RC activity (and of the oxidative phosphorylation) and to reduced ROS scavenging with consequent worsening of the redox balance. RO/NS are finally shown to affect the activity of the Ca^{2+} transporting system (green arrow) with further entry of Ca^{2+} into the mitochondria, thereby fuelling a positive feedback mechanism. Blocking the above-illustrated cycle of alterations constitutes a rationale to develop therapeutic strategies. Accordingly, inhibitors of the ER Ca^{2+} channel(s) (dantrolene), the viroporin p7 (amantadine), the MCU (ruthenium red/Ru360), the PTP (aciclovir) are shown. Reproduced with modifications from Quarato et al. (2013). Copyright (2013), with permission from Elsevier.

both inhibitors of the MCU (Broekemeier et al., 1994; Matlib et al., 1998), the above-reported mitochondrial alterations were fully prevented (Piccoli et al., 2007). A similar protection was observed when these cells were treated with dantrolene, an inhibitor of the ER calcium channels (Piccoli et al., 2007).

Taken together, the results obtained led us to suggest a working model whereby the overload of $mtCa^{2+}$ is the seminal event in the successive alterations (Piccoli et al., 2006, 2009; Quarato et al., 2013). Possibly, overcrowding of HCV proteins at MAMs might affect the overall calcium retention capacity of the ER membranes as a consequence of a mild unfolded protein response (UPR) (Carreras-Sureda et al., 2017) or elicit a specific effect on the Ca^{2+} channels (Deniaud et al., 2008). The MCU-mediated load of Ca^{2+} into the mitochondria drives alterations in the redox homeostasis. This might be achieved by activation of a Ca^{2+}-dependent mitochondrial isoform of the nitric oxide synthase (Dedkova et al., 2004; Ghafourifar and Sen, 2007). NO is known to affect the mitochondrial respiratory chain by competitive inhibition of the cytochrome c oxidase and/or by covalent modification of complex I (Brown and Borutaite, 2004; Sarti et al., 2012). Impairment of the normal electron transfer in the respiratory chain results in enhanced electron leak to O_2, with formation of the superoxide anion ($O_2^{\bullet-}$) (Murphy, 2009), which is further converted to H_2O_2 by the Mn-SOD. To support this model is the evidence provided by confocal microscopy analysis, using specific probes for NO, $O_2^{\bullet-}$, and peroxides, showing a clear compartmentalization of the fluorescent signals resembling the mitochondrial network (Piccoli et al., 2007). Overproduction of ROS has been recurrently reported to enhance $mtCa^{2+}$ uptake likely by modification of redox sensitive cysteines of the ER calcium channels (Feissner et al., 2009; Görlach et al., 2015) and/or of the MCU (Dong et al., 2017). Accordingly, treatment of cells inducibly expressing the HCV polyprotein with the antioxidant N-acetylcysteine (NAC) prevented completely the $mtCa^{2+}$ overload as well as inhibition of the mitochondrial respiratory activity and of the $\Delta\Psi_m$ generation (Piccoli et al., 2007).

The enhanced levels of Ca^{2+} and RO/NS into mitochondria proved to activate a long established feature of the organelle better known as mitochondria permeability transition (MPT) (Giorgio et al., 2017). MPT consists in increased non-specific conductance of the inner mitochondrial membrane to low molecular weight molecules (<1,500 Da). Activation of the MPT is attained by a number of factors promoting binding of cyclophilin D (Cyp D) to the MPT pore (Elrod and Molkentin, 2013). The molecular nature of the MPT pore has been elusive for a long time though recent evidence suggests the F_oF_1-ATP synthase as a plausible candidate (Bernardi et al., 2015; Jonas et al., 2015). Transient opening (i.e., flickering) of the MPT pore works as a relief valve-like system avoiding hyperpolarization of the inner mitochondrial membrane as well as recycling of Ca^{2+} (Aon et al., 2008; Nivala et al., 2011). Conversely, permanent opening of the MPT pore causes exit of low molecular weight antioxidants (like glutathione) and redox coenzymes fostering oxidative stress as well as swelling of mitochondria because of its hyperosmolarity as compared with the cytosol (Di Lisa et al., 2001). This event can lead to autophagy of the organelle, apoptosis or necrosis depending on the prevailing cellular setting (Kroemer et al., 2007).

To verify the involvement of the MPT in the observed HCV-mediated mitochondrial dysfunctions we tested the effect of alisporivir, a robust antiviral drug (Paeshuyse et al., 2006; Coelmont et al., 2009; Gallay and Lin, 2013). Alisporivir is a cyclosporin A analog but without immunosuppressive properties (Gallay and Lin, 2013). It binds to Cyp D, interfering with its opener function of the MPT (Elrod and Molkentin, 2013). When alisporivir was tested on the mitochondrial dysfunctions caused by HCV protein expression we found an impressive capability of the drug to fully prevent (and even reverse) the $\Delta\Psi_m$ collapse, RO/NS production and $mtCa^{2+}$ overload (Quarato et al., 2012).

Combination of all the above reported observations supports a pathogenetic model for HCV infection whereby a self-nourishing mechanism is activated, consisting in positive feed-back loops initiated by the entry of Ca^{2+} into mitochondria and fuelled by the ensuing RO/NS overproduction elicited by impaired activity of the respiratory chain (**Figure 1**). In such a cascade of events an essential role is seemingly played by mitochondrial and ER transporters (i.e., MCU, MPT pore, ER-Ca^{2+} channels) since inhibition of either of them prevents and reverses the HCV protein-mediated mitochondrial alterations.

EXPLORING THE HCV VIROPORIN p7 AS A POTENTIAL THERAPEUTIC TARGET

The impact of Ca^{2+} flux homeostasis in the interplay between HCV and the host cell is also underlined by the presence in the HCV proteins of the viroporin p7 (Madan and Bartenschlager, 2015). p7 is a transmembrane protein constituted by two transmembrane helices which is thought to oligomerize in hexameric structures, forming a channel (Clarke et al., 2006). When inserted into artificial membranes, p7 proved to increase ionic conductance with selectivity toward cations (Griffin et al., 2003; Montserret et al., 2010; Wozniak et al., 2010). It accumulates in ER membranes and is particularly enriched at the MAMs sub-compartment (Griffin et al., 2004). Data obtained *in vitro* suggested a role of the antiviral drug amantadine in inhibiting HCV p7-mediated cation conductance (Griffin et al., 2003; Cook et al., 2013; see also Atoom et al., 2014). Given this premise and in keeping the observed mitochondrial alterations caused by HCV protein expression we tested on those the effects of amantadine, an adamantane-derived compound (**Figure 1**). We found that amantadine not only prevented but also rescued HCV protein-mediated mitochondrial dysfunction in cells inducibly expressing the HCV polyprotein (Quarato et al., 2014). Specifically, amantadine corrected: (i) overload of mitochondrial Ca^{2+}; (ii) inhibition of respiratory chain activity and oxidative phosphorylation; (iii) reduction of membrane potential; (iv) overproduction of reactive oxygen species. The effects of amantadine were observed within 15 min following drug administration and confirmed in Huh-7.5 cells transfected with the infectious full-length HCV genome. However, these effects were also observed in cells expressing subgenomic HCV constructs, indicating that they are not mediated or only in part mediated by p7. Single organelle analyses carried out on isolated mouse liver mitochondria demonstrated that amantadine induces hyperpolarization of the membrane potential (Quarato et al., 2014). Moreover, amantadine treatment increased the calcium threshold required to trigger mitochondrial permeability transition opening (Quarato et al., 2014). These results led to the conclusion that amantadine displays off-target effects likely relatable to Ca^{2+} transporting systems of the host cell.

METABOLIC REWIRING OF HOST CELL BY HCV

Surprisingly, in spite of the overt impairment of the mitochondrial respiratory chain activity and of the concurrent oxidative phosphorylation (OxPhos), HCV-infected cells did not show evident signs of sufferance or bioenergetic failure. Indeed, the difference in growth rate and viability of both HCV-induced U2-OS cells and HCV-infected Huh-7 cells was negligible as compared with control cells. Accordingly, the cellular ATP level was unaffected, if not increased, in HCV-induced U2-OS cells grown in glucose-containing media (Piccoli et al., 2007). Though this is consistent with the non-cytopathic property of HCV, it implies the need to understand how the virus rewires the host cell metabolism (Diamond et al., 2010).

An important factor and regulator of metabolism in cells challenged by stressing conditions is constituted by hypoxia inducible factor 1α (HIF-1α) (Wang and Semenza, 1993). HIF-1α is rapidly degraded under normal oxygen tension following hydroxylation by O_2- and 2-oxo-glutarate-dependent prolyl hydroxylases (PDHs) (Bruick and McKnight, 2001). The hydroxylated HIF-1α is then ubiquitinated and steered toward proteasomal degradation (Mole et al., 2001). Conversely, under hypoxic conditions the hydroxylation of HIF-1α is dampened and it accumulates and moves to the nucleus where promotes transcription of a number of prosurvival genes, including those coding for glycolytic enzymes (Semenza et al., 1994; Wang et al., 1995). However, conditions different from hypoxia, which in turn inhibit PDH activity (i.e., RO/NS and/or competing 2-oxo-acids) result in stabilization of HIF-1α also under normoxia (Déry et al., 2005; Pugh, 2016; **Figure 2A**).

We demonstrated that HIF-1α is stabilized under normoxic conditions both in HCV-induced U2-OS and HCV-infected Huh-7 cells as well as in patients' liver biopsies (Ripoli et al., 2010; see also Nasimuzzaman et al., 2007; Wilson et al., 2012). Consistent with this finding, we showed that the HIF target genes coding for the glycolytic enzymes hexokinases I and II (HKI, HKII) were both upregulated at the transcriptional and protein levels. This would indicate a metabolic shift toward aerobic glycolysis that we supported by an observed higher release of lactate in HCV-induced U2-OS cells (**Figure 2B**). It is worth considering that HKII was shown to interact with the outer mitochondrial membrane at the level of the voltage-dependent anion channel (VDAC) and to prevent MPT activation (Pastorino et al., 2005; Chiara et al., 2008). Also, HKI was found to interact with the outer mitochondrial membrane, thereby blocking apoptotic signals (Abu-Hamad et al., 2008; Schindler and Foley, 2013).

On this basis, we proposed a model, consistent with other reported evidence, whereby the MPT pore oscillates between the closed and open state under the positive influence of HKII, which restrains the effects of RO/NS and $mtCa^{2+}$ (Quarato et al., 2012). Stabilization of HIF-1α, up-regulating the expression of HKII, is likely to be linked to activation of the AKT-mTOR pathway (Land and Tee, 2007; Agani and Jiang, 2013). Indeed it has been suggested that PI3K, the upstream activator of AKT, binds the HCV NS5A protein which activates it permanently (Street et al., 2005). Moreover, the active form of AKT deactivates GSK-3β, which by phosphorylation of VDAC displaces HKII, promoting permanent opening of the MPTP under stressing conditions (Pastorino et al., 2005; see also Chiara et al., 2008). In agreement with this proposal, we found that the phosphorylation state of AKT and GSK-3β was enhanced both in HCV-induced U2-OS and in HCV-transfected Huh 7.5 cells (**Figure 2D**).

We have here a remarkable example of the strategy put in action by HCV which although impairing the most important energetic powerhouse of the cell (i.e., the mitochondrial OxPhos system) at the same time tunes the consequent effects evading premature cell-death signaling of the host cell.

INHIBITORS OF THE ER AND MITOCHONDRIAL CA^{2+} CHANNEL/PORTER DAMPER LIPOGENESIS IN HCV INFECTED CELLS

A recently emerged property of HCV is the enhanced mitophagy in the host cell (Kim et al., 2013, 2014; Ruggieri et al., 2014). Mitophagy is a selective autophagic degradation of mitochondria which is part of a quality control processing of the cell (Anding and Baehrecke, 2017). The main trigger for recognizing damaged mitochondria is a drop in the membrane potential which recruits and activates mitophagic factors like PINK1 and parkin to initiate first the fission of the mitochondrial network and then the engulfment of the isolated mitochondria into isolation membranes to become mitophagosomes (Zimmermann and Reichert, 2017). However, and remarkably in the context of HCV infection, this process appears to be somehow abortive since the mitophagosomes, instead of fusing with lysosomes, have been reported to accumulate, together with lipid droplets, in the membranous web which is the peculiar environment where HCV RNA replication takes place (Hara et al., 2014). Blocking this process results in suppression of the viral replication (Fang et al., 2017). This is possibly another strategy to hinder the MAVS-mediated immune response.

Accumulation of lipid droplets can be easily detected by staining cells with Oil Red O. **Figure 3** shows the impressive accumulation of lipid droplets in HCV-infected Huh 7.5 cells and the co-localization of them with GFP-labeled NS5A HCV protein. Similar results were obtained with HCV-induced U2-OS cells. This observation clearly implies an HCV-mediated deregulation of fatty acid metabolism, which may derive from an inhibition of fatty acid oxidation (FAO) or increased fatty acid synthesis

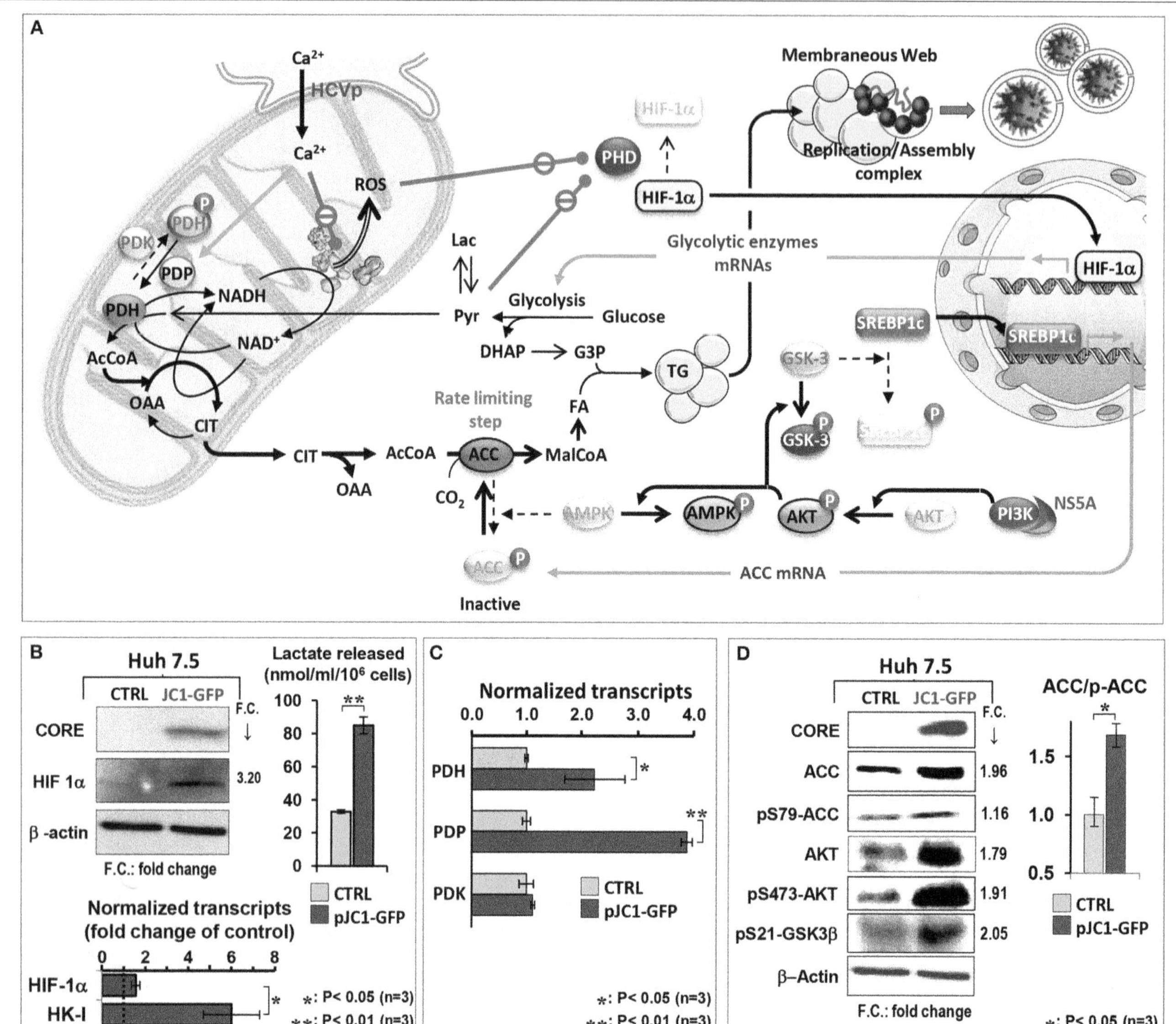

FIGURE 2 | HCV induces rewiring of cell metabolism in infected cells. **(A)** The scheme summarizes major changes in the metabolic pathways induced by HCV infection as supported by evidence reported in the literature and by the unpublished results showed in panels **(B–D)** obtained in HCV Jc1 RNA-transfected Huh-7.5 cells *in vitro*. HCV protein-induced enhanced entry of Ca^{2+} into mitochondria is shown to dampen the respiratory chain activity and oxidative phosphorylation (OxPhos) and to elicit increased reactive oxygen species (ROS) production. These inhibit the prolyl-hydroxylase (PHD) leading to stabilization of the hypoxia induced transcription factor (HIF-1α) which controls the expression of the glycolytic enzymes, thereby shifting cell metabolism toward aerobic glycolysis. **(B)** shows the stabilization of HIF-1α and the consequent metabolic shift evidenced by upregulation of the hexokinase I (HK-I) transcript and by increased lactate release in transfected Huh-7.5 cells. The enhanced glycolytic flux leads to accumulation of pyruvate which proved to further inhibit PHD. Pyruvate enters into mitochondria where it is converted in acetyl-CoA (AcCoA) by the pyruvate dehydrogenase (PDH). The HCV protein-mediated load of Ca^{2+} into mitochondria is shown to activate the pyruvate dehydrogenase phosphate (PDP), which controls the activity of the PDH. To note, at the transcriptional level both PDH and PDP [but not the pyruvate dehydrogenase kinase (PDK)] are significantly up-regulated in HCV RNA-transfected Huh-7.5 cells **(C)**. The enhanced production of AcCoA leads to formation of citrate (CIT), which because of the limited availability of oxidized NAD^+ (caused by impaired respiratory chain activity) is not further transformed *via* the tricarboxylic cycle and exits from mitochondria to shuttle AcCoA in the cytosol. The cytosolic AcCoA functions as precursor for the *de novo* synthesis of fatty acids (FA) that with intermediates of glycolysis forms triglycerides (TG) accumulating as lipid droplets. **(D)** shows that HCV RNA-transfected Huh-7.5 cells displays a two-fold increased expression of the acetyl CoA carboxylase (ACC), the controlling step in FA synthesis. ACC activity is controlled by its inactivating phosphorylation mediated by the AMP-activated protein kinase (AMPK) which is in turn controlled by the phosphorylated state of Akt/protein kinase B. Phosphorylation of AKT is mediated by activation of the phosphatidylinositol 3-kinase (PI3K), which has been reported to interact with HCV NS5A. Notably, the phosphorylated AKT is known to inactivate the glycogen synthase kinase 3β (GSK3β) which inhibits the activity of the transcription factor sterol regulatory element-binding protein 1c (SREBP 1c) controlling the expression of ACC. Consistently, the Western blots in panel **(D)** show enhanced phosphorylation of both AKT and GSK3β. The inability of HCV RNA-transfected to properly oxidize FA by the mitochondrial β-oxidation (requiring efficient respiratory chain) may lead to cytosolic accumulation of acyl-CoA which flow into TG synthesis (not shown). Lipid droplets results in formation of a membraneous web, contributed also by the HCV protein induced extensive rearrangement of host cell membranes, which contains the sites of viral replication and possibly assembly.

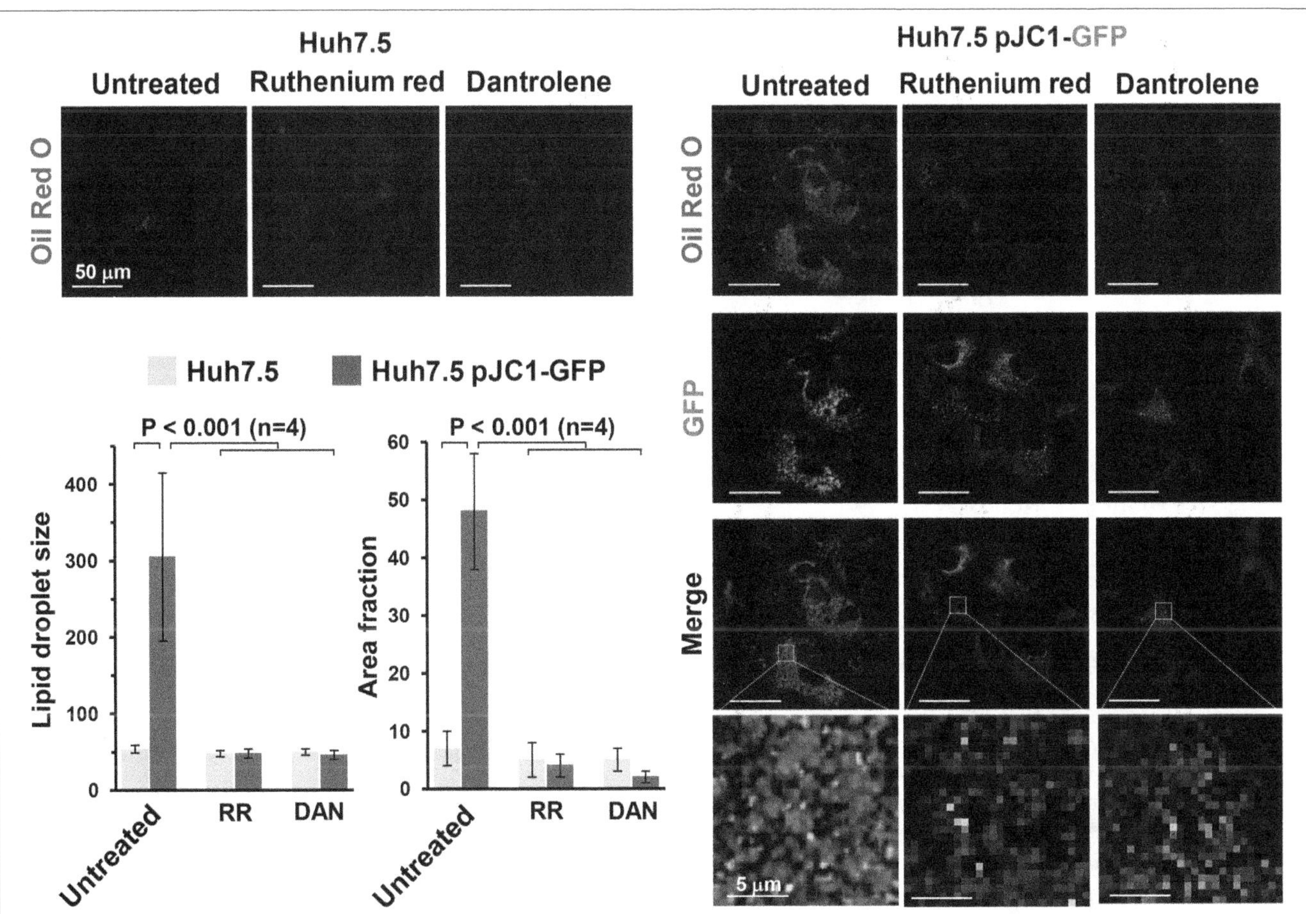

FIGURE 3 | Effect of ruthenium red and dantrolene on lipid droplet formation in transiently HCV RNA-transfected Huh-7.5 cells. Lipid droplets were stained with Oil Red O (3 mg/ml for 60 min) and imaged by laser scanning confocal microscopy. Representative images of control and Jc1-GFP RNA-transfected Huh-7.5 cells are shown illustrating the merge of Oil Red O (red) and GFP-related (green) fluorescence signals; the latter was used to track HCV-transfected cells (>90% of the cell population). Control Huh-7.5 cells were subjected to the transfection protocol but without HCV RNA. The time point after transfection was 72 h (see Ripoli et al., 2010 for further details). Where indicated 5 μM Ruthenium red (RR) or 10 μM dantrolene (DAN) were added soon after transfection. Enlargements of the merged pictures are also shown to better visualize lipid droplets in HCV RNA-transfected Huh-7.5 cells. The histograms of the Oil Red O-related fluorescence in GFP-positive transfected cells comparing untreated and drug-untreated cells are shown and refer to the averaged size and to the occupied cellular area fraction of the lipid droplets. The fluorescence intensity was assessed by averaging 10–20 cells from each of at least 10 optical fields under each condition using ImageJ 1.49v (http://imagej.nih.gov/ij). The average of four independent experiments plus the standard error of the mean (SEM), along with statistical analysis, is shown.

(FAS) or both. Deregulation of peroxisome proliferator-activated receptors (PPARs), the master transcription factors regulating lipid metabolism, is likely to be involved (Agriesti et al., 2012). Notably, treatment of infected cells with either dantrolene or RR prevented lipid droplet accumulation, pointing once again to alteration of the ER-mitochondria calcium flux as a germinal event in HCV infection.

Hampering of FAO can be envisioned as a consequence of the HCV-mediated impairment of respiratory chain function which limits the proper redox recycling of the coenzymes required in fatty acid β-oxidation. In addition, flickering of the MPT would result in progressive leakage from the mitochondrial compartment of factors needed for FAO (like carnitine) (Di Lisa et al., 2001).

However, also an enhanced fatty acid and triglyceride (TG) biosynthesis is likely to occur concurrently with FAO dampening. Consistently, we found up-regulation of the FAS rate-limiting enzyme acetyl CoA carboxylase (Wakil et al., 1983; Kim, 1997) both in terms of enhanced expression and of post-translational activating phosphorylation *via* the PI3K-AKT axis (Hardie, 1989; **Figure 2D**). Activation of the transcription factor SREBP1c, controlling the expression of ACC, is known to be linked to the AKT-mediated inactivation of GSK-3β (Kim et al., 2004; Park et al., 2009; Yecies et al., 2011). Such a signaling pathway was recently found to upregulate HCV RNA translation (Shi et al., 2016). Precursors for FAS and TG are provided by glycolytic metabolites. Acetyl CoA is largely derived by pyruvate oxidative decarboxylation, catalyzed by the pyruvate dehydrogenase (PDH) complex, and *via* the citrate shuttle released in the cytoplasm. The PDH function is tightly controlled by its phosphorylation state, which in turn depends on the balanced activities of a PDH kinase (PDK) and a PDH phosphatase (PDP) (Roche et al., 2001). To note, we found that HCV full-lenght RNA-transfected

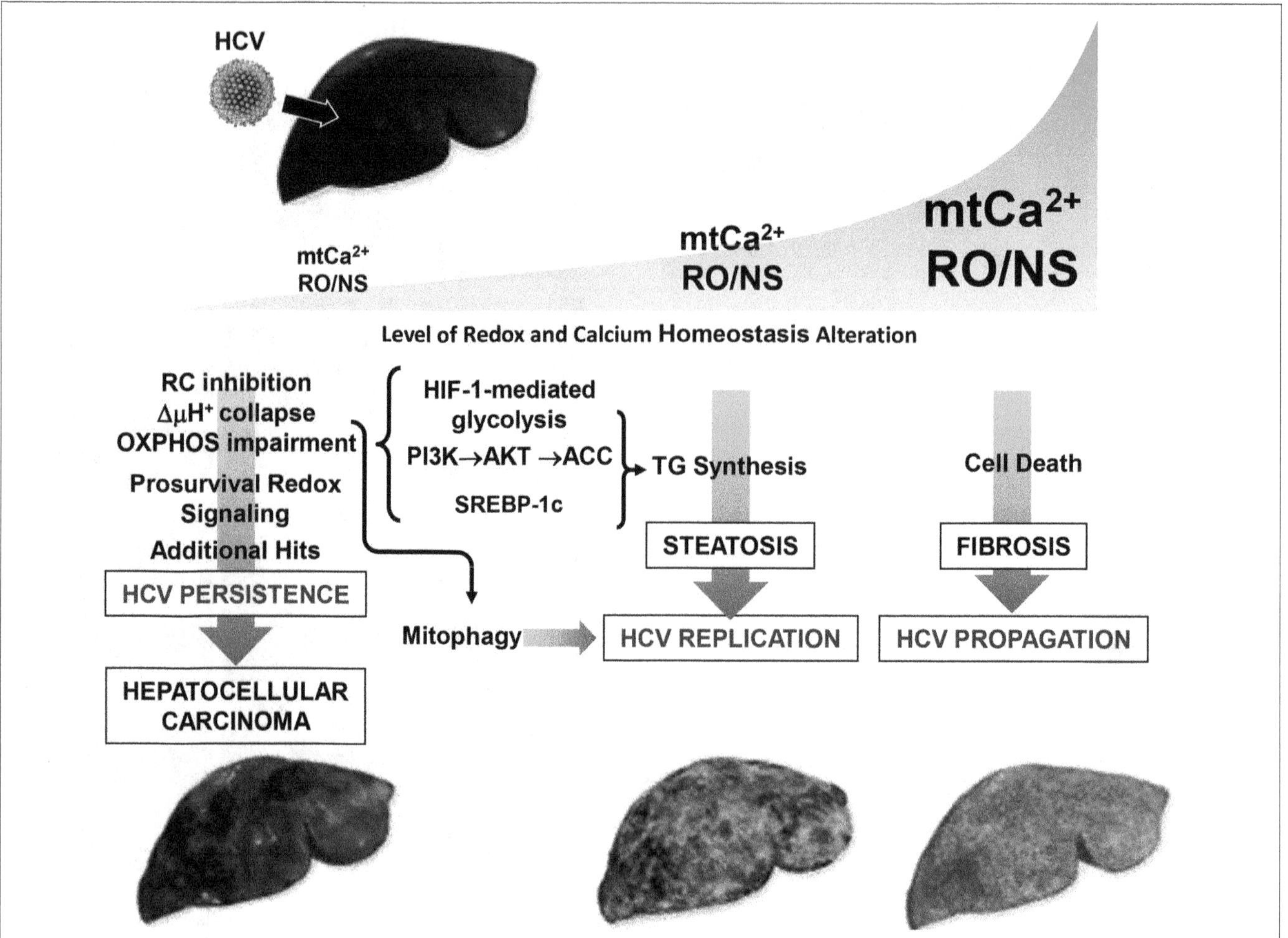

FIGURE 4 | Pathogenetic model of HCV-mediated alterations. The development of disease in patients with chronic hepatitis C is modeled as a function of the level of the oxidative alteration and of the mt-Ca^{2+} load. Three pathogenic settings are presented. Low RO/NS- and mt-Ca^{2+}-dependent stress level activates a pro-survival and proliferative adaptive response by redox signaling. The flickering balance between the mitochondrial PTP closed/open configuration is set to a level that causes collapse of the respiratory chain-mediated protonmotive force (i.e., $\Delta\mu H^+$), with consequent impairment of ATP synthesis by the FoF1-H^+ ATP synthase. This forces the infected cell to shift its energy-supplying metabolism toward glycolysis by activation of the transcription factor HIF-1α. Collapse of the $\Delta\mu H^+$ is a trigger for selective removal of damaged mitochondria by the organelle-specific autophagic machinery (i.e., mitophagy), which is required for HCV replication. Such a prosurvival setting in the host cell facilitates HCV persistence. However, if additional (mutagenic) hits accumulate over the time this may result in clonal expansion, leading to hepatocellular carcinoma. Intermediate levels of RO/NS and mt-Ca^{2+} enhance the closed to open transition of the PTP causing, among others, depletion of low-molecular weight metabolites (i.e., glutathione, NAD^+, carnitine, coenzyme A) needed to guarantee antioxidant capacity and import of long chain acyl-CoA (AcCoA) for β-oxidation. Accumulation of acyl-CoA leads to conversion into triglycerides (TG). Other factors, described in **Figure 2** (i.e., activation of HIF-1α, PI3K-Akt-ACC) and of the sterol regulatory element-binding protein (SREBP-1c) may contribute to enhanced *de novo* lipogenesis. All together this may account for the steatosis which can be observed in HCV-infected hepatocytes. Accumulation of lipid droplets in the cytoplasm is believed to provide an assembly platform for HCV. High intramitochondrial concentrations of Ca^{2+} and ROS induces permanent opening of the PTP causing osmotic swelling and rupture of the outer mitochondria membrane. The consequent release of cytochrome c and other pro-apoptotic factors triggers the caspase cascade. Depending on the intracellular ATP level, this would lead to apoptosis or necrosis activating, in the last case, tissue fibrosis. Reproduced with modifications from Quarato et al. (2013), Copyright (2013), with permission from Elsevier.

Huh 7.5 cells displayed enhanced transcript levels of PDH and PDP (**Figure 2C**). Remarkably, mtCa^{2+} is required to stimulate the PDH phosphatase and consequently the PDH, which is more active in its dephosphorylated state (Huang et al., 1998; Denton, 2009). This notion would explain the observed inhibition of lipid droplet accumulation in HCV-infected cells when treated with inhibitors of either the MCU or ER-calcium channel(s).

CONCLUSIONS

In conclusion, the emerging strategy put in action by HCV is consistent with a fine rewiring of host cell metabolism. This is achieved by depressing mitochondrial OxPhos while fostering glycolysis which provides, in addition to energy, precursors for biosynthetic processes. A major and perhaps germinal event appears to be a deregulation of Ca^{2+} flux homeostasis between the ER and mitochondria at specialized contact sites. This would selectively target mitochondria, avoiding large changes of the Ca^{2+} concentration in the cytosol, thus preserving cell viability. The ensued increase of $mtCa^{2+}$ leads to changes in the mitochondrial redox tone. This results in progressive dysfunction of the respiratory chain activity and the resulting OxPhos failure is bioenergetically compensated by an enhanced glycolytic flux. In this context, concurrent or consequent activation of prosurvival transcription factors contributes to dampen cell death. Realization of a membranous web constituted by accumulation of lipid droplets, and possibly by incomplete mitophagy, provides a suitable platform for HCV replication and virus particles assembly. Depending on the prevailing conditions (i.e., the level of the oxidative alterations and of the $mtCa^{2+}$ load) in such a multistep process, HCV infection can progress to different clinical outcomes including steatosis, fibrosis, HCC (**Figure 4**).

Importantly, the development of drugs selectively targeting ER and/or mitochondrial calcium channels might represent a potential strategy in support of standard HCV therapies.

AUTHOR CONTRIBUTIONS

RS: Carried out the experiments, analyzed the results; CP: Designed and supervised the study, carried out the experiments; DM: Provided expertize, samples and critical feedback, assisted in writing the paper; NC: Designed the study, supervised the project, wrote the paper.

ACKNOWLEDGMENTS

This work wa supported by local grants from the University of Foggia to RS, CP, NC. DM acknowledges support by Swiss National Science Foundation grants 3100A0_122447/1, 31003A_138484/1, and 31003A_156030/1.

REFERENCES

Abu-Hamad, S., Zaid, H., Israelson, A., Nahon, E., and Shoshan-Barmatz, V. (2008). Hexokinase-I protection against apoptotic cell death is mediated via interaction with the voltage-dependent anion channel-1: mapping the site of binding. *J. Biol. Chem.* 283, 13482–13490. doi: 10.1074/jbc.M708216200

Agani, F., and Jiang, B. H. (2013). Oxygen-independent regulation of HIF-1: novel involvement of PI3K/AKT/mTOR pathway in cancer. *Curr. Cancer Drug Targets* 13, 245–251. doi: 10.2174/1568009611313030003

Agriesti, F., Tataranni, T., Ruggieri, V., Capitanio, N., and Piccoli, C. (2012). PPARs and HCV-related hepatocarcinoma: a mitochondrial point of view. *PPAR Res.* 2012:605302. doi: 10.1155/2012/605302

Alter, H. J., and Seeff, L. B. (2000). Recovery, persistence, and sequelae in hepatitis C virus infection: a perspective on long-term outcome. *Semin. Liver Dis.* 20, 17–35. doi: 10.1055/s-2000-9505

Anding, A. L., and Baehrecke, E. H. (2017). Cleaning house: selective autophagy of organelles. *Dev. Cell.* 41, 10–22. doi: 10.1016/j.devcel.2017.02.016

Aon, M. A., Cortassa, S., and O'Rourke, B. (2008). Mitochondrial oscillations in physiology and pathophysiology. *Adv. Exp. Med. Biol.* 641, 98–117. doi: 10.1007/978-0-387-09794-7_8

Atoom, A. M., Taylor, N. G., and Russell, R. S. (2014). The elusive function of the hepatitis C virus p7 protein. *Virology* 462–463, 377–387. doi: 10.1016/j.virol.2014.04.018

Bellecave, P., Sarasin-Filipowicz, M., Donzé, O., Kennel, A., Gouttenoire, J., Meylan, E., et al. (2010). Cleavage of mitochondrial antiviral signaling protein in the liver of patients with chronic hepatitis C correlates with a reduced activation of the endogenous interferon system. *Hepatology* 51, 1127–1136. doi: 10.1002/hep.23426

Bernardi, P., Rasola, A., Forte, M., and Lippe, G. (2015). The mitochondrial permeability transition pore: channel formation by F-ATP synthase, integration in signal transduction, and role in pathophysiology. *Physiol. Rev.* 95, 1111–1155. doi: 10.1152/physrev.00001.2015

Broekemeier, K. M., Krebsbach, R. J., and Pfeiffer, D. R. (1994). Inhibition of the mitochondrial Ca^{2+} uniporter by pure and impure ruthenium red. *Mol. Cell. Biochem.* 139, 33–40. doi: 10.1007/BF00944201

Brown, G. C., and Borutaite, V. (2004). Inhibition of mitochondrial respiratory complex I by nitric oxide, peroxynitrite and S-nitrosothiols. *Biochim. Biophys. Acta* 1658, 44–49. doi: 10.1016/j.bbabio.2004.03.016

Bruick, R. K., and McKnight, S. L. (2001). A conserved family of prolyl-4-hydroxylases that modify HIF. *Science* 294, 1337–1340. doi: 10.1126/science.1066373

Carreras-Sureda, A., Pihán, P., and Hetz, C. (2017). Calcium signaling at the endoplasmi reticulum: fine-tuning stress responses. *Cell Calcium* 70, 24–31. doi: 10.1016/j.ceca.2017.08.004

Chiara, F., Castellaro, D., Marin, O., Petronilli, V., Brusilow, W. S., Juhaszova, M., et al. (2008). Hexokinase II detachment from mitochondria triggers apoptosis through the permeability transition pore independent of voltage-dependent anion channels. *PLoS ONE* 3:e1852. doi: 10.1371/journal.pone.0001852

Choo, Q. L., Kuo, G., Weiner, A. J., Overby, L. R., Bradley, D. W., and Houghton, M. (1989). Isolation of a cDNA clone derived from a blood-borne non-A, non-B viral hepatitis genome. *Science* 244, 359–362. doi: 10.1126/science.2523562

Clarke, D., Griffin, S., Beales, L., Gelais, C. S., Burgess, S., Harris, M., et al. (2006). Evidence for the formation of a heptameric ion channel complex by the hepatitis C virus p7 protein *in vitro*. *J. Biol. Chem.* 281, 37057–37068. doi: 10.1074/jbc.M602434200

Coelmont, L., Kaptein, S., Paeshuyse, J., Vliegen, I., Dumont, J. M., Vuagniaux, G., et al. (2009). Debio 025, a cyclophilin binding molecule, is highly efficient in clearing hepatitis C virus (HCV) replicon-containing cells when used alone or in combination with specifically targeted antiviral therapy for HCV (STAT-C)inhibitors. *Antimicrob. Agents Chemother.* 53, 967–976. doi: 10.1128/AAC.00939-08

Cook, G. A., Dawson, L. A., Tian, Y., and Opella, S. J. (2013). Three-dimensional structure and interaction studies of hepatitis C virus p7 in 1,2-dihexanoyl-sn-glycero-3-phosphocholine by solution nuclear magnetic resonance. *Biochemistry* 52, 5295–5303. doi: 10.1021/bi4006623

De Stefani, D., Raffaello, A., Teardo, E., Szabò, I., and Rizzuto, R. (2011). A forty-kilodalton protein of the inner membrane is the mitochondrial calcium uniporter. *Nature* 476, 336–340. doi: 10.1038/nature10230

Dedkova, E. N., Ji, X., Lipsius, S. L., and Blatter, L. A. (2004). Mitochondrial calcium uptake stimulates nitric oxide production in mitochondria of bovine vascular endothelial cells. *Am. J. Physiol. Cell. Physiol.* 286, 406–415. doi: 10.1152/ajpcell.00155.2003

Deniaud, A., Sharaf el dein, O., Maillier, E., Poncet, D., Kroemer, G., Lemaire, C., et al. (2008). Endoplasmic reticulum stress induces calcium-dependent permeability transition, mitochondrial outer membrane permeabilization and apoptosis. *Oncogene* 27, 285–299. doi: 10.1038/sj.onc.1210638

Denton, R. M. (2009). Regulation of mitochondrial dehydrogenases by calcium ions. *Biochim Biophys. Acta* 1787, 1309–1316. doi: 10.1016/j.bbabio.2009.01.005

Déry, M. A., Michaud, M. D., and Richard, D. E. (2005). Hypoxia-inducible factor 1: regulation of hypoxic and non-hypoxic activators. *Int. J. Biochem. Cell. Biol.* 37, 535–540. doi: 10.1016/j.biocel.2004.08.012

Deryabina, Y. I., Isakova, E. P., Shurubor, E. I., and Zvyagilskaya, R. A. (2004). Mitochondrial calcium transport systems: properties, regulation, and taxonomic features. *Biochemistry* 26, 190–195. doi: 10.1023/B:BIRY.0000016357.17251.7b

Di Bisceglie, A. M. (1998). Hepatitis, C. *Lancet* 351, 351–355. doi: 10.1016/S0140-6736(97)07361-3

Di Lisa, F., Menabò, R., Canton, M., Barile, M., and Bernardi, P. (2001). Opening of the mitochondrial permeability transition pore causes depletion of mitochondrial and cytosolic NAD+ and is a causative event in the death of myocytes in postischemic reperfusion of the heart. *J. Biol. Chem.* 276, 2571–2575. doi: 10.1074/jbc.M006825200

Diamond, D. L., Syder, A. J., Jacobs, J. M., Sorensen, C. M., Walters, K. A., Proll, S. C., et al. (2010). Temporal proteome and lipidome profiles reveal hepatitis C virus-associated reprogramming of hepatocellular metabolism and bioenergetics. *PLoS Pathog.* 6:e1000719. doi: 10.1371/journal.ppat.1000719

Dong, Z., Shanmughapriya, S., Tomar, D., Siddiqui, N., Lynch, S., Nemani, N., et al. (2017). Mitochondrial Ca(2+) uniporter is a mitochondrial luminal redox sensor that augments MCU channel activity. *Mol. Cell* 65, 1014–1028. doi: 10.1016/j.molcel.2017.01.032

Dubuisson, J., Penin, F., and Moradpour, D. (2002). Interaction of hepatitis C virus proteins with host cell membranes and lipids. *Trends Cell Biol.* 12, 517–523. doi: 10.1016/S0962-8924(02)02383-8

Duchen, M. R. (2000). Mitochondria and Ca(2+)in cell physiology and pathophysiology. *Cell Calcium* 28, 339–348. doi: 10.1054/ceca.2000.0170

Elrod, J. W., and Molkentin, J. D. (2013). Physiologic functions of cyclophilin D and the mitochondrial permeability transition pore. *Circ. J.* 77, 1111–1122. doi: 10.1253/circj.CJ-13-0321

Fang, S., Su, J., Liang, B., Li, X., Li, Y., Jiang, J., et al. (2017). Suppression of autophagy by mycophenolic acid contributes to inhibition of HCV replication in human hepatoma cells. *Sci Rep.* 7:44039. doi: 10.1038/srep44039

Feissner, R. F., Skalska, J., Gaum, W. E., and Sheu, S. S. (2009). Crosstalk signaling between mitochondrial Ca^{2+} and ROS. *Front. Biosci.* 14, 1197–1218. doi: 10.2741/3303

Gallay, P. A., and Lin, K. (2013). Profile of alisporivir and its potential in the treatment of hepatitis C. *Drug. Des. Dev. Ther.* 7, 105–115. doi: 10.2147/DDDT.S30946

Ghafourifar, P., and Sen, C. K. (2007). Mitochondrial nitric oxide synthase. *Front. Biosci.* 12, 1072–1078. doi: 10.2741/2127

Giacomello, M., and Pellegrini, L. (2016). The coming of age of the mitochondria-ER contact: a matter of thickness. *Cell Death Differ.* 23, 1417–1427. doi: 10.1038/cdd.2016.52

Giorgi, C., Missiroli, S., Patergnani, S., Duszynski, J., Wieckowski, M. R., and Pinton, P. (2015). Mitochondria-associated membranes: composition, molecular mechanisms, and physiopathological implications. *Antioxid. Redox Signal.* 22, 995–1019. doi: 10.1089/ars.2014.6223

Giorgio, V., Guo, L., Bassot, C., Petronilli, V., and Bernardi, P. (2017). Calcium and regulation of the mitochondrial permeability transition. *Cell Calcium* 70, 56–63. doi: 10.1016/j.ceca.2017.05.004

Görlach, A., Bertram, K., Hudecova, S., and Krizanova, O. (2015). Calcium and ROS: a mutual interplay. *Redox Biol.* 6, 260–271. doi: 10.1016/j.redox.2015.08.010

Granatiero, V., De Stefani, D., and Rizzuto, R. (2017). Mitochondrial calcium handling in physiology and disease. *Adv. Exp. Med. Biol.* 982, 25–47. doi: 10.1007/978-3-319-55330-6_2

Griffin, S. D., Beales, L. P., Clarke, D. S., Worsfold, O., Evans, S. D., Jaeger, J., et al. (2003). The p7 protein of hepatitis C virus forms an ion channel that is blocked by the antiviral drug, Amantadine. *FEBS Lett.* 535, 34–38. doi: 10.1016/S0014-5793(02)03851-6

Griffin, S. D., Harvey, R., Clarke, D. S., Barclay, W. S., Harris, M., and Rowlands, D. J. (2004). A conserved basic loop in hepatitis C virus p7 protein is required for amantadine-sensitive ion channel activity in mammalian cells but is dispensable for localization to mitochondria. *J. Gen. Virol.* 85, 451–461. doi: 10.1099/vir.0.19634-0

Griffin, S., Clarke, D., McCormick, C., Rowlands, D., and Harris, M. (2005). Signal peptide cleavage and internal targeting signals direct the hepatitis C virus p7 protein to distinct intracellular membranes. *J. Virol.* 79, 15525–15536. doi: 10.1128/JVI.79.24.15525-15536.2005

Hamilton, S. L. (2005). Ryanodine receptors. *Cell Calcium* 38, 253–260. doi: 10.1016/j.ceca.2005.06.037

Hara, Y., Yanatori, I., Ikeda, M., Kiyokage, E., Nishina, S., Tomiyama, Y., et al. (2014). Hepatitis C virus core protein suppresses mitophagy by interacting with parkin in the context of mitochondrial depolarization. *Am. J. Pathol.* 184, 3026–3039. doi: 10.1016/j.ajpath.2014.07.024

Hardie, D. G. (1989). Regulation of fatty acid synthesis via phosphorylation of acetyl-CoA carboxylase. *Prog. Lipid Res.* 28, 117–146. doi: 10.1016/0163-7827(89)90010-6

Horner, S. M., Liu, H. M., Park, H. S., Briley, J., and Gale, M. Jr. (2011). Mitochondrial-associated endoplasmic reticulum membranes (MAM) form innate immune synapses and are targeted by hepatitis C virus. *Proc. Natl. Acad. Sci. U.S.A.* 108, 14590–14595. doi: 10.1073/pnas.1110133108

Huang, B. L., Gudi, R., Wu, P., Harris, R. A., Hamilton, J., and Popov, K. M. (1998). Isoenzymes of pyruvate dehydrogenase phosphatase — DNA-derived amino acid sequences, expression, and regulation. *J. Biol. Chem.* 273, 17680–17688. doi: 10.1074/jbc.273.28.17680

Jonas, E. A., Porter, G. A. Jr., Beutner, G., Mnatsakanyan, N., and Alavian, K. N. (2015). Cell death disguised: the mitochondrial permeability transition pore as the c-subunit of the F(1)F(O) ATP synthase. *Pharmacol. Res.* 99, 382–392. doi: 10.1016/j.phrs.2015.04.013

Kasprzak, A., Seidel, J., Biczysko, W., Wysocki, J., Spachacz, R., and Zabel, M. (2005). Intracellular localization of NS3 and C proteins in chronic hepatitis C. *Liver International* 25, 896–903. doi: 10.1111/j.1478-3231.2005.01109.x

Kim, K. H., Song, M. J., Yoo, E. J., Choe, S. S., Park, S. D., and Kim, J. B. (2004). Regulatory role of glycogen synthase kinase 3 for transcriptional activity of ADD1/SREBP1c. *J. Biol. Chem.* 279, 51999–52006. doi: 10.1074/jbc.M405522200

Kim, K.-H. (1997). Regulation of mammalian acetyl-coenzyme A carboxylase. *Annu. Rev. Nutr.* 17, 77–99. doi: 10.1146/annurev.nutr.17.1.77

Kim, S. J., Syed, G. H., and Siddiqui, A. (2013). Hepatitis C virus induces the mitochondrial translocation of Parkin and subsequent mitophagy. *PLoS Pathog.* 9:e1003285. doi: 10.1371/journal.ppat.1003285

Kim, S. J., Syed, G. H., Khan, M., Chiu, W. W., Sohail, M. A., Gish, R. G., et al. (2014). Hepatitis C virus triggers mitochondrial fission and attenuates apoptosis to promote viral persistence. *Proc. Natl. Acad. Sci. U.S.A.* 111, 6413–6418. doi: 10.1073/pnas.1321114111

Kroemer, G., Galluzzi, L., and Brenner, C. (2007). Mitochondrial membrane permeabilization in cell death. *Physiol Rev.* 87, 99–163. doi: 10.1152/physrev.00013.2006

Krols, M., Bultynck, G., and Janssens, S. (2016). ER-Mitochondria contact sites: a new regulator of cellular calcium flux comes into play. *J. Cell Biol.* 214, 367–370. doi: 10.1083/jcb.201607124

Land, S. C., and Tee, A. R. (2007). Hypoxia-inducible factor 1alpha is regulated by the mammalian target of rapamycin (mTOR) via an mTOR signaling motif. *J. Biol. Chem.* 282, 20534–20543. doi: 10.1074/jbc.M611782200

Li, X. D., Sun, L., Seth, R. B., Pineda, G., and Chen, Z. J. (2005). Hepatitis C virus protease NS3/4A cleaves mitochondrial antiviral signaling protein off the mitochondria to evade innate immunity. *Proc. Natl. Acad. Sci. U.S.A.* 102, 17717–17722. doi: 10.1073/pnas.0508531102

Madan, V., and Bartenschlager, R. (2015). Structural and functional properties of the hepatitis C virus p7 viroporin. *Viruses* 7, 4461–4481. doi: 10.3390/v7082826

Mannella, C. A., Buttle, K., Rath, B. K., and Marko, M. (1998). Electron microscopic tomography of rat-liver mitochondria and their interaction with the endoplasmic reticulum. *Biofactors* 8, 225–228. doi: 10.1002/biof.5520080309

Marchi, S., and Pinton, P. (2014). The mitochondrial calcium uniporter complex: molecular components, structure and physiopathological implications. *J. Physiol.* 592, 829–839. doi: 10.1113/jphysiol.2013.268235

Matlib, M. A., Zhou, Z., Knight, S., Ahmed, S., Choi, K. M., Krause-Bauer, J., et al. (1998). Oxygen-bridged dinuclear ruthenium amine complex specifically inhibits Ca^{2+} uptake into mitochondria *in vitro* and *in situ* in single cardiac myocytes. *J. Biol. Chem.* 273, 10223–10231. doi: 10.1074/jbc.273.17.10223

Meylan, E., Curran, J., Hofmann, K., Moradpour, D., Binder, M., Bartenschlager, R., et al. (2005). Cardif is an adaptor protein in the RIG-I antiviral pathway and is targeted by hepatitis C virus. *Nature* 437, 1167–1172. doi: 10.1038/nature04193

Mole, D. R., Maxwell, P. H., Pugh, C. W., and Ratcliffe, P. J. (2001). Regulation of HIF by the von Hippel-Lindau tumour suppressor: implications for cellular oxygen sensing. *IUBMB Life* 52, 43–47. doi: 10.1080/15216540252774757

Montserret, R., Saint, N., Vanbelle, C., Salvay, A. G., Simorre, J. P., Ebel, C., et al. (2010). NMR structure and ion channel activity of the p7 protein from hepatitis C virus. *J. Biol. Chem.* 285, 31446–31461. doi: 10.1074/jbc.M110.122895

Moradpour, D., and Penin, F. (2013). Hepatitis C virus proteins: from structure to function. *Curr Top. Microbiol. Immunol.* 369, 113–142. doi: 10.1007/978-3-642-27340-7_5

Moradpour, D., Evans, M. J., Gosert, R., Yuan, Z., Blum, H. E., Goff, S. P., et al. (2004). Insertion of green fluorescent protein into nonstructural protein 5A allows direct visualization of functional hepatitis C virus replication complexes. *J. Virol.* 78, 7400–7409. doi: 10.1128/JVI.78.14.7400-7409.2004

Moradpour, D., Kary, P., Rice, C. M., and Blum, H. E. (1998). Continuous human cell lines inducibly expressing hepatitis C virus structural and nonstructural proteins. *Hepatology* 28, 192–201. doi: 10.1002/hep.510280125

Moradpour, D., Penin, F., and Rice, C. M. (2007). Replication of hepatitis C virus. *Nat. Rev. Microbiol.* 5, 453–463. doi: 10.1038/nrmicro1645

Mottola, G., Cardinali, G., Ceccacci, A., Trozzi, C., Bartholomew, L., Torrisi, M. R., et al. (2002). Hepatitis C virus nonstructural proteins are localized in a modified endoplasmic reticulum of cells expressing viral subgenomic replicons. *Virology* 293, 31–43. doi: 10.1006/viro.2001.1229

Murphy, M. P. (2009). How mitochondria produce reactive oxygen species. *Biochem. J.* 417, 1–13. doi: 10.1042/BJ20081386

Nasimuzzaman, M., Waris, G., Mikolon, D., Stupack, D. G., and Siddiqui, A. (2007). Hepatitis C virus stabilizes hypoxia-inducible factor 1alpha and stimulates the synthesis of vascular endothelial growth factor. *J. Virol.* 81, 10249–10257. doi: 10.1128/JVI.00763-07

Nivala, M., Korge, P., Nivala, M., Weiss, J. N., and Qu, Z. (2011). Linking flickering to waves and whole-cell oscillations in a mitochondrial network model. *Biophys. J.* 101, 2102–2111. doi: 10.1016/j.bpj.2011.09.038

Nomura-Takigawa, Y., Nagano-Fujii, M., Deng, L., Kitazawa, S., Ishido, S., Sada, K., et al. (2006). Non-structural protein 4A of Hepatitis C virus accumulates on mitochondria and renders the cells prone to undergoing mitochondria-mediated apoptosis. *J. Gen. Virol.* 87, 1935–1945. doi: 10.1099/vir.0.81701-0

Paeshuyse, J., Kaul, A., De Clercq, E., Rosenwirth, B., Dumont, J. M., Scalfaro, P., et al. (2006). The non-immunosuppressive cyclosporin DEBIO-025 is a potent inhibitor of hepatitis C virus replication *in vitro*. *Hepatology* 43, 761–770. doi: 10.1002/hep.21102

Park, C. Y., Jun, H. J., Wakita, T., Cheong, J. H., and Hwang, S. B. (2009). Hepatitis C virus nonstructural 4B protein modulates sterol regulatory element-binding protein signaling via the AKT pathway. *J. Biol. Chem.* 284, 9237–9246. doi: 10.1074/jbc.M808773200

Pastorino, J. G., Hoek, J. B., and Shulga, N. (2005). Activation of glycogen synthase kinase 3beta disrupts the binding of hexokinase II to mitochondria by phosphorylating voltage-dependent anion channel and potentiates chemotherapy-induced cytotoxicity. *Cancer Res.* 65, 10545–10554. doi: 10.1158/0008-5472.CAN-05-1925

Patterson, R. L., Boehning, D., and Snyder, S. H. (2004). Inositol 1,4,5-trisphosphate receptors as signal integrators. *Annu. Rev. Biochem.* 73, 437–465. doi: 10.1146/annurev.biochem.73.071403.161303

Pawlotsky, J. M., Feld, J. J., Zeuzem, S., and Hoofnagle, J. H. (2015). From non-A, non-B hepatitis to hepatitis C virus cure. *J. Hepatol.* 62(1 Suppl.), S87–S99. doi: 10.1016/j.jhep.2015.02.006

Piccoli, C., Quarato, G., Ripoli, M., D'Aprile, A., Scrima, R., Cela, O., et al. (2009). HCV infection induces mitochondrial bioenergetics unbalance: causes and effects. *Biochim. Biophys. Acta* 1787, 539–546. doi: 10.1016/j.bbabio.2008.11.008

Piccoli, C., Scrima, R., D'Aprile, A., Ripoli, M., Lecce, L., Boffoli, D., et al. (2006). Mitochondrial dysfunction in hepatitis C virus infection. *Biochim. Biophys. Acta* 1757, 1429–1437. doi: 10.1016/j.bbabio.2006.05.018

Piccoli, C., Scrima, R., Quarato, G., D'Aprile, A., Ripoli, M., Lecce, L., et al. (2007). Hepatitis C virus protein expression causes calcium-mediated mitochondrial bioenergetic dysfunction and nitro-oxidative stress. *Hepatology* 46, 58–65. doi: 10.1002/hep.21679

Pugh, C. W. (2016). Modulation of the Hypoxic Response. *Adv. Exp. Med. Biol.* 903, 259–271. doi: 10.1007/978-1-4899-7678-9_18

Quarato, G., D'Aprile, A., Gavillet, B., Vuagniaux, G., Moradpour, D., Capitanio, N., et al. (2012). The cyclophilin inhibitor alisporivir prevents hepatitis C virus-mediated mitochondrial dysfunction. *Hepatology* 55, 1333–1343. doi: 10.1002/hep.25514

Quarato, G., Scrima, R., Agriesti, F., Moradpour, D., Capitanio, N., and Piccoli, C. (2013). Targeting mitochondria in the infection strategy of the hepatitis C virus. *Int. J. Biochem. Cell. Biol.* 45, 156–166. doi: 10.1016/j.biocel.2012.06.008

Quarato, G., Scrima, R., Ripoli, M., Agriesti, F., Moradpour, D., Capitanio, N., et al. (2014). Protective role of amantadine in mitochondrial dysfunction and oxidative stress mediated by hepatitis C virus protein expression. *Biochem. Pharmacol.* 89, 545–556. doi: 10.1016/j.bcp.2014.03.018

Raturi, A., and Simmen, T. (2013). Where the endoplasmic reticulum and the mitochondrion tie the knot: the mitochondria-associated membrane (MAM). *Biochim. Biophys. Acta* 1833, 213–224. doi: 10.1016/j.bbamcr.2012.04.013

Ripoli, M., D'Aprile, A., Quarato, G., Sarasin-Filipowicz, M., Gouttenoire, J., Scrima, R., et al. (2010). Hepatitis C virus-linked mitochondrial dysfunction promotes hypoxia-inducible factor 1 alpha-mediated glycolytic adaptation. *J. Virol.* 84, 647–660. doi: 10.1128/JVI.00769-09

Rizzuto, R., and Pozzan, T. (2006). Microdomains of intracellular Ca^{2+}: molecular determinants and functional consequences. *Physiol. Rev.* 86, 369–408. doi: 10.1152/physrev.00004.2005

Rizzuto, R., Pinton, P., Carrington, W., Fay, F. S., Fogarty, K. E., Lifshitz, L. M., et al. (1998). Close contacts with the endoplasmic reticulum as determinants of mitochondrial Ca^{2+} responses. *Science* 280, 1763–1766. doi: 10.1126/science.280.5370.1763

Roche, T. E., Baker, J. C., Yan, X., Hiromasa, Y., Gong, X., Peng, T., et al. (2001). Distinct regulatory properties of pyruvate dehydrogenase kinase and phosphatase isoforms. *Prog. Nucleic Acid Res. Mol. Biol.* 70, 33–75. doi: 10.1016/S0079-6603(01)70013-X

Rouillé, Y., Helle, F., Delgrange, D., Roingeard, P., Voisset, C., Blanchard, E., et al. (2006). Subcellular localization of hepatitis C virus structural proteins in a cell culture system that efficiently replicates the virus. *J. Virol.* 80, 2832–2841. doi: 10.1128/JVI.80.6.2832-2841.2006

Ruggieri, V., Mazzoccoli, C., Pazienza, V., Andriulli, A., Capitanio, N., and Piccoli, C. (2014). Hepatitis C virus, mitochondria and auto/mitophagy: exploiting a host defense mechanism. *World J. Gastroenterol.* 20, 2624–2633. doi: 10.3748/wjg.v20.i10.2624

Sarti, P., Arese, M., Forte, E., Giuffrè, A., and Mastronicola, D. (2012). Mitochondria and nitric oxide: chemistry and pathophysiology. *Adv. Exp. Med. Biol.* 942, 75–92. doi: 10.1007/978-94-007-2869-1_4

Schaller, T., Appel, N., Koutsoudakis, G., Kallis, S., Lohmann, V., Pietschmann, T., et al. (2007). Analysis of hepatitis C virus superinfection *exclusion by using nov*el fluorochrome gene-tagged viral genomes. *J. Virol.* 81, 4591–4603. doi: 10.1128/JVI.02144-06

Schindler, A., and Foley, E. (2013). Hexokinase 1 blocks apoptotic signals at the mitochondria. *Cell Signal.* 25, 2685–2692. doi: 10.1016/j.cellsig.2013.08.035

Schwer, B., Ren, S., Pietschmann, T., Kartenbeck, J., Kaehlcke, K., Bartenschlager, R., et al. (2004). Targeting of hepatitis C virus core protein to mitochondria through a novel C terminal localization motif. *J. Virol.* 78, 7958–7968. doi: 10.1128/JVI.78.15.7958-7968.2004

Semenza, G. L., Roth, P. H., Fang, H. M., and Wang, G. L. (1994). Transcriptional regulation of genes encoding glycolytic enzymes by hypoxia-inducible factor 1. *J. Biol. Chem.* 269, 23757–23763.

Seth, R. B., Sun, L., Ea, C. K., and Chen, Z. J. (2005). Identification and characterization of MAVS, a mitochondrial antiviral signaling protein that activates NF-kappaB and IRF 3. *Cell* 122, 669–682. doi: 10.1016/j.cell.2005.08.012

Shi, Q., Hoffman, B., and Liu, Q. (2016). PI3K-Akt signaling pathway upregulates hepatitis C virus RNA translation through the activation of SREBPs. *Virology* 490, 99–108. doi: 10.1016/j.virol.2016.01.012

Street, A., Macdonald, A., McCormick, C., and Harris, M. (2005). Hepatitis C virus NS5A-mediated activation of phosphoinositide 3-kinase results in stabilization of cellular beta-catenin and stimulation of beta-catenin-responsive transcription. *J. Virol.* 79, 5006–5016. doi: 10.1128/JVI.79.8.5006-5016.2005

Suzuki, R., Sakamoto, S., Tsutsumi, T., Rikimaru, A., Tanaka, K., Shimoike, T., et al. (2005). Molecular determinants for subcellular localization of hepatitis C virus core protein. *J. Virol.* 79, 1271–1281. doi: 10.1128/JVI.79.2.1271-1281.2005

Wakil, S. J., Stoops, J. K., and Joshi, V. C. (1983). Fatty acid synthesis and its regulation. *Annu. Rev. Biochem.* 52, 537–579. doi: 10.1146/annurev.bi.52.070183.002541

Wang, G. L., and Semenza, G. L. (1993). General involvement of hypoxia-inducible factor 1 in transcriptional response to hypoxia. *Proc. Natl. Acad. Sci. U.S.A.* 90, 4304–4308. doi: 10.1073/pnas.90.9.4304

Wang, G. L., Jiang, B.-H., Rue, E. A., and Semenza, G. L. (1995). Hypoxia-inducible factor 1 is a basic-helix-loop-helix-PAS heterodimer regulated by cellular O_2 tension. *Proc. Natl. Acad. Sci. U.S.A.* 92, 5510–5514. doi: 10.1073/pnas.92.12.5510

West, A. P., Shadel, G. S., and Ghosh, S. (2011). Mitochondria in innate immune responses. *Nat. Rev. Immunol.* 11, 389–402. doi: 10.1038/nri2975

Wilson, G. K., Brimacombe, C. L., Rowe, I. A., Reynolds, G. M., Fletcher, N. F., Stamataki, Z., et al. (2012). A dual role for hypoxia inducible factor-1α in the hepatitis C virus lifecycle and hepatoma migration. *J. Hepatol.* 56, 803–809. doi: 10.1016/j.jhep.2011.11.018

Wozniak, A. L., Griffin, S., Rowlands, D., Harris, M., Yi, M., Lemon, S. M., et al. (2010). Intracellular proton conductance of the hepatitis C virus p7 protein and itscontribution to infectious virus production. *PLoS Pathog.* 6:e1001087. doi: 10.1371/journal.ppat.1001087

Yecies, J. L., Zhang, H. H., Menon, S., Liu, S., Yecies, D., Lipovsky, A. I., et al. (2011). Akt stimulates hepatic SREBP1c and lipogenesis through parallel mTORC1-dependent and independent pathways. *Cell Metab.* 14, 21–32. doi: 10.1016/j.cmet.2011.06.002

Zimmermann, M., and Reichert, A. S. (2017). How to get rid of mitochondria: crosstalk and regulation of multiple mitophagy pathways. *Biol. Chem.* 399, 29–45. doi: 10.1515/hsz-2017-0206

13

Aquaporins as Targets of Dietary Bioactive Phytocompounds

Angela Tesse [1†], *Elena Grossini* [2†], *Grazia Tamma* [3], *Catherine Brenner* [4], *Piero Portincasa* [5], *Raul A. Marinelli* [6] *and Giuseppe Calamita* [3*]

[1] *Centre National de La Recherche Scientifique, Institut National de la Santé et de la Recherche Médicale, l'Institut du Thorax, Universitè de Nantes, Nantes, France,* [2] *Laboratory of Physiology, Department of Translational Medicine, University East Piedmont, Novara, Italy,* [3] *Department of Biosciences, Biotecnhologies and Biopharmaceutics, University of Bari "Aldo Moro", Bari, Italy,* [4] *Institut National de la Santé et de la Recherche Médicale UMR-S 1180-LabEx LERMIT, Université Paris-Sud, Université Paris-Saclay, Châtenay Malabry, France,* [5] *Clinica Medica "A. Murri", Department of Biomedical Sciences and Human Oncology, Medical School, University of Bari "Aldo Moro", Bari, Italy,* [6] *Instituto de Fisiología Experimental, CONICET, Facultad de Ciencias Bioquímicas y Farmacéuticas, Universidad Nacional de Rosario, Rosario, Argentina*

Correspondence:
Giuseppe Calamita
giuseppe.calamita@uniba.it

† These authors have contributed equally to this work.

Plant-derived bioactive compounds have protective role for plants but may also modulate several physiological processes of plant consumers. In the last years, a wide spectrum of phytochemicals have been found to be beneficial to health interacting with molecular signaling pathways underlying critical functions such as cell growth and differentiation, apoptosis, autophagy, inflammation, redox balance, cell volume regulation, metabolic homeostasis, and energy balance. Hence, a large number of biologically active phytocompounds of foods have been isolated, characterized, and eventually modified representing a natural source of novel molecules to prevent, delay or cure several human diseases. Aquaporins (AQPs), a family of membrane channel proteins involved in many body functions, are emerging among the targets of bioactive phytochemicals in imparting their beneficial actions. Here, we provide a comprehensive review of this fast growing topic focusing especially on what it is known on the modulatory effects played by several edible plant and herbal compounds on AQPs, both in health and disease. Phytochemical modulation of AQP expression may provide new medical treatment options to improve the prognosis of several diseases.

Keywords: aquaporin membrane channels, functional foods, nutraceutics, epigenetics, gut microbiota, antioxidants, anti-inflammatory, chronic diseases

INTRODUCTION

Growing evidence from epidemiological, *in vivo*, *in vitro*, and clinical trial results indicate that the plant-based food can reduce or prevent the risk of chronic diseases such as cardiovascular disease, arterial hypertension, diabetes mellitus, and cancer due to presence of biologically active plant compounds or phytochemicals. Several classes of phytochemicals from edible plants and herbs exist (Steinmetz and Potter, 1991) and exert beneficial effects in disease prevention and in reducing the incidence of certain chronic diseases. The mechanisms modulate the cell signaling pathways underlying inflammation, oxidative stress, metabolic disorder, apoptosis, and so forth (Maraldi et al., 2014).

This review provides an update on the involvement of Aquaporins (AQPs), a family of membrane channel proteins with important role in many body functions, in the beneficial effects imparted by food polyphenols and herbal phytocompounds, both in health and disease.

AQUAPORINS, A FAMILY OF MEMBRANE CHANNELS WIDELY DISTRIBUTED IN HUMAN TISSUES

Aquaporins (AQPs) are channel proteins largely expressed in living organisms mediating the transport of water and some anaelectrolytes across biological membranes (Agre, 2004). The 13 AQPs (AQP0-12) expressed in mammals are summarily grouped into *orthodox aquaporins* (AQP0, AQP1, AQP2, AQP4, AQP5, AQP6, and AQP8) and *aquaglyceroporins* (AQP3, AQP7, AQP9, AQP10), depending on their ability to conduct only water or water and neutral solutes, particularly glycerol, respectively (**Figure 1**). AQP11 and AQP12 are often grouped as *unorthodox aquaporins* due to their distinct evolutionary pathway and transport properties (Ishibashi et al., 2009). Some AQPs are also able to conduct ammonia (AQP3, AQP4, AQP6, AQP8, and AQP9) and/or hydrogen peroxide (AQP1, AQP3, AQP5, AQP8, and AQP9) and, for these biophysical properties, are also denoted as *ammoniaporins* (or *aquaammoniaporins*) (Jahn et al., 2004) and/or *peroxiporins* (Geyer et al., 2013; Almasalmeh et al., 2014; Rodrigues et al., 2016; Watanabe et al., 2016) (**Figure 2**). Moreover, some AQPs also allow permeation of gases of physiological importance such as CO_2, NO or O_2 (Nakhoul et al., 1998; Herrera et al., 2006; Wang et al., 2007). Expression, transport properties (Agre, 2004), and pharmacological gating (Soveral and Casini, 2017) of AQPs are object of strong interest and intense investigation in all body districts and a number of important roles have been already described, both in health and clinical disorders.

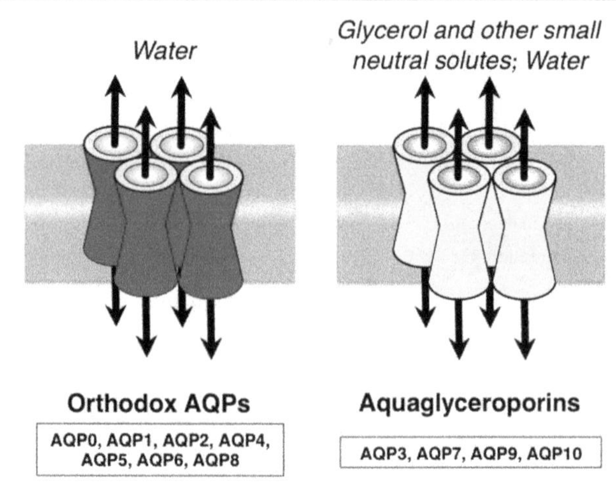

FIGURE 1 | Mammalian aquaporins are grossly subdivided in *orthodox aquaporins* (AQP0, AQP1, AQP2, AQP4, AQP5, AQP6, and AQP8) and *aquaglyceroporins* (AQP3, AQP7, AQP9, and AQP10) depending on their ability to conduct only water or glycerol and some other small neutral solutes, in addition to water, respectively. Two of the 13 AQPs found in mammals, AQP11 and AQP12, are called *unorthodox aquaporins* as they show marked distinctions in terms of evolutionary pathway. Some AQPs also express conductance to gases of physiological relevance.

DIETARY POLYPHENOLS AND AQUAPORINS

The class of polyphenols is characterized by the presence of phenol units in their chemical structure. Polyphenols are the largest group of phytochemicals, and many of them exist in edible plants (Maraldi et al., 2014). Foods enriched in polyphenols were found to exert a wide spectrum of protective effects (i.e., hypolipidemic, anti-oxidative, anti-proliferative, anti-apoptotic, and anti-inflammatory) with the benefit of reducing the prognosis and onset of disease progression (for review see Upadhyay and Dixit, 2015). So far, more than 8,000 phenolic structures have been identified in vegetables, fruits, olive oil, and wine. Due to their diversity and food distribution the latest classification subdivides polyphenols in phenolic acids, curcuminoids, flavonoids, chalcones, stilbenes, lignans, and isoflavonoids (González-Castejón and Rodriguez-Casado, 2011; Upadhyay and Dixit, 2015). Bioactive polyphenols also influence the expression and biophysical properties of mammalian AQPs (Zhang et al., 2014; Fiorentini et al., 2015; Cataldo et al., 2017). The AQPs modulated by polyphenols and related health benefits are summarized in **Table 1**.

Curcuminoids

Curcuminoids (or curcumins) are characterized by a pronounced yellow color composed of linear diarylheptanoids. They are represented by curcumin and its derivatives (i.e., demethoxycurcumin and bisdemethoxycurcumin). Curcuminoids have been tested in particular for their anti-oxidant activity.

Curcumin is a non-flavonoid polyphenol isolated from spice turmeric, and known for playing anti-inflammatory, antioxidant, anti-proliferative, and anti-angiogenic activities (Tsao, 2010). The beneficial effects of curcumin on human health, however, are

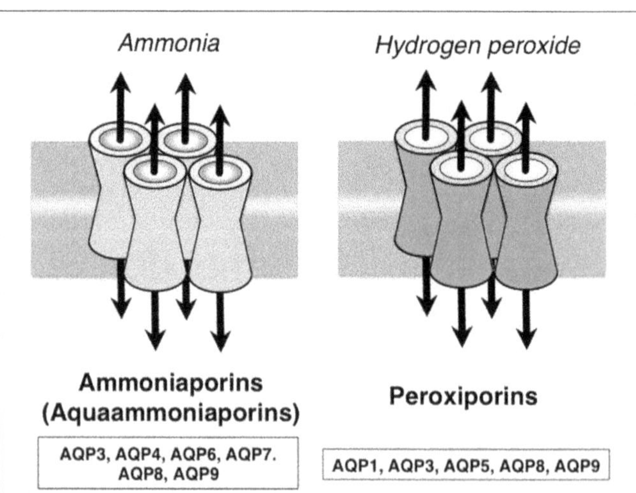

FIGURE 2 | Some AQPs also allow transport of ammonia (AQP3, AQP4, AQP6, AQP7, AQP8, and AQP9), particularly AQP8, and/or hydrogen peroxide (AQP1, AQP3, AQP5, AQP8, and AQP9) and are called *ammoniaporins* (or *aquaammoniaporins*) and *peroxiporins*, respectively.

TABLE 1 | Polyphenolic modulation of AQPs and related beneficial effects.

Polyphenol	Functional derivative	Modulated AQP	Beneficial effect	References
Curcuminoids	Curcumin	Choroid plexus AQP1 ↓ (brain lateral ventricle)	Reduction of intracranial pressure in brain injury (rat model)	Nabiuni et al., 2013
		CaOV3 AQP3 ↓ (ovarian cancer cell line)	Inhibition of ovarian cancer cell migration (*in vitro*)	Ji et al., 2008; Terlikowska et al., 2014
		Brain AQP4 and AQP9 ↓	Reduction of brain edema (rodent model)	Yu et al., 2012; Zhang et al., 2014; Zu et al., 2014; Wang et al., 2015
		HeLa cells AQP (ND)	Hydrogen peroxide elimination (*in vitro*)	Pellavio et al., 2017
Flavonoids	Pinocembrin	Brain AQP4 ↓	Reduction of cerebral edema due to ischemia (rat model)	Gao et al., 2010
	Chrysin	Skin AQP3 ↑	Protection against UV-induced skin damages (*in vitro*)	Wu et al., 2011
	Quercetin	Microglial AQP4 ↓	Amelioration of diabetic retinal edema (rat model)	Kumar et al., 2014
		Salivary gland, lung AQP5 ↑	Amelioration of impaired salivation after irradiation and IAV-induced lung injury (mouse models)	Takahashi et al., 2015; Yu et al., 2016a
		HeLa cells AQP1, AQP3, AQP8, AQP11	Hydrogen peroxide elimination (*in vitro*)	Pellavio et al., 2017
	Hesperetin	Microglial AQP4 ↓	Amelioration of diabetic retinal edema (rat model)	Kumar et al., 2014
	Alpinetin	Lung endothelium AQP1 ↑	Amelioration of SAP-induced acute lung injury (*in vitro*)	Liang et al., 2016
	Naringenin	Mucosal epithelial cells of colon AQP3 ↑	Amelioration of intestinal water absorption	Yin et al., 2018
		HeLa cells AQP(ND)	Hydrogen peroxide elimination (*in vitro*)	Pellavio et al., 2017
	Liquiritigenin	Kidney AQP4 ↓	Reduction of kidney inflammation (rat model)	Hongyan et al., 2016
	Epigallocathechin Gallate	Salivary gland AQP5 ↑	Amelioration of xerostomia in Sjögren syndrome (mouse model)	Saito et al., 2015
		SKOV3 AQP5 ↓ (cancer cell line)	Inhibition of ovarian tumor growth (*in vitro*)	Yan et al., 2012
		Spinal cord AQP4 ↓	Reduced edema in acute SCI (rat model)	Ge et al., 2013
Chalcones	Phloretin	AQP9 (inhibition)	Anti-inflammatory and anti-oxidative action (*in vitro*)	Matsushima et al., 2014
Stilbenes	Resveratrol	Human keratinocyte AQP3 ↓	Inhibition of keratinocyte proliferation (*in vitro*)	Wu et al., 2014
		Brain AQP4 ↓	Amelioration of cerebral I/R injury (rat model)	Li et al., 2015
Isoflavonoids	Genistein and Daidzein	Uterine AQP1 ↑	Uterine responsiveness to estrogens (rat model)	Möller et al., 2010
	Puerarin	Brain AQP4 ↓	Reduction of brain damage and inflammation	Wang et al., 2018

Arrows: ↑, upregulation; ↓, downregulation; SCI, spinal cord injury; ND, specific AQP homolog to be defined.

downplayed by its poor absorption and bioavailability (Anand et al., 2007). Liposomal curcumin or curcumin nanoparticles have increased bioavailability, while structural analogs of curcumin such as EF-24 feature higher stability and faster absorption (Santiago-Vázquez et al., 2016). EF-24 has been demonstrated effective against cancer (Yang et al., 2014; Santiago-Vázquez et al., 2016), Parkinson's (PD), and Alzheimer's (AD) diseases (Pal et al., 2011).

The central nervous system expresses various AQPs (Badaut et al., 2014) and studies using rodent brain have suggested important roles for AQP1, AQP4, and AQP9 in controlling water transport and volume homeostasis (Badaut et al., 2014). AQP1 is highly expressed in choroid plexus, a secretory epithelium which plays a role in cerebrospinal fluid (CSF) formation and secretion (Nabiuni et al., 2013). After brain injury, mice deficient for AQP1 displayed a decreased intracranial pressure and improved survival compared to wild type mice (Oshio et al., 2005). This strongly suggests that AQP1 downregulation might be protective against several neurological disorders characterized by increased intracranial pressure. Notably, curcumin decreases, in a dose-dependent manner, the AQP1 level in choroidal epithelial cells isolated from the lateral ventricle of Wistar rats (Nabiuni et al., 2013). Curcumin could also act inhibiting choroid plexus AQP1 since in a study using Hela cells this phytocompound has been recently suggested to have a direct gating action on some AQPs (Pellavio et al., 2017). AQP4, the most characterized brain water channel, is located mainly on astrocytic endfeets that are in strict contact with blood vessels (Badaut et al., 2014). Curcumin counteracts the brain edema and the effect might include the modulation of the expression of various AQPs, especially AQP4. Indeed, current medical and surgical therapies available for the treatment of intracerebral hemorrhage (ICH) do not adequately control brain edema. Interestingly, curcumin dose-dependently reduced both the gene expression and protein abundance of AQP4 and AQP9 but not those of AQP1 in a mouse model of ICH (Wang et al., 2015). Likely, the protective effects of curcumin may also involve the downregulation of specific water channels.

In a rat model of hypoxic-ischemic brain injury, curcumin significantly reduced the brain edema, and the effect was associated with a relevant morphological amelioration of the damage at the blood-brain barrier, increase of NOS activity and AQP4 expression (Yu et al., 2012). Similarly, in a rat model of hypoxia-hypercapnia, curcumin injection attenuated brain edema and restored the levels of AQP4 expression (Yu et al., 2016b). In the mice model of traumatic brain injury, pre- or post-treatment with curcumin reduced the cerebral edema, the pericontusional expression of IL-1β, and reversed the induction of AQP4 (Zhang et al., 2014). The beneficial effect of curcumin was also observed in an animal model of SCI (impaired motor function and spinal cord edema); curcumin counteracted the abnormal activation of JAK/STAT signaling pathways and reduced the glial fibrillary acidic protein (GFAP) and AQP4 overexpression (Zu et al., 2014). While most available data highlight the beneficial effects of curcumin in neurologic diseases, curcumin could aggravate some CNS manifestations in experimental lupus erythematous. Indeed, curcumin treatment was associated with increased cerebral water content and AQP4 expression in mice with systemic lupus erythematous, likely depending on worsened cerebral atrophy and astrocytosis (Foxley et al., 2013). All together the above-mentioned results suggest that AQP4 is the main target through which curcumin would exert its action on brain edema and SCI.

In cultured human ovarian CaOV3 cells, stimulation with the endothelial growth factor (EGF) promoted AQP3 expression and CaOV3 cell migration. AQP3 knocking down by siRNA was associated with significant impairment of CaOV3 cell migration. Also in this context, curcumin (or a stable analog) proposed for therapeutic treatment of ovarian cancer (Terlikowska et al., 2014), downregulated AQP3 and reduced cell migration in CaOV3, an effect mediated by inhibition of EGFR signaling (Ji et al., 2008).

As shown for quercetin and naringenin (see below), in HeLa cells curcumin elicited antioxidant effects by reducing the hydrogen peroxide cellular content, probably by decreasing its entry into the cell through AQPs-mediated mechanisms (Pellavio et al., 2017). Modulation of AQPs by curcumin in cancer cells resulting in elimination of hydrogen peroxide may not always result beneficial to health when considering that accumulation of hydrogen peroxide (among other ROS) is a mechanism by which a number of conventional anti-cancer treatments govern cancer cells to death.

Curcumin could also influence various physiological functions through interactions with different ion channels and transporters involving several signaling pathways, from the well-known CFTR to voltage-gated potassium channels, volume-regulated anion channel (VRAC), Ca^{2+} release-activated Ca^{2+} channel (CRAC), and glucose transporters (Zhang et al., 2014). More research is needed in this respect, to better highlight the role of curcumin as modulator of various channel functions and pointing to its protective effects in various disease. Moreover, the use of curcumin could be useful also for research purposes since it could help the understanding of the interplay between AQPs system and other membrane transporters (Zhang et al., 2014).

Flavonoids

Flavonoids are the biggest representative subgroup of polyphenols, with more than 4,000 molecules described (Harborne and Williams, 2000; Cheynier, 2005).

Pinocembrin is a natural flavonoid compound, which has been isolated from several plants, such as ginger roots and wild marjoram, honey, and propolis (Massaro et al., 2014; Lan et al., 2016). Pinocembrin exerts pleiotropic effects: reduces reactive oxygen species (ROS) production, apoptosis, and controls mitochondrial functions (Massaro et al., 2014). *In vitro* evidence revealed that pinocembrin can cross the blood-brain-barrier passively indicating possible therapeutic use in nervous system diseases (Yang et al., 2012). In an animal model of focal cerebral ischemia induced by middle cerebral artery occlusion (MCAO), several inflammatory cytokines, tumor necrosis factor-α (TNF-α), and interleukin-1β (IL-1β), inducible nitric synthase (iNOS) and AQP4 were significantly upregulated in the ischemic brain (Gao et al., 2010). Administration of pinocembrin *via* tail vein injection ameliorated the neuronal apoptosis and the edema as well as the typical alterations of endothelial cells and capillaries characterizing ischemia. Pinocembrin treatment decreased the production of cytokines and the expression iNOS and AQP4. These findings suggest that the protective response triggered by the flavonoid might be due to reduced inflammatory signals and decreased level of AQP4, which has been associated with edema subsequent to cerebral ischemia (Gao et al., 2010).

Chrysin is a natural flavonoid occurring in honey and propolis, various fruits, vegetables and mushrooms (Nabavi et al., 2015). Chrysin displays fundamental biological anticancer actions reducing cell proliferation and promoting apoptosis, especially in leukemia cells (Monasterio et al., 2004). In animal studies, UVB and UVA radiation induced skin dehydration and this step was associated with decrease of the expression level of AQP3, one of the main skin AQPs. Other changes included ROS release and apoptosis (Wu et al., 2011). Topical application of chrysin improved the UV-induced skin damage, and significantly increased keratinocyte AQP3, suggesting a chrysin-mediated protection of the deleterious effects exerted by UVs on human skin.

Quercetin is one of the most abundant bioflavonoids in the human diet. It is largely present in different vegetables including onions and broccoli, fruits such as apples, berry crops, and grapes. Quercetin is also found in some herbs, tea, and wine. Similarly to other polyphenols, quercetin displays pleiotropic properties as antioxidant and anti-inflammatory compound. Plant extract of quercetin is the principal ingredient of many potential anti-allergic drugs, supplements, and enriched products, being highly competent in inhibiting IL-8 action, suppressing IL-6 and intracellular calcium level increase (Mlcek et al., 2016). Retinas from streptozotocin-induced diabetic rats showed a remarkable increase of pro-inflammatory cytokines such as TNF-α and IL-1β and a considerable augmentation of AQP4 level, which could mediate the movement of water underlying the retinal edema (Kumar et al., 2014). Changes were accompanied with a significant reduction of retinal glutathione (GSH) and antioxidant enzymes [superoxide dismutase (SOD) and catalase (CAT)]. Oral administration of quercetin leads to an important neuroprotective effect which was characterized by impaired inflammatory cytokines production and release, restoration of GSH, SOD, and CAT levels and significant reduction of AQP4 in Müller cell endfeet and perivascular space with consequent decrease of the edema affecting the retina of diabetic rats. The observed amelioration of retinal edema was suggested as due to quercetin-dependent AQP4 downregulation on Müller cell endfeet and perivascular space. Another orthodox AQP water channel, AQP5, was found to be involved in the beneficial action of quercetin in attenuating the damaged salivary secretion induced in a murine model of impaired salivation by radiation exposure (Takahashi et al., 2015). Quercetin upregulated AQP5 expression and calcium uptake and suppressed the oxidative stress and inflammatory responses induced by the radiation exposure. Increased AQP5 levels were also observed in a mouse model of influenza A virus (IAV)-induced lung injury where AQP5 lung increased after treatment with flavonoid extracts from the Lamiaceae plant *Mosla scabra* (Yu et al., 2016a). The lung AQP5 modulation by the flavonoid was interpreted as a way to restore the normal water permeability alleviating the IAV-induced pulmonary inflammation and apoptosis.

AQP3, 5, 8, and 9 have been reported to facilitate the transmembrane diffusion of hydrogen peroxide in mammalian cells (Almasalmeh et al., 2014; Rodrigues et al., 2016; Watanabe et al., 2016). This is an important aspect since cellular oxidative stress can interfere with water permeability. In HeLa cells, the role of AQPs as target of antioxidant compounds acting on the osmotic water diffusion in the presence of oxidative stress condition has recently been studied (Pellavio et al., 2017). Quercetin appeared to modulate water transport and acted as antioxidant by increasing the expression of AQP3 and AQP8 (together with that of AQP1 and AQP11) at both mRNA and protein level. Particularly, with quercetin, the water permeability decrease caused by oxidative stress was prevented or restored. Furthermore, quercetin significantly reduced the hydrogen peroxide content to levels even lower than those of control cells. Thus, regulation of AQPs gating by antioxidant compounds like quercetin could represent a novel mechanism to modulate exogenously cell signaling and survival during stress, acting on key signaling pathways in cancer and degenerative diseases (see Tamma et al., 2018 for a review).

Hesperetin is a flavanone isolated from several fruits and highly expressed in the *Citrus* species. This flavonoid has different biological properties, including antioxidant, anti-inflammatory, and anticancer effects (Ahmadi et al., 2015; Bodduluru et al., 2015). Its beneficial actions have been showed in different organs including liver, heart, and kidney (Roohbakhsh et al., 2015; Miler et al., 2016). Neuroprotective effects have also been reported, in particular in the treatment of diabetic retinopathy where inflammation, oxidative stress, and neurovascular disorders are involved. Streptozotocin-induced diabetic rats receiving hesperetin for 24 weeks showed restoration of retinal levels of GSH associated to a positive modulation of antioxidant enzyme activities. An inhibition of caspase-3 activity and expression of GFAP was also seen along with reduced inflammatory cytokines (Kumar et al., 2013). Treatment with hesperetin was accompanied by downregulation of AQP4 at Müller cell endfeet and consequent reduction of the edematous state indicating modulation of AQP-associated water permeability.

Alpinetin is a flavanone isolated from the seed of *Alpinia katsumadai* (Zingiberaceae). The compound is widely used in Korean traditional medicine (Lee et al., 2012). Alpinetin has been found to control cell signaling pathways at the base of cell growth, proliferation, and apoptosis (Wang et al., 2013). Alpinetin also causes vasorelaxation (Wang et al., 2001) and counteracts the hydrogen peroxide-induced vascular smooth muscle cell proliferation and migration (Li and Du, 2004). In lipopolysaccharide (LPS)-induced lung injury, alpinetin prevented the LPS-induced TNF-α, IL-6, and IL-1β release and alleviated the inflammatory associated lung hystopathological alterations (Hou et al., 2009). Considerable AQP1 downregulation, a condition negatively correlated with pulmonary edema, has been described in acute lung injury (ALI) and, associated with severe acute pancreatitis (SAP). Interestingly, alpinetin has been found to inhibit TNF-α expression, promote human pulmonary microvascular endothelial cell proliferation and increase the expression level of AQP1 thereby improving the SAP-induced ALI symptoms (Liang et al., 2016). Overall, these findings propose alpinetin as possible therapeutical tool against lung inflammation diseases.

Naringenin is a natural flavonoid widely found in citrus fruits and tomatoes, that has been reported to act as anti-inflammatory, anti-atherogenic, anti-mutagenic, hepatoprotective, and anticancer agent (Yin et al., 2018). Naringenin relieved the loperamide-induced constipation by targeting AQP3. It is known that AQPs are primarily expressed in the mucosal epithelial cells in the colon, in which AQP3 plays a central role in water reabsorption across colonic surface cells. Yin et al. found that naringenin increased the mRNA and protein expression levels of AQP3 in the colon, both in apical and lateral mucosal epithelial cells. Furthermore, a positive correlation was observed between this increase in the AQP3 level and the increase in fecal water content (Yin et al., 2018). As also shown for quercetin, the antioxidant effects elicited by naringenin in HeLa cells have been recently related to its capacity to facilitate hydrogen peroxide elimination through AQPs. These observations would strengthen the role of AQPs as physiologic modulators of hydrogen peroxide diffusion in mammalian cells (Pellavio et al., 2017).

Liquiritigenin belongs to the chiral flavanone family and is an important compound extracted from *Glycyrrhiza uralensis* and found in a variety of plants, including *Glycyrrhiza glabra* (licorice). Liquiritigenin possesses kinds of healthy properties including antioxidation, anti-inflammation, antidiabetes, cardioprotection, and neuroprotection (Hosseinzadeh and Nassiri-Asl, 2015). As regarding the mechanisms, the inhibition of NF-κB and MAPK signaling pathways would be at basis of its antioxidant effects. Liquiritigenin has been shown to exhibit renal protective effects in the animal model of potassium oxonate-induced hyperuricemia, as well, by targeting the AQPs (Hongyan et al., 2016). AQP4 would play an important role in inflammatory responses involving the kidney, also by the regulation of endoplasmic reticulum stress. In the hyperuricemic rat, liquiritigenin has been able to suppress the activation of renal AQP4/NF-κB/IκBα signaling and nod-like receptor protein 3 (NLRP3) inflammasome, resulting in renal inflammation reduction. These findings would suggest that liquiritigenin could act as a potential drug for the treatment of hyperuricemia and renal injury by targeting the AQPs system.

Epigallocatechin gallate (EGCG) is a flavonol esterified with gallic acid mainly found in the green tea *Camellia sinensis* L. EGCG accounts for more than 50% of total green tea polyphenols. This phenolic compound and/or its metabolites exert cardioprotection, neuroprotection, renal protection, osteoprotection, and anticancer actions. Beneficial effects have also been shown in diseases with metabolic disorders such as obesity, metabolic syndrome and type 2 diabetes (Afzal et al., 2015). At a molecular level, EGCG promotes the expression and the activity of several anti-oxidant and anti-inflammatory enzymes. EGCG is also proved to counteract the activation of Toll-like receptor 4 (TLR4) (Marinovic et al., 2015) and nuclear factor-κB (NF-κB) (Albuquerque et al., 2016), pathways associated with the production of inflammatory cytokines. In a mouse model of Sjögren syndrome, treatment with EGCG increased the abundance of AQP5 at the apical plasma membrane of the acinar cells. AQP5 expression resulted upregulated by mechanisms leading to protein kinase A (PKA) activation and NF-κB inhibition (Saito et al., 2015). Conversely, by means of other pathways, EGCG was found to downregulate the expression of AQP5 in the ovarian cancer cell line SKOV3. The lower abundance of AQP5 was suggested to counteract the tumor growth through NF-κB activation (Yan et al., 2012). Considerable decrease of the spinal cord water content was seen in a work employing a rat model of acute SCI where EGCG was administered immediately following the injury (Ge et al., 2013). The anti-edema action exerted by EGCG was ascribed to the marked reduction of spinal cord AQP4 induced by the EGCG administration.

Chalcones

Chalcones are a variety of aromatic ketones, precursors of flavonoids, and isoflavonoids. They are abundant in edible plants and their derivatives have been reported to have an extremely wide variety of biological activities (i.e., anti-bacterial, anti-fungal, anti-neoplastic, anti-inflammatory, anti-diabetic, anti-obesity, immunosuppressant actions) depending on the substitution made on them (Mahapatra et al., 2015).

Phloridzin, one of the most characterized bioactive chalcones, is also a competitive inhibitor of the isoforms 1 and 2 of the sodium glucose cotransporter (SGLT1 and SGLT2, respectively) as it competes with D-glucose in binding the carrier. This action leads to a decrease in glucose absorption and reabsorption by the small intestine and renal proximal tubules, respectively, lowering the glucose level in the blood. However, phloridzin is not an effective drug because when orally consumed, it is nearly entirely converted into phloretin and glucose by hydrolytic enzymes in the small intestine.

Phloretin, an abundant chalcone in apples, is a protective agent with anti-oxidative stress and anti-inflammatory actions (Aliomrani et al., 2016). Phloretin is also known for gating the aquaglyceroporins by inhibiting the AQP-mediated transport of glycerol and urea (Tsukaguchi et al., 1999; Calamita et al., 2008, 2012; Rodriguez et al., 2014), a metabolic intermediate substrate of gluconeogenesis and triacylglycerols (TAG) synthesis (Calamita et al., 2012), and a variety of urea transporters and urea-conducting AQPs such as AQP3, AQP7, and AQP9 (Shayakul et al., 2001; Fenton et al., 2004). AQP9-facilitated urea extrusion out of liver was evoked to explain the loss of urea and diuresis that characterizes mice submitted to high protein diet. This function played by liver AQP9 can be blocked by phloretin (Jelen et al., 2012). It is tempting to think that the anti-inflammatory action exerted by phloretin may also involve the inhibition of AQP9, an AQP that has been suggested to play a role in inflammation (Matsushima et al., 2014).

Stilbenes

Stilbenes belong to the family of phenylpropanoids and are better known as stilbenoids, their hydroxylated derivatives. The most studied stilbenoid is resveratrol, a compound having numerous health benefits.

Trans-resveratrol is a natural hydroxystilbene found in a variety of edible plants including grapes, blueberry, raspberry, and senna leaves. Research on the biological actions of resveratrol on human health has focused on cancer, neurodegenerative, and cardiovascular diseases, and metabolic disorders. At molecular level, resveratrol plays pleiotropic effects including inhibition of kinases, anti-inflammatory, analgesic and anti-cancer activities, and detoxification, by inhibiting the aryl hydrocarbon and dioxin receptor (AhR), (de Medina et al., 2005). AhR stimulation causes oxidative stress, inflammation, apoptosis and immunosuppression, and is associated with an increased risk of osteoporosis, cancers and metabolic disorders such as diabetes (Zollner et al., 2010). As a polyphenol, resveratrol can also act as tyrosine kinases inhibitor and as a modulator of the mitogen activated protein kinase/extracellular signal-regulated kinase 1/2 (MEK-ERK1/2), mitogen-activated protein kinases (MAPK), activator protein 1 (AP-1), and NF-κB pathways in different tissues (Yu et al., 2001; Gao et al., 2004; Kundu et al., 2004). Resveratrol has been reported to influence the gene expression of various AQPs (see Cataldo et al., 2017 for a review). In human keratinocytes, AQP3 has been found to play a pivotal role in skin hydration, although overexpression of AQP3 is also linked with hyperplastic epidermal disorders (Nakahigashi et al., 2011). In normal human epidermal keratinocytes (NHEKs), treatment with resveratrol reduced cell proliferation and the expression of AQP3, the major skin AQP. Particularly, AQP3 downregulation appeared to be secondary to ERK signaling inhibition via upregulation of both Sirtuin 1 (SIRT1) and aryl hydrocarbon receptor AhR (Wu et al., 2014). These novel findings may be important to drug design and development against hyperproliferative skin disorders.

Cerebral ischemia-reperfusion (I/R) is associated with a strong increase of ROS production and brain edema. Resveratrol exerts a beneficial action by modulating the activity of SOD and reducing the iNOS and AQP4 expression levels (Li et al., 2015). More recently, functionalized AQP4 antibody nanoparticles were synthesized to deliver resveratrol in rat optic nerve transection. These engineering nanoparticles displayed high efficacy in reducing oxidative damage and AQP4 immunoreactivity thus preserving the visual function (Lozić et al., 2016).

Isoflavonoids

The isoflavonoids genistein and daidzein are important components of *Leguminosae.* Based on their chemical structure they function as phytoestrogens displaying anti-tumor features. These phytocompounds play an important role in modulating the genes involved in controlling cell-cycle progression.

Genistein and *daidzein* are considered the "sharp edge of balance" between cell survival and cell progression because they control the activation or the inhibition of pivotal signal molecules such as NF-κB. Importantly, they also play a role in reversion of epigenetic events associated with prostate cancer (Adjakly et al., 2013). The bioavailability of these compounds is strongly influenced by gut microbiota, antibiotic administration and individual's age and health status (Franke et al., 2014). A work addressing the effects of lifelong dietary isoflavone on estrogen sensitive tissues was carried out studying the effects of genistein and daidzein on rat uterus (Möller et al., 2010). The effect of genistein either alone or in association with daidzein was compared to that of isoflavone-free diet in rats throughout their whole lifetime. The dietary isoflavone pre-exposure resulted in a much stronger uterine weight increase following external ERα-mediated estrogenic stimuli than that seen in the phytoestrogen-free group. Gene expression analysis showed that the uterine levels of AQP1, and, at a lesser extent, those of AQP3, AQP5, and AQP9, were increased by ovary estrogens. This modulation was considerably influenced by the isoflavone-containing diets, likely by an epigenetic mechanism. Lifelong dietary isoflavone ingestion was suggested to increase the uterine responsiveness to ERα-mediated estrogenic stimuli in female rats where the water homeostasis was highly affected whereas the proliferation rate remained unchanged.

Puerarin is a flavonoid glycoside that is extracted from the root of the leguminous plants *Pueraria lobata* and Thomson Kudzuvine Root. Puerarin displays a series of beneficial activities on hangover, cardiovascular disease, osteoporosis, neurological dysfunction (ischemic stroke, cerebrovascular disease) fever, and liver injury both in clinical treatment and experimental research (Wang et al., 2018). In addition to inhibit inflammation, protective effects elicited by puerarin against cerebral damage would be related to modulation of AQP4 function. Hence, AQP4, which can be mainly found in the primate and rodent perivascular astrocyte end feet, would play a role not only in water movement, but also, as previously reported, in neuroinflammation and brain edema. AQP4 expression would be increased by pro-inflammatory factors like TNF-α. Furthermore, increased phosphorylation of MAPK (p38, ERK1/2, c-Jun N-terminal kinase 1/2) would participate in AQP4 regulation in astrocytes exposed to the inflammatory cytokines released by microglia under the condition of hypoxia, too. Various interventions have been performed to prevent or to treat people rapidly ascending to high altitude. Currently, traditional Chinese medicine has been used to prevent or treat symptoms although the specific mechanisms are still a matter of debate. In rats undergone hypobaric hypoxia, puerarin was able to elicit protective effects against cerebral edema by inhibiting the increase of AQP4 through inhibition of TNF-α release and by counteracting the activation of NF-κB and MAPK pathway (Wang et al., 2018).

CAPSAICINOIDS

Capsaicin is the most representative compound of a group of phytochemicals called capsaicinoids also including dihydrocapsaicin, nordihydrocapsaicin, and some other compounds such capsinoids. In chili peppers, capsaicin, a phenolic amide, gives the sensation of spiciness by acting through the transient receptor potential vanilloid-1 (TRPV1). TRPV1 is a non-selective permeable cation channel expressed in brain, bladder, kidneys, intestines, keratinocytes of epidermis, glial cells, liver, and polymorphonuclear granulocytes, mast cells, and macrophages (Reyes-Escogido Mde et al., 2011). In tumor cells, capsaicin inhibits cell growth and promotes apoptosis by increasing the intracellular calcium concentration and ROS levels, disrupting mitochondrial membrane transition potential and activating NF-κβ transcription factor (Chapa-Oliver and Mejia-Teniente, 2016). In addition, capsaicin stimulates the phosphorylation of p53 at serine-15 and its acetylation through downregulation of SIRT1. Altogether, these posttranslational modifications lead to apoptosis (Ito et al., 2004). Similarly to anti-obesity, anti-diabetic, and anti-inflammatory compounds, capsaicin plays multiple roles in nociceptive heat sensation. Capsaicin can activate sympathetic system to induce brown adipose tissue thermogenesis (Saito, 2015).

Capsaicin upregulated TRPV1 and AQP5 in rabbit salivary glands (**Table 2**). Specifically, in transplanted rabbit submandibular gland cells, capsaicin upregulated and stimulated the translocation of AQP5 from an intracellular pool to the plasma membrane via TRPV1 signaling and ERK phosphorylation (Ding et al., 2010; Zhang et al., 2010). This finding may provide a new therapeutic tool to stimulate submandibular gland hypofunction.

TERPENES

Terpenes are a large and diverse class of organic compounds derived biosynthetically from units of isoprene. They are produced by a variety of plants and even some insects. Terpenoids are compounds related to terpenes characterized by an isoprenoid chemical structure as they may include some oxygen functionality or some rearrangement. Terpenoids are present in a great variety of fruits, vegetables and medicinal plants, representing the largest and most diverse class of chemicals among the myriad of compounds produced by plants. Terpenoids are used extensively for their aromatic qualities and play a role in traditional herbal remedies. The terms terpenes and terpenoids are often used interchangeably. As many other bioactive phytocompounds, terpenes, and terpenoids have been reported to influence the expression of AQPs (**Table 2**).

Monoterpenoids

Carvacrol (or cymophenol) is a monoterpenoid extracted from many plants of the *Lamiaceae* family. Carvacrol has been reported to exert neuroprotective effects in central nervous system diseases such as AD and cerebral ischemia (Zhong et al., 2013). Modulation of brain AQP4 was reported in a preclinical study employing a bacterial collagenase-induced ICH murine model to address the effect of the monoterpenoid on cerebral edema after ICH. Administration of carvacrol improved the neurological deficits following ICH by significantly reducing cerebral edema and AQP4 in perihematomal area (Zhong et al., 2013). It was suggested that carvacrol exerts its protective effect on ICH injury by ameliorating AQP4-mediated cerebral edema.

Marrubiin (MARR) is a terpenoid abundantly found in many Lamiaceae species (i.e., *Marrubium vulgare, Plomis bracteosa, Leonotis nepetifolia*). MARR is a compound featuring high stability and limited catabolism, two properties favoring its bioavailability: MARR is reported to exert cardioprotective, vasorelaxant, gastroprotective, and antidiabetic effects (Popoola et al., 2013). Antioxidant action involving AQPs has been reported in a recent work where pre- or post-treatment of heat-stressed HeLa cells with MARR prevented or reversed, respectively, the intracellular H_2O_2 accumulation induced by the heat (Pellavio et al., 2017).

Triterpenes

Bacopasides are triterpene saponins isolated from the medicinal plant *Bacopa monnieri*. Recently, two structurally related bacopaside compounds, bacopaside I and bacopaside II, have been shown to block differentially the transport activity of AQP1, a finding that fitted with predictions made by *in silico* molecular modeling (Pei et al., 2016). When tested in migration assays using HT29 and SW480 cells, two colon cancer cell lines characterized by high and low expression levels of AQP1, respectively, both bacopasides impaired migration of HT29 cells showing minimal effect on migration of SW480 cells. Based on these results bacopasides were suggested as possible novel lead compounds for pharmaceutical development of selective AQPs blockers in cancer treatment.

The triterpenoid *18β-glycyrrhetinic acid* (β-GA) is a natural compound derived from *Glycyrrhiza glabra* (licorice) root shown to exert antiviral, antitumor and immunosuppressive effects. Studies using rat models of nasal mucosa of allergic rhinitis (AR) showed that intranasal administration of β-GA downregulates AQP1 together with that of eotaxin 1 (CCL11) and eosinophil (EOS) in nasal mucosa of allergic rhinitis rats and cast effects on inhibiting the progress of AR (Li et al., 2015).

Glycyrrhizic acid, a triterpenoid also known as glycyrrhizin, is the main sweet-tasting constituent of licorice root. Based on its inhibiting effect on liver cell injury glycyrrhizin is used for the treatment of chronic viral hepatitis and cirrhosis (van Rossum et al., 1998). Glycyrrhizin is also employed to prevent disease progression in subjects with acute onset autoimmune hepatitis (Yasui et al., 2011). Enoxolone, the aglycone of the glycyrrhizic acid, is used to prevent liver carcinogenesis in patients with chronic hepatitis C. Glycyrrhizin was reported to influence the renal functions by modulating AQP2 and AQP3, two AQPs expressed in the principal cells of the renal distal tubules and collecting ducts where they mediate the antidiuretic hormone (ADH)-induced water reabsorption (Kang et al., 2003). Using a rat model of gentamicin-induced acute renal failure the protective effects of glycyrrhizin downregulated AQP2 in the inner and outer renal medulla, and cortex (Sohn et al., 2003) suggesting that this triterpenoid involves renal AQPs in its beneficial action on renal function.

Ginsenoside Rgl (Rgl) is a triterpenoid saponin known as one of the main compounds harvested from ginseng with pharmaceutical action and potential neuroprotective properties, empirically used in traditional Chinese medicine to treat stroke (Xie et al., 2015). A study using a rat model of cerebral ischemia/reperfusion showed that the neuroprotective effect of Rgl against blood-brain-barrier disruption involves downregulation of brain AQP4 expression (Zhou et al., 2014).

Ginsenoside Rg3 (Rg3), a triterpene saponin, is one of the bioactive extracts contained in ginseng root. Rg3 has been shown to have anticancer activity in various cancer models. Thus, in the highly metastatic prostate cancer cell line PC-3M, treatment with Rg3 was found to lead to a remarkable inhibition of cell migration. In particular, exposure of PC-3M cells to Rg3 suppressed the expression of AQP1, an AQP with a role in cell migration. The anti-metastatic effect of Rg3 was found to occur through the p38 MAPK pathway and some transcription factors acting on the *Aqp1* gene promoter (Pan et al., 2012).

TABLE 2 | Modulation of AQPs by non-polyphenolic phytocompounds and related beneficial effects.

Phytochemical	Functional derivative	Modulated AQP	Beneficial effect	References
Capsaicinoids	Capsaicin	Submandibular salivary gland AQP5 ↑	Amelioration of submandibular salivary gland hypofunction (rabbit model)	Ding et al., 2010; Zhang et al., 2010
Monoterpenoids	Carvacrol	Brain AQP4 ↓	Reduction of ICH-induced brain edema (mouse model)	Zhong et al., 2013
	Marrubin	HeLa cells AQP(ND)	Hydrogen peroxide elimination (*in vitro*)	Pellavio et al., 2017
Triterpenes	Bacopasides I and II	AQP1 (inhibition)	Reduction of cancer cell migration (*in vitro*)	Pei et al., 2016
	18β-glycyrrhetinic acid (β-GA)	Nasal mucosa AQP1 ↓	Treatment against allergic rhinitis (rat model)	Li et al., 2015
	Glycyrrhizic acid	Renal AQP2 ↓	Protection against renal failure (rat model)	Sohn et al., 2003
	Ginsenoside Rg1	Brain AQP4 ↓	Protection against brain ischemia (rat model)	Zhou et al., 2014
	Ginsenodise Rg3	AQP1 ↓	Anti-metastatic effect (*in vitro*)	Pan et al., 2012
Isothiocyanates	Sulphoraphane	AQP4 ↑	Reduction of brain edema (rat model)	Zhao et al., 2005
Tetrahydroanthracene	(R)-Aloesaponol III 8 methyl ether	HeLa cells AQP(ND)	Hydrogen peroxide elimination (*in vitro*)	Pellavio et al., 2017

Arrows: ↑, upregulation; ↓, downregulation; ND, specific AQP homolog to be defined.

SULPHORAPHANE

Sulphoraphane (SUL) is a chemical belonging to isothiocyanates, a group of organosulfur compounds. SUL was identified in broccoli sprouts, which, of the cruciferous vegetables have the highest concentration of this compound (Zhang et al., 1992). Among the reported beneficial effects sulforaphane appears to be a promising phytochemical with neuroprotective properties (Tarozzi et al., 2013).

Using a rodent controlled cortical impact injury model of traumatic brain edema it was observed that post-injury administration of SUL counteracted AQP4 loss in the contusion core and further increased the protein levels of this water channel in the penumbra region compared with injured animals receiving vehicle. This increase in AQP4 expression was accompanied by a significant amelioration of cerebral edema (Zhao et al., 2005). It was suggested that the reduction of the edema in response to SUL administration could be ascribed to water clearance through AQP4 from the injured brain.

TETRAHYDROANTHRACENES

Tetrahydroanthracenes are polycyclic aromatic phytocompounds deriving from the phytochemical hydrogenation of anthracene in *Liliaceae*. This reaction is influenced by light exposition in roots of *Aloe* plants and tetrahydroanthracenes are markers of subterranean anthranoid metabolism. These molecules are used mainly to treat parasitic infections with potential anti-oxidant properties because of their chemical structure.

*(**R**)-Aloesaponol III 8-methyl ether.* The (**R**)-Aloesaponol III 8-methyl ether (ASME) was extracted for the first time from *Eremurus persicus* root but it is contained in other plants such as *Aloe saponaria, Kniphonia foliosa, Eremurus chinensis,* and others. ASME is a tetrahydroanthracene known for having biological activity against *Leishmania* infection. Like the terpenoid MARR, ASME improved the HeLa cells membrane permeability by restoring the AQP-mediated cellular extrusion of H_2O_2 contributing to the reduction in oxidative stress (Pellavio et al., 2017). However, further work is needed to better investigate this preliminary observation since the specific AQP channel responsible for the ASME-induced efflux of H_2O_2 out of the cells is still elusive.

BIOACTIVE EXTRACTS

The beneficial effects of a number of plants are likely due to their original composition and the synergistic action played by the different bioactive phytochemicals they contain rather than to a unique active compound. Here, we review bioactive extracts from plants whose healthy effects have been reported to involve modulation of AQPs (**Table 3**).

Heliotropium indicum is a plant belonging to family of *Boraginaceae* used in folk medicine in many countries. In Ghana, extracts of *H. indicum* are employed as a remedy against cataract formation without any scientific evidence. The

TABLE 3 | Modulation of AQPs by bioactive extracts and related beneficial effects.

Bioactive extract	Modulated AQP	Beneficial effect	References
Extracts of *Heliotropium indicum*	Eye AQP0 ↑	Alleviation of cataract (rat model)	Kyei et al., 2015
Extracts of aged garlic (S-allylmercapto-l-cysteine)	SPC-A1 cell line AQP5 ↑	Anti-inflammatory properties in COPD	Yang et al., 2016
Extracts of Chinese herbs (Isotetrandrine)	Eye AQP4	Amelioration of auto-immune disorders in NMO	Sun et al., 2016

Arrow: ↑, upregulation.

extract of this plant contains an original composition showing numerous bioactive compounds with antibacterial, antitumor, anti-inflammatory and diuretic activities. In a rat model of selenite-induced cataract development, the aqueous total extract of *H. indicum* significantly alleviated cataract at all dose levels tested (0.1–3.0 mg/ml) preserving AQP0, an AQP highly expressed in fiber cells of lenses, and other markers of lens transparency proteins (Kyei et al., 2015).

Garlic has shown versatile therapeutic action in the prevention and treatment of pathologies such as chronic obstructive pulmonary disease (COPD). However, the specific garlic bioactive component underlying this medicinal activity remains elusive. Viscous COPD mucus secretions have been explained also due to a down-regulation to which AQP5, an AQP water channel highly expressed in lungs, undergoes. Interestingly, *S-allylmercapto-l-cysteine* (SAMC), one of the bioactive phytochemicals found in aged garlic, improved the LPS-induced mucus secretion of a COPD cell model, the human airway submucosal gland cell line (SPC-A1), up-regulating AQP5 and mucin 5AC (MUC5AC) *via* NF-κB signaling pathway (Yang et al., 2016).

Isotetrandrine is a biscoclaurine alkaloid, a bioactive compound isolated from traditional Chinese herbs known for reducing the astrocyte cytotoxicity in the neurological autoimmune disorder such as neuromyelitis optica (NMO). This phytochemical was reported to be a small molecule inhibitor of NMO-IgG binding to AQP4 without impairing the expression and water channel activity of AQP4 (Sun et al., 2016).

CONCLUSIONS AND FUTURE PERSPECTIVES

Foods are enriched with myriads of bioactive phytocompounds, and research on their effects on human health is a quickly growing field. The recent recognition that AQPs are among the targets of food phytochemicals paves the way to potentially novel therapeutic options dealing with prognosis and cure of highly prevalent diseases (i.e., metabolic disorders, cancer, neurological diseases, and inflammatory chronic diseases). While the molecular mechanisms by which phytocompounds modulate the expression or gating (i.e., by phloretin, curcumin, and bacopaside II) of AQPs remains to be fully ascertained, there are no doubts that the list of functional food ingredients and herbal phytochemicals influencing AQPs is far from complete. Studies are also warranted to confirm in humans the results that have been obtained *in vitro* or with the use of rodent models also taking into account the gender dimorphism that may exist in terms of AQP expression and localization (Rodríguez et al., 2015). It should also be considered that bioactive phytocompounds are often not active *per se*, while their metabolites are. Thus, new and potentially important translational acquisitions are anticipated in the near future, in this exciting field.

AUTHOR CONTRIBUTIONS

AT and EG contributed to article design, bibliographic search, writing, illustrations, and critical discussion. GT contributed to writing and bibliographic enrichment. CB provided critical discussion; PP contributed to writing and provided critical discussion; RM contributed to article design and writing, and provided critical discussion; GC designed and wrote the first draft of the article and contributed to article refinement, illustrations, bibliographic enrichment, and critical discussion. All authors approved the final version for submission.

REFERENCES

Adjakly, M., Ngollo, M., Boiteux, J. P., Bignon, Y. J., Guy, L., and Bernard-Gallon, D. (2013). Genistein and daidzein: different molecular effects on prostate cancer. *Anticancer Res.* 33, 39–44.

Afzal, M., Safer, A. M., and Menon, M. (2015). Green tea polyphenols and their potential role in health and disease. *Inflammopharmacology* 23, 151–161. doi: 10.1007/s10787-015-0236-1

Agre, P. (2004). Nobel Lecture. Aquaporin water channels. *Biosci. Rep.* 24, 127–163. doi: 10.1007/s10540-005-2577-2

Ahmadi, A., Shadboorestan, A., Nabavi, S. F., Setzer, W. N., and Nabavi, S. M. (2015). The role of hesperidin in cell signal transduction pathway for the prevention or treatment of cancer. *Curr. Med. Chem.* 22, 3462–3471. doi: 10.2174/092986732230151019103810

Albuquerque, K. F., Marinovic, M. P., Morandi, A. C., Bolin, A. P., and Otton, R. (2016). Green tea polyphenol extract *in vivo* attenuates inflammatory features of neutrophils from obese rats. *Eur. J. Nutr.* 55, 1261–1274. doi: 10.1007/s00394-015-0940-z

Aliomrani, M., Sepand, M. R., Mirzaei, H. R., Kazemi, A. R., Nekonam, S., and Sabzevari, O. (2016). Effects of phloretin on oxidative and inflammatory reaction in rat model of cecal ligation and puncture induced sepsis. *Daru* 24:15. doi: 10.1186/s40199-016-0154-9

Almasalmeh, A., Krenc, D., Wu, B., and Beitz, E. (2014). Structural determinants of the hydrogen peroxide permeability of aquaporins. *FEBS J.* 281, 647–656. doi: 10.1111/febs.12653

Anand, P., Kunnumakkara, A. B., Newman, R. A., and Aggarwal, B. B. (2007). Bioavailability of curcumin: problems and promises. *Mol. Pharm.* 4, 807–818. doi: 10.1021/mp700113r

Badaut, J., Fukuda, A. M., Jullienne, A., and Petry, K. G. (2014). Aquaporin and brain diseases. *Biochim. Biophys. Acta* 1840, 1554–1565. doi: 10.1016/j.bbagen.2013.10.032

Bodduluru, L. N., Kasala, E. R., Barua, C. C., Karnam, K. C., Dahiya, V., and Ellutla, M. (2015). Antiproliferative and antioxidant potential of hesperetin against benzo(a)pyrene-induced lung carcinogenesis in Swiss albino mice. *Chem. Biol. Interact.* 242, 345–352. doi: 10.1016/j.cbi.2015.10.020

Calamita, G., Ferri, D., Gena, P., Carreras, F. I., Liquori, G. E., Portincasa, P., et al. (2008). Altered expression and distribution of aquaporin-9 in the liver of rat with obstructive extrahepatic cholestasis. *Am. J. Physiol. Gastrointest. Liver Physiol.* 295, G682–G690. doi: 10.1152/ajpgi.90226.2008

Calamita, G., Gena, P., Ferri, D., Rosito, A., Rojek, A., Nielsen, S., et al. (2012). Biophysical assessment of aquaporin-9 as principal facilitative pathway in mouse liver import of glucogenetic glycerol. *Biol. Cell* 104, 342–351. doi: 10.1111/boc.201100061

Cataldo, I., Maggio, A., Gena, P., de Bari, O., Tamma, G., Portincasa, P., et al. (2017). Modulation of aquaporins by dietary patterns and plant bioactive compounds. *Curr. Med. Chem.* doi: 10.2174/0929867324666170523123010. [Epub ahead of print].

Chapa-Oliver, A. M., and Mejía-Teniente, L. (2016). Capsaicin: from plants to a cancer-suppressing agent. *Molecules* 21:e931. doi: 10.3390/molecules21080931

Cheynier, V. (2005). Polyphenols in foods are more complex than often thought. *Am. J. Clin. Nutr.* 81, 223S–229S. doi: 10.1093/ajcn/81.1.223S

de Medina, P., Casper, R., Savouret, J. F., and Poirot, M. (2005). Synthesis and biological properties of new stilbene derivatives of resveratrol as new selective aryl hydrocarbon modulators. *J. Med. Chem.* 48, 287–291. doi: 10.1021/jm0498194

Ding, Q. W., Zhang, Y., Wang, Y., Wang, Y. N., Zhang, L., Ding, C., et al. (2010). Functional vanilloid receptor-1 in human submandibular glands. *J. Dent. Res.* 89, 711–716. doi: 10.1177/0022034510366841

Fenton, R. A., Chou, C. L., Stewart, G. S., Smith, C. P., and Knepper, M. A. (2004). Urinary concentrating defect in mice with selective deletion of phloretin-sensitive urea transporters in the renal collecting duct. *Proc. Natl. Acad. Sci. U.S.A.* 101, 7469–7474. doi: 10.1073/pnas.0401704101

Fiorentini, D., Zambonin, L., Dalla Sega, F. V., and Hrelia, S. (2015). Polyphenols as modulators of aquaporin family in health and disease. *Oxid. Med. Cell. Longev.* 2015:196914. doi: 10.1155/2015/196914

Foxley, S., Zamora, M., Hack, B., Alexander, R. R., Roman, B., Quigg, R. J., et al. (2013). Curcumin aggravates CNS pathology in experimental systemic lupus erythematosus. *Brain Res.* 1504, 85–96. doi: 10.1016/j.brainres.2013.01.040

Franke, A. A., Lai, J. F., and Halm, B. M. (2014). Absorption, distribution, metabolism, and excretion of isoflavonoids after soy intake. *Arch. Biochem. Biophys.* 559, 24–28. doi: 10.1016/j.abb.2014.06.007

Gao, M., Zhu, S. Y., Tan, C. B., Xu, B., Zhang, W. C., and Du, G. H. (2010). Pinocembrin protects the neurovascular unit by reducing inflammation and extracellular proteolysis in MCAO rats. *J. Asian Nat. Prod. Res.* 12, 407–418. doi: 10.1080/10286020.2010.485129

Gao, S., Liu, G. Z., and Wang, Z. (2004). Modulation of androgen receptor-dependent transcription by resveratrol and genistein in prostate cancer cells. *Prostate* 59, 214–225. doi: 10.1002/pros.10375

Ge, R., Zhu, Y., Diao, Y., Tao, L., Yuan, W., and Xiong, X. C. (2013). Anti-edema effect of epigallocatechin gallate on spinal cord injury in rats. *Brain Res.* 1527, 40–46. doi: 10.1016/j.brainres.2013.06.009

Geyer, R. R., Musa-Aziz, R., Qin, X., and Boron, W. F., (2013). Relative CO(2)/NH(3) selectivities of mammalian aquaporins 0-9. *Am. J. Physiol. Cell Physiol.* 304, C985–C994. doi: 10.1152/ajpcell.00033.2013

González-Castejón, M., and Rodriguez-Casado, A. (2011). Dietary phytochemicals and their potential effects on obesity: a review. *Pharmacol. Res.* 64, 438–455. doi: 10.1016/j.phrs.2011.07.004

Harborne, J. B., and Williams, C. A. (2000). Advances in flavonoid research since 1992. *Phytochemistry* 55, 481–504. doi: 10.1016/S0031-9422(00)00235-1

Herrera, M., Hong, N. J., and Garvin, J. L. (2006). Aquaporin-1 transports NO across cell membranes. *Hypertension* 48, 157–164. doi: 10.1161/01.HYP.0000223652.29338.77

Hongyan, L., Suling, W., Weina, Z., Yajie, Z., and Jie, R. (2016). Antihyperuricemic effect of liquiritigenin in potassium oxonate-induced hyperuricemic rats. *Biomed. Pharmacother.* 84, 1930–1936. doi: 10.1016/j.biopha.2016.11.009

Hosseinzadeh, H., and Nassiri-Asl, M. (2015). Pharmacological effects of *Glycyrrhiza* spp. and its bioactive constituents: update and review. *Phytother. Res.* 29, 1868–1886. doi: 10.1002/ptr.5487

Hou, J. C., Min, L., and Pessin, J. E. (2009). Insulin granule biogenesis, trafficking and exocytosis. *Vitam. Horm.* 80, 473–506. doi: 10.1016/S0083-6729(08)00616-X

Ishibashi, K., Koike, S., Kondo, S., Hara, S., and Tanaka, Y. (2009). The role of a group III AQP, AQP11 in intracellular organelle homeostasis. *J. Med. Invest.* 56(Suppl.), 312–317. doi: 10.2152/jmi.56.312

Ito, K., Nakazato, T., Yamato, K., Miyakawa, Y., Yamada, T., Hozumi, N., et al. (2004). Induction of apoptosis in leukemic cells by homovanillic acid derivative, capsaicin, through oxidative stress: implication of phosphorylation of p53 at Ser-15 residue by reactive oxygen species. *Cancer Res.* 64, 1071–1078. doi: 10.1158/0008-5472.CAN-03-1670

Jahn, T. P., Møller, A. L., Zeuthen, T., Holm, L. M., Klaerke, D. A., Mohsin, B., et al. (2004). Aquaporin homologues in plants and mammals transport ammonia. *FEBS Lett.* 574, 31–36. doi: 10.1016/j.febslet.2004.08.004

Jelen, S., Gena, P., Lebeck, J., Rojek, A., Praetorius, J., Frøkiaer, J., et al. (2012). Aquaporin-9 and urea transporter-A gene deletions affect urea transmembrane passage in murine hepatocytes. *Am. J. Physiol. Gastrointest. Liver Physiol.* 303, G1279–1287. doi: 10.1152/ajpgi.00153.2012

Ji, C., Cao, C., Lu, S., Kivlin, R., Amaral, A., Kouttab, N., et al. (2008). Curcumin attenuates EGF-induced AQP3 up-regulation and cell migration in human ovarian cancer cells. *Cancer Chemother. Pharmacol.* 62, 857–865. doi: 10.1007/s00280-007-0674-6

Kang, D. G., Sohn, E. J., and Lee, H. S. (2003). Effects of glycyrrhizin on renal functions in association with the regulation of water channels. *Am. J. Chin. Med.* 31, 403–413. doi: 10.1142/S0192415X03001089

Kumar, B., Gupta, S. K., Nag, T. C., Srivastava, S., Saxena, R., Jha, K. A., et al. (2014). Retinal neuroprotective effects of quercetin in streptozotocin-induced diabetic rats. *Exp. Eye Res.* 125, 193–202. doi: 10.1016/j.exer.2014.06.009

Kumar, B., Gupta, S. K., Srinivasan, B. P., Nag, T. C., Srivastava, S., Saxena, R., et al. (2013). Hesperetin rescues retinal oxidative stress, neuroinflammation and apoptosis in diabetic rats. *Microvasc. Res.* 87, 65–74. doi: 10.1016/j.mvr.2013.01.002

Kundu, J. K., Chun, K. S., Kim, S. O., and Surh, Y. J. (2004). Resveratrol inhibits phorbol ester-induced cyclooxygenase-2 expression in mouse skin: MAPKs and AP-1 as potential molecular targets. *Biofactors* 21, 33–39. doi: 10.1002/biof.552210108

Kyei, S., Koffuor, G. A., Ramkissoon, P., Afari, C., and Asiamah, E. A. (2015). The claim of anti-cataract potential of *Heliotropium indicum*: a myth or reality? *Ophthalmol. Ther.* 4, 115–128. doi: 10.1007/s40123-015-0042-2

Lan, X., Wang, W., Li, Q., and Wang, J. (2016). The natural flavonoid pinocembrin: molecular targets and potential therapeutic applications. *Mol. Neurobiol.* 53, 1794–1801. doi: 10.1007/s12035-015-9125-2

Lee, M. Y., Seo, C. S., Lee, J. A., Shin, I. S., Kim, S. J., Ha, H., et al. (2012). *Alpinia katsumadai* H(AYATA) seed extract inhibit LPS-induced inflammation by induction of heme oxygenase-1 in RAW264.7 cells. *Inflammation* 35, 746–757. doi: 10.1007/s10753-011-9370-0

Li, W., Tan, C., Liu, Y., Liu, X., Wang, X., Gui, Y., et al. (2015). Resveratrol ameliorates oxidative stress and inhibits aquaporin 4 expression following rat cerebral ischemia-reperfusion injury. *Mol. Med. Rep.* 12, 7756–7762. doi: 10.3892/mmr.2015.4366

Li, Y. J., and Du, G. H. (2004). Effects of alpinetin on rat vascular smooth muscle cells. *J. Asian Nat. Prod. Res.* 6, 87–92. doi: 10.1080/1028602031000135558

Liang, X., Zhang, B., Chen, Q., Zhang, J., Lei, B., Li, B., et al. (2016). The mechanism underlying alpinetin-mediated alleviation of pancreatitis-associated lung injury through upregulating aquaporin-1. *Drug Des. Devel. Ther.* 10, 841–850. doi: 10.2147/DDDT.S97614

Lozić, I., Hartz, R. V., Bartlett, C. A., Shaw, J. A., Archer, M., Naidu, P. S., et al. (2016). Enabling dual cellular destinations of polymeric nanoparticles for treatment following partial injury to the central nervous system. *Biomaterials* 74, 200–216. doi: 10.1016/j.biomaterials.2015.10.001

Mahapatra, D. K., Asati, V., and Bharti, S. K. (2015). Chalcones and their therapeutic targets for the management of diabetes: structural and pharmacological perspectives. *Eur. J. Med. Chem.* 92, 839–865. doi: 10.1016/j.ejmech.2015.01.051

Maraldi, T., Vauzour, D., and Angeloni, C. (2014). Dietary polyphenols and their effects on cell biochemistry and pathophysiology. *Oxid. Med. Cell. Longev.* 2014:576363. doi: 10.1155/2014/576363

Marinovic, M. P., Morandi, A. C., and Otton, R. (2015). Green tea catechins alone or in combination alter functional parameters of human neutrophils via suppressing the activation of TLR-4/NFkappaB p65 signal pathway. *Toxicol. In Vitro* 29, 1766–1778. doi: 10.1016/j.tiv.2015.07.014

Massaro, C. F., Katouli, M., Grkovic, T., Vu, H., Quinn, R. J., Heard, T. A., et al. (2014). Anti-staphylococcal activity of C-methyl flavanones from propolis of Australian stingless bees (*Tetragonula carbonaria*) and fruit resins of *Corymbia torelliana* (*Myrtaceae*). *Fitoterapia* 95, 247–257. doi: 10.1016/j.fitote.2014.03.024

Matsushima, A., Ogura, H., Koh, T., Shimazu, T., and Sugimoto, H. (2014). Enhanced expression of aquaporin 9 in activated polymorphonuclear leukocytes in patients with systemic inflammatory response syndrome. *Shock* 42, 322–326. doi: 10.1097/SHK.0000000000000218

Miler, M., Živanović, J., AjdŽanović, V., Orešcanin-Dušić, Z., Milenković, D., Konić-Ristić, A., et al. (2016). Citrus flavanones naringenin and hesperetin improve antioxidant status and membrane lipid compositions in the liver of old-aged Wistar rats. *Exp. Gerontol.* 84, 49–60. doi: 10.1016/j.exger.2016.08.014

Mlcek, J., Jurikova, T., Skrovankova, S., and Sochor, J. (2016). Quercetin and its anti-allergic immune response. *Molecules* 21:e623. doi: 10.3390/molecules21050623

Möller, F. J., Diel, P., Zierau, O., Hertrampf, T., Maass, J., and Vollmer, G. (2010). Long-term dietary isoflavone exposure enhances estrogen sensitivity of rat uterine responsiveness mediated through estrogen receptor alpha. *Toxicol. Lett.* 196, 142–153. doi: 10.1016/j.toxlet.2010.03.1117

Monasterio, A., Urdaci, M. C., Pinchuk, I. V., López-Moratalla, N., and Martinez-Irujo, J. J. (2004). Flavonoids induce apoptosis in human leukemia U937 cells through caspase- and caspase-calpain-dependent pathways. *Nutr. Cancer* 50, 90–100. doi: 10.1207/s15327914nc5001_12

Nabavi, S. F., Braidy, N., Habtemariam, S., Orhan, I. E., Daglia, M., Manayi, A., et al. (2015). Neuroprotective effects of chrysin: from chemistry to medicine. *Neurochem. Int.* 90, 224–231. doi: 10.1016/j.neuint.2015.09.006

Nabiuni, M., Nazari, Z., Safaeinejad, Z., Delfan, B., and Miyan, J. A. (2013). Curcumin downregulates aquaporin-1 expression in cultured rat choroid plexus cells. *J. Med. Food* 16, 504–510. doi: 10.1089/jmf.2012.0208

Nakahigashi, K., Kabashima, K., Ikoma, A., Verkman, A. S., Miyachi, Y., and Hara-Chikuma, M. (2011). Upregulation of aquaporin-3 is involved in keratinocyte proliferation and epidermal hyperplasia. *J. Invest. Dermatol.* 131, 865–873. doi: 10.1038/jid.2010.395

Nakhoul, N. L., Davis, B. A., Romero, M. F., and Boron, W. F. (1998). Effect of expressing the water channel aquaporin-1 on the CO_2 permeability of Xenopus oocytes. *Am. J. Physiol.* 274, C543–C548. doi: 10.1152/ajpcell.1998.274.2.C543

Oshio, K., Watanabe, H., Song, Y., Verkman, A. S., and Manley, G. T. (2005). Reduced cerebrospinal fluid production and intracranial pressure in mice lacking choroid plexus water channel aquaporin-1. *FASEB J.* 19, 76–78. doi: 10.1096/fj.04-1711fje

Pal, R., Miranda, M., and Narayan, M. (2011). Nitrosative stress-induced Parkinsonian Lewy-like aggregates prevented through polyphenolic phytochemical analog intervention. *Biochem. Biophys. Res. Commun.* 404, 324–329. doi: 10.1016/j.bbrc.2010.11.117

Pan, X. Y., Guo, H., Han, J., Hao, F., An, Y., Xu, Y., et al. (2012). Ginsenoside Rg3 attenuates cell migration via inhibition of aquaporin 1 expression in PC-3M prostate cancer cells. *Eur. J. Pharmacol.* 683, 27–34. doi: 10.1016/j.ejphar.2012.02.040

Pei, J. V., Kourghi, M., De Ieso, M. L., Campbell, E. M., Dorward, H. S., Hardingham, J. E., et al. (2016). Differential inhibition of water and ion channel activities of mammalian aquaporin-1 by two structurally related bacopaside compounds derived from the medicinal plant *Bacopa monnieri*. *Mol. Pharmacol.* 90, 496–507. doi: 10.1124/mol.116.105882

Pellavio, G., Rui, M., Caliogna, L., Martino, E., Gastaldi, G., Collina, S., et al. (2017). Regulation of aquaporin functional properties mediated by the antioxidant effects of natural compounds. *Int. J. Mol. Sci.* 18:2665. doi: 10.3390/ijms18122665

Popoola, O. K., Elbagory, A. M., Ameer, F., and Hussein, A. A. (2013). Marrubiin. *Molecules* 18, 9049–9060. doi: 10.3390/molecules18089049

Reyes-Escogido Mde, L., Gonzalez-Mondragon, E. G., and Vazquez-Tzompantzi, E. (2011). Chemical and pharmacological aspects of capsaicin. *Molecules* 16, 1253–1270. doi: 10.3390/molecules16021253

Rodrigues, C., Mósca, A. F., Martins, A. P., Nobre, T., Prista, C., Antunes, F., et al. (2016). Rat aquaporin-5 Is pH-gated induced by phosphorylation and is implicated in oxidative stress. *Int. J. Mol. Sci.* 17:2090. doi: 10.3390/ijms17122090

Rodríguez, A., Gena, P., Méndez-Giménez, L., Rosito, A., Valentí, V., Rotellar, F., et al. (2014). Reduced hepatic aquaporin-9 and glycerol permeability are related to insulin resistance in non-alcoholic fatty liver disease. *Int. J. Obes.* 38, 1213–1220. doi: 10.1038/ijo.2013.234

Rodríguez, A., Marinelli, R. A., Tesse, A., Frühbeck, G., and Calamita, G. (2015). Sexual dimorphism of adipose and hepatic aquaglyceroporins in health and metabolic disorders. *Front. Endocrinol.* 6:171. doi: 10.3389/fendo.2015.00171

Roohbakhsh, A., Parhiz, H., Soltani, F., Rezaee, R., and Iranshahi, M. (2015). Molecular mechanisms behind the biological effects of hesperidin and hesperetin for the prevention of cancer and cardiovascular diseases. *Life Sci.* 124, 64–74. doi: 10.1016/j.lfs.2014.12.030

Saito, K., Mori, S., Date, F., and Hong, G. (2015). Epigallocatechin gallate stimulates the neuroreactive salivary secretomotor system in autoimmune sialadenitis of MRL-Fas(lpr) mice via activation of cAMP-dependent protein kinase A and inactivation of nuclear factor kappaB. *Autoimmunity* 48, 379–388. doi: 10.3109/08916934.2015.1030617

Saito, M. (2015). Capsaicin and related food ingredients reducing body fat through the activation of TRP and brown fat thermogenesis. *Adv. Food Nutr. Res.* 76, 1–28. doi: 10.1016/bs.afnr.2015.07.002

Santiago-Vázquez, Y., Das, U., Varela-Ramirez, A., Baca, S. T., Ayala-Marin, Y., Lema, C., et al. (2016). Tumor-selective cytotoxicity of a novel pentadiene analogue on human leukemia/lymphoma cells. *Clin. Cancer Drugs* 3, 138–146. doi: 10.2174/2212697X03666160830165250

Shayakul, C., Tsukaguchi, H., Berger, U. V., and Hediger, M. A. (2001). Molecular characterization of a novel urea transporter from kidney inner medullary collecting ducts. *Am. J. Physiol. Renal Physiol.* 280, F487–F494. doi: 10.1152/ajprenal.2001.280.3.F487

Sohn, E. J., Kang, D. G., and Lee, H. S. (2003). Protective effects of glycyrrhizin on gentamicin-induced acute renal failure in rats. *Pharmacol. Toxicol.* 93, 116–122. doi: 10.1034/j.1600-0773.2003.930302.x

Soveral, G., and Casini, A. (2017). aquaporin modulators: a patent review (2010-2015). *Expert Opin. Ther. Pat.* 27, 49–62. doi: 10.1080/13543776.2017.1236085

Steinmetz, K. A., and Potter, J. D. (1991). Vegetables, fruit, and cancer. I. Epidemiology. *Cancer Causes Control* 2, 325–357. doi: 10.1007/BF00051672

Sun, M., Wang, J., Zhou, Y., Wang, Z., Jiang, Y., and Li, M. (2016). Isotetrandrine reduces astrocyte cytotoxicity in neuromyelitis optica by blocking the binding of NMO-IgG to aquaporin 4. *Neuroimmunomodulation* 23, 98–108. doi: 10.1159/000444530

Takahashi, A., Inoue, H., Mishima, K., Ide, F., Nakayama, R., Hasaka, A., et al. (2015). Evaluation of the effects of quercetin on damaged salivary secretion. *PLoS ONE* 10:e0116008. doi: 10.1371/journal.pone.0116008

Tamma, G., Valenti, G., Grossini, E., Donnini, S., Marino, A., Marinelli, R. A., et al. (2018). Aquaporin membrane channels in oxidative stress, cell signaling, and aging: recent advances and research trends. *Oxid. Med. Cell. Longev.* 2018:1501847. doi: 10.1155/2018/1501847

Tarozzi, A., Angeloni, C., Malaguti, M., Morroni, F., and Hrelia, P. (2013). Sulforaphane as a potential protective phytochemical against neurodegenerative diseases. *Oxid. Med. Cell. Longev.* 2013:415078. doi: 10.1155/2013/415078

Terlikowska, K. M., Witkowska, A. M., Zujko, M. E., Dobrzycka, B., and Terlikowski, S. J. (2014). Potential application of curcumin and its analogues in the treatment strategy of patients with primary epithelial ovarian cancer. *Int. J. Mol. Sci.* 15, 21703–21722. doi: 10.3390/ijms151221703

Tsao, R. (2010). Chemistry and biochemistry of dietary polyphenols. *Nutrients* 2, 1231–1246. doi: 10.3390/nu2121231

Tsukaguchi, H., Weremowicz, S., Morton, C. C., and Hediger, M. A. (1999). Functional and molecular characterization of the human neutral solute channel aquaporin-9. *Am. J. Physiol.* 277, F685–F696. doi: 10.1152/ajprenal.1999.277.5.F685

Upadhyay, S., and Dixit, M. (2015). Role of polyphenols and other phytochemicals on molecular signaling. *Oxid. Med. Cell. Longev.* 2015:504253. doi: 10.1155/2015/504253

van Rossum, T. G., Vulto, A. G., De Man, R. A., Brouwer, J. T., and Schalm, S. W. (1998). Review article: glycyrrhizin as a potential treatment for chronic hepatitis C. *Aliment. Pharmacol. Ther.* 12, 199–205. doi: 10.1046/j.1365-2036.1998.00309.x

Wang, B. F., Cui, Z. W., Zhong, Z. H., Sun, Y. H., Sun, Q. F., Yang, G. Y., et al. (2015). Curcumin attenuates brain edema in mice with intracerebral hemorrhage through inhibition of AQP4 and AQP9 expression. *Acta Pharmacol. Sin.* 36, 939–948. doi: 10.1038/aps.2015.47

Wang, C., Yan, M., Jiang, H., Wang, Q., He, S., Chen, J., et al. (2018). Mechanism of aquaporin 4 (AQP 4) up-regulation in rat cerebral edema under hypobaric hypoxia and the preventative effect of puerarin. *Life Sci.* 193, 270–281. doi: 10.1016/j.lfs.2017.10.021

Wang, Y., Cohen, J., Boron, W. F., Schulten, K., and Tajkhorshid, E. (2007). Exploring gas permeability of cellular membranes and membrane channels with molecular dynamics. *J. Struct. Biol.* 157, 534–544. doi: 10.1016/j.jsb.2006.11.008

Wang, Z., Lu, W., Li, Y., and Tang, B. (2013). Alpinetin promotes Bax translocation, induces apoptosis through the mitochondrial pathway and arrests human gastric cancer cells at the G2/M phase. *Mol. Med. Rep.* 7, 915–920. doi: 10.3892/mmr.2012.1243

Wang, Z. T., Lau, C. W., Chan, F. L., Yao, X., Chen, Z. Y., He, Z. D., et al. (2001). Vasorelaxant effects of cardamonin and alpinetin from Alpinia henryi K. *Schum. J. Cardiovasc. Pharmacol.* 37, 596–606. doi: 10.1097/00005344-200105000-00011

Watanabe, S., Moniaga, C. S., Nielsen, S., and Hara-Chikuma, M. (2016). aquaporin-9 facilitates membrane transport of hydrogen peroxide in mammalian cells. *Biochem. Biophys. Res. Commun.* 471, 191–197. doi: 10.1016/j.bbrc.2016.01.153

Wu, N. L., Fang, J. Y., Chen, M., Wu, C. J., Huang, C. C., and Hung, C. F. (2011). Chrysin protects epidermal keratinocytes from UVA- and UVB-induced damage. *J. Agric. Food Chem.* 59, 8391–8400. doi: 10.1021/jf200931t

Wu, Z., Uchi, H., Morino-Koga, S., Shi, W., and Furue, M. (2014). Resveratrol inhibition of human keratinocyte proliferation via SIRT1/ARNT/ERK dependent downregulation of aquaporin 3. *J. Dermatol. Sci.* 75, 16–23. doi: 10.1016/j.jdermsci.2014.03.004

Xie, C. L., Li, J. H., Wang, W. W., Zheng, G. Q., and Wang, L. X. (2015). Neuroprotective effect of ginsenoside-Rg1 on cerebral ischemia/reperfusion injury in rats by downregulating protease-activated receptor-1 expression. *Life Sci.* 121, 145–151. doi: 10.1016/j.lfs.2014.12.002

Yan, C., Yang, J., Shen, L., and Chen, X. (2012). Inhibitory effect of Epigallocatechin gallate on ovarian cancer cell proliferation associated with aquaporin 5 expression. *Arch. Gynecol. Obstet.* 285, 459–467. doi: 10.1007/s00404-011-1942-6

Yang, M., Wang, Y., Zhang, Y., Zhang, F., Zhao, Z., Li, S., et al. (2016). S-allylmercapto-l-cysteine modulates MUC5AC and AQP5 secretions in a COPD model via NF-small ka, CyrillicB signaling pathway. *Int. Immunopharmacol.* 39, 307–313. doi: 10.1016/j.intimp.2016.08.002

Yang, S. J., Lee, S. A., Park, M. G., Kim, J. S., Yu, S. K., Kim, C. S., et al. (2014). Induction of apoptosis by diphenyldifluoroketone in osteogenic sarcoma cells is associated with activation of caspases. *Oncol. Rep.* 31, 2286–2292. doi: 10.3892/or.2014.3066

Yang, Z. H., Sun, X., Qi, Y., Mei, C., Sun, X. B., and Du, G. H. (2012). Uptake characteristics of pinocembrin and its effect on p-glycoprotein at the blood-brain barrier in *in vitro* cell experiments. *J. Asian Nat. Prod. Res.* 14, 14–21. doi: 10.1080/10286020.2011.620393

Yasui, S., Fujiwara, K., Tawada, A., Fukuda, Y., Nakano, M., and Yokosuka, O. (2011). Efficacy of intravenous glycyrrhizin in the early stage of acute onset autoimmune hepatitis. *Dig. Dis. Sci.* 56, 3638–3647. doi: 10.1007/s10620-011-1789-5

Yin, J., Liang, Y., Wang, D., Yan, Z., Yin, H., Wu, D., et al. (2018). Naringenin induces laxative effects by upregulating the expression levels of c-Kit and SCF, as well as those of aquaporin 3 in mice with loperamide-induced constipation. *Int. J. Mol. Med.* 41, 649–658. doi: 10.3892/ijmm.2017.3301

Yu, C. H., Yu, W. Y., Fang, J., Zhang, H. H., Ma, Y., Yu, B., et al. (2016a). *Mosla scabra* flavonoids ameliorate the influenza A virus-induced lung injury and water transport abnormality via the inhibition of PRR and AQP signaling pathways in mice. *J. Ethnopharmacol.* 179, 146–155. doi: 10.1016/j.jep.2015.12.034

Yu, L. S., Fan, Y. Y., Ye, G., Li, J., Feng, X. P., Lin, K., et al. (2016b). Curcumin alleviates brain edema by lowering AQP4 expression levels in a rat model of hypoxia-hypercapnia-induced brain damage. *Exp. Ther. Med.* 11, 709–716. doi: 10.3892/etm.2016.3022

Yu, L., Yi, J., Ye, G., Zheng, Y., Song, Z., Yang, Y., et al. (2012). Effects of curcumin on levels of nitric oxide synthase and AQP-4 in a rat model of hypoxia-ischemic brain damage. *Brain Res.* 1475, 88–95. doi: 10.1016/j.brainres.2012.07.055

Yu, R., Hebbar, V., Kim, D. W., Mandlekar, S., Pezzuto, J. M., and Kong, A. N. (2001). Resveratrol inhibits phorbol ester and UV-induced activator protein 1 activation by interfering with mitogen-activated protein kinase pathways. *Mol. Pharmacol.* 60, 217–224. doi: 10.1124/mol.60.1.217

Zhang, X., Chen, Q., Wang, Y., Peng, W., and Cai, H. (2014). Effects of curcumin on ion channels and transporters. *Front. Physiol.* 5:94. doi: 10.3389/fphys.2014.00094

Zhang, Y., Cong, X., Shi, L., Xiang, B., Li, Y. M., Ding, Q. W., et al. (2010). Activation of transient receptor potential vanilloid subtype 1 increases secretion of the hypofunctional, transplanted submandibular gland. *Am. J. Physiol. Gastrointest. Liver Physiol.* 299, G54–G62. doi: 10.1152/ajpgi.00528.2009

Zhang, Y., Talalay, P., Cho, G. C., and Posner, G. H. (1992). A major inducer of anticarcinogenetic protective enzymes from broccoli: isolation and elucidation of the structure. *Proc. Natl. Acad. Sci. U.S.A.* 89, 2399–2403. doi: 10.1073/pnas.89.6.2399

Zhao, J., Moore, A. N., Clifton, G. L., and Dash, P.-K. (2005). Sulphoraphane enhances aquaporin-4 expression and decreases cerebral edema following traumatic brain injury. *J. Neurosci. Res.* 82, 499–506. doi: 10.1002/jnr.20649

Zhong, Z., Wang, B., Dai, M., Sun, Y., Sun, Q., Yang, G., et al. (2013). Carvacrol alleviates cerebral edema by modulating AQP4 expression after intracerebral hemorrhage in mice. *Neurosci. Lett.* 555, 24–29. doi: 10.1016/j.neulet.2013.09.023

Zhou, Y., Li, H. Q., Lu, L., Fu, D. L., Liu, A. J., Li, J. H., et al. (2014). Ginsenoside Rg1 provides neuroprotection against blood brain barrier disruption and neurological injury in a rat model of cerebral ischemia/reperfusion through downregulation of aquaporin 4 expression. *Phytomedicine* 21, 998–1003. doi: 10.1016/j.phymed.2013.12.005

Zollner, G., Wagner, M., and Trauner, M. (2010). Nuclear receptors as drug targets in cholestasis and drug-induced hepatotoxicity. *Pharmacol. Ther.* 126, 228–243. doi: 10.1016/j.pharmthera.2010.03.005

Zu, J., Wang, Y., Xu, G., Zhuang, J., Gong, H., and Yan, J. (2014). Curcumin improves the recovery of motor function and reduces spinal cord edema in a rat acute spinal cord injury model by inhibiting the JAK/STAT signaling pathway. *Acta Histochem.* 116, 1331–1336. doi: 10.1016/j.acthis.2014.08.004

14

VDAC1 as Pharmacological Target in Cancer and Neurodegeneration: Focus on its Role in Apoptosis

Andrea Magrì[1,2†], *Simona Reina*[1,2†] *and Vito De Pinto*[2*]

[1] *Section of Molecular Biology, Department of Biological, Geological and Environmental Sciences, University of Catania, Catania, Italy,* [2] *Section of Biology and Genetics, Department of Biomedicine and Biotechnology, National Institute for Biomembranes and Biosystems, Section of Catania, Catania, Italy*

***Correspondence:**
Vito De Pinto
vdpbiofa@unict.it

† *These authors have contributed equally to this work.*

Cancer and neurodegeneration are different classes of diseases that share the involvement of mitochondria in their pathogenesis. Whereas the high glycolytic rate (the so-called Warburg metabolism) and the suppression of apoptosis are key elements for the establishment and maintenance of cancer cells, mitochondrial dysfunction and increased cell death mark neurodegeneration. As a main actor in the regulation of cell metabolism and apoptosis, VDAC may represent the common point between these two broad families of pathologies. Located in the outer mitochondrial membrane, VDAC forms channels that control the flux of ions and metabolites across the mitochondrion thus mediating the organelle's cross-talk with the rest of the cell. Furthermore, the interaction with both pro-apoptotic and anti-apoptotic factors makes VDAC a gatekeeper for mitochondria-mediated cell death and survival signaling pathways. Unfortunately, the lack of an evident druggability of this protein, since it has no defined binding or active sites, makes the quest for VDAC interacting molecules a difficult tale. Pharmacologically active molecules of different classes have been proposed to hit cancer and neurodegeneration. In this work, we provide an exhaustive and detailed survey of all the molecules, peptides, and microRNAs that exploit VDAC in the treatment of the two examined classes of pathologies. The mechanism of action and the potential or effectiveness of each compound are discussed.

Keywords: mitochondria, apoptosis, VDAC, peptides, oligos, microRNAs, biological drugs

INTRODUCTION

Mitochondria are crucial organelles for eukaryotic cells since they support the huge demand of energy required to maintain cellular homeostasis. Metabolites and ions are, thus, continuously exchanged with the cytosol through the Mitochondrial Outer Membrane (MOM), which owes its selective permeability mainly to the presence of mitochondrial porins, known as Voltage-Dependent Anion Channel (VDAC) (Shoshan-Barmatz et al., 2010). VDACs are the most abundant pore-forming proteins of the MOM and, differently from other structurally similar proteins such as Tom40 or Sam50, they serve as unspecific channels allowing the exchanges of molecules up to a molecular weight of 1,500 Da. High conserved through evolution, in mammals three distinct genes encode for three different VDAC isoforms, namely VDAC1, VDAC2, and VDAC3. The three isoforms are characterized by similar molecular weight of 28–32 kDa and by about 70% of sequence similarity (Sampson et al., 1997; Messina et al., 2012), all features suggesting a common tridimensional structure. Nevertheless, the three proteins display different roles in physiological and pathological conditions, as well as different expression level and tissue-specificity. Beyond the metabolic functions, the peculiar position of VDACs, at the interface between cytosol and mitochondria, makes porins the mitochondrial docking site for several cytosolic proteins, including molecules involved in the regulation of cell life and death. In this perspective, VDAC proteins appear as regulator of apoptosis, exerting both pro- and/or anti-apoptotic functions in physiological and pathological condition. Many pathologies, such as cancer and neurodegenerative disorders, indeed, show a deregulation of apoptosis pathways that correlates with alteration of VDAC activity, expression and functionality. For this reason, VDAC proteins have quickly become a new pharmacological target, and many molecules and peptides have been developed so far, aimed to modulate VDACs activity and ability to regulate apoptosis, with the final goal to find new therapeutic strategies for many disease treatments. In this review, we have grouped and described molecules and peptides with both pro-apoptotic and pro-survival properties. These molecules have been associated with different pathologies and while several of them are well known and already used in clinical trials, other new molecules, just assayed *in vitro* or at the cellular level, have been surveyed here.

STRUCTURE AND FUNCTION OF VDAC PROTEINS

VDAC proteins are crucial for the metabolic cross talk between cytosol and mitochondria. Through VDACs, the newly synthetized ATP is continuously exchanged with ADP, as well as NAD^+/NADH and many Krebs's cycle intermediates (Benz, 1994; Hodge and Colombini, 1997; Rostovtseva and Colombini, 1997; Lee et al., 1998). VDAC proteins regulate the flux of small ions (Cl^-, K^+, Na^+, and Ca^{2+}), participate in fatty acid transport across the MOM and in cholesterol distribution in mitochondrial membranes (Campbell and Chan, 2008; Lee et al., 2011). Furthermore, VDACs participate in the regulation of calcium concentration, maintaining the physiological level of cytosolic calcium, and are the channels responsible of ROS (superoxide anion) release to the cytosol (Han et al., 2003; Simamura et al., 2008a; De Stefani et al., 2012). Through the interaction with many metabolic enzymes, such as hexokinases, glycerol kinase (Fiek et al., 1982), glucokinase, and creatine kinase (Brdiczka et al., 1994), VDACs take part in the control of glycolytic metabolism. The main VDAC cellular functions are summarized in **Figure 1**.

Among VDAC isoforms, VDAC1 is the most abundant and best characterized one. In 2008, the crystallographic structure of mouse VDAC1 was solved by means of X-ray diffraction and confirmed by NMR in the human protein. As reported in **Figure 2A**, VDAC1 is organized as a transmembrane β-barrel, made by 19 anti-parallel β-strands, while the N-terminal domain, including the first 25 amino acids, is structured in α-helix short stretch, and is localized inside the pore's lumen (Bayrhuber et al., 2008; Hiller et al., 2008; Ujwal et al., 2008). The N-terminal domain is suspected to participate in the stabilization of the pore's structure by its interaction with the channel's wall (Villinger et al., 2010) but, at the same time, it is considered the mobile part of the protein, being exposed to the cytosol under certain conditions (Geula et al., 2012; Tomasello et al., 2013). The 3D structures of the others human VDAC isoforms remain unsolved so far. Recently, VDAC2 from zebrafish was crystalized, showing to have a structure very similar to that of VDAC1 (Schredelseker et al., 2014). Due to the high sequence similarity between the three isoforms, homology modeling studies predict similar 3D structure for VDAC2 and VDAC3. An exception is the N-terminal domain of VDAC2, which is longer than the other two isoforms and cannot be modeled (De Pinto et al., 2010a). Furthermore, homology modeling revealed high similarity also with porins extracted from *Saccharomyces cerevisiae* (Guardiani et al., 2018): the ability of human and mouse VDAC isoforms to complement the lack of the endogenous porin1 in yeast (Reina et al., 2010; Magri et al., 2016a) confirmed that VDACs are made with a common motif.

Electrophysiological techniques are widely used to characterize the electrophysiological features of VDAC channels from many organisms (De Pinto et al., 1989; Palmieri and De Pinto, 1989; Aiello et al., 2004; Reina et al., 2013; Guardiani et al., 2018). Mammalian VDAC1 and VDAC2 easily open pores into an artificial membrane formed in a Planar Lipid Bilayer (PLB) apparatus: the pore-forming activity is studied in terms of conductance increase through the otherwise not conducting phospholipidic membrane (**Figure 2B**). Different VDAC proteins may show differences in their electrophysiological features, in dependence of the sequence of the protein, the phospholipids in the membrane (Brenner and Lemoine, 2014) and the applied voltage. E.g., high cholesterol can impair the activity of many membranes' proteins and, specifically, inhibit VDAC function (Campbell and Chan, 2008). In general, however, they have a typical behavior that can be easily recognized: the formation of the pores is discrete, with a stepwise appearance, and the known VDAC proteins are more or less uniform in this appearance (Benz et al., 1989; Menzel et al., 2009; Guardiani et al., 2018). VDACs are characterized by different conductance values accordingly to the applied voltage. This phenomenon is called voltage-dependence, and it is well known for the channels. *In vitro*, in reconstitution experiments where VDACs are inserted in an artificial membrane, when a low voltage between $\pm$ 20 mV is applied, both VDAC1 and VDAC2 display a high-conductive state (known also as "open" state), with conductance value of about 3.5–4.0 nS in 1 M KCl or NaCl (Colombini, 1980; Xu et al., 1999; Gattin et al., 2015). However, as the voltage increases (in positive or negative sign), VDAC1 and VDAC2 undergo several low-conducting ("closed") states (see **Figures 2C,D**). These features are well conserved in the evolution for many VDAC isoforms: e.g., similar electrophysiological features were found for VDAC1 and, more recently, for VDAC2 from bovine spermatozoa (Menzel et al., 2009) and for VDAC2 extracted from yeast *S. cerevisiae* (Guardiani et al., 2018). On the contrary, human VDAC3 shows a very low propensity to form pores into PLB. VDAC3 channels are characterized by a very low

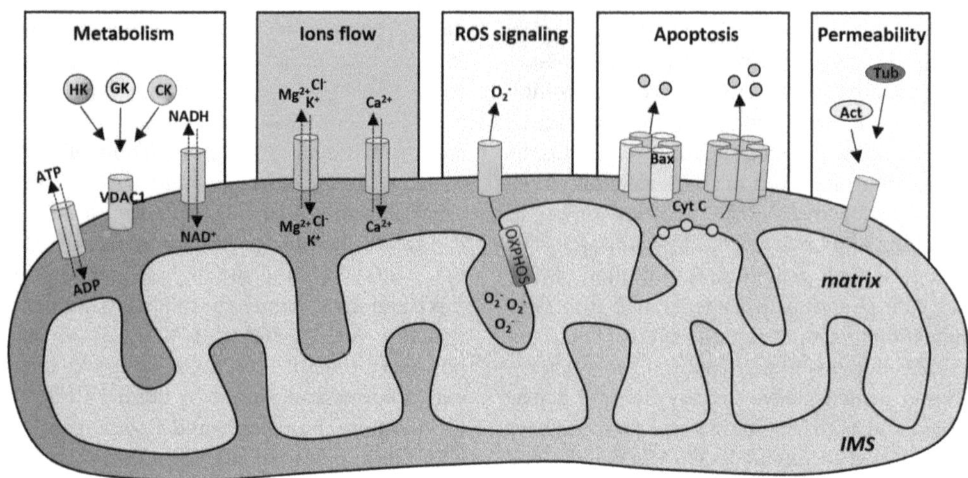

FIGURE 1 | Functional roles of VDAC1 in physiological conditions. Schematic representation of VDAC1 functions in the cell. VDAC1 serves as the main gate in the MOM for metabolites, such as ATP/ADP and NAD^+/NADH, but also Krebs cycle's intermediates, cholesterol and glutamate. Furthermore, by interaction with many cytosolic enzymes, such as Hexokinases (HK), Glucokinase (GK), and Creatine Kinase (CK), VDAC1 provides the ATP source essential for enzyme's activity. VDAC1 controls the flux of magnesium, chloride and potassium ions across the MOM, as well as of calcium, participating in the maintenance of cytosolic Ca^{2+} level in the physiological range. Evidence highlighted that VDAC1 acts as a preferential release channel for the hydrophilic ROS superoxide anion, produced during respiration by OXPHOS. Moreover, VDAC1 is considered a regulator of apoptosis; indeed, under apoptotic stimuli, VDAC1 undergoes oligomerization, by interacting with the pro-apoptotic protein Bax or with other VDAC1 molecules and constituting a channel big enough to promote cytochrome c (CYT C) releases to the cytosol and activation of apoptosis. It has been showed that many cytoskeleton proteins, such as Actin (Act) or Tubulin (Tub) bind VDAC1 participating in the regulation of channel permeability.

conductance (about 100 pS in 1 M KCl) without showing any voltage-dependence (Checchetto et al., 2014; Okazaki et al., 2015). This peculiar behavior of VDAC3 possibly depends from the high oxidation level of cysteines (Reina et al., 2016a), a specific feature which suggests a putative role of VDAC3 in the redox signaling and mitochondrial quality control (De Pinto et al., 2016; Reina et al., 2016b). Accordingly, the analysis of VDAC3 interactome has highlighted the propensity of this isoform to bind redox enzyme and stress-sensor proteins (Messina et al., 2014), supporting this hypothesis.

VDAC IN APOPTOSIS REGULATION

Mitochondria play a key role both in intrinsic and extrinsic pathways of apoptosis. Mitochondria contain a set of apoptogenic factors, including cytochrome c (cyt c), AIF and Smac/Diablo. In physiological conditions, apoptogenic factors are normally located in the intermembrane space of mitochondria (IMS). However, under apoptotic stimuli, they are released into the cytosol, leading to cyt c interaction with APAF-1 and the formation of apoptosome, which in turn activates the caspases cascade (Wang and Youle, 2009; Vaux, 2011). The release of cyt c to the cytosol occurs by the alteration of MOM permeability, a mechanism finely regulated by Bcl-2 proteins. Bcl-2 represents a heterogeneous family of both pro- and anti-apoptotic proteins, characterized by the presence of the common domain BH3. Bcl-2 proteins are mainly cytosolic; however, after certain stimuli, they translocate to the mitochondria, promoting the MOM permeabilization (Martinou and Youle, 2011). Many intrinsic stimuli, such as increased cytoplasmic level of Ca^{2+}, severe oxidative stress, DNA damages and hypoxia (Le Bras et al., 2005; Keeble and Gilmore, 2007; Kroemer and Zitvogel, 2007), promote the mitochondrial translocation of the pro-apoptotic protein Bax and its interaction with the mitochondrial-located Bak, through conformational changes that leads to the formation of hetero-oligomers big enough to allow the passage of apoptogenic factors (Gross et al., 1998; Kroemer et al., 2007). Similarly, an extrinsic signal, e.g., the binding of an extracellular molecule to a specific receptor on the plasma membrane, results in the activation of caspase-8 that, in turn, promotes the cleavage of the pro-apoptotic protein Bid. The truncated Bid form, tBid, translocates into MOM, and interacts with Bak, participating in hetero-oligomers formation (Korsmeyer et al., 2000). In this contest, VDAC proteins participate in the regulation of mitochondrial-mediated apoptosis in different ways. In particular, while VDAC1 is widely considered a pro-apoptotic protein (see below), VDAC2 exerts an anti-apoptotic function. On the contrary, no information about the involvement of VDAC3 in apoptosis regulation is available so far.

Much evidence indeed indicates a specific function as pro-survival protein for VDAC2. This suggests a co-evolution of this mammalian-specific VDAC isoform with Bcl-2 proteins to regulate cell death (Cheng et al., 2003). In fact, VDAC2 specifically binds Bak, sequestrating it into the MOM in an inactive conformer and, thus, inhibiting Bak-dependent mitochondrial apoptosis (Cheng et al., 2003). Only recently, the specific domain of VDAC2 necessary for BAK interaction was identified (Naghdi et al., 2015). A similar mechanism of

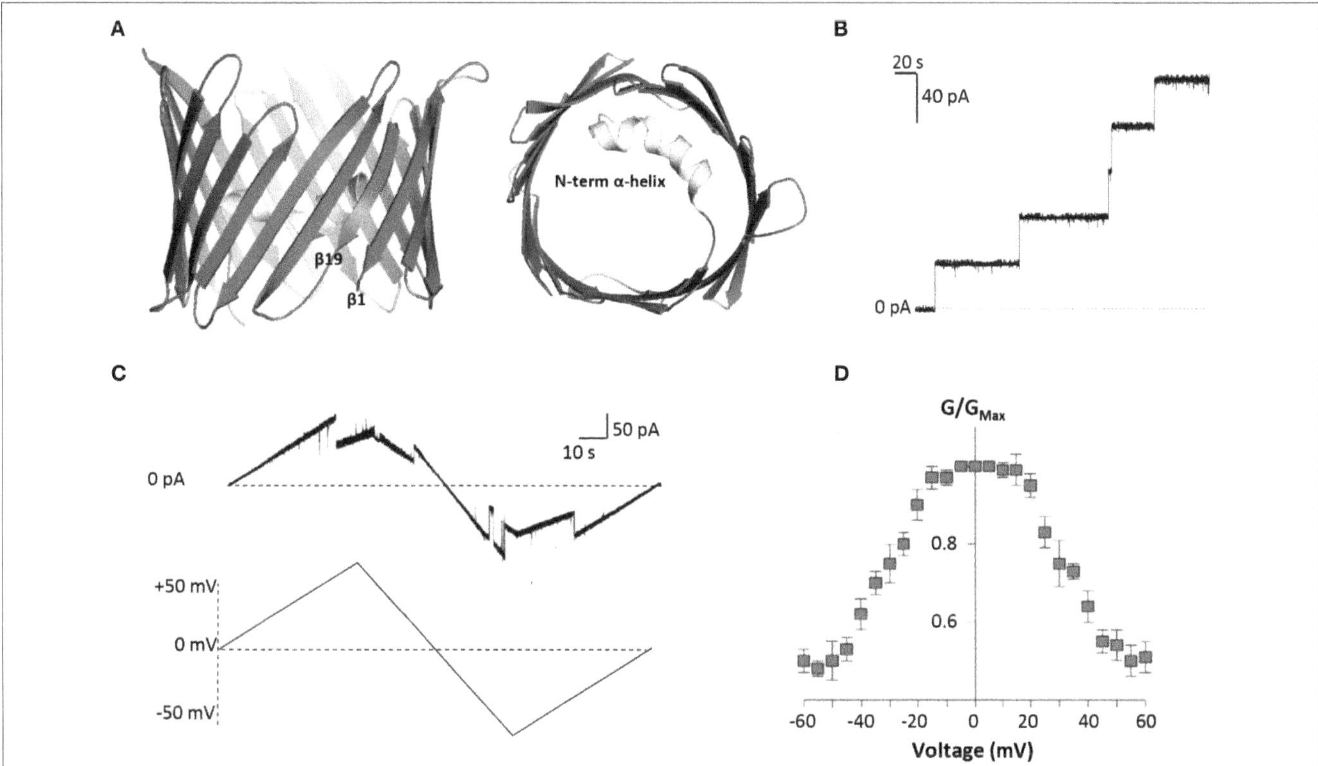

FIGURE 2 | Structure and electrophysiological features of human VDAC1. **(A)** Three-dimensional structure of human VDAC1 from the side or top view. VDAC1 is a β-barrel (in red) formed by 19 anti-parallel β-strands, with the exclusion of β1 and β19 which are parallel. The strands are connected by loops (in purple). The N-terminal domain (in light blue) is arranged in α-helix and it is located inside the pore's lumen. This structure was drawn by PyMol software and is based on the hVDAC1 (PDB 5XDN). **(B)** Representative trace of recombinant hVDAC1 insertion in artificial membrane measured at the PLB. The trace indicates that hVDAC1 can easily form channels of about 4 nS in 1 M KCl. The experiment was performed at the constant voltage of + 10 mV. **(C)** Representative triangular curve of recombinant hVDAC1 showing changes in channel conductance upon application of a voltage ramp between ± 50 mV. As shown, hVDAC1 remains in a stable high-conductive state at low voltages, between ± 30 mV; conversely, at higher voltages, hVDAC1 switches into low-conductive states. The experiment was performed in 1 M KCl. **(D)** Bell-shaped curve of hVDAC1 voltage dependence, showing the channel's open probability (G/G_{Max}) in relation to the voltage applied. Data are expressed as mean of G/G_{Max} ± SEM of $n = 3$ independent experiments, performed in 1 M KCl in a voltage range of ± 60 mV.

VDAC2-mediated inhibition was found also for the cytosolic protein Bax, which was partially found in the MOM and associated to VDAC2 (Ma et al., 2014).

Conversely, VDAC1 is able to bind Bax exerting a pro-apoptotic activity. In particular, the interaction of Bax with VDAC1 not only blocks the ATP/ADP exchange, affecting the channel functioning (Vander Heiden et al., 1999), but leads to the formation of hetero-oligomers VDAC1-Bax involved in cyt c release and caspase cascade activation (Shimizu et al., 1999; Shimizu and Tsujimoto, 2000). Alternatively, apoptotic stimuli are able to induce VDAC1 oligomerization, leading to the formation of channels big enough to allow the passage of cyt c to the cytosol (Keinan et al., 2010).

An early theory indicated that opening of the mitochondrial Permeability Transition Pore (mPTP), led to loss of the mitochondrial membrane potential, mitochondrial swelling, and the rupture of the MOM (Zoratti and Szabò, 1995; Halestrap et al., 1997). In an old model, mPTP was proposed to be formed by VDAC1 in the MOM, adenine nucleotide translocator (ANT) in the IMM, and cyclophilin-D (CyP-D) in the matrix (Marzo et al., 1998; Bernardi, 1999; Green and Evan, 2002; Tsujimoto and Shimizu, 2007). However, mPTP opening in VDAC1- or ANT-null cells (Baines et al., 2007), have challenged the mPTP model, which remains a not completely answered question.

Pro-apoptotic properties of VDAC1 are prevented by its interaction with the metabolic enzymes hexokinases (HKs). The two main HK isoforms, namely HK1 and HK2, are both involved in the first rate-limiting step of glycolysis. Both isoforms bind to VDAC1, obtaining a direct access to mitochondrial ATP, despite HK2 shows a higher affinity for mitochondrial binding (Wilson, 2003). The biological significance of VDAC1-HKs complexes is more profound. Indeed, HKs compete with Bax for binding to VDAC1, reducing the formation of VDAC1-Bax complexes (Vyssokikh et al., 2002); conversely, HKs detachment from VDAC1 induces apoptosis, increasing VDAC1 propensity to bind Bax or to participate in hetero- or homo-oligomeric structure formation (Abu-Hamad et al., 2008). Not coincidentally, VDAC1-HKs complexes are exploited in tumors, since mitochondrial HK2 increases the glycolysis rate, participating to the "Warburg effect," and protects cancer

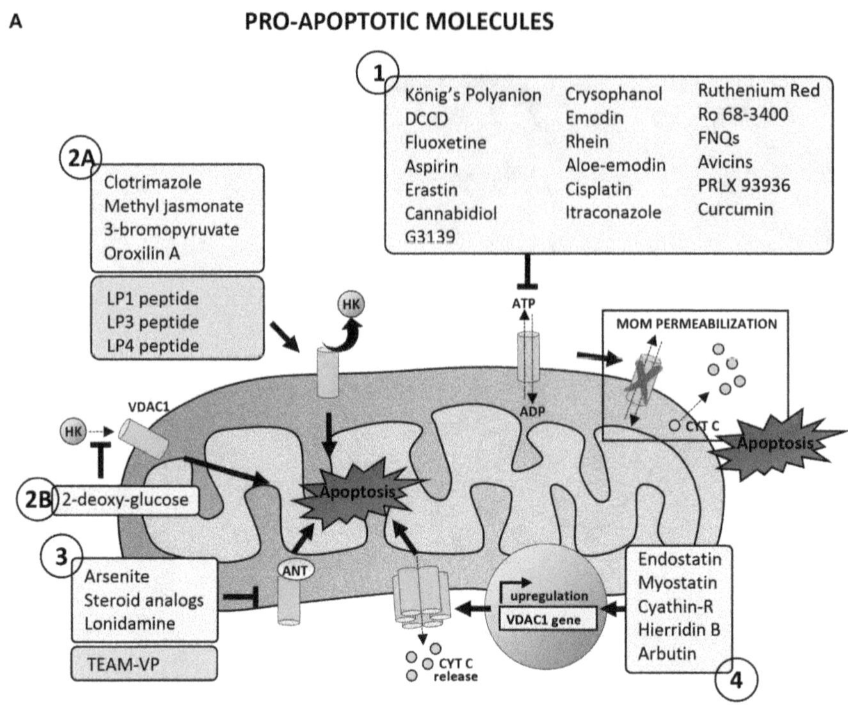

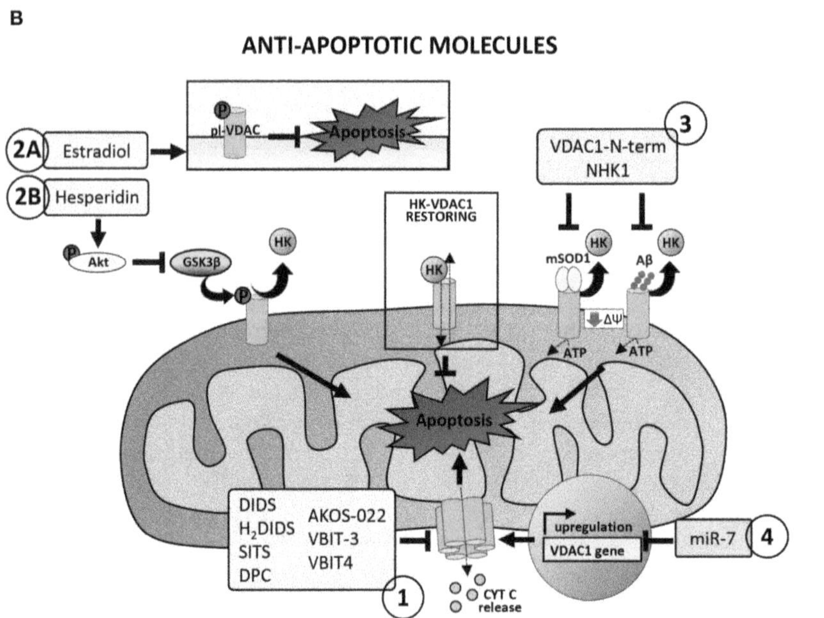

FIGURE 3 | Pro- and anti-apoptotic molecules acting on VDAC1 and putatively involved in pharmacological treatment of cancer and neurodegeneration. **(A)** Pro-apoptotic molecules and peptides acting on VDAC1 with proven or potential role in the pharmacological treatment of cancer phenotype. Group 1 includes molecules acting on VDAC1 channel activity by promoting the impairment of metabolic exchanges between mitochondria and cytosol, leading to MOM permeabilization and activation of apoptosis. Group 2 includes molecules and peptides acting on VDAC1-HKs complexes by promoting HKs detachment from VDAC1 (2A) or preventing HKs binding to VDAC1 (2B). Group 3 includes molecules and peptides acting on ANT-VDAC1 complexes (the precise mechanism is still unclear). Group 4 includes molecules inducing VDAC1 overexpression and the consequent propensity of VDAC1 to form oligomers. **(B)** Anti-apoptotic molecules and peptides acting on VDAC1 and potentially able to reduce mitochondrial dysfunction in neurodegenerative diseases. Group 1 includes peptides with proven ability to bind VDAC1 and to impair the aggregation of misfolded SOD1 mutants or Aβ peptide with VDAC1, restoring VDAC1-HKs complexes, and VDAC1 functionality. Group 2 includes molecules acting on VDAC1 phosphorylation at both plasma membrane (2A) and mitochondrial (2B) level with consequences on VDAC1 channel activity or the ability to bind HKs. Group 3 includes channel blockers, molecules with proven ability to bind specifically VDAC1 and to counteract the VDAC1 oligomerization. Group 4 includes siRNA able to downregulate VDAC1 expression, decreasing in turn the VDAC1 propensity to form oligomers.

cells from apoptosis (Gatenby and Gillies, 2004; Pedersen, 2008).

VDAC-Mediated Apoptosis as a Target for Many Disease's Treatment

VDAC proteins play a crucial role in controlling mitochondrial metabolism and apoptosis. In this perspective, VDACs become interesting from a pharmacological point of view and many molecules targeted to VDAC proteins have been developed so far. Indeed, both alterations of apoptosis and of mitochondrial bioenergetics represent basal molecular mechanisms whose modulation is present in many pathologies.

A cancer hallmark is the apoptosis inhibition. A combination of factors leads to raising cell resistance to death stimuli. In many tumors, several anti-apoptotic proteins are overexpressed (Strasser et al., 1990; Adams and Cory, 2007) and the rapid growth of malignant cells is strongly supported by VDAC1-HKs complexes, which increase glucose metabolism and inhibit apoptosis (Mathupala et al., 2006). Conversely, the detachment of HKs from VDAC1 promotes the channel propensity to interact with the pro-apoptotic Bax and Bak proteins (Majewski et al., 2004) or to form VDAC1 oligomers (Keinan et al., 2010). Therefore, therapeutic approaches aimed to counteract malignant cells proliferation have taken into account strategies directed to induce HKs detachment from VDAC1 and/or to act on VDAC1 expression and channel activity.

In cancer, cell death is significantly inhibited, but in neurodegenerative disease, on the opposite, the early onset of neuron's death is among the causes of the pathologies. Neurodegenerative disorders represent a large group of age-related pathologies, which affect different nervous system's regions. Among disorders affecting brain, the most studied are undoubtedly Alzheimer's disease (AD) and Parkinson's disease (PD), while the most known neuromuscular disorder is Amyotrophic Lateral Sclerosis (ALS), which specifically affects spinal cord. Pathologies such as AD, PD, and ALS are characterized by different etiologies and symptoms. Nevertheless, at the molecular level, they are characterized by accumulation within the cells of misfolded proteins and/or peptide which can directly interact with VDAC1 (Magrì and Messina, 2017). The interaction of misfolded protein with VDAC1 has dramatic consequences for mitochondrial functionality. At the same time, in AD and in PD, a significative alteration of caspase-mediated apoptotic pathways was found (Li et al., 2000; Rohn et al., 2009), which correlated with a reduction of mitochondrial rate of HKs (Israelson et al., 2010; Smilansky et al., 2015; Magrì et al., 2016b). Furthermore, the analysis of post-mortem brain from AD patients and transgenic mice have shown that VDAC1 is over-expressed and that the level of VDAC1 phosphorylation is significantly increased (Cuadrado-Tejedor et al., 2011). In this perspective, molecules able to interfere with misfolded proteins interaction with VDAC1 and/or decrease the pro-apoptotic features due to the overexpression of the channel have been proposed as therapeutic tool. In this review, we grouped molecules that, by acting on VDAC1, exert pro- and anti-apoptotic features, thus putatively able to counteract mitochondrial dysfunction in cancer and neurodegenerative diseases, respectively. However, the targeted delivery of drugs to specific intracellular locations is one of the most challenging obstacle to be overcome. Several chemotherapeutic drug cannot easily cross the protective, physiological barriers in tumor tissues. For this reason, we paid specific attention onto biological molecules like peptides and oligos, which definitely represent a most promising alternative to conventional molecules used nowadays against cancer and neurodegeneration.

VDAC TARGETED MOLECULES THAT AFFECT APOPTOSIS

Pro-apototic Molecules Acting on VDAC1 Channel Activity

Over the years, various anti-cancer molecules able to directly target to VDAC1 were proposed (Reina and De Pinto, 2017). Most of described molecules directly interact with VDAC1, reducing the channel conductance, eventually leading to apoptosis (**Figure 3A**, Group 1). The **König's Polyanion (KPa)**, a 1:2:3 copolymer of methacrylate, maleate, and styrene, is surely one of the first listed compound able to lower VDAC's gating voltage and induce irreversible channel closure *in vitro* (König et al., 1982; Colombini et al., 1987; Tedeschi et al., 1987; Benz et al., 1988; Mannella and Guo, 1990). Nevertheless, the existence of contrasting results that prove both apoptotic and anti-apoptotic effects together with the lack of specificity for VDAC, prevent KPa utilization as an anticancer drug. Likewise, **dicyclohexylcarbodiimide (DCCD)** has been reported to inhibit hexokinase binding by covalently labeling VDAC (Nakashima et al., 1986; Nakashima, 1989; De Pinto et al., 1993; Shafir et al., 1998) and blocking its channel activity (Shafir et al., 1998). The high specificity of this interaction is strengthened by the identification of VDAC-Glu72 amino residue as the binding site of both DCCD and hexokinase (De Pinto et al., 1993; Zaid et al., 2005). In spite of this, the ability of DCCD to inhibit various ATPases prohibits its use in humans.

Several molecules have been intensively tested *in cellulo*. For instance, **fluoxetine**, a drug prescribed for the treatment of major depressive disorders, has been reported to inhibit proliferation of several cancer cells lines (Serafeim et al., 2003; Krishnan et al., 2008; Stepulak et al., 2008; Lee et al., 2010; Mun et al., 2013), although previous studies have associated the administration of this compound to an increased risk of developing tumor (Brandes et al., 1992; Lee et al., 2001). Once penetrated inside the cell, fluoxetine binds mainly to mitochondria (Mukherjee et al., 1998), most likely using VDAC, as demonstrated by PLB assays. In this conditions indeed, fluoxetine interacts with VDAC, altering its channel properties (Nahon et al., 2005; Thinnes, 2005). A recent report, however, questions the specificity of fluoxetine for VDAC, proposing its interaction with the Glutamate receptor 1 (GluR1) to trigger apoptosis in glioma cells (Liu et al., 2015). **Aspirin**, the famous nonsteroidal anti-inflammatory drug used as an antipyretic and analgesic agent, has been lately associated with a pro-apoptotic activity against different cancer cell types, such as colon cancer, chronic lymphocytic leukemia and myeloid leukemia. Tewari et al. demonstrated a direct modulation of membrane-reconstituted VDAC1 by aspirin, suggesting this interaction as responsible for the anticancer effects of the drug (Tewari et al., 2017). Following VDAC1 binding, indeed, aspirin would dissipate mitochondrial membrane potential ($\Delta\psi m$), dissociate HK2 from mitochondria and promote cell death. Accordingly, silencing of VDAC1 protects HeLa cells from aspirin-induced cell death. **Erastin** is another anti-tumor agent that use VDAC as a docking site in mitochondria and induces oxidative, non-apoptotic death in human tumor cells with mutations in the oncogenes HRAS, KRAS, or BRAF. Erastin specifically binds VDAC isoforms 2 and 3 (Yagoda et al., 2007), as confirmed by knockdown experiments, and it also modulates VDAC-tubulin interaction in proliferating cells (Maldonado et al., 2013). VDAC has been also proposed as a target for **cannabidiol (CBD)**, a phytocannabinoid derived from *Cannabis* species and devoid of psychoactive activity. Reconstitution experiments in artificial membranes demonstrated indeed the ability of CBD to directly bind VDAC, markedly decreasing its channel conductance. This interaction, further confirmed by microscale thermophoresis analysis (Rimmerman et al., 2013), may be responsible for the strong anti-tumor effects of cannabidiol observed in numerous cancer cells types (Ligresti et al., 2006; Massi et al., 2013). **Avicins** represent a class of natural compounds reported to target and close VDAC in lipid bilayers, causing the OMM permeabilization and the release of cytochrome *c* (Lemeshko et al., 2006; Haridas et al., 2007). Once again, such a mechanism would explain the pro-apoptotic effect of these triterpenoid saponines in tumor cells (Haridas et al., 2001; Mujoo et al., 2001; Gaikwad et al., 2005). Interestingly, avicins can still trigger cell death via autophagy even when Bax or Bak genes are deleted or caspases are inhibited, suggesting potential therapeutic activity in apoptosis-resistant cancers. Recently, **chrysophanol, emodin, rhein, aloe-emodin,** and **catechin**, the bioactive anti-cancer components of the herb *Rheum officinale Baill*, have been reported to bind VDAC through Thr207 and the N-terminal region of the protein (Li et al., 2017). A survey of literatures shows that these derivatives induce apoptosis in many human cancer cell lines, including lung adenocarcinoma A549, cervical carcinoma HeLa, and hepatoma HepG2 cells (Chu et al., 2012). Given the importance of VDAC as an anti-cancer target, the authors proposed a key role for this interaction in the cytotoxic activity of the compounds. Electrophysiological experiments have demonstrated the ability of **ruthenium Red (RuR)**, a water-soluble *hexavalent* polycation whose effects on apoptosis are debated (Anghileri, 1975; Zaid et al., 2005), to induce channel closure of membrane-reconstituted VDAC1 as well (Israelson et al., 2008). Interestingly, RuR would interact with the same VDAC1 loops responsible for HK1 binding (Israelson et al., 2008). Although with a slightly different mechanism, it is worth mentioning also **furanonaphtoquinones (FNQs)**, a class of highly reactive molecules that induce caspase-dependent apoptosis via ROS production. VDAC was proposed as the pharmacological target of **FNQs**, since their anti-cancer activity was increased upon VDAC1 overexpression and decreased upon VDAC1 silencing by siRNA (Simamura et al., 2006, 2008b). In 2003, Cesura et al. identified VDAC1 as the major molecular target of the PTP inhibitor **Ro 68-3400** in mitochondria prepared from a human neuroblastoma cell line. Later, however, this statement underwent several confutations (Cesura et al., 2003). Initially, single channel analysis revealed that Ro 68-3400 failed to alter the electrophysiological properties of VDAC1 incorporated into lipid membranes and afterwards, Bernardi and coworkers proposed the Mitochondrial Phosphate Carrier (PiC) as the proper interactor (Krauskopf et al., 2006).

Compounds that are already part of clinical trials conclude this list. Among them, **cisplatin** is one of the best known chemotherapeutic drug for the treatment of numerous human cancers (Khan et al., 1982; Scher and Norton, 1992; Abrams et al., 2003; Koch et al., 2013). Several clues about the enhanced sensitivity to cisplatin of cells with increased expression of VDAC1, suggested that this protein may serve as a cisplatin receptor in the apoptotic pathway (Thinnes, 2009). According to Keinan et al. cisplatin would induce cell death through VDAC1 oligomerization (Keinan et al., 2010), albeit discordant data proposed a significantly increased cytotoxicity of this drug in cancer cells silenced for VDAC1 (Wu et al., 2016). Clinical studies performed with **itraconazole**, a common antifungal drug, have demonstrated its potent antiangiogenic and anticancer activity. Again, VDAC would be part of the mechanism of action of this compound. Liu and coworkers, indeed, reported that the binding of itraconazole to VDAC1 causes an increase in the AMP:ATP ratio, which in turn activates AMPK that down-regulates mTOR pathway and thus inhibits cell proliferation (Head et al., 2015). VDAC has been recently proposed as the therapeutic target of **curcumin** as well. Curcumin (diferuloylmethane) is a component of the golden spice turmeric (*Curcuma longa)* with anti-inflammatory and antitumor activity (Aggarwal et al., 2003). Along with reports that claim curcumin capable of binding to Bcl2 proteins (Carroll et al., 2011; Rao et al., 2011; Yang et al., 2015), Tewari et al. firstly demonstrated its interaction with membrane-reconstituted VDAC1 (Tewari et al., 2015). Noteworthy, curcumin has already entered phase II clinical trial for the treatment of advanced pancreatic cancer (Dhillon et al., 2008) and the prevention of colorectal neoplasia (Carroll et al., 2011). Finally, a structural analog of the above mentioned erastin, called **PRLX 93936**, is currently in Phase I/II clinical trial for the treatment of patients with multiple myeloma (*ClinicalTrials.gov* database, NCI). As for erastin, it inhibits VDAC2 and VDAC3 in cells harboring mutations in the oncogenes HRAS, KRAS, and BRAF.

Pro-apoptotic Molecules Counteracting the Interaction of VDAC1 With Hexokinases or the Adenine Nucleotide Transporter

VDAC-hexokinase interaction certainly represents a crucial point in the establishment and maintenance of the cancerous metabolism. For this reason, one of the main classes of anti-cancer drugs targeted to VDAC specifically aims at destroying this bond (**Figure 3A**, Group 2). **Clotrimazole**, an antimycotic drug used in the treatment of fungal infections, is one of the best known molecule able to inhibit glycolysis by inducing the detachment of mitochondrial-bound hexokinase and therefore triggering apoptosis in various mouse models of cancer (Penso and Beitner, 1998; Snajdrova et al., 1998; Palchaudhuri et al., 2008; Kadavakollu et al., 2014). Unfortunately, despite many attempts to increase its bioavailability (Abdel-Moety et al., 2002; Prabagar et al., 2007; Yong et al., 2007), clotrimazole still has limited success in clinical use because of its poor solubility in water. Numerous reports also describe **3-bromopyruvate (3BrPA)** and **methyl jasmonate** as drugs involved in tumor suppression through detachment of hexokinase from VDAC (Galluzzi et al., 2008, 2013; Goldin et al., 2008; Cohen and Flescher, 2009; Cardaci et al., 2012; Ko et al., 2012; Pedersen, 2012; Shoshan, 2012). The first one is a pyruvate analog whose binding probably expose sites previously occupied by HK2 making them available to pro-apoptotic molecules, thus promoting the release of cytochrome *c* from mitochondria (Chen et al., 2009; Nakano et al., 2012). Several *in vitro* studies confirmed the extremely high selectivity of 3BrPA for malignant cells (Pedersen, 2007; Nakano et al., 2011). For many reasons, that we have not the space to discuss here, it has not yet entered in formal clinical trials, albeit human administration of 3BrPA has been reported (Ko et al., 2012; El Sayed et al., 2014). Methyl jasmonate is instead a plant stress hormone of the jasmonate family that showed to be highly selective toward cancer cells and ineffective toward normal cells (Fingrut and Flescher, 2002) and to have the ability to act against drug resistant cells (Fingrut et al., 2005). Although with a somewhat different mechanism, it is also worth mentioning in this context the **2-deoxy glucose (2DG)** that, inhibiting the activity of HK2, indirectly prevents its binding to VDAC. According to Ben Sahra et al., treatment with 2DG would promote cancer cell apoptosis when used in combination with the anti-diabetic drug metformin (Ben Sahra et al., 2010). Currently, 2-deoxy glucose is in phase I/II trial for the treatment of advanced cancer and hormone refractory prostate cancer (ClinicalTrials.gov database, NIH). A potent anti-tumor activity has been as well described for **oroxilin A**, an O-methylated flavone found in *Scutellaria baicalensis* and *Oroxylum indicum*. Besides several studies demonstrating its ability to induce apoptosis (Hu et al., 2006; Li et al., 2009; Zhao et al., 2010), to arrest cell cycle (Yang et al., 2008) and suppress metastasis in many cancer cell types, it was reported that oroxylin A induces dissociation of HK2 from mitochoia in human breast carcinoma cell lines (Wei et al., 2013). Despite conflicting opinions about the essential role for VDAC and adenine nucleotide translocase (ANT) in permeability transition pore (PTP), a channel whose opening leads to mitochondrial depolarization, VDAC-ANT complex is still recognized as an anti-cancer target (Beutner et al., 1998; Neuzil et al., 2013; **Figure 3A**, Group 3). Compounds that act at that level are **lonidamine**, **arsenites,** and **steroid analogs** (Belzacq et al., 2001). Interestingly, the arsenite analog **4-(N-(S-glutathionylacetyl)amino) phenylarsenoxide (GSAO)** was shown to inhibit ANT and to selectively kill proliferating angiogenic endothelial cells, while being non-toxic to growth-arrested endothelial cells (Don et al., 2003).

Pro-apoptotic Molecules Controlling VDAC1 Expression Level

This third class of drugs includes few molecules. They act through less clear mechanisms than those described above, but all culminate in the modulation of VDAC expression levels (**Figure 3A**, Group 4). **Endostatin** is an example. The C-terminal globular domain of collagen XVIII is indeed a potent inhibitor of angiogenesis that promotes apoptosis by up-regulating VDAC1 expression. More specifically, this molecule seems to reduce HK2 expression, which, in turn, would lead to VDAC phosphorylation and accumulation (Yuan et al., 2008). **Myostatin,** a myokine of the transforming growth factor-β (TGF-β) superfamily, influences the expression levels of both HK2 and VDAC as well. Liu et al. proposed impaired VDAC and HK2 expression levels as responsible for HK2 dissociation from VDAC (Liu et al., 2013) and, consequently, for apoptosis induction in cancer cells. As reported in (Huang et al., 2015), **Cyathin-R** attenuates tumor growth and triggers apoptosis in Bax/Bak-deficient cells by modulating VDAC1 expression. This fungal-derived diterpenoid increases VDAC1 protein levels, thus supporting oligomerization that results in cell death. The involvement of VDAC is confirmed by the evidence that its silencing or inhibition of channel conductance and oligomerization completely abrogate Cyathin-R effects. Very recently, the marine metabolite **hierridin B** from *Cyanobium* sp. was proved to induce cytotoxicity selectively in HT-29 adenocarcinoma cells (Leão et al., 2013) through significant changes in VDAC1 mRNA expression and protein content (Freitas et al., 2016). From scarce information available, **arbutin**, a glycosylated hydroquinone extracted from the bearberry plant in the genus *Arctostaphylos* and widely used in cosmetics for its depigmenting effects would induce apoptosis in A375 human malignant melanoma cells by up-regulating VDAC1 (Nawarak et al., 2009).

Anti-apoptotic Molecules Impairing VDAC1 Oligomerization

Alzheimer's disease is characterized by an enanched expression levels of VDAC1 (Yoo et al., 2001; Cuadrado-Tejedor et al., 2011) and by reduced interaction of VDAC1 with the glycolityc enzymes HKs (Smilansky et al., 2015). These conditions increase VDAC1 propensity to form oligomers (Smilansky et al., 2015), promoting in turn the enhancement of apoptosis, with dramatic consequences for the early neuron's death (Mattson, 2000). Therefore, feasible therapeutic strategies to prevent apoptosis in AD include the downregulation of VDAC1 expression and/or the inhibition of VDAC1 oligomerization (**Figure 3B**, Group 1).

The 4,4′-diisothiocyanostilbene-2,2′-disulfonic acid, known as **DIDS**, is a calcium and chloride channel blocker (Cabantchik et al., 1978) which, when added to PLB-reconstituted VDAC1, is able to decrease the channel conductance (Thinnes et al., 1994). It has been demonstrated that DIDS exerts a pro-survival activity in HeLa cells treated with apoptotic inducers by preventing the activation of caspase-3, nuclear DNA fragmentation and cell volume decrease, common hallmarks of apoptosis activation (Benítez-Rangel et al., 2015). Although a direct inhibition of caspase's activity was recently proposed (Benítez-Rangel et al.,

2015), DIDS is able to counteract apoptosis at the early stage, by diminishing VDAC1 oligomerization and thus preventing cyt c release to the cytosol (Keinan et al., 2010). In fact, treatment of HeLa cells with DIDS was able to counteract the toxicity of staurosporine, an established apoptotic inducer, via VDAC1 oligomerization (Keinan et al., 2010). Very similar results were achieved by using DIDS analogs (**H_2DIDS, SITS, DPC**) which successfully counteracted cisplatin- or selenite-induced apoptosis in SH-SY5Y cells (a cell line commonly used as model of neurodegenerative diseases), again by diminishing the oligomerization of VDAC1 (Ben-Hail and Shoshan-Barmatz, 2016). The molecular mechanism correlating the channel block with VDAC1 oligomerization is not completely understood, even though several hypothesis have been proposed. For instance, DIDS binding to VDAC1 could interfere with Bax interaction with VDAC1 and, thus, formation of oligomers (Liu et al., 2008; Tajeddine et al., 2008).

A high-throughput compound screening approach led recently to the identification of other blockers exerting high specificity for VDAC1. One of them, called **AKOS-022**, was able to reduce significantly VDAC1 conductance at the PLB and decrease VDAC1 oligomerization already at micromolar concentration (Ben-Hail et al., 2016). Molecules based on the chemical structure of AKOS-022 were then synthetized, in order to maximize the anti-apoptotic effect. Among them, molecules named **VBIT-3** and **VIBT-4** have shown a pro-survival activity counteracting VDAC1 oligomerization in a pharmacological range of concentration and only in presence of VDAC1 overexpression, suggesting the pharmacological employment in AD (Ben-Hail et al., 2016).

Anti-apoptotic Molecules Modulating Post-translational Modification of VDAC1

VDAC1 is subject of post-translational modifications, such as phosphorylation, oxidation, and acetylation (Kerner et al., 2012; **Figure 3B**, Group 2). In particular, phosphorylation occurs in specific serine, tyrosine or threonine residues and leads to the modulation of the channel activity and the regulation of apoptosis (Bera et al., 1995; Banerjee and Gosh, 2006). Many kinases have been found involved in VDAC1 modification, e.g., the glycogen synthase kinase 3 beta (GSK3β) phosphorylates VDAC1 on threonine 51 (Martel et al., 2013). The phosphorylation of VDAC1 Thr 51 exerts a strong effect on the channel ability to bind HKs: as the phosphorylation extent increases, indeed, the affinity of the glycolytic enzyme for VDAC1 diminishes (Martel et al., 2013). Therefore, activation of GSK3β favors apoptosis by promoting HKs detachment from VDAC1. In AD, the activity of GSK3β is significantly enhanced, resulting in a cascade events which include VDAC1 phosphorylation, detachment of mitochondrial HK1 and activation of apoptosis (Martel et al., 2013). At the same time, the enhanced activity of GSK3β correlated with the accumulation of Aβ peptide and the phosphorylation of Tau (Jope and Johnson, 2004; Jope et al., 2007). **Hesperidin** is a flavonoid found in *citrus* with known anti-inflammatory and anti-oxidant properties. The employment of hesperidin in AD has shown to be protective in different pathological models: e.g., in rat, the flavonoid was able to significantly improve the cognitive impairments typical of the pathology, by decreasing both oxidative stress and apoptosis rate (Justin Thenmozhi et al., 2017). The protective effect of hesperidin in AD is due to the modulation of Akt/GSK-3β pathway, a cascade mechanism that involves VDAC1. Hesperidin, indeed, promotes the phosphorylation of Akt, which once activated, reduces GSK-3β activity (Wang et al., 2013). As consequence, the phosphorylation rate of VDAC1 is significantly reduced while HK1 binding to VDAC1 is improved, supporting cell metabolism and cell growth (Wang et al., 2013).

An analog mechanism was found also for the VDAC1 portion localizing on the plasma membrane (pl-VDAC) (Thinnes et al., 1989). pl-VDAC is particularly abundant in hippocampus and frontal cortex and localizes in specialized membrane regions called lipid rafts (Bàthori et al., 1999; De Pinto et al., 2010b), where together with caveolin-1 and the estrogen receptor α-like (mER), pl-VDAC forms a large protein complex (Ramirez et al., 2009; Herrera et al., 2011). As for the mitochondrial counterpart, pl-VDAC takes part in the control of the extrinsic pathway of apoptosis, by controlling ions transport across the membrane (Akanda et al., 2008; Thinnes, 2010). It has been proposed a key role of pl-VDAC in mediating Aβ-toxicity (Marin et al., 2007; Ramirez et al., 2009). Not coincidentally, pl-VDAC is expressed in brain regions with cognitive functions and thus more susceptible to AD. Experimental evidences have highlighted a protective effect of the estrogen **estradiol** against Aβ-toxicity in different AD models (Sherwin and Henry, 2008; Correia et al., 2010). Estradiol, indeed, modulates the phosphorylation level of pl-VDAC and its channel activity: when phosphorylated by estradiol, pl-VDAC is maintained in a closed and inactive form, which protects cells from apoptosis activation (Herrera et al., 2011). Conversely, the de-phosphorylation of pl-VDAC, operated by the antiestrogen tamoxifen, promotes channel opening, a mechanism which correlates directly with apoptosis (Herrera et al., 2011).

BIOLOGICAL MOLECULES AFFECTING VDAC FUNCTIONS

Pro-apoptotic Peptides Interfering With VDAC1-HKs Interaction

Anti-cancer peptides have primarily been designed to interfere with VDAC binding to some of its major interactors, such as hexokinase. These "interfering" peptides simply mimic VDAC or HK sequences strongly suspected to be involved in the protein-protein interaction: the rationale is to restrict the side effects generally associated to the utilization of chemical drugs. The mechanistic hypothesis behind the pro-apoptotic effects of peptides implies the establishment of a competition between them and the two interacting proteins (**Figure 3A**, Group 2). The first work to lead the way of using anti-tumor peptides was the paper by Arzoine and colleagues. In this report, synthetic peptides mimicking the N-terminal region and two cytoplasmic loops of VDAC, respectively **LP1**, **LP3**, and **LP4**, were found able to detach and even prevent hexokinase binding to VDAC (Arzoine et al., 2009). Subsequently, LP1 and LP4 peptides were further engineered by adding the *Antennapedia* homeodomain (HD*Antp*) from *Drosophila,* in order to increase their intracellular delivery. Interestingly, modified VDAC1-based peptides were proved to reduce the anti-apoptotic effects of Bcl-2 or Bcl-xL (Arbel and Shoshan-Barmatz, 2010; Arbel et al., 2012) and selectively kill Chronic Lymphocytic Leukemia cells (Prezma et al., 2013). Peptides designed on the first 15 amino acid residues of HK1 have been shown to induce apoptosis in different cancer cell types as well (Gelb et al., 1992). Beside those based on VDAC and HK1 sequences, also a peptide from *Lactobacillus casei* peptidoglycan has been reported to exert antitumor activity by detaching mitochondrial-bound hexokinase (Fichera et al., 2016). There are only few information regarding the existence of anticancer peptides able to directly inhibit VDAC activity. An example is **Mastoparan**, a peptide contained in wasp venom and initially considered capable of triggering apoptosis via VDAC binding (Shol'-ts et al., 1984; Pfeiffer et al., 1995). Recently, however, the pro-apoptotic effect of mastoparan has been associated to its ability to interact with the phospholipid phase of the membrane (Yamamoto et al., 2014). The structural analog, the highly cytotoxic **Mitoparan** (MitP) targets mitochondria and induces apoptosis in human cancer cells, with a mechanism in which the involvement of VDAC was not completely demonstrated (Jones et al., 2008). A single report makes the chimeric **TEAM-VP peptide,** composed of a short sequence from HIV-1 Vpr (Viral protein R) fused with a cyclic RGD motif, a member of this class. According to Borgne-Sanchez et al. (2007) indeed, TEAM-VP would induce apoptosis in endothelial cells by binding both ANT and VDAC.

Pro-survival Peptides Contrasting Interaction of Misfolded Protein With VDAC1

A common feature of neurodegenerative diseases is represented by the accumulation of misfolded protein and peptides upon the cytosolic surface of mitochondria or to the VDAC1. Both Aβ peptide and hyper-phosphorylated Tau co-immuno-precipitated with VDAC1 in AD patients and in 3xTg-AD mice (Manczak and Reddy, 2012). Similarly, αSyn was found co-precipitated with VDAC1 in *substantia nigra* of a rat model of PD (Lu et al., 2013). In the neuromuscular disorder ALS, several mutants, but not wild-type, SOD1 were found co-precipitated with VDAC1 exclusively in spinal cord's mitochondria (Israelson et al., 2010). The addition of misfolded proteins to the PLB-reconstituted VDAC1 resulted in a strong inhibition of channel conductance (Israelson et al., 2010; Magrì et al., 2016b), suggesting an impairment of metabolite exchanges through VDAC1. At the same time, as the misfolded proteins interact with VDAC1, the amount of HKs on the mitochondrial surface decreases (Smilansky et al., 2015; Magrì et al., 2016b), possibly altering apoptosis. In this contest, synthetic peptides mimicking specific protein domains can represent a promising therapeutic strategy: they are aimed to bind the bait proteins (for example VDAC1 itself), clogging the docking site normally available for the interaction with other protein(s) (**Figure 3B**, Group 3).

A first strategy consisted in the development of VDAC1-based peptides aimed to bind misfolded proteins. The N-terminal domain of VDAC1, including the first 26 amino acid residues, is commonly considered the mobile part and an exposed moiety of the protein, putatively involved in the binding of cytosolic proteins in physiological conditions (Shi et al., 2003; Geula et al., 2012), as well as of Aβ peptide in AD (Thinnes, 2011). Therefore, a peptide based on the first 26 amino-terminal residues of VDAC1, named VDAC1-N-Term peptide, was recently developed (Smilansky et al., 2015). By exploiting several techniques, such as Surface Plasmon Resonance, the ability of VDAC1-N-Term to bind Aβ peptide was confirmed (Smilansky et al., 2015). Moreover, treatment of PC12 cells with VDAC1-N-Term peptide, in presence of external Aβ, significantly reduces Aβ uptake within the cells as well as the Aβ-induced apoptosis (Smilansky et al., 2015), suggesting a protective role exerted by the peptide against Aβ. As for the mitochondrial VDAC1, the pl-VDAC is suspected to mediate the extracellular Aβ toxicity, possibly promoting the peptide internalization (Thinnes, 2011): in fact, SHSY5Y cells overexpressing pl-VDAC are much sensitive to Aβ peptide toxicity (Smilansky et al., 2015). Therefore, VDAC1-N-Term peptide decreases Aβ internalization and toxicity by binding Aβ, preventing thus its intracellular accumulation (Smilansky et al., 2015).

A second strategy consisted in the development of peptides able to bind VDAC1 and based onto the most known VDAC1 interacting proteins, such as HK1. This strategy was successfully applied in an ALS model, which is characterized by lower HKs expression in affected tissue (Magrì et al., 2016b; Magrì and Messina, 2017). In particular, a small peptide, corresponding to the sequence 2–12 of N-terminal domain of HK1, was developed, since this region is commonly recognized as important for the interaction with VDAC1. Again, *in vitro* techniques were used to prove the interaction of this peptide, named NHK1, with VDAC1 (Magrì et al., 2016b). Furthermore, by binding VDAC1, NHK1 impairs the interaction of SOD1 G93A with the channel as well as accumulation of SOD1 mutant on the cytosolic surface of MOM (Magrì et al., 2016b). Moreover, if expressed in NSC34 cells (a commonly recognized ALS cell line model), NHK1 is able to impair toxicity mediated by SOD1 G93A overexpression (Magrì et al., 2016b). Overall, the results suggest that NHK1 binds VDAC1 and counteracts the binding of SOD1 G93A with a very simple mechanism (Magrì et al., 2016b). Although no experimental evidence are available so far, it is however possible to hypothesize a similar application also in other pathological model, such as PD or AD, in which NHK1 could reduce the affinity of αSyn or Aβ for VDAC1.

Oligonucleotides and microRNAs With Pro- or Anti-apoptotic Features

A pharmacological molecule that appears to exploit VDAC as a mitochondrial target is **G3139**, an 18-mer phosphorothioate anti-sense oligonucleotide complementary to the first six codons of Bcl-2 mRNA. This drug has entered phase III clinical trials in different human cancers (O'Brien et al., 2007; Moulder et al., 2008; Rai et al., 2008) because of its selective and specific down-regulation of Bcl-2 expression. Beside this effect, *in vitro* experiments with PLB indicated the attitude of G3139 to directly bind VDAC1 and to reduce channel conductance (Lai et al., 2006; Tan et al., 2007). Hence, exposure of isolated mitochondria to G3139 results in VDAC closure, accumulation of mitochondrial ROS and onset of cell death (Aggarwal et al., 2003; Tikunov et al., 2010).

Today, microRNAs (miRNAs) definitely represent an emerging tool in the treatment of cancer and neurodegenerative diseases. These molecules are short single-stranded RNAs of 21–24 nucleotides complementary to the 3′-end or, more rarely, to the 5′-end of mRNAs transcribed from target genes. Physiologically, microRNAs regulate gene expression at both transcriptional and post-translational level. Hence, because of their indispensable role in the control of numerous biological processes including cell cycle, cell growth, and apoptosis (Siomi and Siomi, 2010), considerable changes in their expression profiles have been associated with various diseases. In cancer, for instance, the simultaneous expression increase of miRNAs that act as oncogenes and decrease of others functioning like tumor-suppressors has been described (Di Leva et al., 2012). As the main actor in the Warburg metabolism, together with hexokinase, VDAC has been proposed as a target of miRNA modulation (Bargaje et al., 2012; Chaudhuri et al., 2016; Wang et al., 2016). Although there are still very few available data, the small non-coding RNA miR-7 would down-regulate the oncogene VDAC1 in hepatocarcinoma tissues, affecting cell proliferation and metastasis (Wang et al., 2016). Interestingly, Chaudhuri et al. described also a protective effect of miR-7 in cellular models of Parkinson disease, where it prevents depolarization of mitochondria by directly down-regulating VDAC (Chaudhuri et al., 2016) (**Figure 3B**, Group 4).

CONCLUSIONS

This work focused on the significant contribution of VDAC in cancer and neurodegeneration, two types of diseases apparently different from each other. The detailed list reported above shows that all the pharmacological molecules, peptides and mRNAs described in the literature as targeted to VDAC are potentially effective in the therapeutic treatment of these pathologies. It is noticeable that numerous compounds able to induce apoptosis in cancer cells by modulating VDAC are already part of promising clinical trials. Many others, however, have been tested only *in vitro* or *in cellulo* and probably never will be applied in humans because of high toxicity or delivery difficulties. With regard to neurodegenerative diseases, the molecules that proved to suppress apoptosis and thus promote cell survival are still very few. This happens most likely because the molecular mechanisms underlying these disorders are still less characterized than those that define cancer. Although much remains to be to cover and uncover on the physiological role of VDAC in mitochondrial function and dysfunction, the overall data emphasize that targeted drugs and genetic approaches acting on VDAC represent encouraging strategies to treat a wide range of human diseases.

AUTHOR CONTRIBUTIONS

AM and SR: collected the information and reference list for the manuscript. They also draw the figures. VDP: wrote the main part of the text and edited it.

FUNDING

This work was supported by the Italian Ministero dell'Istruzione, dell'Università e della Ricerca, MIUR, (PRIN project 2015795S5W_005) and by the FIR-UNICT project 2014 to VDP. AM is recipient of Fondazione Umberto Veronesi post-doctoral fellowship.

REFERENCES

Abdel-Moety, E. M., Khattab, F. I., Kelani, K. M., and AbouAl- Alamein, A. M. (2002). Chromatographic determination of clotrimazole, ketoconazole and fluconazole in pharmaceutical formulations. *Il Farmaco* 57, 931–938. doi: 10.1016/S0014-827X(02)01270-3

Abrams, T. J., Lee, L. B., Murray, L. J., Pryer, N. K., and Cherrington, J. M. (2003). SU11248 inhibits KIT and platelet-derived growth factor receptor beta in preclinical models of human small cell lung cancer. *Mol. Cancer Ther.* 2, 471–478.

Abu-Hamad, S., Zaid, H., Israelson, A., Nahon, E., and Shoshan-Barmatz, V. (2008). Hexokinase-I protection against apoptotic cell death is mediated via interaction with the voltage-dependent anion channel-1: mapping the site of binding. *J. Biol. Chem.* 283, 13482–13490. doi: 10.1074/jbc.M708216200

Adams, J. M., and Cory, S. (2007). The Bcl-2 apoptotic switch in cancer development and therapy. *Oncogene* 26, 1324–1337. doi: 10.1038/sj.onc.1210220

Aggarwal, B. B., Kumar, A., and Bharti, A. C. (2003). Anticancer potential of curcumin: preclinical and clinical studies. *Anticancer Res.* 23, 363–398.

Aiello, R., Messina, A., Schiffler, B., Benz, R., Tasco, G., Casadio, R., et al. (2004). Functional characterization of a second porin isoform in *Drosophila melanogaster*. DmPorin2 forms voltage-independent cation selective pores. *J. Biol. Chem.* 279, 25364–25373. doi: 10.1074/jbc.M310572200

Akanda, N., Tofighi, R., Brask, J., Tamm, C., Elinder, F., and Ceccatelli, S. (2008). Voltage-dependent anion channels (VDAC) in the plasma membrane play a critical role in apoptosis in differentiated hippocampal neurons but not in neural stem cells. *Cell Cycle* 7, 3225–3234. doi: 10.4161/cc.7.20.6831

Anghileri, L. J. (1975). The *in vivo* inhibition of tumor growth by ruthenium red: its relationship with the metabolism of calcium in the tumor. *Z. Krebsforsch Klin. Onkol. Cancer. Res. Clin. Oncol.* 83, 213–217. doi: 10.1007/BF00304090

Arbel, N., and Shoshan-Barmatz, V. (2010). Voltage-dependent anion channel 1-based peptides interact with bcl-2 to prevent antiapoptotic activity. *J. Biol. Chem.* 285, 6053–6062. doi: 10.1074/jbc.M109.082990

Arbel, N., Ben-Hail, D., and Shoshan-Barmatz, V. (2012). Mediation of the anti-apoptotic activity of BCL-XL upon interaction with VDAC1. *J. Biol. Chem.* 287, 23152–23161. doi: 10.1074/jbc.M112.345918

Arzoine, L., Zilberberg, N., Ben-Romano, R., and Shoshan- Barmatz, V. (2009). Voltage-dependent anion channel 1-based peptides interact with hexokinase to prevent its anti-apoptotic activity. *J. Biol. Chem.* 284, 3946–3955. doi: 10.1074/jbc.M803614200

Baines, C. P., Kaiser, R. A., Sheiko, T., Craigen, W. J., and Molkentin, J. D. (2007). Voltage-dependent anion channels are dispensable for mitochondrial-dependent cell death. *Nat. Cell. Biol.* 9, 550–555. doi: 10.1038/ncb1575

Banerjee, J., and Gosh, S. (2006). Phosphorylation of rat brain mitochondrial voltage-dependent anion as a potential tool to control leakage of cytochrome c. *J. Neurochem.* 98, 670–676. doi: 10.1111/j.1471-4159.2006.03853.x

Bargaje, R., Gupta, S., Sarkeshik, A., Park, R., Xu, T., Sarkar, M., et al. (2012). Identification of novel targets for miR-29a using miRNA proteomics. *PLoS ONE* 7:e43243. doi: 10.1371/journal.pone.0043243

Bàthori, G., Parolini, I., Tombola, F., Szabò, I., Messina, A., Oliva, M., et al. (1999). Porin is present in the plasma membrane where it is concentrated in caveolae and caveolae-related domains. *J. Biol. Chem.* 274, 29607–29612. doi: 10.1074/jbc.274.42.29607

Bayrhuber, M., Meins, T., Habeck, M., Becker, S., Giller, K., Villinger, S., et al. (2008). Structure of the human voltage-dependent anion channel. *Proc. Natl. Acad. Sci. U.S.A.* 105, 15370–15375. doi: 10.1073/pnas.0808115105

Belzacq, A. S., El Hamel, C., Vieira, H. L., Cohen, I., Haouzi, D., Metiviér, D., et al. (2001). Adenine nucleotide translocator mediates the mitochondrial membrane permeabilization induced by lonidamine, arsenite and CD437. *Oncogene* 20, 7579–7587. doi: 10.1038/sj.onc.1204953

Ben Sahra, I., Laurent, K., Giuliano, S., Larbret, F., Ponzio, G., Gounon, P., et al. (2010). Targeting cancer cell metabolism: the combination of metformin and 2-deoxyglucose induces p53-dependent apoptosis in prostate cancer cells. *Cancer Res.* 70, 2465–2475. doi: 10.1158/0008-5472.CAN-09-2782

Ben-Hail, D., and Shoshan-Barmatz, V. (2016). VDAC1-interacting anion transport inhibitors inhibit VDAC1 oligomerization and apoptosis. *Biochim. Biophys. Acta* 1863, 1612–1623. doi: 10.1016/j.bbamcr.2016.04.002

Ben-Hail, D., Begas-Shvartz, R., Shalev, M., Shteinfer-Kuzmine, A., Gruzman, A., Reina, S., et al. (2016). Novel compounds targeting the mitochondrial protein VDAC1 inhibit apoptosis and protect against mitochondria dysfunction. *J. Biol. Chem.* 291, 24986–25003. doi: 10.1074/jbc.M116.744284

Benítez-Rangel, E., López-Méndez, M. C., García, L., and Guerrero-Hernández, A. (2015). DIDS (4,4'-Diisothiocyanatostilbene-2,2'-disulfonate) directly inhibits caspase activity in HeLa cell lysates. *Cell Death Discov.* 1:15037. doi: 10.1038/cddiscovery.2015.37

Benz, R. (1994). Permeation of hydrophilic solutes through mitochondrial outer membranes: review on mitochondrial porins. *Biochim. Biophys. Acta* 1197, 167–196. doi: 10.1016/0304-4157(94)90004-3

Benz, R., Schmid, A., and Dihanik, M. (1989). Pores from mitochondrial outer membranes of yeast and a porin deficient yeast mutant: a comparison. *J. Bioenerg. Biomembr.* 21, 439–450. doi: 10.1007/BF00762516

Benz, R., Wojtczak, L., Bosch, W., and Brdiczka, D. (1988). Inhibition of adenine nucleotide transport through the mitochondrial porin by a synthetic polyanion. *FEBS Lett.* 231, 75–80. doi: 10.1016/0014-5793(88)80706-3

Bera, A. K., Ghosh, S., and Das, S. (1995). Mitochondrial VDAC can be phosphorylated by cyclic AMP-dependent protein kinase. *Biochem. Biophys Res Commun.* 209, 213–217. doi: 10.1006/bbrc.1995.1491

Bernardi, P. (1999). Mitochondrial transport of cations: channels, exchangers, and permeability transition. *Physiol. Rev.* 79, 1127–1155. doi: 10.1152/physrev.1999.79.4.1127

Beutner, G., Rück, A., Riede, B., and Brdiczka, D. (1998). Complexes between porin, hexokinase, mitochondrial creatine kinase and adenylate translocator display properties of the permeability transition pore. Implication for regulation of permeability transition by the kinases. *Biochim. Biophys. Acta* 1368, 7–18. doi: 10.1016/S0005-2736(97)00175-2

Borgne-Sanchez, A., Dupont, S., Langonné, A., Baux, L., Lecoeur, H., Chauvier, D., et al. (2007). Targeted Vpr-derived peptides reach mitochondria to induce apoptosis of alphaVbeta3- expressing endothelial cells. *Cell Death Differ.* 14, 422–435. doi: 10.1038/sj.cdd.4402018

Brandes, L. J., Arron, R. J., Bogdanovic, R. P., Tong, J., Zaborniak, C. L., Hogg, G. R., et al. (1992). Stimulation of malignant growth in rodents by antidepressant drugs at clinically relevant doses. *Cancer Res.* 52, 3796–3800.

Brdiczka, D., Kaldis, P., and Wallimann, T. (1994). *in vitro* complex formation between the octamer of mitochondrial creatine kinase and porin. *J. Biol. Chem.* 269, 27640–27644.

Brenner, C., and Lemoine, A. (2014). Mitochondrial proteins (e.g., VDAC, Bcl-2, HK, ANT) as major control points in oncology. *Front. Oncol.* 4:365. doi: 10.3389/fonc.2014.00365

Cabantchik, Z. I., Knauf, P. A., and Rothstein, A. (1978). The anion transport system of the red blood cell. The role of membrane protein evaluated by the use of probes. *Biochim. Biophys. Acta* 515, 239–302. doi: 10.1016/0304-4157(78)90016-3

Campbell, A. M., and Chan, S. H. (2008). Mitochondrial membrane cholesterol, the voltage dependent anion channel (VDAC), and the Warburg effect. *J. Bioenerg. Biomembr.* 40, 193–197. doi: 10.1007/s10863-008-9138-x

Cardaci, S., Desideri, E., and Ciriolo, M. R. (2012). Targeting aerobic glycolysis: 3-bromopyruvate as a promising anticancer drug. *J. Bioenerg. Biomembr.* 44, 17–29. doi: 10.1007/s10863-012-9422-7

Carroll, R. E., Benya, R. V., Turgeon, D. K., Vareed, S., Neuman, M., Rodriguez, L., et al. (2011). Phase IIa clinical trial of curcumin for the prevention of colorectal neoplasia. *Cancer Prev. Res.* 4, 354–364. doi: 10.1158/1940-6207.CAPR-10-0098

Cesura, A. M., Pinard, E., Schubenel, R., Goetschy, V., Friedlein, A., and Langen, H., et al. (2003). The voltage dependent anion channel is the target for a new class of inhibitors of the mitochondrial Permeability Transition Pore. *J. Biol. Chem.* 278, 49812–49818. doi: 10.1074/jbc.M304748200

Chaudhuri, A. D., Choi, D. C., Kabaria, S., Tran, A., and Junn, E. (2016). MicroRNA-7 Regulates the function of mitochondrial permeability transition pore by targeting VDAC1 expression. *J. Biol. Chem.* 291, 6483–6493. doi: 10.1074/jbc.M115.691352

Checchetto, V., Reina, S., Magrì, A., Szabo, I., and De Pinto, V. (2014). Recombinant human Voltage Dependent Anion selective Channel isoform 3 (hVDAC3) forms pores with a very small conductance. *Cell Physiol. Biochem.* 34, 842–853. doi: 10.1159/000363047

Chen, Z., Zhang, H., Lu, W., and Huang, P. (2009). Role of mitochondria-associated hexokinase II in cancer cell death induced by 3-bromopyruvate. *Biochim. Biophys. Acta* 1787, 553–660. doi: 10.1016/j.bbabio.2009.03.003

Cheng, E. H., Sheiko, T. V., Fisher, J. K., Craigen, W. J., and Korsmeyer, S. J. (2003). VDAC2 inhibits BAK activation and mitochondrial apoptosis. *Science* 301, 513–517. doi: 10.1126/science.1083995

Chu, X., Wei, M., Yang, X., Cao, Q., Xie, X., Guan, M., et al. (2012). Effects of an anthraquinone derivative from Rheum officinale Baill, emodin, on airway responses in a murine model of asthma. *Food Chem. Toxicol.* 50, 2368–2375. doi: 10.1016/j.fct.2012.03.076

Cohen, S., and Flescher, E. (2009). Methyl jasmonate: a plant stress hormone as an anti-cancer drug. *Phytochemistry* 70, 1600–1609. doi: 10.1016/j.phytochem.2009.06.007

Colombini, M. (1980). Structure and mode of action of a voltage dependent anion-selective channel (VDAC) located in the outer mitochondrial membrane. *Ann. N. Y. Acad. Sci.* 341, 552–563. doi: 10.1111/j.1749-6632.1980.tb47198.x

Colombini, M., Yeung, C. L., Tung, J., and König, T. (1987). The mitochondrial outer membrane channel, VDAC, is regulated by a synthetic polyanion. *Biochim. Biophys. Acta* 905, 279–286. doi: 10.1016/0005-2736(87)90456-1

Correia, S. C., Santos, R. X., Cardoso, S., Carvalho, C., Santos, M. S., Oliveira, C. R., et al. (2010). Effects of estrogen in the brain: is it a neuroprotective agent in Alzheimer's disease? *Curr. Aging Sci.* 3, 113–126. doi: 10.2174/1874609811003020113

Cuadrado-Tejedor, M., Vilariño, M., Cabodevilla, F., Del Río, J., Frechilla, D., and Pérez Mediavilla, A. (2011). Enhanced expression of the voltage-dependent anion channel 1 (VDAC1) in Alzheimer's disease transgenic mice: an insight into the pathogenic effects of amyloid-beta. *J. Alzheimers Dis.* 23, 195–206. doi: 10.3233/JAD-2010-100966

De Pinto, V., al Jamal, J. A., and Palmieri, F. (1993). Location of the dicyclohexylcarbodiimide-reactive glutamate residue in the bovine heart mitochondrial porin. *J. Biol. Chem.* 268, 12977–12982.

De Pinto, V., Benz, R., Caggese, C., and Palmieri, F. (1989). Characterization of the mitochondrial porin from *Drosophila melanogaster*. *Biochim. Biophys. Acta* 987, 1–7. doi: 10.1016/0005-2736(89)90447-1

De Pinto, V., Guarino, F., Guarnera, A., Messina, A., Reina, S., Tomasello, F. M., et al. (2010a). Characterization of human VDAC isoforms: a peculiar function for VDAC3? *Biochim. Biophys. Acta* 1797, 1268–1275. doi: 10.1016/j.bbabio.2010.01.031

De Pinto, V., Messina, A., Lane, D. J., and Lawen, A. (2010b). Voltage-dependent anion selective channel (VDAC) in the plasma membrane. *FEBS Lett.* 584, 1793–1799. doi: 10.1016/j.febslet.2010.02.049

De Pinto, V., Reina, S., Gupta, A., Messina, A., and Mahalakshmi, R. (2016). Role of cysteines in mammalian VDAC isoforms' function. *Biochim. Biophys. Acta* 1857, 1219–1227. doi: 10.1016/j.bbabio.2016.02.020

De Stefani, D., Bononi, A., Romagnoli, A., Messina, A., De Pinto, V., Pinton, P., et al. (2012). VDAC1 selectively transfers apoptotic Ca^{2+} signals to mitochondria. *Cell Death Differ.* 19, 267–273. doi: 10.1038/cdd.2011.92

Dhillon, N., Aggarwal, B. B., Newman, R. A., Wolff, R. A., Kunnumakkara, A. B., Abbruzzese, J. L., et al. (2008). Phase II trial of curcumin in patients with advanced pancreatic cancer. *Clin. Cancer Res.* 14, 4491–4499. doi: 10.1158/1078-0432.CCR-08-0024

Di Leva, G., Briskin, D., and Croce, C. M. (2012). MicroRNA in cancer: new hopes for antineoplastic chemotherapy. *Ups. J. Med. Sci.* 117, 202–216. doi: 10.3109/03009734.2012.660551

Don, A. S., Kisker, O., Dilda, P., Donoghue, N., Zhao, X., Decollogne, S., et al. (2003). A peptide trivalent arsenical inhibits tumor angiogenesis by perturbing mitochondrial function in angiogenic endothelial cells. *Cancer Cell* 3, 497–509. doi: 10.1016/S1535-6108(03)00109-0

El Sayed, S. M., Mohamed, W. G., Seddik, M. A., Ahmed, A. S., Mahmoud, A. G., Amer, W. H., et al. (2014). Safety and outcome of treatment of metastatic melanoma using 3- bromopyruvate: a concise literature review and case study. *Chin. J. Cancer* 33, 356–364. doi: 10.5732/cjc.013.10111

Fichera, G. A., Fichera, M., and Milone, G. (2016). Antitumoural activity of a cytotoxic peptide of *Lactobacillus casei* peptidoglycan and its interaction with mitochondrial-bound hexokinase. *Antic. Drugs* 27, 609–619. doi: 10.1097/CAD.0000000000000367

Fiek, C., Benz, R., Roos, N., and Brdiczka, D. (1982). Evidence for identity between the hexokinase-binding protein and the mitochondrial porin in the outer membrane of rat liver mitochondrial. *Biochim. Biophys. Acta* 688, 429–440. doi: 10.1016/0005-2736(82)90354-6

Fingrut, O., and Flescher, E. (2002). Plant stress hormones suppress the proliferation and induce apoptosis in human cancer cells. *Leukemia* 16, 608–616. doi: 10.1038/sj.leu.2402419

Fingrut, O., Reischer, D., Rotem, R., Goldin, N., Altboum, I., Zan-Bar, I., et al. (2005). Jasmonates induce nonapoptotic death in high-resistance mutant p53-expressing Blymphoma cells. *Br. J. Pharmacol.* 146, 800–808. doi: 10.1038/sj.bjp.0706394

Freitas, S., Martins, R., Costa, M., Leão, P. N., Vitorino, R., Vasconcelos, V., et al. (2016). Hierridin B isolated from a marine cyanobacterium alters VDAC1, mitochondrial activity, and cell cycle genes on HT-29 colon adenocarcinoma cells. *Mar. Drugs* 14:E158. doi: 10.3390/md14090158

Gaikwad, A., Poblenz, A., Haridas, V., Zhang, C., Duvic, M., and Gutterman, J. (2005). Triterpenoid electrophiles (avicins) suppress heat shock protein-70 and x-linked inhibitor of apoptosis proteins in malignant cells by activation of ubiquitin machinery: implications for proapoptotic activity. *Clin. Cancer Res.* 11, 1953–1962. doi: 10.1158/1078-0432.CCR-04-1704

Galluzzi, L., Kepp, O., Tajeddine, N., and Kroemer, G. (2008). Disruption of the hexokinase-VDAC complex for tumor therapy. *Oncogene* 27, 4633–4635. doi: 10.1038/onc.2008.114

Galluzzi, L., Kepp, O., Vander Heiden, M. G., and Kroemer, G. (2013). Metabolic targets for cancer therapy. *Nat. Rev. Drug Discov.* 12, 829–846. doi: 10.1038/nrd4145

Gatenby, R. A., and Gillies, R. J. (2004). Why do cancers have high aerobic glycolysis? *Nat. Rev. Cancer* 4, 891–899. doi: 10.1038/nrc1478

Gattin, Z., Schneider, R., Laukat, Y., Giller, K., Maier, E., Zweckstetter, M., et al. (2015). Solid-state NMR, electrophysiology and molecular dynamics characterization of human VDAC2. *J. Biomol. NMR* 61, 311–320. doi: 10.1007/s10858-014-9876-5

Gelb, B. D., Adams, V., Jones, S. N., Griffin, L. D., MacGregor, G. R., and McCabe, E. R. (1992). Targeting of hexokinase 1 to liver and hepatoma mitochondria. *Proc. Natl. Acad. Sci. U.S.A.* 89, 202–206. doi: 10.1073/pnas.89.1.202

Geula, S., Ben-Hail, D., and Shoshan-Barmatz, V. (2012). Structure-based analysis of VDAC1: N-terminus location, translocation, channel gating and association with antiapoptotic proteins. *Biochem. J.* 444, 475–485. doi: 10.1042/BJ20112079

Goldin, N., Arzoine, L., Heyfets, A., Israelson, A., Zaslavsky, Z., Bravman, T., et al. (2008). Methyl jasmonate binds to and detaches mitochondria-bound hexokinase. *Oncogene* 27, 4636–4643. doi: 10.1038/onc.2008.108

Green, D. R., and Evan, G. I. (2002). A matter of life and death. *Cancer Cell* 1, 19–30. doi: 10.1016/S1535-6108(02)00024-7

Gross, A., Jockel, J., Wei, M. C., and Korsmeyer, S. J. (1998). Enforced dimerization of BAX results in its translocation, mitochondrial dysfunction and apoptosis. *EMBO J.* 17, 3878–3885. doi: 10.1093/emboj/17.14.3878

Guardiani, C., Magrì, A., Karachitos, A., Di Rosa, M. C., Reina, S., Bodrenko, I., et al. (2018). yVDAC2, the second mitochondrial porin isoform of *Saccharomyces cerevisiae*. *Biochim. Biophys. Acta* 1859, 270–279. doi: 10.1016/j.bbabio.2018.01.008

Halestrap, A. P., Connern, C. P., Griffiths, E. J., and Kerr, P. M. (1997). Cyclosporin A binding to mitochondrial cyclophilin inhibits the permeability transition pore and protects hearts from ischaemia/reperfusion injury. *Mol. Cell. Biochem.* 174, 167–172. doi: 10.1023/A:1006879618176

Han, D., Antunes, F., Canali, R., Rettori, D., and Cadenas, E. (2003). Voltage-dependent anion channels control the release of the superoxide anion from mitochondria to cytosol. *J. Biol. Chem.* 278, 5557–5563. doi: 10.1074/jbc.M210269200

Haridas, V., Higuchi, M., Jayatilake, G. S., Bailey, D., Mujoo, K., Blake, M. E., et al. (2001). Avicins: triterpenoid saponins from *Acacia victoriae* (Bentham) induce apoptosis by mitochondrial perturbation. *Proc. Natl. Acad. Sci. U.S.A.* 98, 5821–5826. doi: 10.1073/pnas.101619098

Haridas, V., Li, X., Mizumachi, T., Higuchi, M., Lemeshko, V. V., Colombini, M., et al. (2007). Avicins, a novel plant-derived metabolite lowers energy metabolism in tumor cells by targeting the outer mitochondrial membrane. *Mitochondrion* 7, 234–240. doi: 10.1016/j.mito.2006.12.005

Head, S. A., Shi, W., Zhao, L., Gorshkov, K., Pasunooti, K., Chen, Y., et al. (2015). Antifungal drug itraconazole targets VDAC1 to modulate the AMPK/mTOR signaling axis in endothelial cells. *Proc. Natl. Acad. Sci. U.S.A.* 112, 7276–7285. doi: 10.1073/pnas.1512867112

Herrera, J. L., Diaz, M., Hernández-Fernaud, J. R., Salido, E., Alonso, R., Fernández, C., et al. (2011). Voltage-dependent anion channel as a resident protein of lipid rafts: post-transductional regulation by estrogens and involvement in neuronal preservation against Alzheimer's disease. *J. Neurochem.* 116, 820–827. doi: 10.1111/j.1471-4159.2010.06987.x

Hiller, S., Garces, R. G., Malia, T. J., Orekhov, V. Y., Colombini, M., and Wagner, G. (2008). Solution structure of the integral human membrane protein VDAC-1 in detergent micelles. *Science* 321, 1206–1210. doi: 10.1126/science.1161302

Hodge, T., and Colombini, M. (1997). Regulation of metabolite flux through voltage-gating of VDAC channels. *J. Membr. Biol.* 157, 271–279. doi: 10.1007/s002329900235

Hu, Y., Yang, Y., You, Q. D., Liu, W., Gu, H. Y., Zhao, L., et al. (2006). Oroxylin A induced apoptosis of human hepatocellular carcinoma cell line HepG2 was involved in its antitumor activity. *Biochem. Biophys. Res. Commun.* 351, 521–527. doi: 10.1016/j.bbrc.2006.10.064

Huang, L., Han, J., Ben-Hail, D., He, L., Li, B., Chen, Z., et al. (2015). A new fungal diterpene induces VDAC1-dependent apoptosis in Bax/Bak-deficient cells. *J. Biol. Chem.* 290, 23563–23578. doi: 10.1074/jbc.M115.648774

Israelson, A., Arbel, N., Da Cruz, S., Ilieva, H., Yamanaka, K., Shoshan-Barmatz, V., et al. (2010). Misfolded mutant SOD1 directly inhibits VDAC1 conductance in a mouse model of inherited ALS. *Neuron* 67, 575–587. doi: 10.1016/j.neuron.2010.07.019

Israelson, A., Zaid, H., Abu-Hamad, S., Nahon, E., and Shoshan-Barmatz, V. (2008). Mapping the ruthenium red-binding site of the voltage-dependent anion channel-1. *Cell Calcium* 43, 196–204. doi: 10.1016/j.ceca.2007.05.006

Jones, S., Martel, C., Belzacq-Casagrande, A. S., Brenner, C., and Howl, J. (2008). Mitoparan and target-selective chimeric analogs: membrane translocation and intracellular redistribution induces mitochondrial apoptosis. *Biochim. Biophys. Acta* 1783, 849–863. doi: 10.1016/j.bbamcr.2008.01.009

Jope, R. S., and Johnson, G. V. (2004). The glamour and gloom of glycogen synthase kinase-3. *Trends Biochem. Sci.* 29, 95–102. doi: 10.1016/j.tibs.2003.12.004

Jope, R. S., Yuskaitis, C. J., and Beurel, E. (2007). Glycogen synthase kinase-3 (GSK3): inflammation, diseases, and therapeutics. *Neurochem. Res.* 32, 577–595. doi: 10.1007/s11064-006-9128-5

Justin Thenmozhi, A., William Raja, T. R., Manivasagam, T., Janakiraman, U., and Essa, M. M. (2017). Hesperidin ameliorates cognitive dysfunction, oxidative stress and apoptosis against aluminium chloride induced rat model of Alzheimer's disease. *Nutr. Neurosci.* 20, 360–368. doi: 10.1080/1028415X.2016.1144846

Kadavakollu, S., Stailey, C., Kunapareddy, C. S., and White, S. (2014). Clotrimazole as a cancer drug: a short review. *Med. Chem.* 4, 722–724. doi: 10.4172/2161-0444.1000219

Keeble, J. A., and Gilmore, A. P. (2007). Apoptosis commitment-translating survival signals into decisions on mitochondria. *Cell Res.* 17, 976–984. doi: 10.1038/cr.2007.101

Keinan, N., Tyomkin, D., and Shoshan-Barmatz, V. (2010). Oligomerization of the mitochondrial protein voltage-dependent anion channel is coupled to the induction of apoptosis. *Mol. Cell. Biol.* 30, 5698–5709. doi: 10.1128/MCB.00165-10

Kerner, J., Lee, K., Tandler, B., and Hoppel, C. L. (2012). VDAC proteomics: post-translation modifications. *Biochim. Biophys. Acta* 1818, 1520–1525. doi: 10.1016/j.bbamem.2011.11.013

Khan, A. B., D'Souza, B. J., Wharam, M. D., Champion, L. A., Sinks, L. F., Woo, S. Y., et al. (1982). Cisplatin therapy in recurrent childhood brain tumors. *Cancer Treat. Rep.* 66, 2013–2020.

Ko, Y. H., Verhoeven, H. A., Lee, M. J., Corbin, D. J., Vogl, T. J., and Pedersen, P. L. (2012). A translational study "case report" on the small molecule "energy blocker" 3-bromopyruvate (3BP) as a potent anticancer agent: from bench side to bedside. *J. Bioenerg. Biomembr.* 44, 163–170. doi: 10.1007/s10863-012-9417-4

Koch, M., Krieger, M. L., Stölting, D., Brenner, N., Beier, M., Jaehde, U., et al. (2013). Overcoming chemotherapy resistance of ovarian cancer cells by liposomal cisplatin: molecular mechanisms unveiled by gene expression profiling. *Biochem. Pharmacol.* 85, 1077–1090. doi: 10.1016/j.bcp.2013.01.028

König, T., Stipani, I., Horvàth, I., and Palmieri, F. (1982). Inhibition of mitochondrial substrate anion translocators by a synthetic amphipathic polyanion. *J. Bioenerg. Biomembr.* 14, 297–305. doi: 10.1007/BF00743059

Korsmeyer, S. J., Wei, M. C., Saito, M., Weiler, S., Oh, K. J., and Schlesinger, P. H. (2000). Pro-apoptotic cascade activates BID, which oligomerizes BAK or BAX into pores that result in the release of cytochrome c. *Cell Death Differ.* 7, 1166–1173. doi: 10.1038/sj.cdd.4400783

Krauskopf, A., Eriksson, O., Craigen, W. J., Forte, M. A., and Bernardi, P. (2006). Properties of the permeability transition in VDAC1(-/-) mitochondria. *Biochim. Biophys. Acta* 1757, 590–595. doi: 10.1016/j.bbabio.2006.02.007

Krishnan, A., Hariharan, R., Nair, S. A., and Pillai, M. R. (2008). Fluoxetine mediates G0/G1 arrest by inducing functional inhibition of cyclin dependent kinase subunit (CKS)1. *Biochem. Pharmacol.* 75, 1924–1934. doi: 10.1016/j.bcp.2008.02.013

Kroemer, G., and Zitvogel, L. (2007). Death, danger, and immunity: an infernal trio. *Immunol. Rev.* 220, 5–7. doi: 10.1111/j.1600-065X.2007.00576.x

Kroemer, G., Galluzzi, L., and Brenner, C. (2007). Mitochondrial membrane permeabilization in cell death. *Physiol. Rev.* 87, 99–163. doi: 10.1152/physrev.00013.2006

Lai, J. C., Tan, W., Benimetskaya, L., Miller, P., Colombini, M., and Stein, C. A. (2006). A pharmacologic target of G3139 in melanoma cells may be the mitochondrial VDAC. *Proc. Natl. Acad. Sci. U.S.A.* 103, 7494–7499. doi: 10.1073/pnas.0602217103

Le Bras, M., Clément, M. V., Pervaiz, S., and Brenner, C. (2005). Reactive oxygen species and the mitochondrial signaling pathway of cell death. *Histol. Histopathol.* 20, 205–219. doi: 10.14670/HH-20.205

Leão, P. N., Costa, M., Ramos, V., Pereira, A. R., Fernandes, V. C., Domingues, V. F., et al. (2013). Antitumor activity of hierridin B, a cyanobacterial secondary metabolite found in both filamentous and unicellular marine strains. *PLoS ONE* 8:e69562. doi: 10.1371/journal.pone.0069562

Lee, A. C., Xu, X., Blachly-Dyson, E., Forte, M., and Colombini, M. (1998). The role of yeast VDAC genes on the permeability of the mitochondrial outer membrane. *J. Membr. Biol.* 161, 173–181. doi: 10.1007/s002329900324

Lee, C. S., Kim, Y. J., Jang, E. R., Kim, W., and Myung, S. C. (2010). Fluoxetine induces apoptosis in ovarian carcinoma cell line OVCAR-3 through reactive oxygen species-dependent activation of nuclear factor-kappaB. *Basic Clin. Pharmacol. Toxicol.* 106, 446–453. doi: 10.1111/j.1742-7843.2009.00509.x

Lee, H. J., Kim, J. W., Yim, S. V., Kim, M. J., Kim, S. A., Kim, Y. J., et al. (2001). Fluoxetine enhances cell proliferation and prevents apoptosis in dentate gyrus of maternally separated rats. *Mol. Psychiatry* 610, 725- 728. doi: 10.1038/sj.mp.4000947

Lee, K., Kerner, J., and Hoppel, C. L. (2011). Mitochondrial carnitine palmitoyltransferase 1a (CPT1a) is part of an outer membrane fatty acid transfer complex. *J. Biol. Chem.* 286, 25655–25662. doi: 10.1074/jbc.M111.228692

Lemeshko, V. V., Haridas, V., Quijano Pérez, J. C., and Gutterman, J. U. (2006). Avicins, natural anticancer saponins, permeabilize mitochondrial membranes. *Arch. Biochem. Biophys.* 454, 114–122. doi: 10.1016/j.abb.2006.08.008

Li, H. N., Nie, F. F., Liu, W., Dai, Q. S., Lu, N., Qi, Q., et al. (2009). Apoptosis induction of oroxylin A in human cervical cancer HeLa cell line *in vitro* and *in vivo*. *Toxicology* 257, 80–85. doi: 10.1016/j.tox.2008.12.011

Li, M., Ona, V. O., Guégan, C., Chen, M., Jackson-Lewis, V., Andrews, L. J., et al. (2000). Functional role of caspase-1 and caspase-3 in an ALS transgenic mouse model. *Science* 288, 335–339. doi: 10.1126/science.288.5464.335

Li, Q., Qiao, P., Chen, X., Wang, J., Bian, L., and Zheng, X. (2017). Affinity chromatographic methodologies based on immobilized voltage dependent anion channel isoform 1 and application in protein-ligand interaction analysis and bioactive compounds screening from traditional medicine. *J. Chromatogr. A* 1495, 31–45. doi: 10.1016/j.chroma.2017.03.023

Ligresti, A., Moriello, A. S., Starowicz, K., Matias, I., Pisanti, S., De Petrocellis, L., et al. (2006). Antitumor activity of plant cannabinoids with emphasis on the effect of cannabidiol on human breast carcinoma. *J. Pharmacol. Exp. Ther.* 318, 1375–1387. doi: 10.1124/jpet.106.105247

Liu, A. H., Cao, Y. N., Liu, H. T., Zhang, W. W., Liu, Y., Shi, T. W., et al. (2008). DIDS attenuates staurosporine-induced cardiomyocyte apoptosis by PI3K/Akt signaling pathway: activation of eNOS/NO and inhibition of Bax translocation. *Cell. Physiol. Biochem.* 22, 177–186. doi: 10.1159/000149795

Liu, K. H., Yang, S. T., Lin, Y. K., Lin, J. W., Lee, Y. H., Wang, J. Y., et al. (2015). Fluoxetine, an antidepressant, suppresses glioblastoma by evoking AMPAR-mediated calciumdependent apoptosis. *Oncotarget* 6, 5088–5101. doi: 10.18632/oncotarget.3243

Liu, Y., Cheng, H., Zhou, Y., Zhu, Y., Bian, R., Chen, Y., et al. (2013). Myostatin induces mitochondrial metabolic alteration and typical apoptosis in cancer cells. *Cell Death Dis.* 4:e494. doi: 10.1038/cddis.2013.31

Lu, L., Zhang, C., Cai, Q., Lu, Q., Duan, C., Zhu, Y., et al. (2013). Voltage-dependent anion channel involved in the α-synuclein-induced dopaminergic neuron toxicity in rats. *Acta Biochim. Biophys. Sin.* 45, 170–178. doi: 10.1093/abbs/gms114

Ma, S. B., Nguyen, T. N., Tan, I., Ninnis, R., Iyer, S., Stroud, D. A., et al. (2014). Bax targets mitochondria by distinct mechanisms before or during apoptotic cell death: a requirement for VDAC2 or Bak for efficient Bax apoptotic function. *Cell Death Differ.* 21, 1925–1935. doi: 10.1038/cdd.2014.119

Magri, A., Belfiore, R., Reina, S., Tomasello, M. F., Di Rosa, M. C., Guarino, F., et al. (2016a). Hexokinase I N-terminal based peptide prevents the VDAC1-SOD1 G93A interaction and re-establishes ALS cell viability. *Sci. Rep.* 6:34802. doi: 10.1038/srep34802

Magrì, A., Di Rosa, M. C., Tomasello, M. F., Guarino, F., Reina, S., Messina, A., et al. (2016b). Overexpression of human SOD1 in VDAC1-less yeast restores mitochondrial functionality modulating beta-barrel outer membrane protein genes. *Biochim. Biophys. Acta* 1857, 789–798. doi: 10.1016/j.bbabio.2016.03.003

Magrì, A., and Messina, A. (2017). Interactions of VDAC with proteins involved in neurodegenerative aggregation: an opportunity for advancement on therapeutic molecules. *Curr. Med. Chem.* 24, 4470–4487. doi: 10.2174/0929867324666170601073920

Majewski, N., Nogueira, V., Bhaskar, P., Coy, P. E., Skeen, J. E., Gottlob, K., et al. (2004). Hexokinase-mitochondria interaction mediated by Akt is required to inhibit apoptosis in the presence or absence of Bax and Bak. *Mol. Cell* 16, 819–830. doi: 10.1016/j.molcel.2004.11.014

Maldonado, E. N., Sheldon, K. L., DeHart, D. N., Patnaik, J., Manevich, Y., Townsend, D. M., et al. (2013). Voltage-dependent anion channels modulate mitochondrial metabolism in cancer cells: regulation by free tubulin and erastin. *J. Biol. Chem.* 288, 11920–11929. doi: 10.1074/jbc.M112.433847

Manczak, M., and Reddy, P. H. (2012). Abnormal interaction of VDAC1 with amyloid beta and phosphorylated tau causes mitochondrial dysfunction in Alzheimer's disease. *Hum. Mol. Genet.* 21, 5131–5146. doi: 10.1093/hmg/dds360

Mannella, C. A., and Guo, X. W. (1990). Interaction between the VDAC channel and a polyanionic effector. An electron microscopic study. *Biophys. J.* 57, 23–31. doi: 10.1016/S0006-3495(90)82503-0

Marin, R., Ramírez, C. M., González, M., González-Muñoz, E., Zorzano, A., Camps, M., et al. (2007). Voltage-dependent anion channel (VDAC) participates in amyloid beta induced toxicity and interacts with plasma membrane estrogen receptor alpha in septal and hippocampal neurons. *Mol. Membr. Biol.* 24, 148–160. doi: 10.1080/09687860601055559

Martel, C., Allouche, M., Esposti, D. D., Fanelli, E., Boursier, C., Henry, C., et al. (2013). Glycogen synthase kinase 3-mediated voltage-dependent anion channel phosphorylation controls outer mitochondrial membrane permeability during lipid accumulation. *Hepatology* 57, 93–102. doi: 10.1002/hep.25967

Martinou, J. C., and Youle, R. J. (2011). Mitochondria in apoptosis: Bcl-2 family members and mitochondrial dynamics. *Dev. Cell* 21, 92–101. doi: 10.1016/j.devcel.2011.06.017

Marzo, I., Brenner, C., Zamzami, N., Jürgensmeier, J. M., Susin, S. A., Vieira, H. L., et al. (1998). Bax and adenine nucleotide translocator cooperate in the mitochondrial control of apoptosis. *Science* 281, 2027–2031. doi: 10.1126/science.281.5385.2027

Massi, P., Solinas, M., Cinquina, V., and Parolaro, D. (2013). Cannabidiol as potential anticancer drug. *Br. J. Clin. Pharmacol.* 75, 303 312. doi: 10.1111/j.1365-2125.2012.04298.x

Mathupala, S. P., Ko, Y. H., and Pedersen, P. L. (2006). Hexokinase II: cancer's double-edged sword acting as both facilitator and gatekeeper of malignancy when bound to mitochondria. *Oncogene* 25, 4777–4786. doi: 10.1038/sj.onc.1209603

Mattson, M. P. (2000). Apoptosis in neurodegenerative disorders. *Nat. Rev. Mol. Cell Biol.* 1, 120–129. doi: 10.1038/35040009

Menzel, V. A., Cassará, M. C., Benz, R., de Pinto, V., Messina, A., Cunsolo, V., et al. (2009). Molecular and functional characterization of VDAC2 purified from mammal spermatozoa. *Biosci. Rep.* 29, 351–362. doi: 10.1042/BSR20080123

Messina, A., Reina, S., Guarino, F., and De Pinto, V. (2012). VDAC isoforms in mammals. *Biochim. Biophys. Acta* 1818, 1466–1476. doi: 10.1016/j.bbamem.2011.10.005

Messina, A., Reina, S., Guarino, F., Magrì, A., Tomasello, M. F., Clark, R. E., et al. (2014). Live cell interactome of the human Voltage Dependent Anion Channel 3 (VDAC3) revealed in HeLa cells by Affinity Purification Tag Technique. *Mol. BioSyst.* 10, 2134–2145. doi: 10.1039/C4MB00237G

Moulder, S. L., Symmans, W. F., Booser, D. J., Madden, T. L., Lipsanen, C., Yuan, L., et al. (2008). Phase I/II study of G3139 (Bcl-2 antisense oligonucleotide) in combination with doxorubicin and docetaxel in breast cancer. *Clin. Cancer Res.* 14, 7909–7916. doi: 10.1158/1078-0432.CCR-08-1104

Mujoo, K., Haridas, V., Hoffmann, J. J., Wächter, G. A., Hutter, L. K., Lu, Y., et al. (2001). Triterpenoid saponins from *Acacia victoriae* (Bentham) decrease tumor cell proliferation and induce apoptosis. *Cancer Res.* 61, 5486–5490.

Mukherjee, J., Das, M. K., Yang, Z. Y., and Lew, R. (1998). Evaluation of the binding of the radiolabeled antidepressant drug, 18Ffluoxetine in the rodent brain: an *in vitro* and *in vivo* study. *Nucl. Med. Biol.* 25, 605–610. doi: 10.1016/S0969-8051(98)00043-2

Mun, A. R., Lee, S. J., Kim, G. B., Kang, H. S., Kim, J. S., and Kim, S. J. (2013). Fluoxetine-induced apoptosis in hepatocellular carcinoma cells. *Anticancer Res.* 33, 3691–3697.

Naghdi, S., Várnai, P., and Hajnóczky, G. (2015). Motifs of VDAC2 required for mitochondrial Bak import and tBid-induced apoptosis. *Proc. Natl. Acad. Sci. U.S.A.* 112, 5590–5599. doi: 10.1073/pnas.1510574112

Nahon, E., Israelson, A., Abu-Hamad, S., and Shoshan Barmatz, V. (2005). Fluoxetine (Prozac) interaction with the mitochondrial voltage-dependent anion channel and protection against apoptotic cell death. *FEBS Lett.* 579, 5105–5110. doi: 10.1016/j.febslet.2005.08.020

Nakano, A., Miki, H., Nakamura, S., Harada, T., Oda, A., Amou, H., et al. (2012). Up-regulation of hexokinase II in myeloma cells: targeting myeloma cells with 3-bromopyruvate. *J. Bioenerg. Biomembr.* 44, 31–38. doi: 10.1007/s10863-012-9412-9

Nakano, A., Tsuji, D., Miki, H., Cui, Q., El Sayed, S. M., Ikegame, A., et al. (2011). Glycolysis inhibition inactivates ABC transporters to restore drug sensitivity in malignant cells. *PLoS ONE* 6:e27222. doi: 10.1371/journal.pone.0027222

Nakashima, R. A. (1989). Hexokinase-binding properties of the mitochondrial VDAC protein: inhibition by DCCD and location of putative DCCD-binding sites. *J. Bioenerg. Biomembr.* 21, 461–470. doi: 10.1007/BF00762518

Nakashima, R. A., Mangan, P. S., Colombini, M., and Pedersen, P. L. (1986). Hexokinase receptor complex in hepatoma mitochondria: evidence from N, N'-dicyclohexylcarbodiimide labeling studies for the involvement of the pore-forming protein VDAC. *Biochemistry* 25, 1015–1021. doi: 10.1021/bi00353a010

Nawarak, J., Huang-Liu, R., Kao, S. H., Liao, H. H., Sinchaikul, S., Chen, S. T., et al. (2009). Proteomics analysis of A375 human malignant melanoma cells in response to arbutin treatment. *Biochim. Biophys. Acta* 1794, 159–167. doi: 10.1016/j.bbapap.2008.09.023

Neuzil, J., Dong, L. F., Rohlena, J., Truksa, J., and Ralph, S. J. (2013). Classification of mitocans, anti-cancer drugs acting on mitochondria. *Mitochondrion* 13, 199–208. doi: 10.1016/j.mito.2012.07.112

O'Brien, S., Moore, J. O., Boyd, T. E., Larratt, L. M., Skotnicki, A., Koziner, B., et al. (2007). Randomized phase III trial of fludarabine plus cyclophosphamide with or without oblimersen sodium (Bcl-2 antisense) in patients with relapsed or refractory chronic lymphocytic leukemia. *J. Clin. Oncol.* 25, 1114–1120. doi: 10.1200/JCO.2006.07.1191

Okazaki, M., Kurabayashi, K., Asanuma, M., Saito, Y., Dodo, K., and Sodeoka, M. (2015). VDAC3 gating is activated by suppression of disulfide-bond formation between the N terminal region and the bottom of the pore. *Biochim. Biophys. Acta* 1848, 3188–3196. doi: 10.1016/j.bbamem.2015.09.017

Palchaudhuri, R., Nesterenko, V., and Hergenrother, P. J. (2008). The complex role of the triphenylmethyl motif in anticancer compounds. *J. Am. Chem. Soc.* 130, 10274–10281. doi: 10.1021/ja8020999

Palmieri, F., and De Pinto, V. (1989). Purification and properties of the voltage dependent anion channel of the outer mitochondrial membrane. *J. Bioenerg. Biomembr.* 21, 417–425. doi: 10.1007/BF00762514

Pedersen, P. L. (2007). The cancer cell's "power plants" as promising therapeutic targets: an overview. *J. Bioenerg. Biomembr.* 39, 1–12. doi: 10.1007/s10863-007-9070-5

Pedersen, P. L. (2008). Voltage dependent anion channels (VDACs): a brief introduction with a focus on the outer mitochondrial compartment's roles to get her with hexokinase-2 in the "Warburg effect" in cancer. *J. Bioenerg. Biomembr.* 40, 123–126. doi: 10.1007/s10863-008-9165-7

Pedersen, P. L. (2012). 3-Bromopyruvate (3BP) a fast acting, promising, powerful, specific, and effective "small molecule" anti-cancer agent taken from labside to bedside: introduction to a special issue. *J. Bioenerg. Biomembr.* 44, 1–6. doi: 10.1007/s10863-012-9425-4

Penso, J., and Beitner, R. (1998). Clotrimazole and bifonazole detach hexokinase from mitochondria of melanoma cells. *Eur. J. Pharmacol.* 342, 113–117. doi: 10.1016/S0014-2999(97)01507-0

Pfeiffer, D. R., Gudz, T. I., Novgorodov, S. A., and Erdahl, W. L. (1995). The peptide mastoparan is a potent facilitator of the mitochondrial permeability transition. *J. Biol. Chem.* 270, 4923–4932. doi: 10.1074/jbc.270.9.4923

Prabagar, B., Yoo, B. K., Woo, J. S., Kim, J. A., Rhee, J. D., Piao, M. G., et al. (2007). Enhanced bioavailability of poorly water-soluble clotrimazole by inclusion with beta-cyclodextrin. *Arch. Pharm. Res.* 30, 249–254. doi: 10.1007/BF02977701

Prezma, T., Shteinfer, A., Admoni, L., Raviv, Z., Sela, I., Levi, I., et al. (2013). VDAC1-based peptides: novel pro-apoptotic agents and potential therapeutics for Bcell chronic lymphocytic leukemia. *Cell Death Dis.* 4:e809. doi: 10.1038/cddis.2013.316

Rai, K. R., Moore, J., Wu, J., Novick, S. C., and O'Brien, S. M. (2008). Effect of the addition of oblimersen (Bcl-2 antisense) to fludarabine/cyclophosphamide for relapsed/refractory chronic lymphocytic leukemia (CLL) on survival in patients who achieve CR/nPR: five-year follow-up from a randomized phase III study. *J. Clin. Oncol.* 26, (Suppl. 15), 7008–7008. doi: 10.1200/jco.2008.26.15_suppl.7008

Ramirez, C. M., Gonzalez, M., Diaz, M., Alonso, R., Ferrer, I., Santpere, G., et al. (2009). VDAC and ER interaction in caveolae from human cortex is altered in Alzheimer's disease. *Mol. Cell Neurosci.* 42, 172–183. doi: 10.1016/j.mcn.2009.07.001

Rao, J., Xu, D. R., Zheng, F. M., Long, Z. J., Huang, S. S., Wu, X., et al. (2011). Curcumin reduces expression of Bcl-2, leading to apoptosis in daunorubicin-insensitive CD34+ acute myeloid leukemia cell lines and primary sorted CD34+ acute myeloid leukemia cells. *J. Transl. Med.* 9:71. doi: 10.1186/1479-5876-9-71

Reina, S., and De Pinto, V. (2017). Anti-cancer compound targeted to VDAC: potential and perspectives. *Curr. Med. Chem.* 24, 4447–4469. doi: 10.2174/0929867324666170530074039

Reina, S., Checchetto, V., Saletti, R., Gupta, A., Chaturvedi, D., Guardiani, C., et al. (2016a). VDAC3 as a sensor of oxidative state of the intermembrane space of mitochondria: the putative role of cysteine residue modifications. *Oncotarget* 7, 2249–2268. doi: 10.18632/oncotarget.6850

Reina, S., Guarino, F., Magrì, A., and De Pinto, V. (2016b). VDAC3 as a potential marker of mitochondrial status is involved in cancer and pathology. *Front. Oncol.* 6:264. doi: 10.3389/fonc.2016.00264

Reina, S., Palermo, V., Guarnera, A., Guarino, F., Messina, A., Mazzoni, C., et al. (2010). Swapping of the N-terminus of VDAC1 with VDAC3 restores full activity of the channel and confers anti aging features to the cell. *FEBS Lett.* 584, 2837–2844. doi: 10.1016/j.febslet.2010.04.066

Reina, S., Magrì, A., Lolicato, M., Guarino, F., Impellizzeri, A., Maier, E., et al. (2013). Deletion of β strands 9 and 10 converts VDAC1 voltage dependence in an asymmetrical process. *Biochim. Biophys. Acta* 1827, 793–805. doi: 10.1016/j.bbabio.2013.03.007

Rimmerman, N., Ben-Hail, D., Porat, Z., Juknat, A., Kozela, E., Daniels, M. P., et al. (2013). Direct modulation of the outer mitochondrial membrane channel, voltage-dependent anion channel 1 (VDAC1) by cannabidiol: a novel mechanism for cannabinoid-induced cell death. *Cell Death Dis.* 4:e949. doi: 10.1038/cddis.2013.471

Rohn, T. T., Kokoulina, P., Eaton, C. R., and Poon, W. W. (2009). Caspase activation in transgenic mice with Alzheimer-like pathology: results from a pilot study utilizing the caspase inhibitor Q-VD-OPh. *Int. J. Clin. Exp. Med.* 2, 300–308.

Rostovtseva, T., and Colombini, M. (1997). VDAC channels mediate and gate the flow of ATP: implications for the regulation of mitochondrial function. *Biophys. J.* 72, 1954–1962. doi: 10.1016/S0006-3495(97)78841-6

Sampson, M. J., Lovell, R. S., and Craigen, W. J. (1997). The murine voltage-dependent anion channel gene family. Conserved structure and function. *J. Biol. Chem.* 272, 18966–18973. doi: 10.1074/jbc.272.30.18966

Scher, H. I., and Norton, L. (1992). Chemotherapy for urothelial tract malignancies: breaking the deadlock. *Semin. Surg. Oncol.* 8, 316–341. doi: 10.1002/ssu.2980080511

Schredelseker, J., Paz, A., López, C. J., Altenbach, C., Leung, C. S., Drexler, M. K., et al. (2014). High resolution structure and double electron-electron resonance of the zebrafish voltage-dependent anion channel 2 reveal an oligomeric population. *J. Biol. Chem.* 289, 12566–12577. doi: 10.1074/jbc.M113.497438

Serafeim, A., Holder, M. J., Grafton, G., Chamba, A., Drayson, M. T., Luong, Q. T., et al. (2003). Selective serotonin reuptake inhibitors directly signal for apoptosis in biopsy-like Burkitt lymphoma cells. *Blood* 101, 3212–3219. doi: 10.1182/blood-2002-07-2044

Shafir, I., Feng, W., and Shoshan-Barmatz, V. (1998). Dicyclohexylcarbodiimide interaction with the voltage-dependent anion channel from sarcoplasmic reticulum. *Eur. J. Biochem.* 253, 627–636. doi: 10.1046/j.1432-1327.1998.2530627.x

Sherwin, B. B., and Henry, J. F. (2008). Brain aging modulates the neuroprotective effects of estrogen on selective aspects of cognition in women: a critical review. *Front. Neuroendocrinol.* 29, 88–113. doi: 10.1016/j.yfrne.2007.08.002

Shi, Y., Chen, J., Weng, C., Chen, R., Zheng, Y., Chen, Q., et al. (2003). Identification of the protein-protein contact site and interaction mode of human VDAC1 with Bcl-2 family proteins. *Biochem. Biophys. Res. Commun.* 305, 989–996. doi: 10.1016/S0006-291X(03)00871-4

Shimizu, S., and Tsujimoto, Y. (2000). Proapoptotic BH3-only Bcl-2 family members induce cytochrome c release, but not mitochondrial membrane potential loss, and do not directly modulate voltage-dependent anion channel activity. *Proc. Natl. Acad. Sci. U.S.A.* 97, 577–582. doi: 10.1073/pnas.97.2.577

Shimizu, S., Narita, M., and Tsujimoto, Y. (1999). Bcl-2 family proteins regulate the release of apoptogenic cytochrome c by the mitochondrial channel VDAC. *Nature* 399, 483–487. doi: 10.1038/20959

Shol'-ts, K. F., Aliverdieva, D. A., Snezhkova, L. G., Miroshnikov, A. I., and Kotel'-Nikova, A. V. (1984). Effects of mastoparan from hornet venom on mitochondria. *Doklady* 273, 398–400.

Shoshan, M. C. (2012). 3-Bromopyruvate: targets and outcomes. *J. Bioenerg. Biomembr.* 44, 7–15. doi: 10.1007/s10863-012-9419-2

Shoshan-Barmatz, V., De Pinto, V., Zweckstetter, M., Raviv, Z., Keinan, N., and Arbel, N. (2010). VDAC, a multi-functional mitochondrial protein regulating cell life and death. *Mol. Aspects Med.* 31, 227–285. doi: 10.1016/j.mam.2010.03.002

Simamura, E., Hirai, K., Shimada, H., Koyama, J., Niwa, Y., and Shimizu, S. (2006). Furanonaphthoquinones cause apoptosis of cancer cells by inducing the production of reactive oxygen species by the mitochondrial voltage-dependent anion channel. *Cancer Biol. Ther.* 5, 1523–1529. doi: 10.4161/cbt.5.11.3302

Simamura, E., Shimada, H., Hatta, T., and Hirai, K. (2008a). Mitochondrial voltage-dependent anion channels (VDACs) as novel pharmacological targets for anti-cancer agents. *J. Bioenerg. Biomembr.* 40, 213–217. doi: 10.1007/s10863-008-9158-6

Simamura, E., Shimada, H., Ishigaki, Y., Hatta, T., Higashi, N., and Hirai, K. (2008b). Bioreductive activation of quinone antitumor drugs by mitochondrial voltage-dependent anion channel 1. *Anat. Sci. Int.* 83, 261–266. doi: 10.1111/j.1447-073X.2008.00241.x

Siomi, H., and Siomi, M. C. (2010). Posttranscriptional regulation of microRNA biogenesis in animals. *Mol. Cell* 38, 323–332. doi: 10.1016/j.molcel.2010.03.013

Smilansky, A., Dangoor, L., Nakdimon, I., Ben-Hail, D., Mizrachi, D., and Shoshan-Barmatz, V. (2015). The Voltage-dependent Anion Channel 1 mediates amyloid β toxicity and represents a potential target for Alzheimer Disease therapy. *J. Biol. Chem.* 290, 30670–30683. doi: 10.1074/jbc.M115.691493

Snajdrova, L., Xu, A., and Narayanan, N. (1998). Clotrimazole, an antimycotic drug, inhibits the sarcoplasmic reticulum calcium pump and contractile function in heart muscle. *J. Biol. Chem.* 273, 28032–28039. doi: 10.1074/jbc.273.43.28032

Stepulak, A., Rzeski, W., Sifringer, M., Brocke, K., Gratopp, A., Kupisz, K., et al. (2008). Fluoxetine inhibits the extracellular signal regulated kinase pathway and suppresses growth of cancer cells. *Cancer Biol. Ther.* 7, 1685–1693. doi: 10.4161/cbt.7.10.6664

Strasser, A., Harris, A. W., Bath, M. L., and Cory, S. (1990). Novel primitive lymphoid tumors induced in transgenic mice by cooperation between *myc* and *bcl-2*. *Nature* 348, 331–333. doi: 10.1038/348331a0

Tajeddine, N., Galluzzi, L., Kepp, O., Hangen, E., Morselli, E., Senovilla, L., et al. (2008). Hierarchical involvement of Bak, VDAC1 and Bax in cisplatin-induced cell death. *Oncogene* 27, 4221–4232. doi: 10.1038/onc.2008.63

Tan, W., Loke, Y. H., Stein, C. A., Miller, P., and Colombini, M. (2007). Phosphorothioate oligonucleotides block the VDAC channel. *Biophys. J.* 93, 1184–1191. doi: 10.1529/biophysj.107.105379

Tedeschi, H., Mannella, C. A., and Bowman, C. L. (1987). Patch clamping the outer mitochondrial membrane. *J. Membr. Biol.* 97, 21–29. doi: 10.1007/BF01869611

Tewari, D., Ahmed, T., Chirasani, V. R., Singh, P. K., Maji, S. K., Senapati, S., et al. (2015). Modulation of the mitochondrial voltage dependent anion channel (VDAC) by curcumin. *Biochim. Biophys. Acta* 1848, 151–158. doi: 10.1016/j.bbamem.2014.10.014

Tewari, D., Majumdar, D., Vallabhaneni, S., and Bera, A. K. (2017). Aspirin induces cell death by directly modulating mitochondrial voltage-dependent anion channel (VDAC). *Sci. Rep.* 7:45184. doi: 10.1038/srep45184

Thinnes, F. P. (2005). Does fluoxetine (Prozak) block mitochondrial permeability transition by blocking VDAC as part of permeability transition pores? *Mol. Genet. Metab.* 84:378. doi: 10.1016/j.ymgme.2004.12.008

Thinnes, F. P. (2009). Human type-1 VDAC, a cisplatin target involved in either apoptotic pathway. *Mol. Genet. Metab.* 97:163. doi: 10.1016/j.ymgme.2009.01.014

Thinnes, F. P. (2010). Amyloid Aß, cut from APP by ß-secretase BACE1 and γ-secretase, induces apoptosis via opening type-1 porin/VDAC in cell membranes of hypometabolic cells - A basic model for the induction of apoptosis!? *Mol. Genet. Metab.* 101, 301–303. doi: 10.1016/j.ymgme.2010.07.007

Thinnes, F. P. (2011). Apoptogenic interactions of plasmalemmal type-1 VDAC and Aβ peptides via GxxxG motifs induce Alzheimer's disease - a basic model of apoptosis? *Wien Med. Wochenschr.* 161, 274–276. doi: 10.1007/s10354-011-0887-5

Thinnes, F. P., Florke, H., Winkelbach, H., Stadtmuller, U., Heiden, M., Karabinos, A., et al. (1994). Channel active mammalian porin, purified from crude membrane fractions of human B lymphocytes or bovine skeletal muscle, reversibly binds the stilbene-disulfonate group of the chloride channel blocker DIDS. *Biol. Chem. Hoppe Seyler* 375, 315–322. doi: 10.1515/bchm3.1994.375.5.315

Thinnes, F. P., Gota, H., Kayser, H., Benz, R., Schmidt, W. E., Kratzin, H. D., et al. (1989). Identification of human porins. I. Purification of a porin from human B-lymphocytes (Porin 31HL) and the topochemical prof of its expression on the plasmalemma of the progenitor cells. *Biol. Chem. Hoppe Seyler* 370, 1253–1264.

Tikunov, A., Johnson, C. B., Pediaditakis, P., Markevich, N., Macdonald, J. M., Lemasters, J. J., et al. (2010). Closure of VDAC causes oxidative stress and accelerates the Ca($^{2+}$)-induced mitochondrial permeability transition in rat liver mitochondria. *Arch. Biochem. Biophys.* 495, 174–181. doi: 10.1016/j.abb.2010.01.008

Tomasello, M. F., Guarino, F., Reina, S., Messina, A., and De Pinto, V. (2013). The Voltage-Dependent Anion selective Channel 1 (VDAC1) topography in the mitochondrial outer membrane as detected in intact cell. *PLoS ONE* 8:e81522. doi: 10.1371/journal.pone.0081522

Tsujimoto, Y., and Shimizu, S. (2007). Role of the mitochondrial membrane permeability transition in cell death. *Apoptosis* 12, 835–840. doi: 10.1007/s10495-006-0525-7

Ujwal, R., Cascio, D., Colletier, J. P., Faham, S., Zhang, J., Toro, L., et al. (2008). The crystal structure of mouse VDAC1 at 2.3 A resolution reveals mechanistic insights into metabolite gating. *Proc. Natl. Acad. Sci. U.S.A.* 105, 17742–17747. doi: 10.1073/pnas.0809634105

Vander Heiden, M. G., Chandel, N. S., Schumacker, P. T., and Thompson, C. B. (1999). Bcl xL prevents cell death following growth factor withdrawal by facilitating mitochondrial ATP/ADP exchange. *Mol. Cell* 3, 159–167. doi: 10.1016/S1097-2765(00)80307-X

Vaux, D. L. (2011). Apoptogenic factors released from mitochondria. *Biochim. Biophys. Acta* 1813, 546–550. doi: 10.1016/j.bbamcr.2010.08.002

Villinger, S., Briones, R., Giller, K., Zachariae, U., Lange, A., de Groot, B. L., et al. (2010). Functional dynamics in the voltage-dependent anion channel. *Proc. Natl. Acad. Sci. U.S.A.* 107, 22546–22551. doi: 10.1073/pnas.1012310108

Vyssokikh, M. Y., Zorova, L., Zorov, D., Heimlich, G., Jürgensmeier, J. J., and Brdiczka, D. (2002). Bax releases cytochrome c preferentially from a complex between porin and adenine nucleotide translocator. Hexokinase activity suppresses this effect. *Mol. Biol. Rep.* 29, 93–96. doi: 10.1023/A:1020383108620

Wang, C., and Youle, R. J. (2009). The role of mitochondria in apoptosis. *Annu. Rev. Genet.* 43, 95–118. doi: 10.1146/annurev-genet-102108-134850

Wang, D. M., Li, S. Q., Zhu, X. Y., Wang, Y., Wu, W. L., and Zhang, X. J. (2013). Protective effects of Hesperidin against Amyloid-b (Ab) induced neurotoxicity through the Voltage Dependent Anion Channel 1 (VDAC1)-mediated mitochondrial apoptotic pathway in PC12 Cells. *Neurochem. Res.* 38, 1034–1044. doi: 10.1007/s11064-013-1013-4

Wang, F., Qiang, Y., Zhu, L., Jiang, Y., Wang, Y., Shao, X., et al. (2016). MicroRNA-7 downregulates the oncogene VDAC1 to influence hepatocellular carcinoma proliferation and metastasis. *Tumour Biol.* 37, 10235–10246. doi: 10.1007/s13277-016-4836-1

Wei, L., Zhou, Y., Dai, Q., Qiao, C., Zhao, L., Hui, H., et al. (2013). Oroxylin A induces dissociation of hexokinase II from the mitochondria and inhibits glycolysis by SIRT3-mediated deacetylation of cyclophilin D in breast carcinoma. *Cell Death Dis.* 4:e601. doi: 10.1038/cddis.2013.131

Wilson, J. E. (2003). Isozymes of mammalian hexokinase: structure, subcellular localization and metabolic functions. *J. Exp. Biol.* 206, 2049–2057. doi: 10.1242/jeb.00241

Wu, C. H., Lin, Y. W., Wu, T. F., Ko, J. L., and Wang, P. H. (2016). Clinical implication of voltage-dependent anion channel 1 in uterine cervical cancer and its action on cervical cancer cells. *Oncotarget* 7, 4210–4225. doi: 10.18632/oncotarget.6704

Xu, X., Decker, W., Sampson, M. J., Craigen, W. J., and Colombini, M. (1999). Mouse VDAC isoforms expressed in yeast: channel properties and their roles in mitochondrial outer membrane permeability. *J. Membr. Biol.* 170, 89–102. doi: 10.1007/s002329900540

Yagoda, N., von Rechenberg, M., Zaganjor, E., Bauer, A. J., Yang, W. S., Fridman, D. J., et al. (2007). RAS-RAF-MEKdependent oxidative cell death involving voltage-dependent anion channels. *Nature* 447, 864–868. doi: 10.1038/nature05859

Yamamoto, T., Ito, M., Kageyama, K., Kuwahara, K., Yamashita, K., Takiguchi, Y., et al. (2014). Mastoparan peptide causes mitochondrial permeability transition not by interacting with specific membrane proteins but by interacting with the phospholipid phase. *FEBS J.* 281, 3933–3944. doi: 10.1111/febs.12930

Yang, J., Ning, J., Peng, L., and He, D. (2015). Effect of curcumin on Bcl-2 and Bax expression in nude mice prostate cancer. *Int. J. Clin. Exp. Pathol.* 8, 9272–9278.

Yang, Y., Hu, Y., Gu, H. Y., Lu, N., Liu, W., Qi, Q., et al. (2008). Oroxylin A induces G2/M phase cell-cycle arrest via inhibiting Cdk7-mediated expression of Cdc2/p34 in human gastric carcinoma BGC- 823 cells. *J. Pharm. Pharmacol.* 60, 1459–1463. doi: 10.1211/jpp.60.11.0006

Yong, C. S., Li, D. X., Prabagar, B., Park, B. C., Yi, S. J., Yoo, B. K., et al. (2007). The effect of beta-cyclodextrin complexation on the bioavailability and hepatotoxicity of clotrimazole. *Pharmazie* 62, 756–759. doi: 10.1691/ph.2007.10.7018

Yoo, B. C., Fountoulakis, M., Cairns, N., and Lubec, G. (2001). Changes of voltage-dependent anion-selective channel proteins VDAC1 and VDAC2 brain levels in patients with Alzheimer's disease and Down syndrome. *Electrophoresis* 22, 172–179. doi: 10.1002/1522-2683(200101)22:1<172::AID-ELPS172>3.0.CO;2-P

Yuan, S., Fu, Y., Wang, X., Shi, H., Huang, Y., Song, X., et al. (2008). Voltage-dependent anion channel 1 is involved in endostatin-induced endothelial cell apoptosis. *FASEB J.* 22, 2809–2820. doi: 10.1096/fj.08-107417

Zaid, H., Abu-Hamad, S., Israelson, A., Nathan, I., and Shoshan-Barmatz, V. (2005). The voltage-dependent anion channel-1 modulates apoptotic cell death. *Cell Death Differ.* 12, 751–760. doi: 10.1038/sj.cdd.4401599

Zhao, L., Chen, Z., Wang, J., Yang, L., Zhao, Q., Wang, J., et al. (2010). Synergistic effect of 5-fluorouracil and the flavanoid oroxylin A on HepG2 human hepatocellular carcinoma and on H22 transplanted mice. *Cancer Chemother. Pharmacol.* 65, 481–489. doi: 10.1007/s00280-009-1053-2

Zoratti, M., and Szabò, I. (1995). The mitochondrial permeability transition. *Biochim. Biophys. Acta* 1241, 139–176. doi: 10.1016/0304-4157(95)00003-A

15

Mechanisms of Aquaporin-Facilitated Cancer Invasion and Metastasis

*Michael L. De Ieso and Andrea J. Yool**

Department of Physiology, Adelaide Medical School, University of Adelaide, Adelaide, SA, Australia

***Correspondence:**
Andrea J. Yool
andrea.yool@adelaide.edu.au

Cancer is a leading cause of death worldwide, and its incidence is rising with numbers expected to increase 70% in the next two decades. The fact that current mainline treatments for cancer patients are accompanied by debilitating side effects prompts a growing demand for new therapies that not only inhibit growth and proliferation of cancer cells, but also control invasion and metastasis. One class of targets gaining international attention is the aquaporins, a family of membrane-spanning water channels with diverse physiological functions and extensive tissue-specific distributions in humans. Aquaporins−1,−2,−3,−4,−5,−8, and−9 have been linked to roles in cancer invasion, and metastasis, but their mechanisms of action remain to be fully defined. Aquaporins are implicated in the metastatic cascade in processes of angiogenesis, cellular dissociation, migration, and invasion. Cancer invasion and metastasis are proposed to be potentiated by aquaporins in boosting tumor angiogenesis, enhancing cell volume regulation, regulating cell-cell and cell-matrix adhesions, interacting with actin cytoskeleton, regulating proteases and extracellular-matrix degrading molecules, contributing to the regulation of epithelial-mesenchymal transitions, and interacting with signaling pathways enabling motility and invasion. Pharmacological modulators of aquaporin channels are being identified and tested for therapeutic potential, including compounds derived from loop diuretics, metal-containing organic compounds, plant natural products, and other small molecules. Further studies on aquaporin-dependent functions in cancer metastasis are needed to define the differential contributions of different classes of aquaporin channels to regulation of fluid balance, cell volume, small solute transport, signal transduction, their possible relevance as rate limiting steps, and potential values as therapeutic targets for invasion and metastasis.

Keywords: aquaporin, cell migration, metastasis, cancer, invasion, pharmacology, drug

INTRODUCTION

Aquaporins

Aquaporins (AQPs) are a family of water channels that also include a subset of classes shown to mediate transport of glycerol, ions, and other molecules (Li and Wang, 2017). The first aquaporin to be cloned, aquaporin-1 (AQP1), was identified in red blood cells and renal proximal tubules (Denker et al., 1988; Preston and Agre, 1991). In the *Xenopus laevis* expression system, introduced AQP1 channels enabled high osmotic water flux across the plasma membrane as compared to non-AQP control oocytes (Preston et al., 1992), explaining the mechanism enabling rapid transmembrane passage of water in certain types of cells. To date, 15 classes of aquaporin genes have been identified in mammals (AQP0–AQP14), with AQPs 13 and 14 found in older lineages of mammals (Metatheria and Prototheria) (Ishibashi et al., 2009; Finn et al., 2014; Finn and Cerda, 2015). The first 13 aquaporins (AQP0–AQP12) have been divided into categories based on functional properties (Li and Wang, 2017). One comprises the classical aquaporins (AQP0,−1,−2,−4,−5,−6,−8), which were thought initially to transport only water, though some also transport gases, urea, hydrogen peroxide, ammonia, and charged particles (Ehring and Hall, 1988; Preston et al., 1992; Fushimi et al., 1993; Hasegawa et al., 1994; Raina et al., 1995; Ma et al., 1996, 1997a; Chandy et al., 1997; Ishibashi et al., 1997b; Yasui et al., 1999; Anthony et al., 2000; Nakhoul et al., 2001; Bienert et al., 2007; Herrera and Garvin, 2011; Almasalmeh et al., 2014; Rodrigues et al., 2016). A second category consists of the aquaglyceroporins (AQP3,−7,−9, and−10), which are permeable to water and glycerol, with some also exhibiting urea, arsenite, and hydrogen peroxide permeability (Ishibashi et al., 1997a, 1998, 2002; Yang and Verkman, 1997; Liu et al., 2002; Lee et al., 2006; Rojek et al., 2008; Miller et al., 2010; Watanabe et al., 2016). A possible third category consists of AQP11 and AQP12, distantly related paralogs with only 20% homology with other mammalian AQPs (Ishibashi, 2009), which appear to carry both water and glycerol (Yakata et al., 2011; Bjørkskov et al., 2017). The permeability of AQP11 to glycerol could be important for its function in human adipocytes, in which it is natively expressed (Madeira et al., 2014). Aquaporins assemble as homo-tetramers, with monomers ranging 26–34 kDa (Verkman and Mitra, 2000). In most AQPs, each monomer is composed of six transmembrane domains and intracellular amino and carboxyl termini, with highly conserved asparagine-proline-alanine (NPA) motifs in cytoplasmic loop B and in extracellular loop E (Jung et al., 1994). The NPA motifs in loops B and E contribute to a monomeric pore structure that mediates selective, bidirectional, single-file transport of water in the classical aquaporins (Sui et al., 2001), and water and glycerol in aquaglyceroporins (Jensen et al., 2001).

Intracellular signaling processes regulate AQP channels by altering functional activity, intracellular localization, and levels of expression in different cells and tissues. For example, the peptide hormone vasopressin regulates excretion of water in the kidney by augmenting water permeability of collecting duct cells. Vasopressin induces phosphorylation of AQP2 (Hoffert et al., 2006), stimulating the reversible translocation of AQP2 from intracellular vesicles to the apical plasma membrane (Nielsen et al., 1995). Guanosine triphosphate (GTP) stimulates AQP1-induced swelling of secretory vesicles in the exocrine pancreas (Cho et al., 2002), with functional implications in pancreatic exocrine secretions. Additionally, AQP1 ion channel activity is activated by intracellular cGMP (Anthony et al., 2000), and phosphorylation of Y253 in the carboxyl terminal domain regulates responsiveness of AQP1 ion channels to cGMP (Campbell et al., 2012). Given the diverse array of functional properties, mechanisms of regulation, and tissue-specific distributions being discovered for aquaporins, it is not surprising that different classes of aquaporins (AQP-1,−2,−3,−4,−5,−8, and−9) have been implicated specifically in the complex steps associated with cancer invasion and metastasis (**Table 1**), suggesting specialized roles for these channels have been arrogated into the pathological processes.

Cancer Invasion and Metastasis

Cancer is a leading cause of death worldwide, accounting for 8.2 million deaths in 2012 (Ferlay et al., 2015). The incidence of cancer is rising steadily in an aging population, with numbers expected to increase 70% in the next two decades (Ferlay et al., 2015). Current treatments involve chemotherapy, radiation therapy, and surgery (Miller et al., 2016), associated with an array of side effects including nausea (Koeller et al., 2002), impaired fertility and premature menopause (Howard-Anderson et al., 2012; Wasilewski-Masker et al., 2014), painful neuropathy (Gamelin et al., 2002; Rivera and Cianfrocca, 2015), increased risk of cardiovascular disease (Monsuez et al., 2010; Willemse et al., 2013), and loss of bone density (Gralow et al., 2013). Inhibiting proliferation remains the primary focus of cancer treatments, although the predominant cause of death is cancer metastasis (Yamaguchi et al., 2005; Spano et al., 2012). Less devastating cancer therapies might be achievable via a combination of strategies that not only inhibit proliferation, but also control metastasis of tumor cells from their primary site to distant organs (Friedl and Wolf, 2003). Cancer cell migration through the body exploits pathways including blood stream, lymphatic system, and transcoelomic movement across body cavities (Wyckoff et al., 2000; Pepper et al., 2003; Tan et al., 2006). The hierarchical nature of the metastatic cascade suggests it should be vulnerable to intervention at multiple levels including angiogenesis, detachment of cells from the primary tumor, and infiltration of dissociated tumor cells into and out of circulatory pathways via intravasation and extravasation, respectively (**Figure 1**). AQPs that serve as rate-limiting steps in the metastatic cascade should have substantial value as prognostic markers and pharmacological targets for treatments.

ANGIOGENESIS

Both cancer invasion and metastasis are enhanced by angiogenesis. Angiogenesis, activated in response to inadequate oxygen perfusion, triggers extracellular matrix breakdown; endothelial cell proliferation, differentiation, and migration; and recruitment of periendothelial cells (Clapp and de la Escalera, 2006) which form discontinuous layers around vessels and exert developmental and homeostatic control (Njauw et al., 2008). Under physiological conditions, angiogenesis is seen in the proliferative phase of the menstrual cycle (Demir et al., 2010), development of fetal and placental vasculature (Demir et al., 2007), and skeletal muscle following physical activity (Egginton, 2009). In pathological scenarios such as tumorigenesis, tissue hypoxia stimulates the formation of new vasculature, enabling tumors to better obtain nutrients, exchange gases, and excrete waste (Nishida et al., 2006). Folkman et al. (1966) showed that tumors up to 2 mm in diameter could survive via passive diffusion from surrounding tissue; but angiogenesis was essential for support of larger tumors.

TABLE 1 | Key roles of AQPs involved in cancer invasion and metastasis.

AQP	Permeable to:	Key physiological role(s)	Cancer(s) up-regulated	Key role(s) in cancer invasion and metastasis
AQP1	• Water (Preston et al., 1992), monovalent cations (Anthony et al., 2000), CO_2 (Nakhoul et al., 1998), H_2O_2 (Almasalmeh et al., 2014), NO (Herrera et al., 2006), and NH_3 (Nakhoul et al., 2001)	• Water reabsorption in proximal tubule of the kidney for concentrating urine (Ma et al., 1998; Schnermann et al., 1998) • Secretion of aqueous fluid from ciliary epithelium in the eye, and cerebrospinal fluid from the choroid plexus (Zhang et al., 2002; Oshio et al., 2005) • Perception of thermal inflammatory pain and cold-induced pain (Zhang and Verkman, 2010)	Glioma (Saadoun et al., 2002a; El Hindy et al., 2013), mammary carcinoma (Endo et al., 1999), lung adenocarcinoma (Hoque et al., 2006), colorectal carcinoma (Moon et al., 2003), hemangioblastoma (Chen et al., 2006), and multiple myeloma (microvessels) (Vacca et al., 2001)	• Upregulated in response to tumor tissue hypoxia. Enables recruitment of new tumor vasculature by enhancing endothelial cell migration • Polarizes to leading and trailing edge of migrating cell, and enhances tumor cell migration and invasion by enabling rapid membrane protrusion formation via cell volume regulation and interaction with cytoskeletal dynamics • Enhances mesenchymal stem cell migration via FAK and β-catenin pathways • Might contribute to EMT • Possible interaction with ECM-degrading proteases
AQP2	• Water (Fushimi et al., 1993)	• Water reabsorption in collecting duct of the kidney to concentrate urine (Rojek et al., 2006)	Endometrial carcinoma (Zou et al., 2011)	• Enables "traction" for migrating cell by contributing to the regulation and recycling of focal adhesion proteins (e.g., integrin) • Necessary in estradiol-induced invasion and adhesion of endometrial carcinoma cells, through reorganization of F-actin
AQP3	• Water (Echevarria et al., 1994), glycerol, urea (Ishibashi et al., 1994), H_2O_2 (Miller et al., 2010), arsenite (Lee et al., 2006), and NH_3 (Holm et al., 2005)	• Water reabsorption in collecting duct of the kidney to concentrate urine (Ma et al., 2000) • Skin hydration (Ma et al., 2002) • Skin wound healing (Hara-Chikuma and Verkman, 2008a)	Lung cancer (Liu et al., 2007), hepatocellular carcinoma (Guo et al., 2013), gastric cancer (Shen et al., 2010), prostate cancer (Hwang et al., 2012), oesophageal and oral squamous cell carcinoma (Kusayama et al., 2011), colorectal carcinoma (Moon et al., 2003), skin squamous cell carcinoma (Hara-Chikuma and Verkman, 2008b), ovarian cancer (Ji et al., 2008), pancreatic cancer (Direito et al., 2017), and breast cancer (Mobasheri and Barrett-Jolley, 2014)	• Upregulated by EGF, and contributes to EGF-induced EMT and cancer migration • Contributes to chemokine-dependent cancer migration via enabling H_2O_2 influx and its downstream cell signaling • Interacts with ECM-degrading proteases • Might enhance tumor cell migration and invasion via regulation of cell protrusion formation
AQP4	• Water (Hasegawa et al., 1994)	• Water reabsorption in collecting duct of the kidney to concentrate urine (Ma et al., 1997b) • Transport of water into and out of the brain and spinal cord via blood-brain barrier (Manley et al., 2000) • Neuroexcitation (Binder et al., 2006) • Enables astrocyte cell migration following injury (Saadoun et al., 2005b)	Glioma (Saadoun et al., 2002b) and meningioma (Ng et al., 2009)	• Co-localizes with ion channels at leading and trailing edges of migrating cancer cells • Enhances tumor cell migration and invasion by enabling rapid membrane protrusion formation via cell volume regulation and interaction with cytoskeletal dynamics • Might interact with ECM-degrading proteases
AQP5	• Water (Raina et al., 1995) and H_2O_2 (Rodrigues et al., 2016)	• Secretion of saliva (Ma et al., 1999) and airway mucus (Song and Verkman, 2001)	Prostate cancer (Li et al., 2014), chronic myelogenous leukemia (Chae et al., 2008a), colorectal carcinoma (Wang et al., 2012), hepatocellular carcinoma (Guo et al., 2013), lung cancer (Chae et al., 2008b), cervical cancer (Zhang et al., 2012), pancreatic cancer (Direito et al., 2017), and breast cancer (Jung et al., 2011)	• Promotes EMT • Co-localizes with ion channels at leading and trailing edges of migrating cancer cells • Enhances tumor cell migration and invasion by enabling rapid membrane protrusion formation via cell volume regulation • Might interact with EGFR/ERK1/2 signaling pathway
AQP8	• Water, urea (Ma et al., 1997a), H_2O_2 (Bienert et al., 2007), and NH_3 (Holm et al., 2005; Saparov et al., 2007)	• Canalicular bile water secretion (Calamita et al., 2005) • Colonic water reabsorption (Yamamoto et al., 2007)	Cervical cancer (Shi et al., 2012, 2014)	• Not yet known

(Continued)

TABLE 1 | Continued

AQP	Permeable to:	Key physiological role(s)	Cancer(s) up-regulated	Key role(s) in cancer invasion and metastasis
AQP9	• Water, urea (Ishibashi et al., 1998), glycerol (Tsukaguchi et al., 1998), arsenite (Liu et al., 2002), and H_2O_2 (Watanabe et al., 2016)	• Hepatic glycerol uptake and metabolism for glucose production (Kuriyama et al., 2002; Rojek et al., 2007; Maeda et al., 2009) • Route for excretion of arsenic by the liver (Carbrey et al., 2009) and modulates arsenic sensitivity in leukemia (Bhattacharjee et al., 2004; Leung et al., 2007)	Glioblastoma (Fossdal et al., 2012), astrocytoma (Tan et al., 2008), prostate cancer (Chen et al., 2016)	• Overexpression might correspond with reduced EMT and growth in hepatocellular carcinoma • Might interact with ERK1/2 and MMP9 to enhance prostate cancer invasion and migration

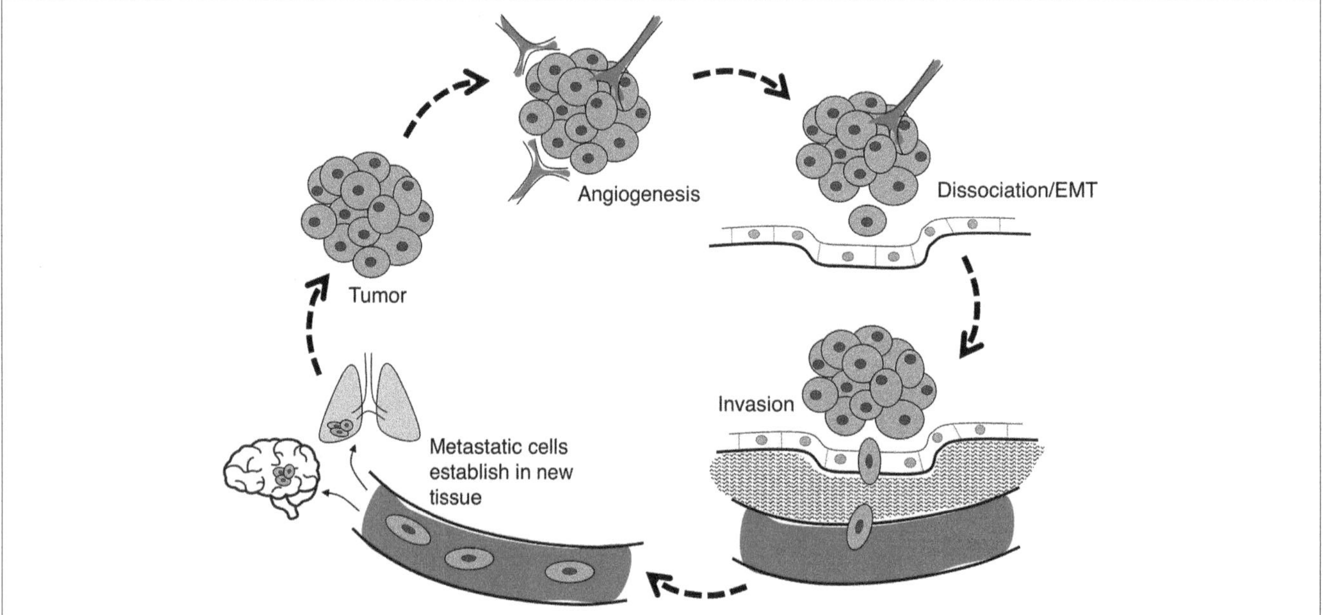

FIGURE 1 | Flow diagram summarizing the steps in cancer metastasis. Metastasis involves the migration of cells from the primary tumor to distant organs. Large tumors with tissue hypoxia rely on angiogenesis for vascular exchange of nutrients and waste. Primary tumor cells undergo phenotypic changes including loss of cell-cell adhesions which enables cells to dissociate from primary tumor, invade the adjacent extracellular matrix (ECM), and intravasate into the blood or lymph systems. Circulating tumor cells extravasate to seed secondary sites at which the process can reoccur.

AQP1, expressed in peripheral vascular endothelial cells, is involved in tumor angiogenesis (Nielsen et al., 1993; Endo et al., 1999; Saadoun et al., 2002a; El Hindy et al., 2013; Verkman et al., 2014). AQP1 knock-down in chick embryo chorioallantoic membrane resulted in a dramatic inhibition of angiogenesis (Camerino et al., 2006). Saadoun et al. (2005a) found AQP1-deficient mice exhibited reduced tumor growth and angiogenesis as compared to wild type, following subcutaneous or intracranial B16F10 melanoma cell implantation. Their work showed AQP1-null endothelial cells from mouse aorta had reduced motility as compared to wild-type, suggesting AQP1 was needed to facilitate cell migration for angiogenesis. Monzani et al. (2009) confirmed a reduced migration capacity in human microvascular endothelial cells (HMEC-1) after AQP1 knockdown by siRNA. AQP1 mRNA and protein levels are increased in response to tissue hypoxia (Kaneko et al., 2008; Abreu-Rodríguez et al., 2011). AQP1 facilitates hypoxia-induced angiogenesis by enhancing endothelial cell migration.

Angiogenesis is regulated by growth factors such as vascular endothelial growth factor (VEGF), which stimulates endothelial cell proliferation and angiogenesis in response to hypoxia (Suzuki et al., 2006), through processes that could augment AQP1 activity indirectly. Pan et al. (2008) found a positive correlation between levels of AQP1 expression, intratumoral microvascular density, and VEGF in endometrial adenocarcinoma. Similarly, AQP1 gene deletion correlated with reduced VEGF receptor expression in mouse primary breast tumor cells (Esteva-Font et al., 2014), and knockdown of AQP1 in human retinal vascular endothelial cells with concurrent inhibition of VEGF caused an additive inhibition of hypoxia-induced angiogenesis (Kaneko et al., 2008). However, application of VEGF-neutralizing antibodies did not alter AQP1 expression (Kaneko et al., 2008), and levels of VEGF in primary breast tumors were not different between AQP1-null and wild-type mice (Esteva-Font et al., 2014), supporting the idea that VEGF is regulated independently of AQP1 expression or activity.

Other angiogenic factors, such as hypoxia-inducible factor 1-alpha (HIF-1α), induce AQP1 expression in low oxygen conditions (Abreu-Rodríguez et al., 2011). The AQP1 gene promoter carries a HIF-1α binding site which drives AQP1 expression in response to hypoxia in cultured human retinal vascular endothelial cells (HRVECs) (Tanaka et al., 2011), and involves phosphorylation of p38 mitogen-activated protein kinase (MAPK) (Tie et al., 2012). Estrogen signaling also targets the promoter region of the AQP1 gene to increase transcription, inducing enhanced tubulogenesis of vascular endothelial cells as a model for angiogenesis (Zou et al., 2013). In summary, AQP1 is upregulated by angiogenic factors in response to hypoxia, and necessary for endothelial cell migration and angiogenesis. Therapies aimed at blocking transcriptional activation of AQP1 could impede cancer angiogenesis, if the treatment could be spatially limited to the tumor site without impacting normal cell functions.

CELLULAR DISSOCIATION AND EPITHELIAL-MESENCHYMAL TRANSITION

Epithelial-mesenchymal transition (EMT) occurs in normal physiological conditions such as implantation, embryogenesis, and organ development, as well as pathological processes such as cancer invasion and metastasis (Vićovac and Aplin, 1996; Thiery, 2002). During EMT, polarized epithelial cells undergo biochemical changes to adopt a mesenchymal phenotype, characterized by a loss of cell polarity, reduced cell-cell adhesiveness, and enhanced invasive capacity (Thiery, 2002, 2003; Cavallaro and Christofori, 2004; Kalluri and Weinberg, 2009; van Zijl et al., 2011). Epithelial cadherin (E-cadherin), a transmembrane glycoprotein, enables calcium-dependent tight adhesions between epithelial cells and links to cytoskeletal elements (Angst et al., 2001; Alizadeh et al., 2014). Downregulation of E-cadherin is a hallmark feature of EMT (Cano et al., 2000; Chua et al., 2007; Korpal et al., 2008). EMT in cancer is induced by signals from the tumor-associated stroma, including epidermal growth factor (EGF), platelet-derived growth factor (PDGF), hepatocyte-derived growth factor (HGF), and transforming growth factor beta (TGF-β) (Miettinen et al., 1994; Pagan et al., 1999; Lo et al., 2007; Kong et al., 2009; Xu et al., 2009). These signals stimulate transcription factors such as SNAI1 (SNAIL), SNAI2 (SLUG), zinc finger E-box binding homeobox 1 (ZEB1), Mothers against decapentaplegic homolog 2 (SMAD-2) and Twist, which are all E-cadherin transcription repressors (Yang et al., 2004; Medici et al., 2008).

Classes of aquaporins such as AQP3 have been implicated in the EMT process. AQP3 up-regulation in response to EGF in colorectal, gastric, and pancreatic cancers, is associated with augmented cell migration, invasion, and metastasis (Huang et al., 2010; Liu et al., 2012; Li et al., 2013). In gastric cancer, EGF-induced AQP3 upregulation enhances the mesenchymal transformation (Chen et al., 2014). Chen et al. (2014) determined that mRNA and protein levels of vimentin and fibronectin (proteins associated with mesenchymal phenotype) were significantly increased in cells with high levels of AQP3 expression but decreased in AQP3-deficient cells. Conversely, E-cadherin expression was significantly lower in cells with high AQP3 and increased in AQP3-knockdown cells. The mechanisms for AQP3-facilitated pancreatic and colorectal cancer cell migration have not yet been determined. It will be interesting to investigate whether AQP3 promotes EMT in these cancers.

In addition to AQP3, AQPs 1, 4, 5, and 9 also have been linked to EMT in different types of cancer cells. In lung adenocarcinoma cells, AQP1 overexpression correlated with the down-regulation of E-cadherin, and up-regulation of vimentin (Yun et al., 2016). AQP4 knockdown in human breast cancer was associated with increased levels of E-cadherin, and in glioma cells with increased β-catenin (involved in actin reorganization and cell-cell adhesion) and connexin-43 (a gap junction protein that contributes to cell-cell signaling and adhesion) (Ding et al., 2011; Li Y. et al., 2016), suggesting AQP4 might enhance cell detachment from primary tumors. However, opposing evidence showed knockdown of AQP4 in primary human astrocytes correlated with down-regulation of connexin-43 (Nicchia et al., 2005); and transfection of wild type AQP4 into glioma cell lines caused enhanced adhesion (McCoy and Sontheimer, 2007). In primary glial cells, AQP4 expression levels had no appreciable effect on cell-cell adhesion under the conditions tested (Zhang and Verkman, 2008). In human non-small cell lung cancer cells (NSCLCs), AQP5 increased invasiveness; conversely, expression of AQP5 mutant channels lacking membrane targeting signals or the S156 phosphorylation site did not augment invasiveness (Chae et al., 2008b). Overexpression of AQP5 in NSCLCs was associated with a reduction in epithelial cell markers such as E-cadherin, α-catenin, and γ-catenin, and an increase in mesenchymal cell markers such as fibronectin and vimentin, concomitant with a mesenchymal change in morphology. Similarly, AQP3 and AQP5 overexpression in pancreatic ductal adenocarcinoma is accompanied by downregulation of E-cadherin and upregulation of vimentin (Direito et al., 2017). The invasion-promoting properties of AQP5 expression appear to depend on the c-Src signaling pathway, a potent trigger of EMT (Guarino et al., 2007; Chae et al., 2008b). High AQP5 expression correlated with an increase in phosphorylated SMAD2, promoting EMT in colorectal cancer, whereas AQP5 silencing was associated with a down-regulation of phosphorylated SMAD2, and a repressed EMT response (Chen et al., 2017). AQP9 is downregulated in hepatocellular carcinoma; overexpression corresponds to reduced growth and EMT, thus reducing cancer invasion and metastasis (Li C. F et al., 2016; Zhang et al., 2016). Evidence suggests that AQPs have different effects depending on the type of cancer. Moreover, the state of cancer progression, environmental factors, and the types of assays used will be complicating factors; nevertheless, AQPs have clear potential as diagnostic and prognostic biomarkers, and as therapeutic targets for modulation of EMT, cell-cell adhesion, and dissociation phases of cancer progression.

INVASION AND CELL MIGRATION

Cell migration involves the translocation of individual and collective groups of cells through fluid or tissues, relevant for survival in multicellular and single-celled organisms (Klausen et al., 2003; Friedl et al., 2004). Migration enables physiological morphogenesis, immunity, and tissue repair (Friedl et al., 2004; Friedl and Weigelin, 2008). In most mammalian cells, migration is highest during development and morphogenesis and decreases after terminal differentiation. In pathological circumstances such as cancer, migration machinery can be reactivated. AQPs−1,−3,−4, and−5,−8, and−9 are known to contribute to cancer cell migration and invasion. Translocation of cancer cells can be initiated by chemokines released from host tissues, and growth factors such as EGF secreted by stromal cells (Dittmar et al., 2008; Roussos et al., 2011).

AQP3 has been suggested to increase EGF-induced cancer growth and migration by mediating H_2O_2 flux (Miller et al., 2010; Hara-Chikuma et al., 2016). H_2O_2 is known as an oxidative stressor, but is also a second messenger in cell proliferation, differentiation and migration (Thannickal and Fanburg, 2000; Rhee, 2006). AQP3 knockdown in skin and lung cancer cell lines reduced EGF-induced H_2O_2 influx, and attenuated EGF signaling cascades (Hara-Chikuma et al., 2016), reducing migration and growth. H_2O_2 also influenced chemokine-dependent migration of T-cells and breast cancer cells (Hara-Chikuma et al., 2012; Satooka and Hara-Chikuma, 2016). AQP1,−3,−5,−8, and−9 have all been suggested to transport H_2O_2 (Bienert et al., 2007; Miller et al., 2010; Almasalmeh et al., 2014; Rodrigues et al., 2016; Watanabe et al., 2016). All of these classes also have been linked with cancer cell migration (Hu and Verkman, 2006; Shi et al., 2013; Li et al., 2014; Chen et al., 2015; Zhang et al., 2016); however, H_2O_2 transport has thus far been linked only to AQP3 as a control mechanism in cancer cell migration. Further work might show H_2O_2 transport in other classes of AQPs regulates cell motility and invasion.

Polarization

Key molecular and cellular events involved in cell migration can be classified into five inter-dependent stages, which are polarization, protrusion, cell-matrix adhesion, extracellular matrix (ECM) degradation and retraction (**Figure 2**). Cell polarization provides functionally specialized domains in the membrane and cytoplasm (Drubin and Nelson, 1996), typified by asymmetric distributions of organelles, signaling mechanisms, and membrane channels, transporters and receptors (Swaney et al., 2010). In movement, changes in cell polarization generate leading and trailing edges, predominantly regulated by small GTPases such as CDC42 (Johnson and Pringle, 1990; Allen et al., 1998), which controls the recruitment of partitioning-defective (PAR) proteins, atypical protein kinase C (aPKC), and actin polymerization machinery (Etienne-Manneville and Hall, 2003; Goldstein and Macara, 2007). AQPs−1,−4,−5, and−9 have been shown to show polarized localization at the leading edges of migrating cells. Specific co-distributions with ion transporters such as the Na^+/H^+ exchanger, the Cl^-/HCO_3^- exchanger, and the $Na^+/\text{-}HCO_3$ co-transporter, suggest sophisticated mechanisms for regulation of fluid influx and efflux (Loitto et al., 2002; Verkman, 2005; Hara-Chikuma and Verkman, 2006; Papadopoulos et al., 2008; Stroka et al., 2014), potentially driving membrane protrusions for cell locomotion (Schwab et al., 2007).

Protrusion

A migrating cell extends its leading edge into the ECM by assembling a branched network of intracellular actin filaments, predicted to yield a physical force that dynamically pushes the membrane out, alternating with relaxation and actin depolymerization (Wang, 1985; Theriot and Mitchison, 1991; Pollard and Borisy, 2003). Membrane expansion requires the vesicle fusion to support the increase in surface area (Bretscher and Aguado-Velasco, 1998; Pierini et al., 2000; Fletcher and Rappoport, 2010). Three types of protrusions found in motile cells are lamellipodia, filopodia, and invadopodia. Lamellipodia are broad, flat, actin-rich protrusions that extend in the direction of locomotion and provide a foundation on which the cell moves forward (Cramer et al., 1997). Filopodia are long, thin protrusions of the membrane thought to be exploratory, "sensing" the local environment (Mattila and Lappalainen, 2008). Lamellipodial and filopodial formations are modulated by small GTPases in the Rho family, such as Rac1 and CDC42 (Ridley et al., 1992; Allen et al., 1997; Hall, 1998; Machesky, 2008), which stimulate actin polymerization in response to growth factor (Hall, 1998) and integrin receptor activations (Price et al., 1998). Interestingly, AQP9-facilitated water flux appears to critical for filopodial protrusion formation in fibroblasts, via the CDC42 pathway (Loitto et al., 2007). The Arp2/3 (actin-related protein 2/3) complex regulates the formation of new actin filaments in migrating cancer cells, and is regulated by Scar/WAVE complex (otherwise known as WANP), which interacts with the small GTPase Rac1 for lamellipodial assembly (Ibarra et al., 2005). Invadopodia are actin-rich, matrix-degrading protrusions that appear when ECM degradation and cell adhesion are needed to create space for movement, involving proteases such as MMP2, MMP9, and MT1-MMP and src tyrosine kinase (Weaver, 2006). Changes in cell volume during protrusion are assumed to require rapid water flow (Condeelis, 1993), and could occur in part in response to osmotic gradients governed by ion transport and actin polymerization state (Diez et al., 2005; Disanza et al., 2005; Schwab et al., 2007).

AQPs at the leading edges of migrating cells are well positioned to facilitate cell volume changes and cytoskeletal modifications during protrusion formation (Monzani et al., 2009; Jiang and Jiang, 2010; Klebe et al., 2015; Wei and Dong, 2015; Pelagalli et al., 2016). AQP1 overexpression in B16F10 melanoma cells and 4T1 mammary gland tumor cells enhanced cell migration and lamellipodial width *in vitro*, and augmented metastasis in a mouse model (Hu and Verkman, 2006). AQP1 is proposed to enhance lamellipodial formation by increasing membrane osmotic water permeability (Verkman, 2005; Hu

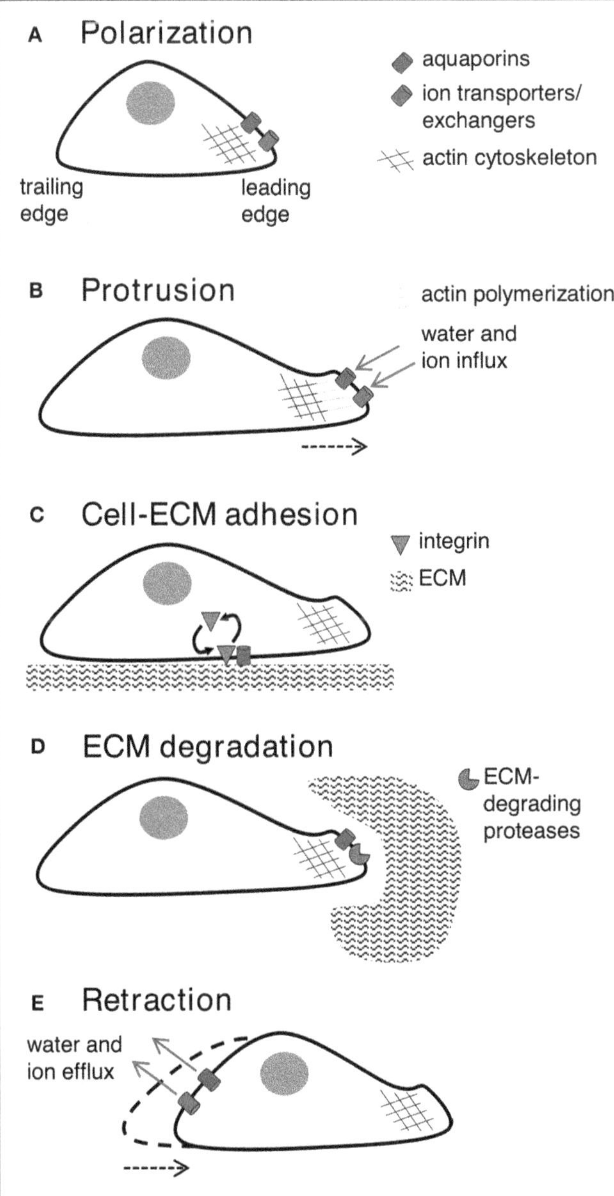

FIGURE 2 | Key contributions of aquaporins in cell migration. **(A)** Forward movement is preceded by establishing specialized loci within the cell, with redistribution of aquaporins, ion transporters/exchangers, and actin polymerization machinery to the leading edge. AQP-1,–4,–5, or–9 can be found on leading edges of migrating cancer cells. **(B)** Protrusions of the membrane might use water influx (down an osmotic gradient established by ion transporters/exchangers) and actin polymerization beneath the plasma membrane to dynamically push the membrane forward. AQP-1,–4, and–5 are implicated in water influx for protrusion extension in cancer cells; AQPs-1 and–4 also appear to interact with actin cytoskeleton. **(C)** Protrusions adhere to the ECM using integrin to generate "traction" for cellular movement. AQP2 might modulate turnover of integrin at adhesion sites, enabling forward cellular movement. **(D)** ECM degradation by enzymes can widen gaps through which the cell body can penetrate. AQP-1,–3,–4 and–9 are suggested to interact with ECM-degrading enzymes. **(E)** The final step is retraction of the cell trailing edge, thought to use aquaporins for water efflux following by K^+ export.

and Verkman, 2006; Jiang, 2009), allowing water entry at the leading edge to impose hydrostatic pressure, drive membrane extension, and create space for actin polymerization. In addition to water channel activity, AQP1 is also thought to be an ion channel, proposed to allow gated conduction of monovalent cations through the central tetrameric pore (Anthony et al., 2000; Yu et al., 2006). The dual water and ion conductance of AQP1 is essential for colon cancer cell migration *in vitro* (Kourghi et al., 2015). Conversely, in clinical cases of cholangiocarcinoma, high AQP1 expression has been correlated with low metastasis (Aishima et al., 2007; Sekine et al., 2016), suggesting that AQP1 might play different roles in different types of cancers.

Other classes of AQP water channels are not necessarily interchangeable with AQP1 in facilitating cell migration (McCoy and Sontheimer, 2007), suggesting features of AQP1 other than simple osmotic water permeability are involved. AQP1-enhanced cell migration might also be due to interactions with cytoskeletal proteins. For example, Monzani et al. (2009) demonstrated that AQP1 knockdown dramatically impeded actin cytoskeletal organization in migrating human melanoma and endothelial cell lines via interaction with Lin-7/β-catenin. The Lin-7/β-catenin complex enables asymmetrical organization of filamentous actin (F-actin). AQP1 might act as a scaffolding protein at the leading edges. Jiang (2009) found that knocking down AQP1 was associated with re-localization of actin in migrating HT20 colon cancer cells, and a reduction in the activity of actin regulatory factors RhoA and Rac. A PDZ domain in Lin-7 could mediate interaction with rhotekin protein, which inhibits Rho GTPase signaling that is involved in cell migration, invasion, and cytoskeletal reorganization (Sudo et al., 2006). Rhotekin merits further evaluation in models of AQP1-dependent cytoskeletal organization.

A role for AQP4 in glioma cell migration has similarly been proposed to occur through regulation of cell volume and cytoskeletal interactions. Protein kinase C (PKC)-mediated phosphorylation of AQP4 at serine 180 correlated with a decreased glioma cell invasion (McCoy et al., 2010). AQP4-facilitated glioma invasion is dependent on co-expression of chloride channels (ClC2) and the potassium-chloride co-transporter 1 (KCC1) in invadopodia, which could provide the ionic driving force for water efflux leading to cell shrinkage that could augment invasiveness through ECM (Mcferrin and Sontheimer, 2006; McCoy et al., 2010). AQP4 effects on actin cytoskeleton suggest a role for α-syntrophin, interacting with the C-terminal domain of AQP4 at a PDZ-binding site (Neely et al., 2001). In human glioma and primary astrocytes, reduced AQP4 expression correlated with dramatic morphological elongation, reduced invasiveness, and impaired F-actin polymerization (Nicchia et al., 2005; Ding et al., 2011).

AQP5 facilitates protrusion formation, volume regulation, cell migration, and metastasis. AQP5 expression is correlated with cell invasiveness and metastasis of human prostate cancer (Li et al., 2014), lymph node metastasis in patients with colon cancer (Kang et al., 2015), and metastatic potential of lung cancer cells (Zhang et al., 2010). Moreover, Jung et al. (2011) showed that a shRNA-induced reduction in AQP5 expression in MCF7 breast cancer cells was associated with significantly reduced cell proliferation and migration. The mechanism of AQP5-facilitated cancer cell invasion and metastasis might be due to its direct or indirect interaction with the epidermal growth factor receptor/extracellular signal-regulated kinase (ERK1/2) pathway (Kang et al., 2008; Zhang et al., 2010), known to be important in cancer metastasis and aggressiveness (Vicent et al., 2004). Additionally, AQP5 mediates lung cancer cell membrane osmotic water permeability, and has been suggested to contribute to cancer cell migration and invasion by enabling rapid cell volume regulation and subsequent protrusion formation (Chen et al., 2011). The complementary role of ion transport for migration in AQP5-expressing cells was supported by Stroka et al. (2014), who found that cell migration through physically confined spaces occurred despite block of actin polymerization and myosin contraction, but relied on co-expression of the Na^+/H^+ exchanger with AQP5, supporting AQP5-induced cell volume regulation and its importance in cell motility.

AQP8 expression influences migration and invasion of cervical cancer cells, and AQP3 expression enhances pancreatic and colorectal cancer cell invasion and metastasis (Liu et al., 2012; Li et al., 2013; Shi et al., 2013). Further work is needed to investigate whether mechanisms of AQP3- and AQP8-facilitated cancer cell migration and invasion involve cell volume regulation, protrusion formation, cytoskeletal interaction, or other functional properties of the AQP channels that remain to be defined.

Cell-Matrix Adhesion

Cell-matrix adhesions, first observed in cultured fibroblasts, connect the extracellular matrix to the actin cytoskeleton (Curtis, 1964). During migration, contacts with substratum must form to facilitate extension, and must detach to allow forward displacement of the cell. Insufficient anchoring causes protrusions to collapse, leading to a "membrane ruffling" phenomenon (Vicente-Manzanares and Horwitz, 2011). Protrusions adhere to ECM via integrin receptors, in turn linked to intracellular actin filaments (Ridley et al., 2003). The extracellular binding of integrin receptors to ECM ligands initiates integrin clustering, and activates protein tyrosine kinases and small GTPases. The organization of actin cytoskeleton and cell polarity controls the positions of focal adhesions for cell locomotion (Geiger et al., 2001; Martin et al., 2002). Cell-matrix adhesions create the focal points for generation of traction to pull the cell forward over the substratum.

Classes of aquaporins (AQP1-4) have been shown to interact with adhesion molecules and to influence adhesive properties of migrating cells. Increased AQP1 in mesenchymal stem cells enhances migration by a mechanism involving β-catenin and the focal adhesion kinase (FAK) (Meng et al., 2014), which regulates integrin signaling at focal adhesion sites (Schaller et al., 1992; McLean et al., 2005; Zhao and Guan, 2011). Whether AQP1 and FAK also interact in cancer cell migration remains to be tested. AQP2 appears to promote cell migration by modulating integrin β1 at focal adhesion sites, by a mechanism thought to involve an arginine-glycine-aspartate (RGD) motif in the second extracellular loop of AQP2 (Chen et al., 2012). When AQP2 is absent, integrin β1 is retained at focal adhesion sites, delaying recycling of focal adhesions, thus reducing migration rate. AQP2 also enables estradiol-induced migration and adhesion of endometrial carcinoma cells by mechanisms involving annexin-2 and reorganization of F-actin (Zou et al., 2011). Knockdown of AQP3 in human esophageal and oral squamous cell carcinoma with siRNA correlated with reduced phosphorylation of FAK, impaired cell adhesion and cell death (Kusayama et al., 2011); these effects would be predicted to impair cancer cell migration. AQP4 expression has been suggested to enhance cell-matrix adhesion in cancer cells (McCoy and Sontheimer, 2007). More research is needed to identify the intracellular signaling mechanisms and to determine whether other AQP classes alter cell migration via modulation of cell adhesion.

ECM Degradation

Extracellular matrix degradation widens pathways through which cells can penetrate tissues, and reduces the distortion of the rounded cell body needed for physical progress (Brinckerhoff and Matrisian, 2002; Mott and Werb, 2004). Invadopodia sprout from leading edge filopodia, extending through tiny channels in the ECM, and adhere to ECM collagen fibers (Weaver, 2006; Friedl and Wolf, 2009). To accommodate displacement of the cell body, constraining ECM fibers are cleared by local proteolysis, using surface proteases such as zinc-dependent matrix metalloproteinases (MMP) and serine proteases (Nagase and Woessner, 1999; Netzel-Arnett et al., 2003; Wolf et al., 2007). AQPs−1,−3,−4, and−9 have been shown to interact with specific MMPs to facilitate ECM degradation and invasion.

In lung cancer cells, migration was facilitated by AQP1 expression, linked to expression of MMP2 and MMP9 (Wei and Dong, 2015). In gastric cancer cells (SGC7901), AQP3 levels were correlated with MMP2, MMP9, and MT1-MMP levels, and enhanced invasiveness via phosphoinositide 3-kinase signaling (Xu et al., 2011). Positive correlations between AQP3, MMP2, and MMP9 and cancer invasiveness also occur in lung cancer (Xia et al., 2014; Xiong et al., 2017). In prostate cancer, AQP3 expression is correlated with up-regulation of MMP3 via ERK1/2 signaling, with increased cell motility and invasion (Chen et al., 2015). In glioma, AQP4 levels correlated with migration and invasiveness *in vitro* and *in vivo* through a mechanism involving MMP2 (Ding et al., 2011). AQP9 upregulation in prostate cancer could enhance growth, migration, and invasion involving ERK1/2 signaling; reduced levels of phosphorylated ERK1/2 and MMP9 were observed in AQP9-deficient cell lines (Chen et al., 2016). These studies suggest one of the key components of AQP-mediated facilitation of cancer cell invasion is the regulation of MMP proteases needed for degradation of ECM.

Retraction

Following integrin-ligand binding, cross-linking proteins such as myosin II contract the actin filament strands (Vicente-Manzanares et al., 2009), developing tension against the intact adhesion points (Chrzanowska-Wodnicka and Burridge, 1996). The final step in the cycle of cell movement is retraction of the trailing edge. A working model is that membrane tension opens stretch-activated Ca^{2+} channels, activating calpain and triggering disassembly of focal adhesion proteins on the trailing edge, while concurrent K^+ efflux drives volume loss at the cell rear, resulting in detachment and net translocation along the substrate. In this model, the role of AQP channels is to facilitate osmotic water efflux in response to K^+ efflux (Huttenlocher et al., 1997; Palecek et al., 1998; Schwab et al., 2007) presumably in parallel with electroneutral efflux of chloride ions.

AQP PHARMACOLOGY AND THERAPEUTIC IMPLICATIONS IN CANCER INVASION AND METASTASIS

Aquaporin pharmacological agents have attracted keen interest for their potential therapeutic uses in diseases involving impaired fluid homeostasis. Aquaporins in cancer metastasis are new translational targets for AQP modulators. Known and proposed inhibitors of AQPs include cysteine-reactive metals such as mercury (II) chloride ($HgCl_2$) (Preston et al., 1993), gold-based compounds (Martins et al., 2013), carbonic anhydrase inhibitor acetazolamide (Ma et al., 2004a; Gao et al., 2006), and small molecule inhibitors such as tetraethylammonium (TEA^+) (Brooks et al., 2000), although the small molecule blockers vary in efficacy between preparations. The pharmacological panel for AQPs has been expanding steadily, with new compounds being discovered around the world, including for example the University of Niigata, Japan (Huber et al., 2009), Radboud University, Netherlands (Detmers et al., 2006), the Faculty of Pharmacy, University of Lisbon, Portugal (Martins et al., 2012), the Institute of Food and Agricultural Research and Technology, Barcelona, Spain (Seeliger et al., 2012), the University of Adelaide, Australia (Niemietz and Tyerman, 2002; Yool, 2007), the University of Groningen, Netherlands (Martins et al., 2013), the University of Kiel, Germany (Wu et al., 2008), and others. This review focuses specifically on selected AQP pharmacological agents that to date have been tested in models of cancer cell migration and metastasis (**Table 2**).

Acetazolamide and Topiramate

Acetazolamide and topiramate are FDA-approved drugs that inhibit carbonic anhydrase. Acetazolamide at 100 μM was reported to inhibit water channel activity by 39% for AQP1 expressed in human embryonic kidney (HEK293) cells (Gao et al., 2006), and by 81% at 10 μM in the *Xenopus* oocyte expression system (Ma et al., 2004a). AQP4 activity was inhibited by 47% at 1,250 μM in proteoliposomes (Tanimura et al., 2009). However, acetazolamide (at doses up to 10,000 μM) did not block water flux in erythrocytes with native AQP1 expression, or epithelial cells transfected with AQP1 (Yang et al., 2006; Søgaard and Zeuthen, 2008). Acetazolamide inhibited angiogenesis in a chick chorioallantoic membrane assay, and tumor growth and metastasis in mice with Lewis lung carcinoma (Xiang et al., 2002, 2004), perhaps as a result of reduced AQP1 expression (Bin and Shi-Peng, 2011). Topiramate reduces Lewis lung carcinoma growth and metastasis, with effects similarly attributed to suppression of AQP1 expression (Ma et al., 2004b). It will be of interest to compare the effects of acetazolamide and topiramate on angiogenesis, tumor growth, and metastasis with those of AQP1 channel inhibitors.

Tetraethylammonium

TEA^+ is an inhibitor of voltage-gated potassium channels, calcium-dependent potassium channels, the nicotinic acetylcholine receptor, and it has also been shown to block AQP-1,−2, and−4 water permeability in *Xenopus laevis* oocytes and kidney derived cell lines (Brooks et al., 2000; Yool et al., 2002; Detmers et al., 2006). However, inhibition of AQP1 water permeability by TEA^+ is variable, having been confirmed by some groups (Detmers et al., 2006), and challenged by others (Søgaard and Zeuthen, 2008). Yang et al. (2006) reported no block of water flux by TEA^+ in erythrocytes with native AQP1, or in epithelial cells transfected with AQP1, and suggested previous positive results might have been due to inhibition of K^+ channels and altered baseline cell volume; however, the observation that site-directed mutation of AQP1 altered TEA sensitivity (Brooks et al., 2000) ruled out this alternative explanation. TEA^+ block of AQP1 water permeability reduced cell migration and invasion in *in vitro* models of osteosarcoma and hepatocellular carcinoma (Pelagalli et al., 2016), with outcomes interpreted as consistent with action of TEA^+ as a possible AQP1 inhibitor. However, given the variability in efficacy and cross-talk with other channels, TEA^+ is not an ideal candidate for clinical development, although the targets causing the observed block of cancer cell migration and invasion might merit further investigation.

Bumetanide Derivatives

Bumetanide is a sulfamoylanthranilic acid derivative used clinically to increase diuresis by blocking sodium cotransporter activity at the loop of Henle in the nephron. Molecular derivatives of bumetanide have been synthesized and found to exhibit inhibitory effects on classes of AQP channels. For example, the bumetanide derivative AqB013 blocks osmotic water fluxes mediated by mammalian AQP1 and AQP4 channels expressed in *Xenopus laevis* oocytes (Migliati et al., 2009). The water channel blocker AqB013 was shown to inhibit endothelial tube formation and colon cancer cell migration and invasion *in vitro* (Dorward et al., 2016). Other bumetanide derivatives, AqB011 and AqB007, block the AQP1 ion conductance, but not water flux (Kourghi et al., 2015). In AQP1, the central tetrameric pore is thought to be permeable to monovalent cations, CO_2, and NO (Nakhoul et al., 1998; Herrera et al., 2006; Yu et al., 2006; Musa-Aziz et al., 2009), although some work questioned AQP1-mediated CO_2 and cation transport properties (Yang et al., 2000; Fang et al., 2002; Tsunoda et al., 2004). An ionic conductance in AQP1-expressing *Xenopus* oocytes stimulated with forskolin was first reported in 1996 (Yool et al., 1996); however, the forskolin response proved to be inconsistent when repeated by other groups (Agre et al., 1997). Further work showed the forskolin effect was indirect; the direct regulation of the AQP1 cation conductance depended on cGMP binding (Anthony et al., 2000). The reason that AQP1 cation channels have low opening probability (Saparov et al., 2001) or are not detectable (Tsunoda et al., 2004) reflects the availability of AQP1 to be gated by cGMP, which depends on tyrosine phosphorylation status of the carboxyl terminal domain, suggesting the AQP1 ion channel function is highly regulated (Campbell et al., 2012). With the discovery of AQP1

TABLE 2 | Summary of AQP pharmacology used in cancer invasion and metastasis.

Molecule name	Molecular structure	AQP activity	Effect
TEA^+	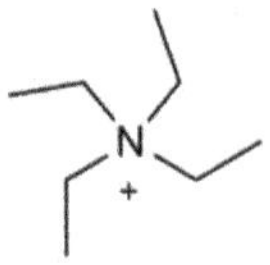	• Inhibits AQP1, AQP2, and AQP4 water flux (Brooks et al., 2000; Yool et al., 2002; Detmers et al., 2006)	• Inhibits osteosarcoma and hepatocellular carcinoma cell migration and invasion (*in vitro*) (Pelagalli et al., 2016)
Acetazolamide	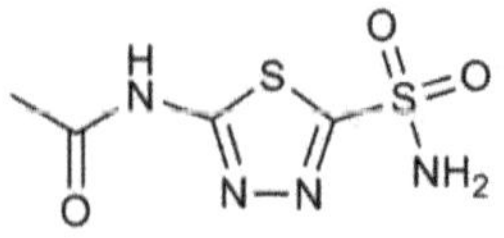	• Inhibits AQP1 and AQP4 water flux (Ma et al., 2004a; Tanimura et al., 2009) • Suppresses AQP1 expression (Xiang et al., 2004)	• Inhibits angiogenesis and metastasis in Lewis lung carcinoma (*in vivo*) (Xiang et al., 2002, 2004) • Suppresses tumor growth in colon cancer (*in vivo*) (Bin and Shi-Peng, 2011)
Topiramate	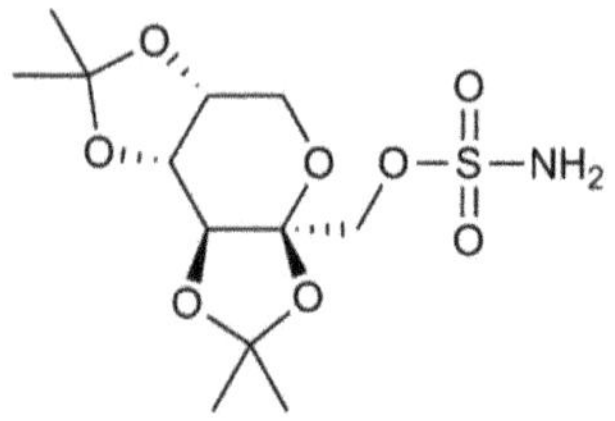	• Suppresses AQP1 expression (Ma et al., 2004b)	• Suppresses Lewis lung carcinoma growth and metastasis (*in vivo*) (Ma et al., 2004b)
AqB007	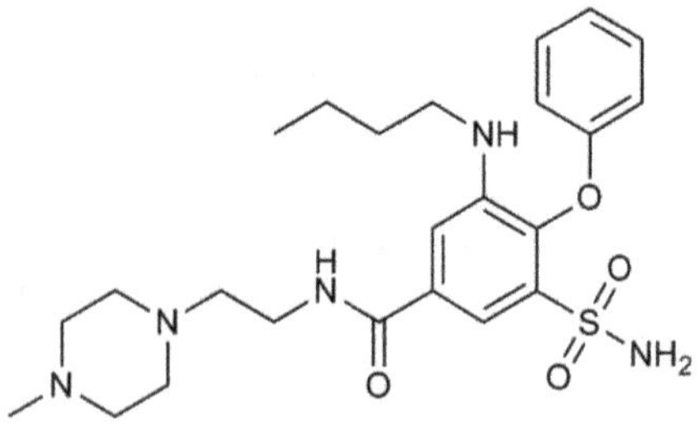	• Inhibits AQP1 ion flux (Kourghi et al., 2015)	• Inhibits colon cancer cell migration (*in vitro*) (Kourghi et al., 2015)
AqB011	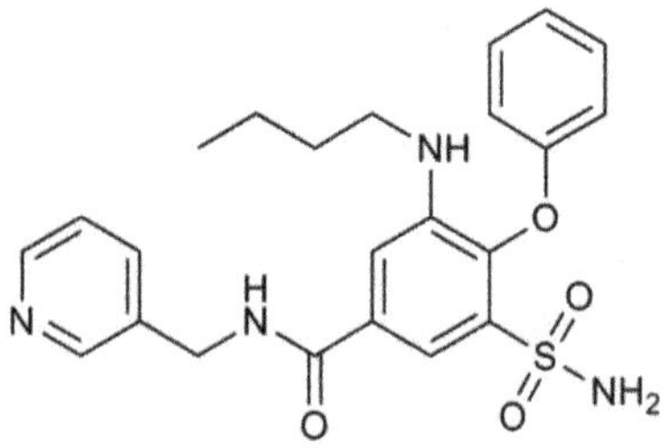	• Inhibits AQP1 ion flux (Kourghi et al., 2015)	• Inhibits colon cancer cell migration (*in vitro*) (Kourghi et al., 2015)
AqB013	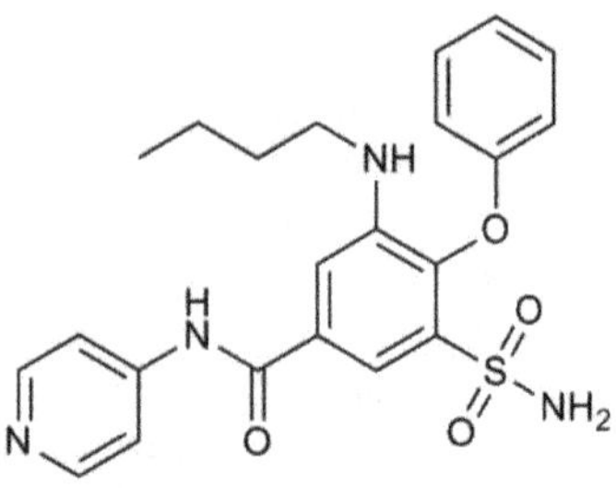	• Inhibits AQP1 and AQP4 water flux (Migliati et al., 2009)	• Inhibits endothelial tube formation and colon cancer cell migration (*in vitro*) (Dorward et al., 2016)

(Continued)

TABLE 1 | Continued

Molecule name	Molecular structure	AQP activity	Effect
Bacopaside I	HO-S(=O)(=O)-O…; HO; OH; OH; HO; HO; OH; HO; OH; O; H; H; HO; H	• Inhibits AQP1 water flux (Pei et al., 2016)	• Inhibits colon cancer cell migration (*in vitro*) (Pei et al., 2016)
Curcumin	H_3CO; HO; OH; OCH_3	• Inhibits EGF-induced AQP3 upregulation (Ji et al., 2008)	• Inhibits ovarian cancer cell migration (*in vitro*) (Ji et al., 2008)
Bacopaside II	HO; HO; OH; OH; HO; HO; OH; HO; OH; O; H; H; HO; H	• Inhibits AQP1 water flux (Pei et al., 2016)	• Inhibits colon cancer cell migration (*in vitro*) (Pei et al., 2016)
Ginsenoside Rg3	HO; OH; HO OH; OH; HO; OH; OH; OH; H; H; H; H	• Suppresses AQP1 expression (Pan et al., 2012)	• Inhibits prostate cancer cell migration (*in vitro*) (Pan et al., 2012)

ion blocking agents, AqB011 and AqB007, the physiological function of the ion channel activity could finally be addressed. When applied to AQP1-expressing HT29 colon cancer cells, these inhibitory compounds significantly reduced cancer cell motility (Kourghi et al., 2015), suggesting a physiological role of AQP1 ion conductance in cell migration. Mutation of the candidate binding site in the AQP1 intracellular loop D domain removed sensitivity to AqB011, showing that the inhibitory mechanism directly involved the AQP1 channel and could not readily be attributed to off-target actions on other channels or transporters (Kourghi et al., 2018). Another bumetanide derivative AqB050 was shown to inhibit mesothelioma cell motility and metastatic potential *in vitro*, but not *in vivo* (Klebe et al., 2015). The mechanism of action of AqB050 in blocking mesothelioma cell motility *in vitro* remains to be determined.

Plant-Based Derivatives

Plant-based derivatives that reduce cancer cell migration and invasion include agents that have also have been found to inhibit AQPs. Bacopa monnieri is a perennial herb native to the wetlands of India that is used in alternative medicinal therapies. Chemical constituents bacopaside-I and bacopaside-II, were shown to block AQP1 but not AQP4 water channels (Pei et al., 2016). Pei and colleagues also found that bacopaside-I and bacopaside-II attenuated migration of colon cancer cell lines expressing high levels of AQP1, but had no effect on lines with low AQP1, suggesting the inhibitory effects were AQP1-specific. Ginsenoside Rg3 from a traditional Asian medicinal plant Panax ginseng is an intriguing candidate for possible anti-metastatic therapies. Ginsenoside Rg3 inhibited prostate cancer cell migration and was associated with downregulation of AQP1 expression via the p38 MAPK pathway and transcription factors (Pan et al., 2012). Effects of Ginsenoside Rg3 directly on water channel activity, or on expression levels of other aquaporins, remain unknown. Curcumin is a naturally occurring ingredient in turmeric, used as therapeutic tool for pathologies including cancer (Gupta et al., 2013). Curcumin was found to inhibit EGF-induced upregulation of AQP3 and migration in human ovarian cancer cells, via inhibition of AKT/ERK and PI3K pathways (Ji et al., 2008); however, curcumin affects a number of biochemical pathways and might not be suited when AQP-specific modulation is required (Aggarwal et al., 2003). Research on the effects of curcumin in other cancers such as gastric cancer, in which EGF-induced AQP3 up-regulation occurs, might further understanding of the role of AQP3 in cell migration and invasion (Huang et al., 2010).

Metal-Based Inhibitors

Mercury has classically been used as an AQP1 inhibitor. In the human AQP1 monomer, the NPA motif in loop E is near cysteine 189, which is the site at which mercury inhibits osmotic water permeability (Preston et al., 1993). Lack of a cysteine in the corresponding position is consistent with mercury insensitivity in mammalian AQP4 (Preston et al., 1993). However, mercury is not a promising candidate for AQP-specific modulation or therapeutic application due to its toxicity and non-specific side-effects. Metal-based inhibitors that have been tested in models of cancer include AQP3 inhibitors such as $NiCl_2$ (Zelenina et al., 2003) and $CuSO_4$ (Zelenina et al., 2004), which inhibited EGF-induced cell migration in human ovarian cancer cells. Auphen is a gold-based compound which, when administered at concentrations of 100 μM, blocks AQP3 glycerol transport by 90%, and water transport by 20% in human red blood cells (Martins et al., 2012). Auphen also blocks proliferation in various mammalian cell lines, including human epidermoid carcinoma, by inhibiting AQP3 glycerol transport (Serna et al., 2014). This merits more research into the importance of AQP3-facilitated glycerol transport in cancer invasiveness, and whether gold-based compounds such as auphen can also be used to suppress cancer invasion and metastasis.

CONCLUSION

Aquaporin-dependent mechanisms serve as key steps throughout the process of metastasis, in angiogenesis, cellular dissociation, cell migration and invasion. AQPs−1,−2,−3,−4,−5,−8, and−9 contribute to one or more processes, generally potentiating cancer invasion and metastasis by boosting tumor angiogenesis, enhancing cell volume regulation, regulating cell-cell and cell-matrix adhesions, interacting with the actin cytoskeleton, regulating proteases and ECM degrading molecules, contributing to the regulation of epithelial-mesenchymal transition in cancer cells, and interacting with specific signaling pathways important in cancer cell motility and invasions. Pharmacological agents for aquaporin channels have therapeutic promise for improving cancer treatment, and include derivatives of bumetanide, organic metal compounds, plant medicinal agents, and other small molecule compounds. Although conflicting evidence has been raised for some compounds, there is nevertheless a compelling need to continue identifying novel candidates for AQP-specific modulators relevant not only for the treatment of cancer, but other pathological conditions. In conclusion, although much remains to be defined for molecular mechanisms in cancer invasion and metastasis, the roles of AQP channel function in cancer progression will inspire new therapeutic targets for improving treatment of malignant and invasive carcinomas.

AUTHOR CONTRIBUTIONS

MD: wrote the manuscript; AY: reviewed and edited the manuscript.

FUNDING

This work was supported by a Discovery Project grant from Australian Research Council (ARC DP160104641).

ACKNOWLEDGMENTS

Thanks to Dr. Jinxin Pei for assisting with molecular structure diagrams (**Table 2**).

REFERENCES

Abreu-Rodríguez, I., Silva, R. S., Martins, A. P., Soveral, G., Toledo-Aral, J. J., López-Barneo, J., et al. (2011). Functional and transcriptional induction of aquaporin-1 gene by hypoxia; analysis of promoter and role of Hif-1α. *PLoS ONE* 6:e28385. doi: 10.1371/journal.pone.0028385

Aggarwal, B. B., Kumar, A., and Bharti, A. C. (2003). Anticancer potential of curcumin: preclinical and clinical studies. *Anticancer Res.* 23, 363–398.

Agre, P., Lee, M. D., Devidas, S., and Guggino, W. B. (1997). Aquaporins and ion conductance. *Science* 275:1490; author reply 1492. doi: 10.1126/science.275.5305.1490

Aishima, S., Kuroda, Y., Nishihara, Y., Taguchi, K., Iguchi, T., Taketomi, A., et al. (2007). Down-regulation of aquaporin-1 in intrahepatic cholangiocarcinoma is related to tumor progression and mucin expression. *Hum. Pathol.* 38, 1819–1825. doi: 10.1016/j.humpath.2007.04.016

Alizadeh, A. M., Shiri, S., and Farsinejad, S. (2014). Metastasis review: from bench to bedside. *Tumor Biol.* 35, 8483–8523. doi: 10.1007/s13277-014-2421-z

Allen, W. E., Jones, G. E., Pollard, J. W., and Ridley, A. J. (1997). Rho, Rac and Cdc42 regulate actin organization and cell adhesion in macrophages. *J. Cell Sci.* 110, 707–720.

Allen, W. E., Zicha, D., Ridley, A. J., and Jones, G. E. (1998). A role for Cdc42 in macrophage chemotaxis. *J. Cell Biol.* 141, 1147–1157. doi: 10.1083/jcb.141.5.1147

Almasalmeh, A., Krenc, D., Wu, B., and Beitz, E. (2014). Structural determinants of the hydrogen peroxide permeability of aquaporins. *FEBS J.* 281, 647–656. doi: 10.1111/febs.12653

Angst, B. D., Marcozzi, C., and Magee, A. I. (2001). The cadherin superfamily: diversity in form and function. *J. Cell Sci.* 114, 629–641.

Anthony, T. L., Brooks, H. L., Boassa, D., Leonov, S., Yanochko, G. M., Regan, J. W., et al. (2000). Cloned human aquaporin-1 is a cyclic GMP-gated ion channel. *Mol. Pharmacol.* 57, 576–588. doi: 10.1124/mol.57.3.576

Bhattacharjee, H., Carbrey, J., Rosen, B. P., and Mukhopadhyay, R. (2004). Drug uptake and pharmacological modulation of drug sensitivity in leukemia by AQP9. *Biochem. Biophys. Res. Commun.* 322, 836–841. doi: 10.1016/j.bbrc.2004.08.002

Bienert, G. P., Møller, A. L., Kristiansen, K. A., Schulz, A., Møller, I. M., Schjoerring, J. K., et al. (2007). Specific aquaporins facilitate the diffusion of hydrogen peroxide across membranes. *J. Biol. Chem.* 282, 1183–1192. doi: 10.1074/jbc.M603761200

Bin, K., and Shi-Peng, Z. (2011). Acetazolamide inhibits aquaporin-1 expression and colon cancer xenograft tumor growth. *Hepatogastroenterology* 58, 1502–1506. doi: 10.5754/hge11154

Binder, D. K., Yao, X., Zador, Z., Sick, T. J., Verkman, A. S., and Manley, G. T. (2006). Increased seizure duration and slowed potassium kinetics in mice lacking aquaporin-4 water channels. *Glia* 53, 631–636. doi: 10.1002/glia.20318

Bjørkskov, F. B., Krabbe, S. L., Nurup, C. N., Missel, J. W., Spulber, M., Bomholt, J., et al. (2017). Purification and functional comparison of nine human Aquaporins produced in *Saccharomyces cerevisiae* for the purpose of biophysical characterization. *Sci. Rep.* 7:16899. doi: 10.1038/s41598-017-17095-6

Bretscher, M. S., and Aguado-Velasco, C. (1998). Membrane traffic during cell locomotion. *Curr. Opin. Cell Biol.* 10, 537–541. doi: 10.1016/S0955-0674(98)80070-7

Brinckerhoff, C. E., and Matrisian, L. M. (2002). Matrix metalloproteinases: a tail of a frog that became a prince. *Nat. Rev. Mol. Cell Biol.* 3, 207–214. doi: 10.1038/nrm763

Brooks, H. L., Regan, J. W., and Yool, A. J. (2000). Inhibition of aquaporin-1 water permeability by tetraethylammonium: involvement of the loop E pore region. *Mol. Pharmacol.* 57, 1021–1026.

Calamita, G., Ferri, D., Bazzini, C., Mazzone, A., Botta, G., Liquori, G. E., et al. (2005). Expression and subcellular localization of the AQP8 and AQP1 water channels in the mouse gall-bladder epithelium. *Biol. Cell* 97, 415–423. doi: 10.1042/BC20040137

Camerino, G., Nicchia, G., Dinardo, M., Ribatti, D., Svelto, M., and Frigeri, A. (2006). *In vivo* silencing of aquaporin-1 by RNA interference inhibits angiogenesis in the chick embryo chorioallantoic membrane assay. *Cell. Mol. Biol.* 52, 51–56.

Campbell, E. M., Birdsell, D. N., and Yool, A. J. (2012). The activity of human aquaporin 1 as a cGMP-gated cation channel is regulated by tyrosine phosphorylation in the carboxyl-terminal domain. *Mol. Pharmacol.* 81, 97–105. doi: 10.1124/mol.111.073692

Cano, A., Pérez-Moreno, M. A., Rodrigo, I., Locascio, A., Blanco, M. J., del Barrio, M. G., et al. (2000). The transcription factor snail controls epithelial–mesenchymal transitions by repressing E-cadherin expression. *Nat. Cell Biol.* 2, 76–83. doi: 10.1038/35000025

Carbrey, J. M., Song, L., Zhou, Y., Yoshinaga, M., Rojek, A., Wang, Y., et al. (2009). Reduced arsenic clearance and increased toxicity in aquaglyceroporin-9-null mice. *Proc. Natl. Acad. Sci. U.S.A.* 106, 15956–15960. doi: 10.1073/pnas.0908108106

Cavallaro, U., and Christofori, G. (2004). Cell adhesion and signalling by cadherins and Ig-CAMs in cancer. *Nat. Rev. Cancer* 4, 118–132. doi: 10.1038/nrc1276

Chae, Y. K., Kang, S. K., Kim, M. S., Woo, J., Lee, J., Chang, S., et al. (2008a). Human AQP5 plays a role in the progression of chronic myelogenous leukemia (CML). *PLoS ONE* 3:e2594. doi: 10.1371/journal.pone.0002594

Chae, Y. K., Woo, J., Kim, M.-J., Kang, S. K., Kim, M. S., Lee, J., et al. (2008b). Expression of aquaporin 5 (AQP5) promotes tumor invasion in human non small cell lung cancer. *PLoS ONE* 3:e2162. doi: 10.1371/journal.pone.0002162

Chandy, G., Zampighi, G. A., Kreman, M., and Hall, J. E. (1997). Comparison of the water transporting properties of MIP and AQP1. *J. Membr. Biol.* 159, 29–39. doi: 10.1007/s002329900266

Chen, C., Ma, T., Zhang, C., Zhang, H., Bai, L., Kong, L., et al. (2017). Down-regulation of aquaporin 5-mediated epithelial-mesenchymal transition and anti-metastatic effect by natural product Cairicoside E in colorectal cancer. *Mol. Carcinog.* 56, 2692–2705. doi: 10.1002/mc.22712

Chen, J., Wang, T., Zhou, Y.-C., Gao, F., Zhang, Z.-H., Xu, H., et al. (2014). Aquaporin 3 promotes epithelial-mesenchymal transition in gastric cancer. *J. Exp. Clin. Cancer Res.* 33:38. doi: 10.1186/1756-9966-33-38

Chen, J., Wang, Z., Xu, D., Liu, Y., and Gao, Y. (2015). Aquaporin 3 promotes prostate cancer cell motility and invasion via extracellular signal-regulated kinase 1/2-mediated matrix metalloproteinase-3 secretion. *Mol. Med. Rep.* 11, 2882–2888. doi: 10.3892/mmr.2014.3097

Chen, Q., Zhu, L., Zheng, B., Wang, J., Song, X., Zheng, W., et al. (2016). Effect of AQP9 expression in androgen-independent prostate cancer cell PC3. *Int. J. Mol. Sci.* 17:738. doi: 10.3390/ijms17050738

Chen, Y., Rice, W., Gu, Z., Li, J., Huang, J., Brenner, M. B., et al. (2012). Aquaporin 2 promotes cell migration and epithelial morphogenesis. *J. Am. Soc. Nephrol.* 23, 1506–1517. doi: 10.1681/ASN.2012010079

Chen, Y., Tachibana, O., Oda, M., Xu, R., Hamada, J.-I, Yamashita, J., et al. (2006). Increased expression of aquaporin 1 in human hemangioblastomas and its correlation with cyst formation. *J. Neurooncol.* 80, 219–225. doi: 10.1007/s11060-005-9057-1

Chen, Z., Zhang, Z., Gu, Y., and Bai, C. (2011). Impaired migration and cell volume regulation in aquaporin 5-deficient SPC-A1 cells. *Respir. Physiol. Neurobiol.* 176, 110–117. doi: 10.1016/j.resp.2011.02.001

Cho, S.-J., Sattar, A. A., Jeong, E.-H., Satchi, M., Cho, J. A., Dash, S., et al. (2002). Aquaporin 1 regulates GTP-induced rapid gating of water in secretory vesicles. *Proc. Natl. Acad. Sci. U.S.A.* 99, 4720–4724. doi: 10.1073/pnas.072083499

Chrzanowska-Wodnicka, M., and Burridge, K. (1996). Rho-stimulated contractility drives the formation of stress fibers and focal adhesions. *J. Cell Biol.* 133, 1403–1415. doi: 10.1083/jcb.133.6.1403

Chua, H., Bhat-Nakshatri, P., Clare, S., Morimiya, A., Badve, S., and Nakshatri, H. (2007). NF-κB represses E-cadherin expression and enhances epithelial to mesenchymal transition of mammary epithelial cells: potential involvement of ZEB-1 and ZEB-2. *Oncogene* 26, 711–724. doi: 10.1038/sj.onc.1209808

Clapp, C., and de la Escalera, G. M. (2006). Aquaporin-1: a novel promoter of tumor angiogenesis. *Trends Endocrinol. Metab.* 17, 1–2. doi: 10.1016/j.tem.2005.11.009

Condeelis, J. (1993). Life at the leading edge: the formation of cell protrusions. *Annu. Rev. Cell Biol.* 9, 411–444. doi: 10.1146/annurev.cb.09.110193.002211

Cramer, L. P., Siebert, M., and Mitchison, T. J. (1997). Identification of novel graded polarity actin filament bundles in locomoting heart fibroblasts: implications for the generation of motile force. *J. Cell Biol.* 136, 1287–1305. doi: 10.1083/jcb.136.6.1287

Curtis, A. (1964). The mechanism of adhesion of cells to glass A study by interference reflection microscopy. *J. Cell Biol.* 20, 199–215. doi: 10.1083/jcb.20.2.199

Demir, R., Seval, Y., and Huppertz, B. (2007). Vasculogenesis and angiogenesis in the early human placenta. *Acta Histochem.* 109, 257–265. doi: 10.1016/j.acthis.2007.02.008

Demir, R., Yaba, A., and Huppertz, B. (2010). Vasculogenesis and angiogenesis in the endometrium during menstrual cycle and implantation. *Acta Histochem.* 112, 203–214. doi: 10.1016/j.acthis.2009.04.004

Denker, B. M., Smith, B. L., Kuhajda, F. P., and Agre, P. (1988). Identification, purification, and partial characterization of a novel Mr 28,000 integral membrane protein from erythrocytes and renal tubules. *J. Biol. Chem.* 263, 15634–15642.

Detmers, F. J., de Groot, B. L., Müller, E. M., Hinton, A., Konings, I. B., Sze, M., et al. (2006). Quaternary ammonium compounds as water channel blockers. Specificity, potency, and site of action. *J. Biol. Chem.* 281, 14207–14214. doi: 10.1074/jbc.M513072200

Diez, S., Gerisch, G., Anderson, K., Müller-Taubenberger, A., and Bretschneider, T. (2005). Subsecond reorganization of the actin network in cell motility and chemotaxis. *Proc. Natl. Acad. Sci. U.S.A.* 102, 7601–7606. doi: 10.1073/pnas.0408546102

Ding, T., Ma, Y., Li, W., Liu, X., Ying, G., Fu, L., et al. (2011). Role of aquaporin-4 in the regulation of migration and invasion of human glioma cells. *Int. J. Oncol.* 38, 1521–1531. doi: 10.3892/ijo.2011.983

Direito, I., Paulino, J., Vigia, E., Brito, M. A., and Soveral, G. (2017). Differential expression of aquaporin-3 and aquaporin-5 in pancreatic ductal adenocarcinoma. *J. Surg. Oncol.* 115, 980–996. doi: 10.1002/jso.24605

Disanza, A., Steffen, A., Hertzog, M., Frittoli, E., Rottner, K., and Scita, G. (2005). Actin polymerization machinery: the finish line of signaling networks, the starting point of cellular movement. *Cell. Mol. Life Sci.* 62, 955–970. doi: 10.1007/s00018-004-4472-6

Dittmar, T., Heyder, C., Gloria-Maercker, E., Hatzmann, W., and Zänker, K. S. (2008). Adhesion molecules and chemokines: the navigation system for circulating tumor (stem) cells to metastasize in an organ-specific manner. *Clin. Exp. Metastasis* 25, 11–32. doi: 10.1007/s10585-007-9095-5

Dorward, H. S., Du, A., Bruhn, M. A., Wrin, J., Pei, J. V., Evdokiou, A., et al. (2016). Pharmacological blockade of aquaporin-1 water channel by AqB013 restricts migration and invasiveness of colon cancer cells and prevents endothelial tube formation *in vitro*. *Nat. Rev. Cancer* 35:36. doi: 10.1186/s13046-016-0310-6

Drubin, D. G., and Nelson, W. J. (1996). Origins of cell polarity. *Cell* 84, 335–344. doi: 10.1016/S0092-8674(00)81278-7

Echevarria, M., Windhager, E. E., Tate, S. S., and Frindt, G. (1994). Cloning and expression of AQP3, a water channel from the medullary collecting duct of rat kidney. *Proc. Natl. Acad. Sci. U.S.A.* 91, 10997–11001. doi: 10.1073/pnas.91.23.10997

Egginton, S. (2009). Invited review: activity-induced angiogenesis. *Pflügers Arch. Eur. J. Physiol.* 457:963. doi: 10.1007/s00424-008-0563-9

Ehring, G. R., and Hall, J. E. (1988). "Single channel properties of lens MIP 28 reconstituted into planar lipid bilayers," in *Proceedings of the Western Pharmacology Society*, 251.

El Hindy, N., Bankfalvi, A., Herring, A., Adamzik, M., Lambertz, N., Zhu, Y., et al. (2013). Correlation of aquaporin-1 water channel protein expression with tumor angiogenesis in human astrocytoma. *Anticancer Res.* 33, 609–613.

Endo, M., Jain, R. K., Witwer, B., and Brown, D. (1999). Water channel (aquaporin 1) expression and distribution in mammary carcinomas and glioblastomas. *Microvasc. Res.* 58, 89–98. doi: 10.1006/mvre.1999.2158

Esteva-Font, C., Jin, B.-J., and Verkman, A. S. (2014). Aquaporin-1 gene deletion reduces breast tumor growth and lung metastasis in tumor-producing MMTV-PyVT mice. *FASEB J.* 28, 1446–1453. doi: 10.1096/fj.13-245621

Etienne-Manneville, S., and Hall, A. (2003). Cell polarity: Par6, aPKC and cytoskeletal crosstalk. *Curr. Opin. Cell Biol.* 15, 67–72. doi: 10.1016/S0955-0674(02)00005-4

Fang, X., Yang, B., Matthay, M. A., and Verkman, A. (2002). Evidence against aquaporin-1-dependent CO2 permeability in lung and kidney. *J. Physiol.* 542, 63–69. doi: 10.1113/jphysiol.2001.013813

Ferlay, J., Soerjomataram, I., Dikshit, R., Eser, S., Mathers, C., Rebelo, M., et al. (2015). Cancer incidence and mortality worldwide: sources, methods and major patterns in GLOBOCAN 2012. *Int. J.Cancer* 136, E359–E386. doi: 10.1002/ijc.29210

Finn, R. N., and Cerdà, J. (2015). Evolution and functional diversity of aquaporins. *Biol. Bull.* 229, 6–23. doi: 10.1086/BBLv229n1p6

Finn, R. N., Chauvign,é, F., Hlidberg, J. B., Cutler, C. P., and Cerdà J. (2014). The lineage-specific evolution of aquaporin gene clusters facilitated tetrapod terrestrial adaptation. *PLoS ONE* 9:e113686. doi: 10.1371/journal.pone.0113686

Fletcher, S. J., and Rappoport, J. Z. (2010). Moving forward: polarised trafficking in cell migration. *Trends Cell Biol.* 20, 71–78. doi: 10.1016/j.tcb.2009.11.006

Folkman, J., Cole, P., and Zimmerman, S. (1966). Tumor behavior in isolated perfused organs: *in vitro* growth and metastases of biopsy material in rabbit thyroid and canine intestinal segment. *Ann. Surg.* 164:491. doi: 10.1097/00000658-196609000-00012

Fossdal, G., Vik-Mo, E. O., Sandberg, C., Varghese, M., Kaarbø, M., Telmo, E., et al. (2012). Aqp 9 and brain tumour stem cells. *Sci. World J.* 2012:915176. doi: 10.1100/2012/915176

Friedl, P., and Weigelin, B. (2008). Interstitial leukocyte migration and immune function. *Nat. Immunol.* 9, 960–969. doi: 10.1038/ni.f.212

Friedl, P., and Wolf, K. (2003). Tumour-cell invasion and migration: diversity and escape mechanisms. *Nat. Rev. Cancer* 3, 362–374. doi: 10.1038/nrc1075

Friedl, P., and Wolf, K. (2009). Proteolytic interstitial cell migration: a five-step process. *Cancer Metastasis Rev.* 28, 129–135. doi: 10.1007/s10555-008-9174-3

Friedl, P., Hegerfeldt, Y., and Tusch, M. (2004). Collective cell migration in morphogenesis and cancer. *Int. J. Dev. Biol.* 48, 441–450. doi: 10.1387/ijdb.041821pf

Fushimi, K., Uchida, S., Hara, Y., Hirata, Y., Marumo, F., and Sasaki, S. (1993). Cloning and expression of apical membrane water channel of rat kidney collecting tubule. *Nature* 361:549. doi: 10.1038/361549a0

Gamelin, E., Gamelin, L., Bossi, L., and Quasthoff, S. (2002). Clinical aspects and molecular basis of oxaliplatin neurotoxicity: current management and development of preventive measures. *Semin. Oncol.* 29(5Suppl. 15), 21–33. doi: 10.1053/sonc.2002.35525

Gao, J., Wang, X., Chang, Y., Zhang, J., Song, Q., Yu, H., et al. (2006). Acetazolamide inhibits osmotic water permeability by interaction with aquaporin-1. *Anal. Biochem.* 350, 165–170. doi: 10.1016/j.ab.2006.01.003

Geiger, B., Bershadsky, A., Pankov, R., and Yamada, K. M. (2001). Transmembrane crosstalk between the extracellular matrix and the cytoskeleton. *Nat. Rev. Mol. Cell Biol.* 2, 793–805. doi: 10.1038/35099066

Goldstein, B., and Macara, I. G. (2007). The PAR proteins: fundamental players in animal cell polarization. *Dev. Cell* 13, 609–622. doi: 10.1016/j.devcel.2007.10.007

Gralow, J. R., Biermann, J. S., Farooki, A., Fornier, M. N., Gagel, R. F., Kumar, R., et al. (2013). NCCN task force report: bone health in cancer care. *J. Natl. Comp. Cancer Netw.* 11, S1–S50. doi: 10.6004/jnccn.2013.0215

Guarino, M., Rubino, B., and Ballabio, G. (2007). The role of epithelial-mesenchymal transition in cancer pathology. *Pathology* 39, 305–318. doi: 10.1080/00313020701329914

Guo, X., Sun, T., Yang, M., Li, Z., Li, Z., and Gao, Y. (2013). Prognostic value of combined aquaporin 3 and aquaporin 5 overexpression in hepatocellular carcinoma. *Biomed Res. Int.* 2013:206525. doi: 10.1155/2013/206525

Gupta, S. C., Patchva, S., and Aggarwal, B. B. (2013). Therapeutic roles of curcumin: lessons learned from clinical trials. *AAPS J.* 15, 195–218. doi: 10.1208/s12248-012-9432-8

Hall, A. (1998). Rho GTPases and the actin cytoskeleton. *Science* 279, 509–514. doi: 10.1126/science.279.5350.509

Hara-Chikuma, M., and Verkman, A. (2008a). Aquaporin-3 facilitates epidermal cell migration and proliferation during wound healing. *J. Mol. Med.* 86, 221–231. doi: 10.1007/s00109-007-0272-4

Hara-Chikuma, M., and Verkman, A. (2008b). Prevention of skin tumorigenesis and impairment of epidermal cell proliferation by targeted aquaporin-3 gene disruption. *Mol. Cell. Biol.* 28, 326–332. doi: 10.1128/MCB.01482-07

Hara-Chikuma, M., and Verkman, A. S. (2006). Aquaporin-1 facilitates epithelial cell migration in kidney proximal tubule. *J. Am. Soc. Nephrol.* 17, 39–45. doi: 10.1681/ASN.2005080846

Hara-Chikuma, M., Chikuma, S., Sugiyama, Y., Kabashima, K., Verkman, A. S., Inoue, S., et al. (2012). Chemokine-dependent T cell migration requires aquaporin-3–mediated hydrogen peroxide uptake. *J. Exp. Med.* 209, 1743–1752. doi: 10.1084/jem.20112398

Hara-Chikuma, M., Watanabe, S., and Satooka, H. (2016). Involvement of aquaporin-3 in epidermal growth factor receptor signaling via hydrogen peroxide transport in cancer cells. *Biochem. Biophys. Res. Commun.* 471, 603–609. doi: 10.1016/j.bbrc.2016.02.010

Hasegawa, H., Ma, T., Skach, W., Matthay, M. A., and Verkman, A. (1994). Molecular cloning of a mercurial-insensitive water channel expressed in selected water-transporting tissues. *J. Biol. Chem.* 269, 5497–5500.

Herrera, M., and Garvin, J. L. (2011). Aquaporins as gas channels. *Pflügers Arch. Eur. J. Physiol.* 462:623. doi: 10.1007/s00424-011-1002-x

Herrera, M., Hong, N. J., and Garvin, J. L. (2006). Aquaporin-1 transports NO across cell membranes. *Hypertension* 48, 157–164. doi: 10.1161/01.HYP.0000223652.29338.77

Hoffert, J. D., Pisitkun, T., Wang, G., Shen, R.-F., and Knepper, M. A. (2006). Quantitative phosphoproteomics of vasopressin-sensitive renal cells: regulation of aquaporin-2 phosphorylation at two sites. *Proc. Natl. Acad. Sci. U.S.A.* 103, 7159–7164. doi: 10.1073/pnas.0600895103

Holm, L. M., Jahn, T. P., Møller, A. L., Schjoerring, J. K., Ferri, D., Klaerke, D. A., et al. (2005). NH3 and NH4+ permeability in aquaporin-expressing Xenopus oocytes. *Pflügers Arch.* 450, 415–428. doi: 10.1007/s00424-005-1399-1

Hoque, M. O., Soria, J.-C., Woo, J., Lee, T., Lee, J., Jang, S. J., et al. (2006). Aquaporin 1 is overexpressed in lung cancer and stimulates NIH-3T3 cell proliferation and anchorage-independent growth. *Am. J. Pathol.* 168, 1345–1353. doi: 10.2353/ajpath.2006.050596

Howard-Anderson, J., Ganz, P. A., Bower, J. E., and Stanton, A. L. (2012). Quality of life, fertility concerns, and behavioral health outcomes in younger breast cancer survivors: a systematic review. *J. Natl. Cancer Inst.* 104, 386–405. doi: 10.1093/jnci/djr541

Hu, J., and Verkman, A. S. (2006). Increased migration and metastatic potential of tumor cells expressing aquaporin water channels. *FASEB J.* 20, 1892–1894. doi: 10.1096/fj.06-5930fje

Huang, Y., Zhu, Z., Sun, M., Wang, J., Guo, R., Shen, L., et al. (2010). Critical role of aquaporin-3 in the human epidermal growth factor-induced migration and proliferation in the human gastric adenocarcinoma cells. *Cancer Biol. Ther.* 9, 1000–1007. doi: 10.4161/cbt.9.12.11705

Huber, V. J., Tsujita, M., Kwee, I. L., and Nakada, T. (2009). Inhibition of aquaporin 4 by antiepileptic drugs. *Bioorg. Med. Chem.* 17, 418–424. doi: 10.1016/j.bmc.2007.12.038

Huttenlocher, A., Palecek, S. P., Lu, Q., Zhang, W., Mellgren, R. L., Lauffenburger, D. A., et al. (1997). Regulation of cell migration by the calcium-dependent protease calpain. *J. Biol. Chem.* 272, 32719–32722. doi: 10.1074/jbc.272.52.32719

Hwang, I., Jung, S.-I., Hwang, E.-C., Song, S. H., Lee, H.-S., Kim, S.-O., et al. (2012). Expression and localization of aquaporins in benign prostate hyperplasia and prostate cancer. *Chonnam Med. J.* 48, 174–178. doi: 10.4068/cmj.2012.48.3.174

Ibarra, N., Pollitt, A., and Insall, R. (2005). Regulation of actin assembly by SCAR/WAVE proteins. *Biochem. Soc. Trans.* 33(Pt 6), 1243–1246. doi: 10.1042/BST0331243

Ishibashi, K. (2009). New members of mammalian aquaporins: AQP10–AQP12. *Aquaporins* 190, 251–262. doi: 10.1007/978-3-540-79885-9_13

Ishibashi, K., Hara, S., and Kondo, S. (2009). Aquaporin water channels in mammals. *Clin. Exp. Nephrol.* 13, 107–117. doi: 10.1007/s10157-008-0118-6

Ishibashi, K., Kuwahara, M., Gu, Y., Kageyama, Y., Tohsaka, A., Suzuki, F., et al. (1997a). Cloning and functional expression of a new water channel abundantly expressed in the testis permeable to water, glycerol, and urea. *J. Biol. Chem.* 272, 20782–20786. doi: 10.1074/jbc.272.33.20782

Ishibashi, K., Kuwahara, M., Gu, Y., Tanaka, Y., Marumo, F., and Sasaki, S. (1998). Cloning and functional expression of a new aquaporin (AQP9) abundantly expressed in the peripheral leukocytes permeable to water and urea, but not to glycerol. *Biochem. Biophys. Res. Commun.* 244, 268–274. doi: 10.1006/bbrc.1998.8252

Ishibashi, K., Kuwahara, M., Kageyama, Y., Tohsaka, A., Marumo, F., and Sasaki, S. (1997b). Cloning and functional expression of a second new aquaporin abundantly expressed in testis. *Biochem. Biophys. Res. Commun.* 237, 714–718. doi: 10.1006/bbrc.1997.7219

Ishibashi, K., Morinaga, T., Kuwahara, M., Sasaki, S., and Imai, M. (2002). Cloning and identification of a new member of water channel (AQP10) as an aquaglyceroporin. *Biochim. Biophys. Acta* 1576, 335–340. doi: 10.1016/S0167-4781(02)00393-7

Ishibashi, K., Sasaki, S., Fushimi, K., Uchida, S., Kuwahara, M., Saito, H., et al. (1994). Molecular cloning and expression of a member of the aquaporin family with permeability to glycerol and urea in addition to water expressed at the basolateral membrane of kidney collecting duct cells. *Proc. Natl. Acad. Sci. U.S.A.* 91, 6269–6273. doi: 10.1073/pnas.91.14.6269

Jensen, M. Ø., Tajkhorshid, E., and Schulten, K. (2001). The mechanism of glycerol conduction in aquaglyceroporins. *Structure* 9, 1083–1093. doi: 10.1016/S0969-2126(01)00668-2

Ji, C., Cao, C., Lu, S., Kivlin, R., Amaral, A., Kouttab, N., et al. (2008). Curcumin attenuates EGF-induced AQP3 up-regulation and cell migration in human ovarian cancer cells. *Cancer Chemother. Pharmacol.* 62, 857–865. doi: 10.1007/s00280-007-0674-6

Jiang, Y. (2009). Aquaporin-1 activity of plasma membrane affects HT20 colon cancer cell migration. *IUBMB Life* 61, 1001–1009. doi: 10.1002/iub.243

Jiang, Y., and Jiang, Z.-B. (2010). Aquaporin 1-expressing MCF-7 mammary carcinoma cells show enhanced migration *in vitro*. *J. Biomed. Sci. Eng.* 3:95. doi: 10.4236/jbise.2010.31014

Johnson, D. I., and Pringle, J. R. (1990). Molecular characterization of CDC42, a Saccharomyces cerevisiae gene involved in the development of cell polarity. *J. Cell Biol.* 111, 143–152. doi: 10.1083/jcb.111.1.143

Jung, H. J., Park, J.-Y., Jeon, H.-S., and Kwon, T.-H. (2011). Aquaporin-5: a marker protein for proliferation and migration of human breast cancer cells. *PLoS ONE* 6:e28492. doi: 10.1371/journal.pone.0028492

Jung, J. S., Preston, G. M., Smith, B. L., Guggino, W. B., and Agre, P. (1994). Molecular structure of the water channel through aquaporin CHIP. The hourglass model. *J. Biol. Chem.* 269, 14648–14654.

Kalluri, R., and Weinberg, R. A. (2009). The basics of epithelial-mesenchymal transition. *J. Clin. Invest.* 119:1420. doi: 10.1172/JCI39104

Kaneko, K., Yagui, K., Tanaka, A., Yoshihara, K., Ishikawa, K., Takahashi, K., et al. (2008). Aquaporin 1 is required for hypoxia-inducible angiogenesis in human retinal vascular endothelial cells. *Microvasc. Res.* 75, 297–301. doi: 10.1016/j.mvr.2007.12.003

Kang, B. W., Kim, J. G., Lee, S. J., Chae, Y. S., Jeong, J. Y., Yoon, G. S., et al. (2015). Expression of aquaporin-1, aquaporin-3, and aquaporin-5 correlates with nodal metastasis in colon cancer. *Oncology* 88, 369–376. doi: 10.1159/000369073

Kang, S. K., Chae, Y. K., Woo, J., Kim, M. S., Park, J. C., Lee, J., et al. (2008). Role of human aquaporin 5 in colorectal carcinogenesis. *Am. J. Pathol.* 173, 518–525. doi: 10.2353/ajpath.2008.071198

Klausen, M., Aaes-Jørgensen, A., Molin, S., and Tolker-Nielsen, T. (2003). Involvement of bacterial migration in the development of complex multicellular structures in Pseudomonas aeruginosa biofilms. *Mol. Microbiol.* 50, 61–68. doi: 10.1046/j.1365-2958.2003.03677.x

Klebe, S., Griggs, K., Cheng, Y., Driml, J., Henderson, D. W., and Reid, G. (2015). Blockade of aquaporin 1 inhibits proliferation, motility, and metastatic potential of mesothelioma *in vitro* but not in an *in vivo* model. *Dis. Markers* 2015:286719. doi: 10.1155/2015/286719

Koeller, J. M., Aapro, M. S., Gralla, R. J., Grunberg, S. M., Hesketh, P. J., Kris, M. G., et al. (2002). Antiemetic guidelines: creating a more practical treatment approach. *Support. Care Cancer* 10, 519–522. doi: 10.1007/s00520-001-0335-y

Kong, D., Li, Y., Wang, Z., Banerjee, S., Ahmad, A., Kim, H. R. C., et al. (2009). miR-200 Regulates PDGF-D-mediated epithelial–mesenchymal transition, adhesion, and invasion of prostate cancer cells. *Stem Cells* 27, 1712–1721. doi: 10.1002/stem.101

Korpal, M., Lee, E. S., Hu, G., and Kang, Y. (2008). The miR-200 family inhibits epithelial-mesenchymal transition and cancer cell migration by direct targeting of E-cadherin transcriptional repressors ZEB1 and ZEB2. *J. Biol. Chem.* 283, 14910–14914. doi: 10.1074/jbc.C800074200

Kourghi, M., De Ieso, M. L., Nourmohammadi, S., Pei, J. V., and Yool, A. J. (2018). Identification of loop D domain amino acids in the human Aquaporin-1 channel involved in activation of the ionic conductance and inhibition by AqB011. *Front. Chem.* 6:142. doi: 10.3389/fchem.2018.00142

Kourghi, M., Pei, J. V., De Ieso, M. L., Flynn, G., and Yool, A. J. (2015). Bumetanide derivatives AqB007 and AqB011 selectively block the Aquaporin-1 ion channel conductance and slow cancer cell migration. *Mol. Pharmacol.* 115:101618. doi: 10.1124/mol.115.101618

Kuriyama, H., Shimomura, I., Kishida, K., Kondo, H., Furuyama, N., Nishizawa, H., et al. (2002). Coordinated regulation of fat-specific and liver-specific glycerol channels, aquaporin adipose and aquaporin 9. *Diabetes* 51, 2915–2921. doi: 10.2337/diabetes.51.10.2915

Kusayama, M., Wada, K., Nagata, M., Ishimoto, S., Takahashi, H., Yoneda, M., et al. (2011). Critical role of aquaporin 3 on growth of human esophageal and oral squamous cell carcinoma. *Cancer Sci.* 102, 1128–1136. doi: 10.1111/j.1349-7006.2011.01927.x

Lee, T.-C., Ho, I.-C., Lu, W.-J., and Huang, J.-D. (2006). Enhanced expression of multidrug resistance-associated protein 2 and reduced expression of aquaglyceroporin 3 in an arsenic-resistant human cell line. *J. Biol. Chem.* 281, 18401–18407. doi: 10.1074/jbc.M601266200

Leung, J., Pang, A., Yuen, W.-H., Kwong, Y.-L., and Tse, E. W. C. (2007). Relationship of expression of aquaglyceroporin 9 with arsenic uptake and sensitivity in leukemia cells. *Blood* 109, 740–746. doi: 10.1182/blood-2006-04-019588

Li, A., Lu, D., Zhang, Y., Li, J., Fang, Y., Li, F., et al. (2013). Critical role of aquaporin-3 in epidermal growth factor-induced migration of colorectal carcinoma cells and its clinical significance. *Oncol. Rep.* 29, 535–540. doi: 10.3892/or.2012.2144

Li, C., and Wang, W. (2017). Molecular biology of aquaporins. *Adv. Exp. Med. Biol.* 969, 1–34. doi: 10.1007/978-94-024-1057-0_1

Li, C.-F., Zhang, W.-G., Liu, M., Qiu, L.-W., Chen, X.-F., Lv, L., et al. (2016). Aquaporin 9 inhibits hepatocellular carcinoma through up-regulating FOXO1 expression. *Oncotarget* 7, 44161–44170. doi: 10.18632/oncotarget.10143

Li, J., Wang, Z., Chong, T., Chen, H., Li, H., Li, G., et al. (2014). Over-expression of a poor prognostic marker in prostate cancer: AQP5 promotes cells growth and local invasion. *World J. Surg. Oncol.* 12:284. doi: 10.1186/1477-7819-12-284

Li, Y. B., Sun, S. R., and Han, X. H. (2016). Down-regulation of AQP4 inhibits proliferation, migration and invasion of human breast cancer cells. *Folia Biol.* 62, 131–137.

Liu, W., Wang, K., Gong, K., Li, X., and Luo, K. (2012). Epidermal growth factor enhances MPC-83 pancreatic cancer cell migration through the upregulation of aquaporin 3. *Mol. Med. Rep.* 6, 607–610. doi: 10.3892/mmr.2012.966

Liu, Y. L., Matsuzaki, T., Nakazawa, T., Murata, S., Nakamura, N., Kondo, T., et al. (2007). Expression of aquaporin 3 (AQP3) in normal and neoplastic lung tissues. *Hum. Pathol.* 38, 171–178. doi: 10.1016/j.humpath.2006.07.015

Liu, Z., Shen, J., Carbrey, J. M., Mukhopadhyay, R., Agre, P., and Rosen, B. P. (2002). Arsenite transport by mammalian aquaglyceroporins AQP7 and AQP9. *Proc. Natl. Acad. Sci. U.S.A.* 99, 6053–6058. doi: 10.1073/pnas.092131899

Lo, H.-W., Hsu, S.-C., Xia, W., Cao, X., Shih, J.-Y., Wei, Y., et al. (2007). Epidermal growth factor receptor cooperates with signal transducer and activator of transcription 3 to induce epithelial-mesenchymal transition in cancer cells via up-regulation of TWIST gene expression. *Cancer Res.* 67, 9066–9076. doi: 10.1158/0008-5472.CAN-07-0575

Loitto, V. M., Huang, C., Sigal, Y. J., and Jacobson, K. (2007). Filopodia are induced by aquaporin-9 expression. *Exp. Cell Res.* 313, 1295–1306. doi: 10.1016/j.yexcr.2007.01.023

Loitto, V.-M., Forslund, T., Sundqvist, T., Magnusson, K.-E., and Gustafsson, M. (2002). Neutrophil leukocyte motility requires directed water influx. *J. Leukoc. Biol.* 71, 212–222. doi: 10.1189/jlb.71.2.212

Ma, B., Xiang, Y., Mu, S.-M., Li, T., Yu, H.-M., and Li, X.-J. (2004a). Effects of acetazolamide and anordiol on osmotic water permeability in AQP1-cRNA injected Xenopus oocyte. *Acta pharmacol. Sin.* 25, 90–97.

Ma, B., Xiang, Y., Li, T., Yu, H.-M., and Li, X.-J. (2004b). Inhibitory effect of topiramate on Lewis lung carcinoma metastasis and its relation with AQP1 water channel. *Acta pharmacol. Sin.* 25, 54–60.

Ma, T., Hara, M., Sougrat, R., Verbavatz, J.-M., and Verkman, A. (2002). Impaired stratum corneum hydration in mice lacking epidermal water channel aquaporin-3. *J. Biol. Chem.* 277, 17147–17153. doi: 10.1074/jbc.M200925200

Ma, T., Song, Y., Gillespie, A., Carlson, E. J., Epstein, C. J., and Verkman, A. (1999). Defective secretion of saliva in transgenic mice lacking aquaporin-5 water channels. *J. Biol. Chem.* 274, 20071–20074. doi: 10.1074/jbc.274.29.20071

Ma, T., Song, Y., Yang, B., Gillespie, A., Carlson, E. J., Epstein, C. J., et al. (2000). Nephrogenic diabetes insipidus in mice lacking aquaporin-3 water channels. *Proc. Natl. Acad. Sci. U.S.A.* 97, 4386–4391. doi: 10.1073/pnas.080499597

Ma, T., Yang, B., and Verkman, A. (1997a). Cloning of a novel water and urea-permeable aquaporin from mouse expressed strongly in colon, placenta, liver, and heart. *Biochem. Biophys. Res. Commun.* 240, 324–328. doi: 10.1006/bbrc.1997.7664

Ma, T., Yang, B., Gillespie, A., Carlson, E. J., Epstein, C. J., and Verkman, A. (1997b). Generation and phenotype of a transgenic knockout mouse lacking the mercurial-insensitive water channel aquaporin-4. *J. Clin. Invest.* 100:957. doi: 10.1172/JCI231

Ma, T., Yang, B., Gillespie, A., Carlson, E. J., Epstein, C. J., and Verkman, A. S. (1998). Severely impaired urinary concentrating ability in transgenic mice lacking aquaporin-1 water channels. *J. Biol. Chem.* 273, 4296–4299. doi: 10.1074/jbc.273.8.4296

Ma, T., Yang, B., Kuo, W.-L., and Verkman, A. S. (1996). cDNA cloning and gene structure of a novel water channel expressed exclusively in human kidney: evidence for a gene cluster of aquaporins at chromosome locus 12q13. *Genomics* 35, 543–550. doi: 10.1006/geno.1996.0396

Machesky, L. M. (2008). Lamellipodia and filopodia in metastasis and invasion. *FEBS Lett.* 582, 2102–2111. doi: 10.1016/j.febslet.2008.03.039

Madeira, A., Fernández-Veledo, S., Camps, M., Zorzano, A., Moura, T. F., Ceperuelo-Mallafré, V., et al. (2014). Human aquaporin-11 is a water and glycerol channel and localizes in the vicinity of lipid droplets in human adipocytes. *Obesity* 22, 2010–2017. doi: 10.1002/oby.20792

Maeda, N., Hibuse, T., and Funahashi, T. (2009). Role of aquaporin-7 and aquaporin-9 in glycerol metabolism; involvement in obesity. *Handb. Exp. Pharmacol.* 2009, 233–249. doi: 10.1007/978-3-540-79885-9_12

Manley, G. T., Fujimura, M., Ma, T., Noshita, N., Filiz, F., Bollen, A. W., et al. (2000). Aquaporin-4 deletion in mice reduces brain edema after acute water intoxication and ischemic stroke. *Nat. Med.* 6, 159–163. doi: 10.1038/72256

Martin, K. H., Slack, J. K., Boerner, S. A., Martin, C. C., and Parsons, J. T. (2002). Integrin connections map: to infinity and beyond. *Science* 296, 1652–1653. doi: 10.1126/science.296.5573.1652

Martins, A. P., Ciancetta, A., de Almeida, A., Marrone, A., Re, N., Soveral, G., et al. (2013). Aquaporin inhibition by gold (III) compounds: new insights. *ChemMedChem* 8, 1086–1092. doi: 10.1002/cmdc.201300107

Martins, A. P., Marrone, A., Ciancetta, A., Cobo, A. G., Echevarría, M., Moura, T. F., et al. (2012). Targeting aquaporin function: potent inhibition of aquaglyceroporin-3 by a gold-based compound. *PLoS ONE* 7:e37435. doi: 10.1371/journal.pone.0037435

Mattila, P. K., and Lappalainen, P. (2008). Filopodia: molecular architecture and cellular functions. *Nat. Rev. Mol. Cell Biol.* 9, 446–454. doi: 10.1038/nrm2406

McCoy, E. S., Haas, B. R., and Sontheimer, H. (2010). Water permeability through aquaporin-4 is regulated by protein kinase C and becomes rate-limiting for glioma invasion. *Neuroscience* 168, 971–981. doi: 10.1016/j.neuroscience.2009.09.020

McCoy, E., and Sontheimer, H. (2007). Expression and function of water channels (aquaporins) in migrating malignant astrocytes. *Glia* 55, 1034–1043. doi: 10.1002/glia.20524

Mcferrin, M. B., and Sontheimer, H. (2006). A role for ion channels in glioma cell invasion. *Neuron Glia Biol.* 2, 39–49. doi: 10.1017/S1740925X06000044

McLean, G. W., Carragher, N. O., Avizienyte, E., Evans, J., Brunton, V. G., and Frame, M. C. (2005). The role of focal-adhesion kinase in cancer—a new therapeutic opportunity. *Nat. Rev. Cancer* 5:505. doi: 10.1038/nrc1647

Medici, D., Hay, E. D., and Olsen, B. R. (2008). Snail and Slug promote epithelial-mesenchymal transition through β-catenin–T-cell factor-4-dependent expression of transforming growth factor-β3. *Mol. Biol. Cell* 19, 4875–4887. doi: 10.1091/mbc.E08-05-0506

Meng, F., Rui, Y., Xu, L., Wan, C., Jiang, X., and Li, G. (2014). Aqp1 enhances migration of bone marrow mesenchymal stem cells through regulation of FAK and beta-catenin. *Stem Cells Dev.* 23, 66–75. doi: 10.1089/scd.2013.0185

Miettinen, P. J., Ebner, R., Lopez, A. R., and Derynck, R. (1994). TGF-beta induced transdifferentiation of mammary epithelial cells to mesenchymal cells: involvement of type I receptors. *J. Cell Biol.* 127, 2021–2036. doi: 10.1083/jcb.127.6.2021

Migliati, E., Meurice, N., DuBois, P., Fang, J. S., Somasekharan, S., Beckett, E., et al. (2009). Inhibition of aquaporin-1 and aquaporin-4 water permeability by a derivative of the loop diuretic bumetanide acting at an internal pore-occluding binding site. *Mol. Pharmacol.* 76, 105–112. doi: 10.1124/mol.108.053744

Miller, E. W., Dickinson, B. C., and Chang, C. J. (2010). Aquaporin-3 mediates hydrogen peroxide uptake to regulate downstream intracellular signaling. *Proc. Natl. Acad. Sci. U.S.A.* 107, 15681–15686. doi: 10.1073/pnas.1005776107

Miller, K. D., Siegel, R. L., Lin, C. C., Mariotto, A. B., Kramer, J. L., Rowland, J. H., et al. (2016). Cancer treatment and survivorship statistics, 2016. *CA. Cancer J. Clin.* 66, 271–289. doi: 10.3322/caac.21349

Mobasheri, A., and Barrett-Jolley, R. (2014). Aquaporin water channels in the mammary gland: from physiology to pathophysiology and neoplasia. *J. Mamm. Gland Biol. Neoplasia* 19, 91–102. doi: 10.1007/s10911-013-9312-6

Monsuez, J.-J., Charniot, J.-C., Vignat, N., and Artigou, J.-Y. (2010). Cardiac side-effects of cancer chemotherapy. *Int. J. Cardiol.* 144, 3–15. doi: 10.1016/j.ijcard.2010.03.003

Monzani, E., Bazzotti, R., Perego, C., and La Porta, C. A. (2009). AQP1 is not only a water channel: it contributes to cell migration through Lin7/beta-catenin. *PLoS ONE* 4:e6167. doi: 10.1371/journal.pone.0006167

Moon, C., Soria, J.-C., Jang, S. J., Lee, J., Hoque, M., Sibony, M., et al. (2003). Involvement of aquaporins in colorectal carcinogenesis. *Oncogene* 22, 6699–6703. doi: 10.1038/sj.onc.1206762

Mott, J. D., and Werb, Z. (2004). Regulation of matrix biology by matrix metalloproteinases. *Curr. Opin. Cell Biol.* 16, 558–564. doi: 10.1016/j.ceb.2004.07.010

Musa-Aziz, R., Chen, L.-M., Pelletier, M. F., and Boron, W. F. (2009). Relative CO2/NH3 selectivities of AQP1, AQP4, AQP5, AmtB, and RhAG. *Proc. Natl. Acad. Sci. U.S.A.* 106, 5406–5411. doi: 10.1073/pnas.0813231106

Nagase, H., and Woessner, J. F. (1999). Matrix metalloproteinases. *J. Biol. Chem.* 274, 21491–21494. doi: 10.1074/jbc.274.31.21491

Nakhoul, N. L., Davis, B. A., Romero, M. F., and Boron, W. F. (1998). Effect of expressing the water channel aquaporin-1 on the CO_2 permeability of *Xenopus oocytes. Am. J. Physiol. Cell Physiol.* 274, C543–C548. doi: 10.1152/ajpcell.1998.274.2.C543

Nakhoul, N. L., Hering-Smith, K. S., Abdulnour-Nakhoul, S. M., and Hamm, L. L. (2001). Transport of NH3/NH 4+ in oocytes expressing aquaporin-1. *Am. J. Physiol. Renal Physiol.* 281, F255–F263. doi: 10.1152/ajprenal.2001.281.2.F255

Neely, J. D., Amiry-Moghaddam, M., Ottersen, O. P., Froehner, S. C., Agre, P., and Adams, M. E. (2001). Syntrophin-dependent expression and localization of Aquaporin-4 water channel protein. *Proc. Natl. Acad. Sci. U.S.A.* 98, 14108–14113. doi: 10.1073/pnas.241508198

Netzel-Arnett, S., Hooper, J. D., Szabo, R., Madison, E. L., Quigley, J. P., Bugge, T. H., et al. (2003). Membrane anchored serine proteases: a rapidly expanding group of cell surface proteolytic enzymes with potential roles in cancer. *Cancer Metastasis Rev.* 22, 237–258. doi: 10.1023/A:1023003616848

Ng, W. H., Hy, J. W., Tan, W. L., Liew, D., Lim, T., Ang, B. T., et al. (2009). Aquaporin-4 expression is increased in edematous meningiomas. *J. Clin. Neurosci.* 16, 441–443. doi: 10.1016/j.jocn.2008.04.028

Nicchia, G. P., Srinivas, M., Li, W., Brosnan, C. F., Frigeri, A., and Spray, D. C. (2005). New possible roles for aquaporin-4 in astrocytes: cell cytoskeleton and functional relationship with connexin43. *FASEB J.* 19, 1674–1676. doi: 10.1096/fj.04-3281fje

Nielsen, S., Chou, C.-L., Marples, D., Christensen, E. I., Kishore, B. K., and Knepper, M. A. (1995). Vasopressin increases water permeability of kidney collecting duct by inducing translocation of aquaporin-CD water channels to plasma membrane. *Proc. Natl. Acad. Sci. U.S.A.* 92, 1013–1017. doi: 10.1073/pnas.92.4.1013

Nielsen, S., Smith, B. L., Christensen, E. I., and Agre, P. (1993). Distribution of the aquaporin CHIP in secretory and resorptive epithelia and capillary endothelia. *Proc. Natl. Acad. Sci. U.S.A.* 90, 7275–7279. doi: 10.1073/pnas.90.15.7275

Niemietz, C. M., and Tyerman, S. D. (2002). New potent inhibitors of aquaporins: silver and gold compounds inhibit aquaporins of plant and human origin. *FEBS Lett.* 531, 443–447. doi: 10.1016/S0014-5793(02)03581-0

Nishida, N., Yano, H., Nishida, T., Kamura, T., and Kojiro, M. (2006). Angiogenesis in cancer. *Vasc. Health Risk Manag.* 2, 213–219. doi: 10.2147/vhrm.2006.2.3.213

Njauw, C.-N., Yuan, H., Zheng, L., Yao, M., and Martins-Green, M. (2008). Origin of periendothelial cells in microvessels derived from human microvascular endothelial cells. *Int. J. Biochem. Cell Biol.* 40, 710–720. doi: 10.1016/j.biocel.2007.10.012

Oshio, K., Watanabe, H., Song, Y., Verkman, A., and Manley, G. T. (2005). Reduced cerebrospinal fluid production and intracranial pressure in mice lacking choroid plexus water channel Aquaporin-1. *FASEB J.* 19, 76–78. doi: 10.1096/fj.04-1711fje

Pagan, R., Sánchez, A., Martin, I., Llobera, M., Fabregat, I., and Vilar,ó S. (1999). Effects of growth and differentiation factors on the epithelial-mesenchymal transition in cultured neonatal rat hepatocytes. *J. Hepatol.* 31, 895–904. doi: 10.1016/S0168-8278(99)80292-X

Palecek, S. P., Huttenlocher, A., Horwitz, A. F., and Lauffenburger, D. A. (1998). Physical and biochemical regulation of integrin release during rear detachment of migrating cells. *J. Cell Sci.* 111, 929–940.

Pan, H., Sun, C. C., Zhou, C. Y., and Huang, H. F. (2008). Expression of aquaporin - 1 in normal, hyperplasic, and carcinomatous endometria. *Int. J. Gynecol. Obstet.* 101, 239–244. doi: 10.1016/j.ijgo.2007.12.006

Pan, X. Y., Guo, H., Han, J., Hao, F., An, Y., Xu, Y., et al. (2012). Ginsenoside Rg3 attenuates cell migration via inhibition of aquaporin 1 expression in PC-3M prostate cancer cells. *Eur. J. Pharmacol.* 683, 27–34. doi: 10.1016/j.ejphar.2012.02.040

Papadopoulos, M. C., Saadoun, S., and Verkman, A. S. (2008). Aquaporins and cell migration. *Pflug Arch. Eur. J. Phys.* 456, 693–700. doi: 10.1007/s00424-007-0357-5

Pei, J. V., Kourghi, M., De Ieso, M. L., Campbell, E. M., Dorward, H. S., Hardingham, J. E., et al. (2016). Differential Inhibition of water and ion channel activities of mammalian aquaporin-1 by two structurally related bacopaside compounds derived from the medicinal plant *Bacopa monnieri*. *Mol. Pharmacol.* 90, 496–507. doi: 10.1124/mol.116.105882

Pelagalli, A., Nardelli, A., Fontanella, R., and Zannetti, A. (2016). Inhibition of AQP1 hampers osteosarcoma and hepatocellular carcinoma progression mediated by bone marrow-derived mesenchymal stem cells. *Int. J. Mol. Sci.* 17, 1102. doi: 10.3390/ijms17071102

Pepper, M. S., Tille, J.-C., Nisato, R., and Skobe, M. (2003). Lymphangiogenesis and tumor metastasis. *Cell Tissue Res.* 314, 167–177. doi: 10.1007/s00441-003-0748-7

Pierini, L. M., Lawson, M. A., Eddy, R. J., Hendey, B., and Maxfield, F. R. (2000). Oriented endocytic recycling of α5β1 in motile neutrophils. *Blood* 95, 2471–2480.

Pollard, T. D., and Borisy, G. G. (2003). Cellular motility driven by assembly and disassembly of actin filaments. *Cell* 112, 453–465. doi: 10.1016/S0092-8674(03)00120-X

Preston, G. M., and Agre, P. (1991). Isolation of the cDNA for erythrocyte integral membrane protein of 28 kilodaltons: member of an ancient channel family. *Proc. Natl. Acad. Sci. U.S.A.* 88, 11110–11114. doi: 10.1073/pnas.88.24.11110

Preston, G. M., Carroll, T. P., Guggino, W. B., and Agre, P. (1992). Appearance of water channels in *Xenopus oocytes* expressing red cell CHIP28 protein. *Science* 256, 385–387. doi: 10.1126/science.256.5055.385

Preston, G. M., Jung, J. S., Guggino, W. B., and Agre, P. (1993). The mercury-sensitive residue at cysteine 189 in the CHIP28 water channel. *J. Biol. Chem.* 268, 17–20.

Price, L. S., Leng, J., Schwartz, M. A., and Bokoch, G. M. (1998). Activation of Rac and Cdc42 by integrins mediates cell spreading. *Mol. Biol. Cell* 9, 1863–1871. doi: 10.1091/mbc.9.7.1863

Raina, S., Preston, G. M., Guggino, W. B., and Agre, P. (1995). Molecular cloning and characterization of an aquaporin cDNA from salivary, lacrimal, and respiratory tissues. *J. Biol. Chem.* 270, 1908–1912. doi: 10.1074/jbc.270.4.1908

Rhee, S. G. (2006). H_2O_2, a necessary evil for cell signaling. *Science* 312, 1882–1883. doi: 10.1126/science.1130481

Ridley, A. J., Paterson, H. F., Johnston, C. L., Diekmann, D., and Hall, A. (1992). The small GTP-binding protein rac regulates growth factor-induced membrane ruffling. *Cell* 70, 401–410. doi: 10.1016/0092-8674(92)90164-8

Ridley, A. J., Schwartz, M. A., Burridge, K., Firtel, R. A., Ginsberg, M. H., Borisy, G., et al. (2003). Cell migration: integrating signals from front to back. *Science* 302, 1704–1709. doi: 10.1126/science.1092053

Rivera, E., and Cianfrocca, M. (2015). Overview of neuropathy associated with taxanes for the treatment of metastatic breast cancer. *Cancer Chemother. Pharmacol.* 75, 659–670. doi: 10.1007/s00280-014-2607-5

Rodrigues, C., Mósca, A. F., Martins, A. P., Nobre, T., Prista, C., Antunes, F., et al. (2016). Rat Aquaporin-5 is pH-Gated induced by phosphorylation and is implicated in oxidative stress. *Int. J. Mol. Sci.* 17:2090. doi: 10.3390/ijms17122090

Rojek, A. M., Skowronski, M. T., Füchtbauer, E.-M., Füchtbauer, A. C., Fenton, R. A., Agre, P., et al. (2007). Defective glycerol metabolism in aquaporin 9 (AQP9) knockout mice. *Proc. Natl. Acad. Sci. U.S.A.* 104, 3609–3614. doi: 10.1073/pnas.0610894104

Rojek, A., Füchtbauer, E.-M., Kwon, T.-H., Frøkiaer, J., and Nielsen, S. (2006). Severe urinary concentrating defect in renal collecting duct-selective AQP2 conditional-knockout mice. *Proc. Natl. Acad. Sci. U.S.A.* 103, 6037–6042. doi: 10.1073/pnas.0511324103

Rojek, A., Praetorius, J., Frøkiaer, J., Nielsen, S., and Fenton, R. A. (2008). A current view of the mammalian aquaglyceroporins. *Annu. Rev. Physiol.* 70, 301–327. doi: 10.1146/annurev.physiol.70.113006.100452

Roussos, E. T., Condeelis, J. S., and Patsialou, A. (2011). Chemotaxis in cancer. *Nat. Rev. Cancer* 11:573. doi: 10.1038/nrc3078

Saadoun, S., Papadopoulos, M. C., Hara-Chikuma, M., and Verkman, A. (2005a). Impairment of angiogenesis and cell migration by targeted aquaporin-1 gene disruption. *Nature* 434:786. doi: 10.1038/nature03460

Saadoun, S., Papadopoulos, M. C., Watanabe, H., Yan, D., Manley, G. T., and Verkman, A. (2005b). Involvement of aquaporin-4 in astroglial cell migration and glial scar formation. *J. Cell Sci.* 118, 5691–5698. doi: 10.1242/jcs.02680

Saadoun, S., Papadopoulos, M. C., Davies, D. C., Bell, B., and Krishna, S. (2002a). Increased aquaporin 1 water channel expression inhuman brain tumours. *Br. J. Cancer* 87, 621–623. doi: 10.1038/sj.bjc.6600512

Saadoun, S., Papadopoulos, M. C., Davies, D. C., Krishna, S., and Bell, B. A. (2002b). Aquaporin-4 expression is increased in oedematous human brain tumours. *J. Neurol. Neurosurg. Psychiatr.* 72, 262–265. doi: 10.1136/jnnp.72.2.262

Saparov, S. M., Kozono, D., Rothe, U., Agre, P., and Pohl, P. (2001). Water and ion permeation of aquaporin-1 in planar lipid bilayers. Major differences in structural determinants and stoichiometry. *J. Biol. Chem.* 276, 31515–31520. doi: 10.1074/jbc.M104267200

Saparov, S. M., Liu, K., Agre, P., and Pohl, P. (2007). Fast and selective ammonia transport by aquaporin-8. *J. Biol. Chem.* 282, 5296–5301. doi: 10.1074/jbc.M609343200

Satooka, H., and Hara-Chikuma, M. (2016). Aquaporin-3 controls breast cancer cell migration by regulating hydrogen peroxide transport and its downstream cell signaling. *Mol. Cell. Biol.* 36, 1206–1218. doi: 10.1128/MCB.00971-15

Schaller, M. D., Borgman, C. A., Cobb, B. S., Vines, R. R., Reynolds, A. B., and Parsons, J. T. (1992). pp125FAK a structurally distinctive protein-tyrosine kinase associated with focal adhesions. *Proc. Natl. Acad. Sci. U.S.A.* 89, 5192–5196. doi: 10.1073/pnas.89.11.5192

Schnermann, J., Chou, C.-L., Ma, T., Traynor, T., Knepper, M. A., and Verkman, A. S. (1998). Defective proximal tubular fluid reabsorption in transgenic aquaporin-1 null mice. *Proc. Natl. Acad. Sci. U.S.A.* 95, 9660–9664. doi: 10.1073/pnas.95.16.9660

Schwab, A., Nechyporuk-Zloy, V., Fabian, A., and Stock, C. (2007). Cells move when ions and water flow. *Pflug. Arch. Eur. J. Phys.* 453, 421–432. doi: 10.1007/s00424-006-0138-6

Seeliger, D., Zapater, C., Krenc, D., Haddoub, R., Flitsch, S., Beitz, E., et al. (2012). Discovery of novel human aquaporin-1 blockers. *ACS Chem. Biol.* 8, 249–256. doi: 10.1021/cb300153z

Sekine, S., Okumura, T., Nagata, T., Shibuya, K., Yoshioka, I., Matsui, K., et al. (2016). Expression analysis of aquaporin-1 (Aqp-1) in human biliary tract carcinoma. *J. Cancer Ther.* 7:17. doi: 10.4236/jct.2016.71003

Serna, A., Galán-Cobo, A., Rodrigues, C., Sánchez-Gomar, I., Toledo-Aral, J. J., Moura, T. F., et al. (2014). Functional inhibition of Aquaporin-3 with a gold-based compound induces blockage of cell proliferation. *J. Cell. Physiol.* 229, 1787–1801. doi: 10.1002/jcp.24632

Shen, L., Zhu, Z., Huang, Y., Shu, Y., Sun, M., Xu, H., et al. (2010). Expression profile of multiple aquaporins in human gastric carcinoma and its clinical significance. *Biomed. Pharmacother.* 64, 313–318. doi: 10.1016/j.biopha.2009.12.003

Shi, Y.-H., Chen, R., Talafu, T., Nijiati, R., and Lalai, S. (2012). Significance and expression of aquaporin 1, 3, 8 in cervical carcinoma in Xinjiang Uygur women of China. *Asian Pac. J. Cancer Prev.* 13, 1971–1975. doi: 10.7314/APJCP.2012.13.5.1971

Shi, Y.-H., Rehemu, N., Ma, H., Tuokan, T., Chen, R., and Suzuke, L. (2013). Increased migration and local invasion potential of SiHa cervical cancer cells expressing Aquaporin 8. *Asian Pac. J. Cancer Prev.* 14, 1825–1828. doi: 10.7314/APJCP.2013.14.3.1825

Shi, Y.-H., Tuokan, T., Lin, C., and Chang, H. (2014). Aquaporin 8 involvement in human cervical cancer SiHa migration via the EGFR-Erk1/2 pathway. *Asian Pac. J. Cancer Prev.* 15, 6391–6395. doi: 10.7314/APJCP.2014.15.15.6391

Søgaard, R., and Zeuthen, T. (2008). Test of blockers of AQP1 water permeability by a high-resolution method: no effects of tetraethylammonium ions or acetazolamide. *Pflüg. Arch. Eur. J. Physiol.* 456, 285–292. doi: 10.1007/s00424-007-0392-2

Song, Y., and Verkman, A. (2001). Aquaporin-5 dependent fluid secretion in airway submucosal glands. *J. Biol. Chem.* 276, 41288–41292. doi: 10.1074/jbc.M107257200

Spano, D., Heck, C., De Antonellis, P., Christofori, G., and Zollo, M. (2012). Molecular networks that regulate cancer metastasis. *Semin. Cancer Biol.* 22, 234–249. doi: 10.1016/j.semcancer.2012.03.006

Stroka, K. M., Jiang, H., Chen, S.-H., Tong, Z., Wirtz, D., Sun, S. X., et al. (2014). Water permeation drives tumor cell migration in confined microenvironments. *Cell* 157, 611–623. doi: 10.1016/j.cell.2014.02.052

Sudo, K., Ito, H., Iwamoto, I., Morishita, R., Asano, T., and Nagata, K.-,i (2006). Identification of a cell polarity-related protein, Lin-7B, as a binding partner for a Rho effector, Rhotekin, and their possible interaction in neurons. *Neurosci. Res.* 56, 347–355. doi: 10.1016/j.neures.2006.08.003

Sui, H., Han, B.-G., Lee, J. K., Walian, P., and Jap, B. K. (2001). Structural basis of water-specific transport through the AQP1 water channel. *Nature* 414, 872–878. doi: 10.1038/414872a

Suzuki, R., Okuda, M., Asai, J., Nagashima, G., Itokawa, H., Matsunaga, A., et al. (2006). Astrocytes co-express aquaporin-1,-4, and vascular endothelial growth factor in brain edema tissue associated with brain contusion. *Acta Neurochir. Suppl.* 96, 398–401. doi: 10.1007/3-211-30714-1_82

Swaney, K. F., Huang, C.-H., and Devreotes, P. N. (2010). Eukaryotic chemotaxis: a network of signaling pathways controls motility, directional sensing, and polarity. *Annu. Rev. Biophys.* 39:265. doi: 10.1146/annurev.biophys.093008.131228

Tan, D. S., Agarwal, R., and Kaye, S. B. (2006). Mechanisms of transcoelomic metastasis in ovarian cancer. *Lancet Oncol.* 7, 925–934. doi: 10.1016/S1470-2045(06)70939-1

Tan, G., Sun, S. Q., and Yuan, D. L. (2008). Expression of the water channel protein aquaporin-9 in human astrocytic tumours: correlation with pathological grade. *J. Int. Med. Res.* 36, 777–782. doi: 10.1177/147323000803600420

Tanaka, A., Sakurai, K., Kaneko, K., Ogino, J., Yagui, K., Ishikawa, K., et al. (2011). The role of the hypoxia-inducible factor 1 binding site in the induction of aquaporin-1 mRNA expression by hypoxia. *DNA Cell Biol.* 30, 539–544. doi: 10.1089/dna.2009.1014

Tanimura, Y., Hiroaki, Y., and Fujiyoshi, Y. (2009). Acetazolamide reversibly inhibits water conduction by aquaporin-4. *J. Struct. Biol.* 166, 16–21. doi: 10.1016/j.jsb.2008.11.010

Thannickal, V. J., and Fanburg, B. L. (2000). Reactive oxygen species in cell signaling. *Am. J. Physiol. Lung Cell. Mol. Physiol.* 279, L1005–L1028. doi: 10.1152/ajplung.2000.279.6.L1005

Theriot, J. A., and Mitchison, T. J. (1991). Actin microfilament dynamics in locomoting cells. *Nature* 352, 126–131. doi: 10.1038/352126a0

Thiery, J. P. (2002). Epithelial–mesenchymal transitions in tumour progression. *Nat. Rev. Cancer* 2, 442–454. doi: 10.1038/nrc822

Thiery, J. P. (2003). Epithelial–mesenchymal transitions in development and pathologies. *Curr. Opin. Cell Biol.* 15, 740–746. doi: 10.1016/j.ceb.2003.10.006

Tie, L., Lu, N., Pan, X.-Y., Pan, Y., An, Y., Gao, J.-W., et al. (2012). Hypoxia-induced up-regulation of aquaporin-1 protein in prostate cancer cells in a p38-dependent manner. *Cell. Physiol. Biochem.* 29, 269–280. doi: 10.1159/000337608

Tsukaguchi, H., Shayakul, C., Berger, U. V., Mackenzie, B., Devidas, S., Guggino, W. B., et al. (1998). Molecular characterization of a broad selectivity neutral solute channel. *J. Biol. Chem.* 273, 24737–24743. doi: 10.1074/jbc.273.38.24737

Tsunoda, S. P., Wiesner, B., Lorenz, D., Rosenthal, W., and Pohl, P. (2004). Aquaporin-1, nothing but a water channel. *J. Biol. Chem.* 279, 11364–11367. doi: 10.1074/jbc.M310881200

Vacca, A., Frigeri, A., Ribatti, D., Nicchia, G. P., Nico, B., Ria, R., et al. (2001). Microvessel overexpression of aquaporin 1 parallels bone marrow angiogenesis in patients with active multiple myeloma. *Br. J. Haematol.* 113, 415–421. doi: 10.1046/j.1365-2141.2001.02738.x

van Zijl, F., Krupitza, G., and Mikulits, W. (2011). Initial steps of metastasis: cell invasion and endothelial transmigration. *Mutat.Res.* 728, 23–34. doi: 10.1016/j.mrrev.2011.05.002

Verkman, A. (2005). More than just water channels: unexpected cellular roles of aquaporins. *J. Cell Sci.* 118, 3225–3232. doi: 10.1242/jcs.02519

Verkman, A. S., Anderson, M. O., and Papadopoulos, M. C. (2014). Aquaporins: important but elusive drug targets. *Nat. Rev. Drug Discov.* 13, 259–277. doi: 10.1038/nrd4226

Verkman, A. S., and Mitra, A. K. (2000). Structure and function of aquaporin water channels. *Am. J. Physiol. Renal Physiol.* 278, F13–F28. doi: 10.1152/ajprenal.2000.278.1.F13

Vicent, S., López-Picazo, J. M., Toledo, G., Lozano, M. D., Torre, W., Garcia-Corchón, C., et al. (2004). ERK1/2 is activated in non-small-cell lung cancer and associated with advanced tumours. *Br. J. Cancer* 90:1047. doi: 10.1038/sj.bjc.6601644

Vicente-Manzanares, M., and Horwitz, A. R. (2011). Cell migration: an overview. *Methods Mol. Biol.* 769, 1–24. doi: 10.1007/978-1-61779-207-6_1

Vicente-Manzanares, M., Ma, X., Adelstein, R. S., and Horwitz, A. R. (2009). Non-muscle myosin II takes centre stage in cell adhesion and migration. *Nat. Rev. Mol. Cell Biol.* 10, 778–790. doi: 10.1038/nrm2786

Vićovac, L., and Aplin, J. (1996). Epithelial-mesenchymal transition during trophoblast differentiation. *Cells Tissues Organs* 156, 202–216. doi: 10.1159/000147847

Wang, W., Li, Q., Yang, T., Bai, G., Li, D., Li, Q., et al. (2012). Expression of AQP5 and AQP8 in human colorectal carcinoma and their clinical significance. *World J. Surg. Oncol.* 10:242. doi: 10.1186/1477-7819-10-242

Wang, Y.-L. (1985). Exchange of actin subunits at the leading edge of living fibroblasts: possible role of treadmilling. *J. Cell Biol.* 101, 597–602. doi: 10.1083/jcb.101.2.597

Wasilewski-Masker, K., Seidel, K. D., Leisenring, W., Mertens, A. C., Shnorhavorian, M., Ritenour, C. W., et al. (2014). Male infertility in long-term survivors of pediatric cancer: a report from the childhood cancer survivor study. *J. Cancer Survivorship* 8, 437–447. doi: 10.1007/s11764-014-0354-6

Watanabe, S., Moniaga, C. S., Nielsen, S., and Hara-Chikuma, M. (2016). Aquaporin-9 facilitates membrane transport of hydrogen peroxide in mammalian cells. *Biochem. Biophys. Res. Commun.* 471, 191–197. doi: 10.1016/j.bbrc.2016.01.153

Weaver, A. M. (2006). Invadopodia: specialized cell structures for cancer invasion. *Clin. Exp. Metastasis* 23, 97–105. doi: 10.1007/s10585-006-9014-1

Wei, X., and Dong, J. (2015). Aquaporin 1 promotes the proliferation and migration of lung cancer cell *in vitro*. *Oncol. Rep.* 34, 1440–1448. doi: 10.3892/or.2015.4107

Willemse, P., Burggraaf, J., Hamdy, N., Weijl, N., Vossen, C., Van Wulften, L., et al. (2013). Prevalence of the metabolic syndrome and cardiovascular disease risk in chemotherapy-treated testicular germ cell tumour survivors. *Br. J. Cancer* 109, 60–67. doi: 10.1038/bjc.2013.226

Wolf, K., Wu, Y. I., Liu, Y., Geiger, J., Tam, E., Overall, C., et al. (2007). Multi-step pericellular proteolysis controls the transition from individual to collective cancer cell invasion. *Nat. Cell Biol.* 9, 893–904. doi: 10.1038/ncb1616

Wu, B., Altmann, K., Barzel, I., Krehan, S., and Beitz, E. (2008). A yeast-based phenotypic screen for aquaporin inhibitors. *Pflüg. Arch. Eur. J. Physiol.* 456, 717–720. doi: 10.1007/s00424-007-0383-3

Wyckoff, J. B., Jones, J. G., Condeelis, J. S., and Segall, J. E. (2000). A critical step in metastasis: *in vivo* analysis of intravasation at the primary tumor. *Cancer Res.* 60, 2504–2511.

Xia, H., Ma, Y. F., Yu, C. H., Li, Y. J., Tang, J., Li, J. B., et al. (2014). Aquaporin 3 knockdown suppresses tumour growth and angiogenesis in experimental non-small cell lung cancer. *Exp. Physiol.* 99, 974–984. doi: 10.1113/expphysiol.2014.078527

Xiang, Y., Ma, B., Li, T., Gao, J.-W., Yu, H.-M., and Li, X.-J. (2004). Acetazolamide inhibits aquaporin-1 protein expression and angiogenesis. *Acta Pharmacol. Sin.* 25, 812–816.

Xiang, Y., Ma, B., Li, T., Yu, H.-M., and Li, X.-J. (2002). Acetazolamide suppresses tumor metastasis and related protein expression in mice bearing Lewis lung carcinoma. *Acta Pharmacol. Sin.* 23, 745–751.

Xiong, G., Chen, X., Zhang, Q., Fang, Y., Chen, W., Li, C., et al. (2017). RNA interference influenced the proliferation and invasion of XWLC-05 lung cancer cells through inhibiting aquaporin 3. *Biochem. Biophys. Res. Commun.* 485, 627–634. doi: 10.1016/j.bbrc.2017.02.013

Xu, H., Xu, Y., Zhang, W., Shen, L., Yang, L., and Xu, Z. (2011). Aquaporin-3 positively regulates matrix metalloproteinases via PI3K/AKT signal pathway in human gastric carcinoma SGC7901 cells. *Nat. Rev. Cancer* 30:86. doi: 10.1186/1756-9966-30-86

Xu, J., Lamouille, S., and Derynck, R. (2009). TGF-β-induced epithelial to mesenchymal transition. *Cell Res.* 19, 156–172. doi: 10.1038/cr.2009.5

Yakata, K., Tani, K., and Fujiyoshi, Y. (2011). Water permeability and characterization of aquaporin-11. *J. Struct. Biol.* 174, 315–320. doi: 10.1016/j.jsb.2011.01.003

Yamaguchi, H., Wyckoff, J., and Condeelis, J. (2005). Cell migration in tumors. *Curr. Opin. Cell Biol.* 17, 559–564. doi: 10.1016/j.ceb.2005.08.002

Yamamoto, T., Kuramoto, H., and Kadowaki, M. (2007). Downregulation in aquaporin 4 and aquaporin 8 expression of the colon associated with the induction of allergic diarrhea in a mouse model of food allergy. *Life Sci.* 81, 115–120. doi: 10.1016/j.lfs.2007.04.036

Yang, B., and Verkman, A. (1997). Water and glycerol permeabilities of aquaporins 1–5 and MIP determined quantitatively by expression of epitope-tagged constructs inXenopus oocytes. *J. Biol. Chem.* 272, 16140–16146. doi: 10.1074/jbc.272.26.16140

Yang, B., Fukuda, N., van Hoek, A., Matthay, M. A., Ma, T., and Verkman, A. (2000). Carbon dioxide permeability of aquaporin-1 measured in erythrocytes and lung of aquaporin-1 null mice and in reconstituted proteoliposomes. *J. Biol. Chem.* 275, 2686–2692. doi: 10.1074/jbc.275.4.2686

Yang, B., Kim, J. K., and Verkman, A. (2006). Comparative efficacy of HgCl2 with candidate aquaporin-1 inhibitors DMSO, gold, TEA+ and acetazolamide. *FEBS Lett.* 580, 6679–6684. doi: 10.1016/j.febslet.2006.11.025

Yang, J., Mani, S. A., Donaher, J. L., Ramaswamy, S., Itzykson, R. A., Come, C., et al. (2004). Twist, a master regulator of morphogenesis, plays an essential role in tumor metastasis. *Cell* 117, 927–939. doi: 10.1016/j.cell.2004.06.006

Yasui, M., Hazama, A., Kwon, T.-H., Nielsen, S., Guggino, W. B., and Agre, P. (1999). Rapid gating and anion permeability of an intracellular aquaporin. *Nature* 402, 184–187. doi: 10.1038/46045

Yool, A. J. (2007). Functional domains of aquaporin-1: keys to physiology, and targets for drug discovery. *Curr. Pharm. Des.* 13, 3212–3221. doi: 10.2174/138161207782341349

Yool, A. J., Brokl, O. H., Pannabecker, T. L., Dantzler, W. H., and Stamer, W. D. (2002). Tetraethylammonium block of water flux in Aquaporin-1 channels expressed in kidney thin limbs of Henle's loop and a kidney-derived cell line. *BMC Physiol.* 2:4. doi: 10.1186/1472-6793-2-4

Yool, A. J., Stamer, W. D., and Regan, J. W. (1996). Forskolin stimulation of water and cation permeability in aquaporin-1 water channels. *Science* 273, 1216–1218. doi: 10.1126/science.273.5279.1216

Yu, J., Yool, A. J., Schulten, K., and Tajkhorshid, E. (2006). Mechanism of gating and ion conductivity of a possible tetrameric pore in aquaporin-1. *Structure* 14, 1411–1423. doi: 10.1016/j.str.2006.07.006

Yun, S., Sun, P.-L., Jin, Y., Kim, H., Park, E., Park, S. Y., et al. (2016). Aquaporin 1 is an independent marker of poor prognosis in lung adenocarcinoma. *J. Pathol. Transl. Med.* 50:251. doi: 10.4132/jptm.2016.03.30

Zelenina, M., Bondar, A. A., Zelenin, S., and Aperia, A. (2003). Nickel and extracellular acidification inhibit the water permeability of human aquaporin-3 in lung epithelial cells. *J. Biol. Chem.* 278, 30037–30043. doi: 10.1074/jbc.M302206200

Zelenina, M., Tritto, S., Bondar, A. A., Zelenin, S., and Aperia, A. (2004). Copper inhibits the water and glycerol permeability of aquaporin-3. *J. Biol. Chem.* 279, 51939–51943. doi: 10.1074/jbc.M407645200

Zhang, D., Vetrivel, L., and Verkman, A. (2002). Aquaporin deletion in mice reduces intraocular pressure and aqueous fluid production. *J. Gen. Physiol.* 119:561–569. doi: 10.1085/jgp.20028597

Zhang, H., and Verkman, A. (2008). Evidence against involvement of aquaporin-4 in cell–cell adhesion. *J. Mol. Biol.* 382, 1136–1143. doi: 10.1016/j.jmb.2008.07.089

Zhang, H., and Verkman, A. S. (2010). Aquaporin-1 tunes pain perception by interaction with Nav1. 8 Na+ channels in dorsal root ganglion neurons. *J. Biol. Chem.* 285, 5896–5906. doi: 10.1074/jbc.M109.090233

Zhang, T., Zhao, C., Chen, D., and Zhou, Z. (2012). Overexpression of AQP5 in cervical cancer: correlation with clinicopathological features and prognosis. *Med. Oncol.* 29, 1998–2004. doi: 10.1007/s12032-011-0095-6

Zhang, W.-G, Li, C.-F, Liu, M., Chen, X.-F, Shuai, K., Kong, X., et al. (2016). Aquaporin 9 is down-regulated in hepatocellular carcinoma and its over-expression suppresses hepatoma cell invasion through inhibiting epithelial-to-mesenchymal transition. *Cancer Lett.* 378, 111–119. doi: 10.1016/j.canlet.2016.05.021

Zhang, Z., Chen, Z., Song, Y., Zhang, P., Hu, J., and Bai, C. (2010). Expression of aquaporin 5 increases proliferation and metastasis potential of lung cancer. *J. Pathol.* 221, 210–220. doi: 10.1002/path.2702

Zhao, X., and Guan, J.-L. (2011). Focal adhesion kinase and its signaling pathways in cell migration and angiogenesis. *Adv. Drug Deliv. Rev.* 63, 610–615. doi: 10.1016/j.addr.2010.11.001

Zou, L.-B., Shi, S., Zhang, R.-J., Wang, T.-T., Tan, Y.-J., Zhang, D., et al. (2013). Aquaporin-1 plays a crucial role in estrogen-induced tubulogenesis of vascular endothelial cells. *J. Clin. Endocrinol. Metab.* 98, E672–E682. doi: 10.1210/jc.2012-4081

Zou, L.-B., Zhang, R.-J., Tan, Y.-J., Ding, G.-L., Shi, S., Zhang, D., et al. (2011). Identification of estrogen response element in theaquaporin-2 gene that mediates estrogen-induced cell migration and invasion in human endometrial carcinoma. *J. Clin. Endocrinol. Metab.* 96, E1399–E1408. doi: 10.1210/jc.2011-0426

16

The Expression of AQP1 is Modified in Lung of Patients with Idiopathic Pulmonary Fibrosis: Addressing a Possible New Target

Ana Galán-Cobo [1], Elena Arellano-Orden [1], Rocío Sánchez Silva [1], José Luis López-Campos [2,3], César Gutiérrez Rivera [2], Lourdes Gómez Izquierdo [4], Nela Suárez-Luna [1], María Molina-Molina [3,5], José A. Rodríguez Portal [2] and Miriam Echevarría [1*]*

[1] Departamento de Fisiología Médica y Biofísica, Instituto de Biomedicina de Sevilla, Hospital Universitario Virgen del Rocío, CSIC, Universidad de Sevilla, Sevilla, Spain, [2] Unidad Médico-Quirúrgica de Enfermedades Respiratorias, Hospital Universitario Virgen del Rocio, Sevilla, Spain, [3] Centro de Investigación Biomédica en Red sobre Enfermedades Respiratorias (CIBERES), Madrid, Spain, [4] Servicio Anatomía Patológica, HU Virgen del Rocío Sevilla, Seville, Spain, [5] Laboratorio de Neumologia Experimental, Servicio de Neumologia, Institut d'Investigació Biomédica de Bellvitge, Hospital Universitario de Bellvitge, Barcelona, Spain

***Correspondence:**
Ana Galán-Cobo
agalan@mdanderson.org
Miriam Echevarría
irusta@us.es

Activation of the epithelial-mesenchymal transition process (EMT) by which alveolar cells in human lung tissue undergo differentiation giving rise to a mesenchymal phenotype (fibroblast/miofibroblasts) has been well recognized as a key element in the origin of idiopathic pulmonary fibrosis (IPF). Here we analyzed expression of AQP1 in lung biopsies of patients diagnosed with IPF, and compared it to biopsies derived from patients with diverse lung pneumonies, such as hypersensitivity pneumonitis, sarcoidosis or normal lungs. Immunostaining for AQP1 showed a clear increment of AQP1 localized in the alveolar epithelium in biopsies from IPF patients alone. Moreover, to examine the possible participation of AQP1 in the pathophysiology of IPF, we evaluated its role in the pro-fibrotic transformation induced by transforming growth factor (TGF-β) *in vitro.* Human alveolar epithelial cells (A549), and fibroblasts derived from an IPF patient (LL29), or fibroblasts from healthy normal lung tissue (MRC-5), were treated with TGF-β, and levels of expression of AQP1, as well as those of E-cadherin, vimentin, α-SMA and collagen were analyzed by RT-qPCR, western blot and immunohistochemistry. An increase of AQP1 mRNA and protein after TGF-β treatment (4–72h) was observed either in A549 or IPF fibroblast-LL29 but not in MRC-5 fibroblasts. A gradual reduction of E-cadherin, and increased expression of vimentin, with no changes in α-SMA levels were observed in A549. Whereas in LL29 and MRC-5, TGF-β1 elicited a large production of collagen and α-SMA that was significantly greater in IPF fibroblast-LL29. Changes observed are consistent with activation of EMT by TGF-β, but whether modifications in AQP1 expression are responsible or independent events occurring at the same time is still unknown. Our results suggest that AQP1 plays a role in the pro-fibrotic TGF-β action and contributes to the etiology and pathophysiology of IPF. Understanding AQP1's role will help us comprehend the fate of this disease.

Keywords: interstitial lung disease (ILD), fibrosis, sarcoidosis, aquaporins (AQPs), inflamation, type II pneumocytes, IPF, AQP1

INTRODUCTION

Idiopathic pulmonary fibrosis (IPF) is the most widely found interstitial lung disease. IPF is a progressive disease usually fatal, characterized by inability of the alveolar epithelium to repair a lesion. The re-epithelialization fails and transformation to fibroblast/myofibroblast persist, with increase in extracellular matrix deposition and alteration of functional lung architecture, which will finally produce a respiratory failure (Lynch et al., 2006; Raghu et al., 2011). Clinical IPF is normally associated in surgical lung biopsy with a histopathological pattern of usual interstitial pneumonia (UIP). Though the origin of this pathology remains not fully understood, (Willis and Borok, 2007; Spagnolo et al., 2015) it is postulated that following alveolar epithelial injury, a process of repair and scar formation is initiated that implicates important changes and cell activation. However, in some cases, an alteration of the healing process occurs and lung fibrosis develops (Willis et al., 2006). In IPF, activated epithelial cells and recruited inflammatory cells release potent fibrogenic growth factors and cytokines that favor fibroblasts proliferation and its transformation to myofibroblasts (Khalil et al., 2005; Takai et al., 2013). The activation of an epithelial-mesenchymal transition (EMT) process by which alveolar epithelial cells (AEC) undergo a transition or trans-differentiation process to mesenchymal like cells, such as fibroblasts or myofibroblasts, is gaining acceptance as a key element in the origin of this pathology. Both pathological alternative pathways do not exclude each other and may likely coexist in the origin of IPF.

Different fibrogenic growth factors have been clearly implicated as inducers of lung fibrosis, among them the transforming growth factor (TGF-β) is perhaps the most relevant factor associated to lung fibrosis. Furthermore, a crucial role for TGF-β has been indicated in the induction of EMT in many physiological scenarios, including for instances in tissue fibrosis (Chapman, 2011; Tirino et al., 2013). It has been demonstrated that TGF-β induces *in vitro* EMT in AEC, and that epithelial and mesenchymal markers co-localize in hyperplastic alveolar type II cells in interstitial pulmonary fibrosis (IPF) tissue, indicating that AEC could show great plasticity and function as a source for new fibro- and myofibroblasts cells in lung fibrosis (Chapman, 2011; Tirino et al., 2013).

Several aquaporins (AQP1, AQP3, AQP4, and AQP5) have been recognized in the respiratory system. Each one presents in a particular location, probably indicating different physiological roles in the pulmonary tissue (Guarino et al., 2009; Camelo et al., 2014). AQP1 is expressed in both membranes, apical and basolateral, of the microvascular endothelium, besides of being expressed in the visceral pleura. AQP3 and AQP4 are expressed in the airway epithelium. AQP5 is expressed in the apical membrane of type-I pneumocytes, and also in the apical side of acinar cells in the submucosal glands of nasopharynx and rest of airways.

In previous studies, we demonstrated that Aquaporin-1 (AQP1) up-regulates its expression in the lung of animals exposed to hypoxia for 24–48 h (Echevarría et al., 2007). We also demonstrated that the transcription factor inducible by hypoxia HIF-1a, partially participates in this process along with other factors in the inflammatory pathway (Abreu-Rodríguez et al., 2011). We then became interested if the regulation by hypoxia would occur in patients suffering hypoxemic diseases and whether the remodeling of AQP1 expression may play a role in developing pathologies, such as chronic obstructive pulmonary disease (EPOC) (Calero et al., 2014) and IPF (Gutiérrez et al., 2013).

A clear association between expression of AQP1 and increment of cell proliferation in different cellular models has been recently demonstrated (Galán-Cobo et al., 2015, 2016). Moreover, in a murine model of acute lung injury a relationship between ANGII and AQP1 expression was indicated (Cao et al., 2010) and up-regulation of pulmonary AQP1 expression was observed in mice with pulmonary fibrosis induced by bleomycin (Gao et al., 2013), leading authors to propose a possible role for AQP1 in the pathogenesis of lung fibrosis.

Thus, with all these precedents in mind we decided to look for alternative pathways that may explain connections between changes in the AQP1 expression pattern in lung cellular types of patients with IPF and the pathophysiology of the disease. Lung biopsies of patients with different interstitial lung disorders were analyzed by immunohistochemistry for AQP1 expression and experiments in cell lines treated with the pro-fibrotic agent TGF-β1 were performed *in vitro*. The human alveolar epithelial cell line A549, and two different cell lines of human fibroblast, one derived from an IPF patient (LL-29) and the other from healthy fibroblast (MRC5), were treated with TGF-β1, and the correlation between expression of AQP1 and other proteins were analyzed to determine their role in the induced EMT or fibroblast-myofibroblast transition process.

MATERIALS AND METHODS

Human Tissue Samples

All paraffin-embedded samples were acquired from the Department of Pathology, HUVR of Seville, Spain. Originally, samples were obtained by pulmonary biopsy corresponding to IPF and other fibrotic and non-fibrotic interstitial lung diseases (ILD). For the control group we took samples of patients undergoing surgery for spontaneous pneumothorax otherwise healthy. The number of groups, as well as the number of samples included per group in the analysis are indicated in **Table 1**, and are as follow: (20) idiopatic pulmonary fibrosis-usual interstitial pneumonia (IPF-UIP), (2) non-specific interstitial pneumonia (NSIP), (1) cryptogenic organizing pneumonia (COP), (5) IPF-not otherwise specified, (6) hypersensitivity pneumonitis, (4) sarcoidosis and (7) control lungs. Written informed consent was obtained from all participants. The study followed the tenets of the WMA Declaration of Helsinki for research involving human subjects and was approved by the ethics committee of the University Hospital Virgen del Rocío (HUVR).

Immunohistochemistry of Biopsies

All samples examined were obtained from formalin-fixed, paraffin-embedded pieces. Slices of 5 μm were cut with a microtome and mounted on microscope slides. Immunohistochemical samples were obtained from paraffin sections that were immersed in xylene and rehydrated through a series of decreasing dilutions of ethanol. Blocking of endogenous peroxidase, epitope retrieval and immunostaining procedure were done as previously reported (López-Campos et al., 2011). Primary antibody, rabbit polyclonal anti-AQP1, (1:500 dilution, Abcam, Cambridge, UK) was used overnight, for the developing of brown precipitates we then used the two steps system EnVision + Dual Link System-HRP (DakoCytomation, Dako Denmark). Qualitative analysis was made by two independent observers. We assigned zero for no staining on the sample, low positive (<25% of the sample stained), medium positive (50% of the sample stained) and high positive (>75% of the sample stained) values (**Tables 1, 2**). Immunoreactivity was analyzed in terms of surface and type of cells showing AQP1 on their surface. Samples were photographed using an AX70-Olympus microscope equipped with an Olympus DP10 camera (Denmark).

Cell Culture

A549 cells (Human lung alveolar epithelial) and LL29 (Human idiopathic pulmonary fibrosis) were purchased from the American Type Culture Collection (ATCC, Rockville, USA); MRC-5 (Human lung fibroblast cell line) cells were obtained from the European Collection of Cell Culture (ECACC, Salisbury, UK). A549 cells were cultured as monolayers in DMEM:F12 (F12K Nut Mix) supplemented with 10% heat-inactivated fetal bovine serum, 100 U/mL penicillin-streptomycin (Invitrogen, Carlsbad, CA, USA). MRC-5 cells were cultured as monolayers in MEM supplemented with 10% heat-inactivated fetal bovine serum, 100 U/mL penicillin-streptomycin, and 2 mM L-glutamine (Invitrogen, Carlsbad, CA, USA). LL-29 cells were cultured in Ham's F12K medium supplemented with 15% heat-inactive fetal bovine serum, 100 U/mL penicillin-streptomycin, and 2 mM L-glutamine (Invitrogen, Carlsbad, CA, USA). Cells were cultured at 5% CO_2 at 37°C.

TABLE 1 | Summary of interstitial lung diseases (pneumonias) included in the study.

	N	(%)
Idiopathic Pulmonary Fibrosis (IPF)/Usual interstitial pneumonia (IPF-UIP)	20	44.4
Non-specific interstitial pneumonia (NSIP)	2	4.4
Cryptogenic organizing pneumonia (COP)	1	2.2
Idiopathic interstitial pneumonia not otherwise specified	5	11.1
Hypersensitivity pneumonia	6	13.3
Sarcoidosis	4	8.9
Controls	7	15.6
Total	45	100

TGF-β1 Assays

A549 (2.4×10^5), MRC-5 (3×10^5), and LL-29 (2.5×10^5) cells were plated on 60 mm dishes (Nunc, Roskilde, Denmark), when the cells reached 80% of confluence we added fresh medium 1% FBS for 24 h and then we added 10 ng/ml of TGF-β1 (R&D System, Minneapolis, MN, USA) for 4, 16, 24, 48, or 72 h. We used untreated cells as control.

Morphological changes in A549, MRC-5 and LL-29 cells were examined by inverted fluorescence microscopy (Zeiss Axiovert 25, Carl Zeiss Co. Oberkochen, Germany) and photographed using a CCD Canon camera.

Indirect Immunocytochemistry Staining of Cultures Cell

Cells were seeded into 24-well plates at a concentration of 2×10^4 cells/well. After treatment with 10 ng/ml TGF-β1 for 24 h the culture medium was discarded and cells were washed with Ca^{++}-Mg^{++} PBS 1x and fixed with 3% paraformaldehyde for 10 min at room temperature. Cells were

TABLE 2 | Association between AQP1 staining and interstitial pneumonias.

	Type II pneumocytes AQP1 immunoreactivity				*P*-value*
	Negative	Low positive	Medium positive	High positive	
Usual interstitial pneumonia (*n* = 20)	2 (10%)	1 (5%)	8 (40%)	9 (45%)	0.001
Non-specific interstitial pneumonia (*n* = 2)	–	–	1 (50%)	1 (50%)	0.087
Cryptogenic organizing pneumonia (*n* = 1)	–	–	1 (100%)	–	0.249
Idiopathic interstitial pneumonia not otherwise specified (*n* = 5)	4 (80%)	–	1 (20%)	–	0.685
Hypersensivity pneumonia (*n* = 6)	3 (50%)	3 (50%)	–	–	0.266
Sarcoidosis (*n* = 4)	4 (100%)	–	–	–	1
Control (*n* = 7)	6 (85.7%)	1 (14.3%)	–	–	–

*Two independent observers gave negative value for no stain, low positive for <25% of the sample stained, medium positive for 50% of the sample stained and high positive for >75% of the sample stained. *P-value was calculated by χ2 with Monte Carlo method for association between AQP1 staining and interstitial pneumonias comparing each interstitial pneumonia against the control group and using the Bonferroni correction for multiple comparisons (p < 0.008) only the group of usual interstitial pneumonia resulted different from control (p = 0.001).*

washed and permeabilized/blocked with 0.1% Triton X-100 in 10% Fetal Calf Serum (FCS) solution for 10 min at room temperature and incubated with primary antibodies; 1:200 of E-cadherin (BD Biosciences, San Jose, CA, USA) and 1:100 of AQP1 (Abcam, Cambridge, UK) overnight at 4°C. After washing with PBS cells were then incubated with Alexa 488 donkey anti-mouse (Invitrogen, Carlsbad, CA, USA) 1:200 in blocking solution for AQP1 and E-cadherin staining for 1 h at room temperature. F-actin was labeled with red-fluorescent Alexa Fluor 594 Phalloidin (Thermo Fisher Scientific, Waltham, MA, USA) 1:1000 for 10 min at room temperature. Samples were washed with PBS and then mounted with DAKO (Invitrogen, Carlsbad, CA, USA) and preserved at 4°C. Immunocytochemestries were photographed using a fluorescence microscope Olympus BX 71 with a refrigerated camera DP70.

Western Blotting

Plated cells were washed with cold PBS, collected by scraping in 1 ml of cold PBS and centrifuged at 300 g for 5 min at 4°C. For whole-cell protein extract, the pellet was lysed in a variable volume of homogenization buffer containing: 50 mM Hepes (pH 7.3); 5 mM EDTA; 250 mM NaCl; 5 mM DTT; 0.2% (v/v) NP40 (Sigma–Aldrich); and 1% (v/v) Complete Protease Inhibitors Cocktail (Sigma–Aldrich). The resuspended pellet was left on ice for 5–15 min, vortexed, and then centrifuged at 16,000 g for 15 min at 4°C, and proteins contained in the supernatant were stored. Protein concentration was analyzed using the Bradford method (BioRad Protein Assay, BioRad, Berkeley, CA) and kept at −20°C until Western blot analysis (Galán-Cobo et al., 2016). For all proteins analyzed, 30 μg of whole-cell extracts were resolved by SDS-PAGE on 10–12% gels. After electrophoresis, proteins were transferred onto PVDF membranes (Hybond-P, Amersham Biosciences, Pittsburgh, PA) using a Novex apparatus (Novel Experimental Technology, San Diego, CA). Membranes were probed with 1:700 anti-AQP1 (Abcam, Cambridge, UK), 1:2500 anti-E-Cadherin (BD Biosciences, San Jose, CA, USA), 1:1500 anti-Vimentin (Abcam, Cambridge, UK), 1:1000 anti-α-SMA (Abcam, Cambridge, UK) and 1:10000 anti-cyclophilin A (Abcam, Cambridge, UK) antibodies. Immunoreactive bands were developed with the ECL Prime system (Amersham Biosciences) and visualized using a digital imaging system (ImageQuant LAS 4000 Mini, GE Healthcare, Buckinghamshire, UK).

RNA Isolation and Quantitative PCR

RNA was extracted from cells using TRIzol reagent (Invitrogen, Carlsbad, CA, USA) according with manufacturer protocol. After mRNA isolation, reverse transcription (RT) was performed for 5 μg of RNA using SuperScript II RNase-H reverse transcriptase (Invitrogen, Carlsbad, CA, USA). Real-time quantitative PCR (qPCR) analysis was carried out in an ABI Prism 7500 Sequence Detection System using SYBR Green PCR Master Mix (Applied Biosystems, Warrington, UK) and the thermocycler conditions recommended by the manufacturer. The expression of HPRT1 was used to normalize for differences in amounts of input DNA between samples. Primers were designed using the Primer Express software (version 2.0, Applied Biosystems, Warrington, UK) and their sequences are indicated in **Table 3**. Melting curve analysis showed a single sharp peak with the expected melting temperature for all samples.

Statistical Analysis

Data analysis was performed using SPSS Advanced Statistics (SPSS Inc., Chicago, Illinois), version 19.0. For the statistical analysis of data derived from analysis by immunohistochemistry of patient biopsies, the "p" value for comparative analysis of association between AQP1 staining and interstitial pneumonias was calculated by χ^2 with Monte Carlo method. The Bonferroni correction was used for multiple comparisons and the Fisher exact test when comparing each interstitial pneumonia against the control group. For all experiments performed in cells in culture the data are expressed as mean ± standard error of the mean from at least four different experiments. The statistical significance for normal distribution data was estimated using one-way ANOVA followed by Bonferroni's *post-hoc* test to compare more than two groups. Data with non-normal distribution were analyzed using Mann-Whitney U or Kruskal-Wallis H-test for two or more than two groups, respectively. Values of $p \leq 0.05$ were considered significant.

TABLE 3 | Primer sequences used for the amplification of cDNAs by qPCR.

Genes	Forward sequence	Reverse sequence
Aquoporin 1 (*AQP1*)	GGACACCTCCTGGCTATTGACTAC	GTTGCTGAAGTTGTGTGTGATCAC
E-Cadherin (*CDH1*)	TCGACACCCGATTCAAAGTG	GTCCCAGGCGTAGACCAAGA
Vimentin (*VIM*)	TGCCCTTAAAGGAACCAATGAG	AGGCGGCCAATAGTGTCTTG
α-SMA (*ACTA2*)	CTGTTCCAGCCATCCTTCAT	CCGTGATCTCCTTCTGCATT
Collagen Type I Alpha 1 (*COL1A1*)	TGACCGAGACGTGTGGAAAC	CAGATCACGTCATCGCACAAC
Hypoxanthine Phosphoribosyltransferase 1 (*HPRT1*)	ACTGAACGTCTTGCTCGAGATG	AGCAGGTCAGCAAAGAATTTATAGC

Primers were designed using the Primer Express software (Applied-Biosystems). qPCR: quantitative PCR.

RESULTS

AQP1 Is Specifically Expressed in Hyperplasic Cuboidal Type II Pneumocytes in the Alveolar Epithelium in Patients With Idiopathic Pulmonary Fibrosis

In the present study we analyzed expression of AQP1 in lung biopsies of patients diagnosed with IPF, and compare it to biopsies derived from diverse interstitial lung diseases such as others pneumonias, hypersensitivity pneumonitis, sarcoidosis, or normal lungs (**Table 1**). Conditions for AQP1 antibody immunohistochemistry in human lung biopsies were determined in a previous study (López-Campos et al., 2011). A summary of results from the analysis of biopsies is presented in **Table 2**. Normal lung tissues is consistent with previous reports (López-Campos et al., 2011; Calero et al., 2014) in that AQP1 immunostaining was detected predominantly in endothelial cells of alveoli capillaries and the rest of blood vessels; faint labeling was also detected on neumocytes of the alveolar wall (**Figure 1**). No labeling was detected in absence of the primary antibody (data not shown).

Compared to the rest of pathologies analyzed, the immunohistochemistry assays revealed that only biopsies from IPF show a clear increment of AQP1 staining that localizes remarkably over hyperplasic cuboidal type II pneumocytes in the alveolar epithelium, and to a much lesser grade over few planar, hyperplasic or metaplasic type I cells (**Figure 1**). A more detailed observation over the fibrosis focus of IPF patients, where the transition from fibroblasts to miofibroblasts occurred, showed that type I epithelial cells lining the fibrotic focus are totally deprived of AQP1 expression. In the rest of the samples basal AQP1 expression was limited to erythrocytes and endothelial cells. Absence of AQP1 labeling was observed over the interstitial lung or in myoepithelial cells. Changes in the expression pattern of β-catenin and E-cadherin were also studied but need further analysis of the immunoassays. In conclusion, the analysis demonstrates a possible role for AQP1 expression in the reactive process occurring over fibrotic focus of the alveoli epithelium of IPF patients.

AQP1 Is Overexpressed Along Epithelial Mesenchymal Transition (EMT) Induced by TGF-β

To further investigate the implication of AQP1 in the initiation and progression of IPF we examined epithelial cells as central to the pathogenesis of IPF. Experiments performed in the human lung epithelial cell line A549 has shown that treatment with the pro-fibrotic agent TGF-β1 (10 ng/ml) produces a time course (24, 48, 72, and 96 h) differentiation of the epithelial cells toward a fibroblastic-like phenotype, together with an increase of mRNA levels of the mesenchymal markers vimentin (5-fold) and α-SMA (2.5-fold). Consequently, a decrease in the levels of the epithelial marker E-cadherin was found after TGF-β1 treatment. Interestingly, levels of AQP1-mRNA were also measured and a

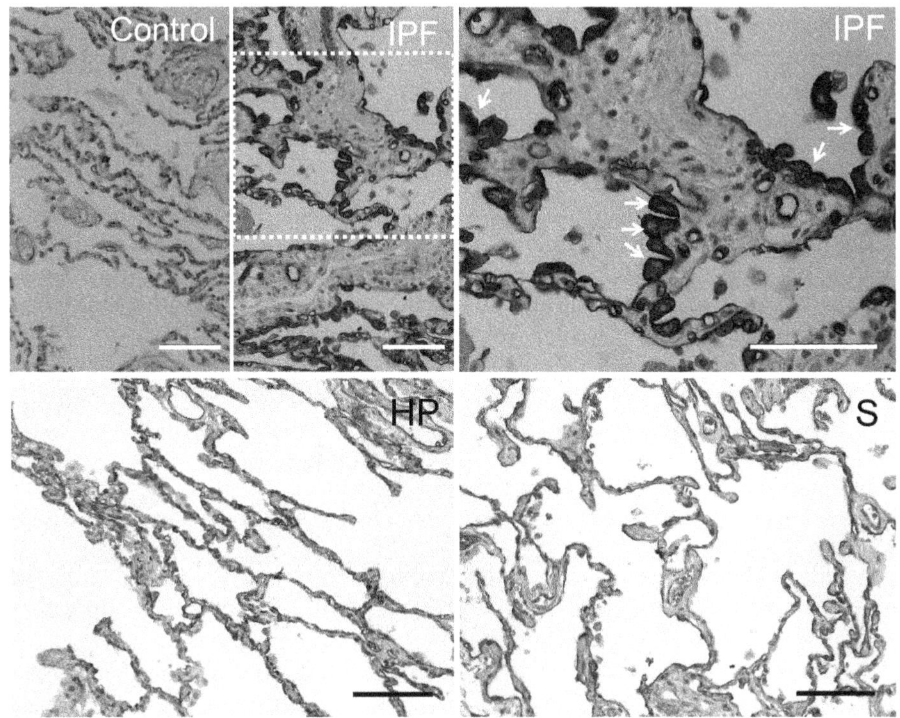

FIGURE 1 | Immunostaining of AQP1 in lung biopsies of patients. Pulmonary parenchyma of a healthy patient is shown as control. In the pulmonary parenchyma of patients with usual intersticial pneumonia (IPF) reactive type II pneumocytes of alveolus showed intense expression of AQP1 (see the arrows in the IPF at larger magnification). In biopsies of patients with hypersensitivity pneumonia (HP) or sarcoidosis (S), the staining of AQP1 was mainly located in capillaries endothelia. Scale bar represents 100 μm in each case. Note the different size of bar in each case.

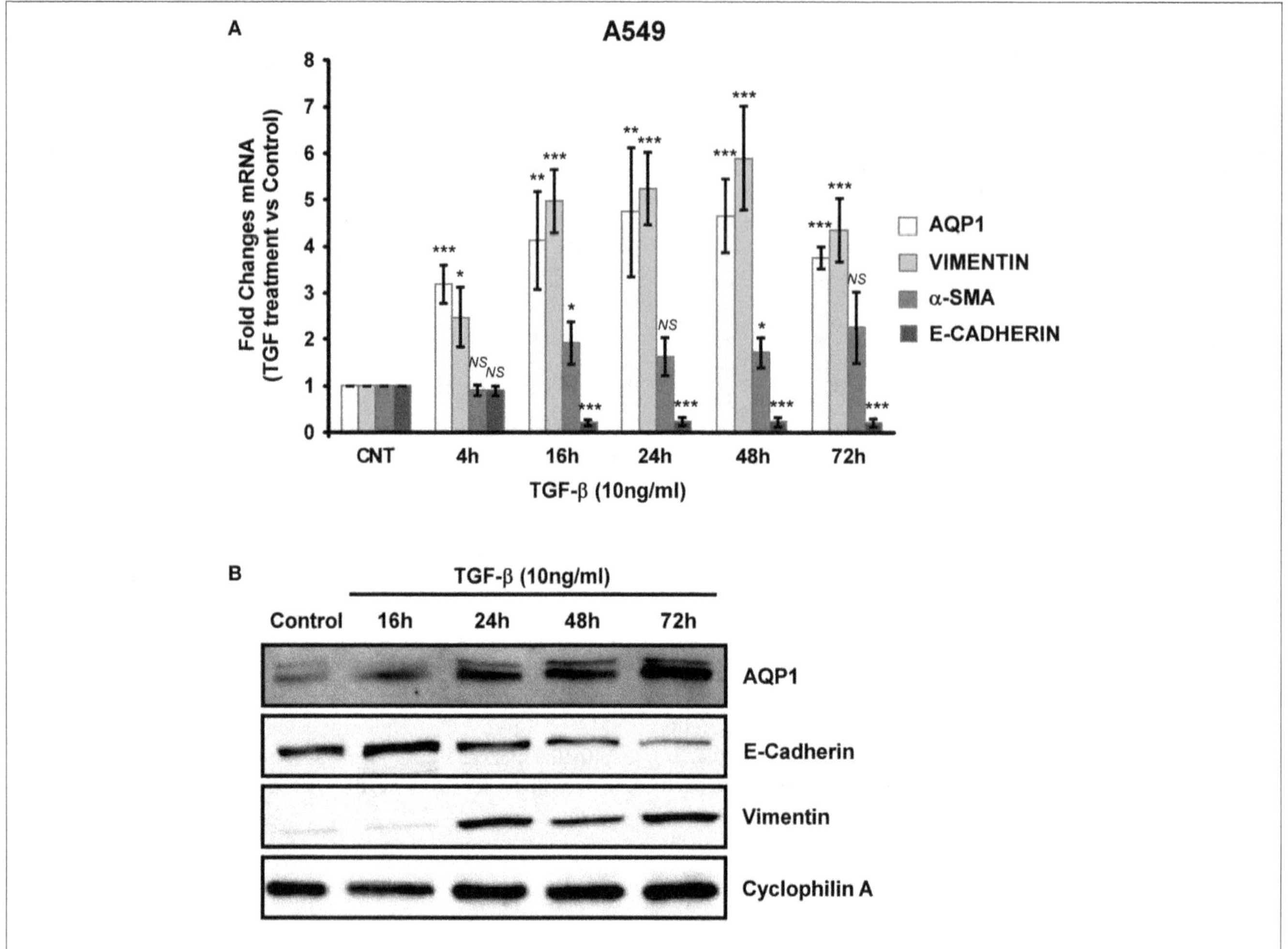

FIGURE 2 | Analysis of EMT induction in A549 cell lines. Cells were treated with TGF-β1 (10 ng/ml) for 4, 16, 24, 48, and 72 hours and the mRNA levels of AQP1, E-cadherin, Vimentin and α-SMA where quantified by real time RT-PCR analysis **(A)** and the protein levels by Western blot **(B)**.

substantial increase of AQP1 expression (5-fold) was observed in parallel to the changes described before for vimentin and α-SMA (**Figure 2A**). Similar results to those described for the mRNA, were found for the protein levels of E-cadherin, vimentin and AQP1 (**Figure 2B**). Immunostaining for AQP1 again showed higher expression levels of AQP1 in the lung epithelial cells A549 after TGF-β1 treatment (**Figure 3**), supporting previous data and indicating a possible role of AQP1 in the EMT process in lung tissue.

We then repeated similar experiments with TGF-β1 using two different fibroblast cell lines. A cell line of fibroblasts derived from patients with IPF (LL29) and a cell line of healthy fibroblasts (MRC-5). An increment of the capacity for extracellular matrix production was found in LL29 cells after TGF-β1 treatment indicated by higher levels of type I collagen (10-fold) and of α-SMA (5-fold). In parallel a strong and stable induction of AQP1 mRNA and protein levels were observed in this cell line obtained from an IPF patient (**Figure 4**) unlike, in the healthy fibroblast cell line MRC-5. Although similar induction of α-SMA and type I collagen were found, AQP1 levels remained unchanged after TGF-β1 treatment (**Figure 5**).

Altogether, these results support the hypothesis that increments of AQP1 expression induced by TGF-β1 occur in the lung tissue of patients with IPF. As a result of rising AQP1 in the alveolar epithelia, the cells undergo EMT or fibroblast-myofibroblast transition, thereby contributing to formation of fibroblastic foci and subsequent fibroblast and extracellular matrix accumulation.

DISCUSSION

Immunohistochemical studies in rats and mice have shown that AQP1 is present in the capillaries and in the sub-epithelial connective tissue of the animal's respiratory tract. Alveolar cells do not express AQP1 on its surface and expression of AQP1 is restricted to the capillary endothelium (Nielsen et al., 1997). At present, the idea remains that AQP1 provides the principal pathway for osmotic transport of water between airspace and lung capillary compartments. Nevertheless, neither alveolar fluid clearance in neonatal and adult lung nor lung fluid accumulation in experimental models of lung injury have reported being affected by AQP1 deletion.

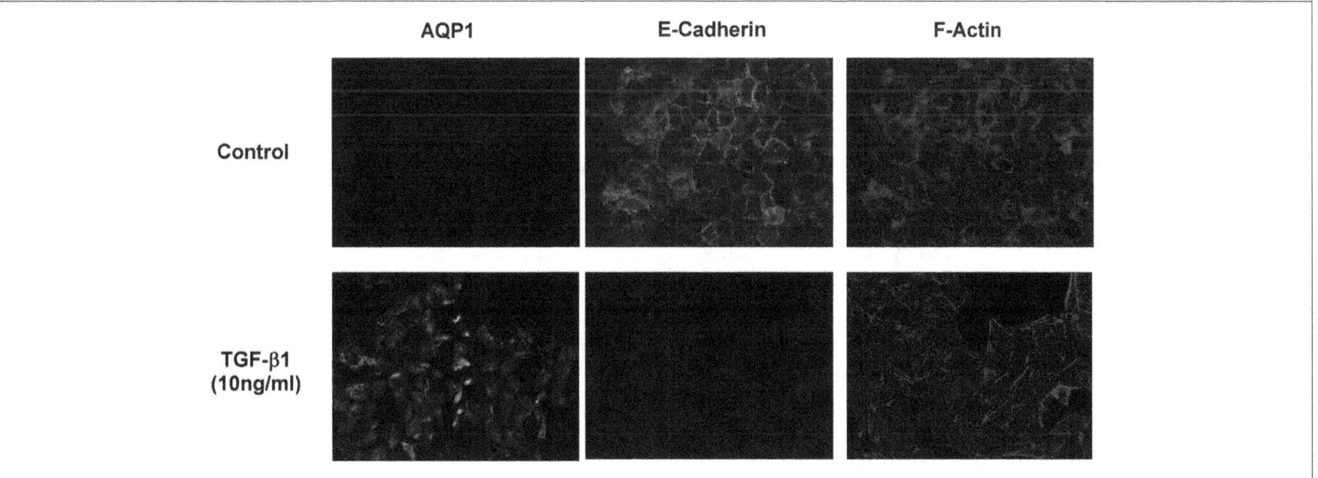

FIGURE 3 | Immunostaining showing AQP1, E-cadherin and F-actin expression in A549 cells without TGF-β1 treatment (Control) and after TGF-β1 (10 ng/ml) treatment.

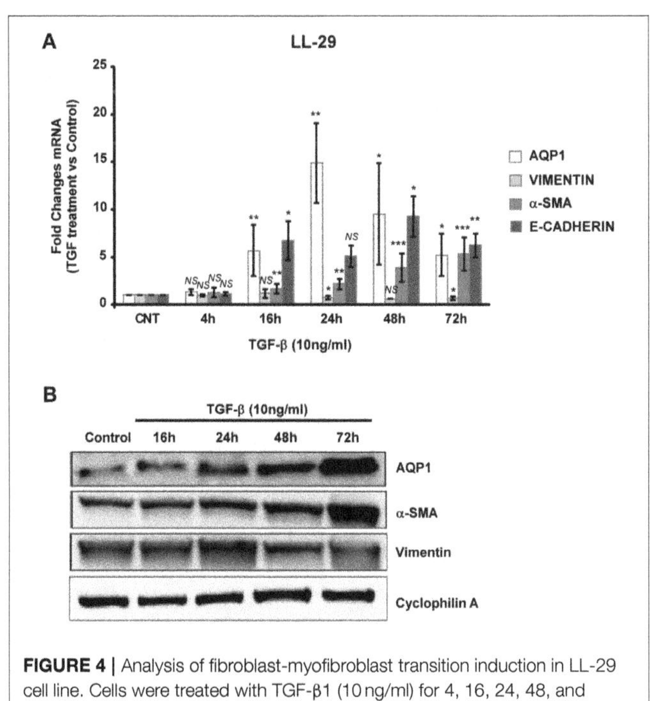

FIGURE 4 | Analysis of fibroblast-myofibroblast transition induction in LL-29 cell line. Cells were treated with TGF-β1 (10 ng/ml) for 4, 16, 24, 48, and 72 hours and the mRNA levels of AQP1, Vimentin, α-SMA and Collagen type I where quantified by real time RT-PCR analysis **(A)** and the protein levels of AQP1, Vimentin and α-SMA were quantified by Western blot **(B)**.

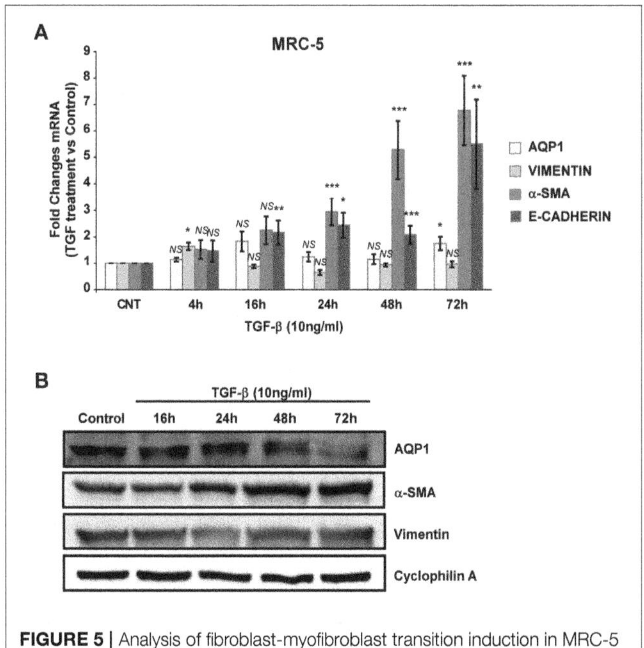

FIGURE 5 | Analysis of fibroblast-myofibroblast transition induction in MRC-5 cell line. Cells were treated with TGF-β1 (10 ng/ml) for 4, 16, 24, 48, and 72 hours and the mRNA levels of AQP1, Vimentin, α-SMA and Collagen type I where quantified by real time RT-PCR analysis **(A)** and the protein levels of AQP1, Vimentin and α-SMA were quantified by Western blot **(B)**.

In the present work, we have shown for the first time a large expression of AQP1 in human lung tissue from IPF patients, not only in endothelial cells but also in the alveolar epithelial surface. Alveolar surface is covered by two types of epithelial cells, alveolar cells called type I (AT I) and type II (AT II), also called pneumocytes type I and type II. AT I cells represent 90% of the alveolar border and are responsible for making gas exchange. AT II cells are characterized by synthesizing and secreting pulmonary surfactant which actives alveolar surface and prevent its collapse among other important functions such as immune defense (Chroneos et al., 2010). AT II cells are progenitors of AT I cells and therefore are responsible for repairing the alveolar epithelium after damage. Under normal conditions, the alveolar epithelial repair occurs through the proliferation of AT II cells and their differentiation into AT I cells. However, IPF is characterized by the fact that both alveolar type II cells and the type I undergo apoptosis and are replaced by fibroblasts (Barbas-Filho et al., 2001) contributing to the disappearance and transformation of the alveolar epithelium. As previously described, ATI cells do not express AQP1 (Nielsen et al., 1997). Interestingly, our data shows that expression of AQP1 in the alveolar epithelium was exclusively found in ATII cells.

Analysis performed in different diseases other than IPF show that AQP1 expression is not uniform. This water channel is not expressed in normal lung alveolar cells and is expressed to a much lesser extent in AT II cells from samples obtained from various interstitial lung diseases other than IPF. Even in cases of intense inflammatory activity like hypersensitivity pneumonitis or sarcoidosis, there is not expression of AQP1 in alveolar epithelial cells. The highest expression of AQP1 in type II alveolar epithelial cells occurs significantly in IPF samples. IPF is a progressive disease of unknown etiology (Crystal et al., 2002) that classically presents a histopathological pattern of UIP. The primary characteristics are areas of conventional fibrosis with variable regions of fibroblastic foci, scattered with zones of normal or almost normal lung. Additionally, IPF is also typified by ATII cell hyperplasia (Selman and Pardo, 2003). Although initial studies gave special attention and prevalent role to inflammation on fibrogenesis, the present hypothesis proposes a principal role of the epithelium in the pathogenesis and progression of this disease. Thus, IPF is likely the result of an initial epithelial injury to which the natural repair process fail to repair setting an initial focus of cell activation and damage (Chilosi et al., 2003). Identification of cells in which markers of epithelial and mesenchymal phenotypes are co-expressed, seen both in human lung and in cultures *in vitro,* sustain the paradigm by which alveolar epithelial cells may serve as a supply of myofibroblasts in lung fibrosis (Willis et al., 2005). Currently, activation and apoptosis of epithelial cells is considered one of the initial events in the development of IPF (Sisson et al., 2010).

In IPF, proliferation and migration are two important events in the alveolar epithelium transformation. Interestingly, AQP1 has been implicated in cell proliferation and migration promotion in lung among other proliferative tissue models (Saadoun et al., 2005; Wei and Dong, 2015; Wu et al., 2015; Galán-Cobo et al., 2016; Tomita et al., 2017; Wang et al., 2017; Yun et al., 2017). On the other hand, EMT is a key event in the IPF progression, which promotes accumulation of fibroblasts and deposition of extracellular matrix in response to epithelial injury. TGF-β signaling is considered a key activator of EMT and fibroblast activation in this disease (Chapman, 2011; Tirino et al., 2013). Migration is an essential process during EMT, and although AQP1 has not been directly related with EMT, it is well know that this protein helps the cell migration process by facilitating water influx at the tip of the lamellipodium, resulting in a membrane protusion (Saadoun et al., 2005), and by interacting with β-catenin (Monzani et al., 2009; Yun et al., 2017). Other AQPs, such as AQP3 and AQP5, activate this process as well (Chen et al., 2014, 2017). Therefore, the large increase in expression of AQP1 we observed on AT II cells in IPF patient biopsies may be crucial in supporting the high proliferation and migration events during the alveolar epithelium transformation. The strong induction by TGF-β1 of AQP1 expression specially observed in AECs (A549) in transition to a myofibroblast-like phenotype cell, or in the fibroblasts derived from an IPF patient (LL29), might be among the initial actions triggered by this potent fibrotic agent.

The initial injury which causes lesions in epithelial cells that lead to pulmonary fibrosis are unknown. For the very first time, we have demonstrated increased expression of AQP1 in type II alveolar epithelial cells in IPF patient samples. The increased expression of AQP1, its possible relationship with hyperplasia, and the subsequent insult of ATII remains unclear. Although deeper analysis are required to elucidate the role of AQP1 in the origin of IPF, our findings suggest AQP1 plays an important role in disease progression of IPF patients and should be further explored.

CONCLUSIONS

The alveolar epithelium of a normal human lung does not express AQP1. However, our studies indicate that IPF patient's hyperplasic type II pneumocytes show an increase in AQP1 expression on their surface. We investigated the role of TGF-β1, in the epithelial to mesenchymal transition of alveolar epithelial cells and lung fibroblast in IPF patient samples and also confirmed the induction of AQP1 expression. Therefore, the appearance of hyperplastic cells and regulation of AQP1 are implicated in the physiopathology of IPF.

AUTHOR CONTRIBUTIONS

AG-C and EA-O: Made all molecular biology experiments with culture cells; RS-S and NS-L: Carried out the immunoassays over patient's biopsies; JL-C, CG, MM-M, and JR: Selected, treated and diagnosed the patients included in the analysis; LG: Revised and interpreted immune results in patient's biopsies; ME and AG-C: Conceived and designed the experiments and wrote the manuscript; ME and JR: Contributed reagents, materials, and analysis tools. All authors read and approved the final manuscript.

ACKNOWLEDGMENTS

We are thankful to all patients which samples were included in this work. This study has been supported by the grants PI12/01882 and PI16/00493 from the Spanish Ministry of Economy and Competitiveness, co-funded by ISCIII and FEDER funds, conceded to ME, and grants from Neumosur and SEPAR foundations given to JR. We thank Juan Manuel Praena for his help with statistical analysis of data.

REFERENCES

Abreu-Rodríguez, I., Sánchez Silva, R., Martins, A. P., Soveral, G., Toledo-Aral, J. J., López-Barneo, J., et al. (2011). Functional and transcriptional induction of aquaporin-1 gene by hypoxia; analysis of promoter and role of Hif-1α. *PLoS ONE* 6:e28385. doi: 10.1371/journal.pone.0028385

Barbas-Filho, J. V., Ferreira, M. A., Sesso, A., Kairalla, R. A., Carvalho, C. R., and Capelozzi, V. L. (2001). Evidence of type II pneumocyte apoptosis in the pathogenesis of idiopathic pulmonary fibrosis (IFP)/usual interstitial pneumonia (UIP). *J. Clin. Pathol.* 54, 132–138. doi: 10.1136/jcp.54.2.132

Calero, C., López-Campos, J. L., Izquierdo, L. G., Sánchez-Silva, R., López-Villalobos, J. L., Sáenz-Coronilla, F. J., et al. (2014). Expression of aquaporins in bronchial tissue and lung parenchyma of patients with chronic obstructive pulmonary disease. *Multidiscip. Respir. Med.* 9:29. doi: 10.1186/2049-6958-9-29

Camelo, A., Dunmore, R., Sleeman, M. A., and Clarke, D. (2014). The epithelium in idiopathic pulmonary fibrosis: breaking the barrier. *Front. Pharmacol.* 4:173. doi: 10.3389/fphar.2013.00173

Cao, C. S., Yin, Q., Huang, L., Zhan, Z., Yang, J. B., and Xiong, H. W. (2010). Effect of angiotensin II on the expression of aquaporin 1 in lung of rats following acute lung injury. *Zhongguo Wei Zhong Bing Ji Jiu Yi Xue* 22, 426–429.

Chapman, H. A. (2011). Epithelial-mesenchymal interactions in pulmonary fibrosis. *Annu. Rev. Physiol.* 73, 413–435. doi: 10.1146/annurev-physiol-012110-142225

Chen, C., Ma, T., Zhang, C., Zhang, H., Bai, L., Kong, L., et al. (2017). Down-regulation of aquaporin 5-mediated epithelial-mesenchymal transition and anti-metastatic effect by natural product Cairicoside E in colorectal cancer. *Mol. Carcinog.* 56, 2692–2705. doi: 10.1002/mc.22712

Chen, J., Wang, T., Zhou, Y. C., Gao, F., Zhang, Z.-H., Xu, H., et al. (2014). Aquaporin 3 promotes epithelial-mesenchymal transition in gastric cancer. *J. Exp. Clin. Cancer Res.* 33:38. doi: 10.1186/1756-9966-33-38

Chilosi, M., Poletti, V., Zamò, A., Lestani, M., Montagna, L., Piccoli, P., et al. (2003). Aberrant Wnt/β-catenin pathway activation in idiopathic pulmonary fibrosis. *Am. J. Pathol.* 162, 1495–1502. doi: 10.1016/S0002-9440(10)64282-4

Chroneos, Z. C., Sever-Chroneos, Z., and Shepherd, V. L. (2010). Pulmonary surfactant: an immunological perspective. *Cell. Physiol. Biochem.* 25, 13–26. doi: 10.1159/000272047

Crystal, R. G., Bitterman, P. B., Mossman, B., Schwarz, M. I., Sheppard, D., Almasy, L., et al. (2002). Future research directions in idiopathic pulmonary fibrosis. *Am. J. Respir. Crit. Care Med.* 166, 236–246. doi: 10.1164/rccm.2201069

Echevarría, M., Muñoz-Cabello, A. M., Sánchez-Silva, R., Toledo-Aral, J. J., and López-Barneo, J. (2007). Development of cytosolic hypoxia and hypoxia-inducible factor stabilization are facilitated by aquaporin-1 expression. *J. Biol. Chem.* 282, 30207–30215. doi: 10.1074/jbc.M702639200

Galán-Cobo, A., Ramírez-Lorca, R., Serna, A., and Echevarría, M. (2015). Overexpression of AQP3 modifies the cell cycle and the proliferation rate of mammalian cells in culture. *PLoS ONE* 10:e0137692. doi: 10.1371/journal.pone.0137692

Galán-Cobo, A., Ramírez-Lorca, R., Toledo-Aral, J. J., and Echevarría, M. (2016). Aquaporin-1 plays important role in proliferation by affecting cell cycle progression. *J. Cell. Physiol.* 231, 243–256. doi: 10.1002/jcp.25078

Gao, X., Wang, G., Zhang, W., Peng, Q., Xue, M., and Jinhong, H. (2013). Expression of pulmonary aquaporin 1 is dramatically upregulated in mice with pulmonary fibrosis induced by bleomycin. *Arch. Med. Sci.* 9, 916–921. doi: 10.5114/aoms.2012.31011

Guarino, M., Tosoni, A., and Nebuloni, M. (2009). Direct contribution of epithelium to organ fibrosis: epithelial-mesenchymal transition. *Hum. Pathol.* 40, 1365–1376. doi: 10.1016/j.humpath.2009.02.020

Gutiérrez, C., Donate, Á., Gómez Izquierdo, L., Molina-Molina, M., Echevarría, M., and Rodriguez Portal, J. A. (2013). Aquoaporin-1 expression in idiopathic pulmonary fibrosis. *Eur. Respir. J.* 42(Suppl. 57):P2337.

Khalil, N., Xu, Y. D., O'Connor, R., and Duronio, V. (2005). Proliferation of pulmonary interstitial fibroblasts is mediated by transforming growth factor-β1-induced release of extracellular fibroblast growth factor-2 and phosphorylation of p38 MAPK and JNK. *J. Biol. Chem.* 280, 43000–43009. doi: 10.1074/jbc.M510441200

López-Campos, J. L., Sánchez Silva, R., Gómez Izquierdo, L., Márquez, E., Ortega Ruiz, F., Cejudo, P., et al. (2011). Overexpression of aquaporin-1 in lung adenocarcinomas and pleural mesotheliomas. *Histol. Histopathol.* 26, 451–459. doi: 10.14670/HH-26.451

Lynch, J. P., Saggar, R., Weigt, S. S., Zisman, D. A., and White, E. S. (2006). Usual interstitial pneumonia. *Semin. Respir. Crit. Care Med.* 27, 634–651. doi: 10.1055/s-2006-957335

Monzani, E., Bazzotti, R., Perego, C., and La Porta, C. A. M. (2009). AQP1 is not only a water channel: it contributes to cell migration through Lin7/Beta-catenin. *PLoS ONE* 4:e6167. doi: 10.1371/journal.pone.0006167

Nielsen, S., King, L. S., Christensen, B. M., and Agre, P. (1997). Aquaporins in complex tissues. II. Subcellular distribution in respiratory and glandular tissues of rat. *Am. J. Physiol.* 273(5 Pt 1), C1549-61.

Raghu, G., Collard, H. R., Egan, J. J., Martinez, F. J., Behr, J., Brown, K. K., et al. (2011). An official ATS/ERS/JRS/ALAT statement: idiopathic pulmonary fibrosis: evidence-based guidelines for diagnosis and management. *Am. J. Respir. Crit. Care Med.* 183, 788–824. doi: 10.1164/rccm.2009-040GL

Saadoun, S., Papadopoulos, M. C., Hara-Chikuma, M., and Verkman, A. S. (2005). Impairment of angiogenesis and cell migration by targeted aquaporin-1 gene disruption. *Nature* 434, 786. doi: 10.1038/nature03460

Selman, M., and Pardo, A. (2003). The epithelial/fibroblastic pathway in the pathogenesis of idiopathic pulmonary fibrosis. *Am. J. Respir. Cell Mol. Biol.* 29, S93–S97.

Sisson, T. H., Mendez, M., Choi, K., Subbotina, N., Courey, A., Cunningham, A., et al. (2010). Targeted injury of type II alveolar epithelial cells induces pulmonary fibrosis. *Am. J. Respir. Crit. Care Med.* 181, 254–263. doi: 10.1164/rccm.200810-1615OC

Spagnolo, P., Sverzellati, N., Rossi, G., Cavazza, A., Tzouvelekis, A., Crestani, B., et al. (2015). Idiopathic pulmonary fibrosis: an update. *Ann. Med.* 47, 15–27. doi: 10.3109/07853890.2014.982165

Takai, E., Tsukimoto, M., and Kojima, S. (2013). TGF-β1 Downregulates COX-2 expression leading to decrease of PGE2 production in human lung cancer A549 cells, which is involved in fibrotic response to TGF-β1. *PLOS ONE* 8:e76346. doi: 10.1371/journal.pone.0076346

Tirino, V., Camerlingo, R., Bifulco, K., Irollo, E., Montella, R., Paino, F., et al. (2013). TGF-β1 exposure induces epithelial to mesenchymal transition both in CSCs and non-CSCs of the A549 cell line, leading to an increase of migration ability in the CD133+ A549 cell fraction. *Cell Death Dis.* 4:e620. doi: 10.1038/cddis.2013.144

Tomita, Y., Dorward, H., Yool, J. A., Smith, E., Townsend, R. A., Price, J. T., et al. (2017). Role of aquaporin 1 signalling in cancer development and progression. *Int. J. Mol. Sci.* 18:299. doi: 10.3390/ijms18020299

Wang, Y., Fan, Y., Zheng, C., and Zhang, X. (2017). Knockdown of AQP1 inhibits growth and invasion of human ovarian cancer cells. *Mol. Med. Rep.* 16, 5499–5504. doi: 10.3892/mmr.2017.7282

Wei, X., and Dong, J. (2015). Aquaporin 1 promotes the proliferation and migration of lung cancer cell *in vitro*. *Oncol. Rep.* 34, 1440–1448. doi: 10.3892/or.2015.4107

Willis, B. C., and Borok, Z. (2007). TGF-β-induced EMT: mechanisms and implications for fibrotic lung disease. *Am. J. Physiol. Lung Cell. Mol. Physiol.* 293, L525–L534. doi: 10.1152/ajplung.00163.2007

Willis, B. C., duBois, R. M., and Borok, Z. (2006). Epithelial origin of myofibroblasts during fibrosis in the lung. *Proc. Am. Thorac. Soc.* 3, 377–382. doi: 10.1513/pats.200601-004TK

Willis, B. C., Liebler, J. M., Luby-Phelps, K., Nicholson, A. G., Crandall, E. D., du Bois, R. M., et al. (2005). Induction of epithelial-mesenchymal transition in alveolar epithelial cells by transforming growth factor-β1: potential role in idiopathic pulmonary fibrosis. *Am. J. Pathol.* 166, 1321–1332. doi: 10.1016/S0002-9440(10)62351-6

Wu, Z., Li, S., Liu, J., Shi, Y., Wang, J., Chen, D., et al. (2015). RNAi-mediated silencing of AQP1 expression inhibited the proliferation, invasion and tumorigenesis of osteosarcoma cells. *Cancer Biol. Ther.* 16, 1332–1340. doi: 10.1080/15384047.2015.1070983

Yun, X., Jiang, H., Lai, N., Wang, J., and Shimoda, L. A. (2017). Aquaporin 1-mediated changes in pulmonary arterial smooth muscle cell migration and proliferation involve β-catenin. *Am. J. Physiol. Lung Cell. Mol. Physiol.* 313, L889–L898. doi: 10.1152/ajplung.00247.2016

17

Identification of Loop D Domain Amino Acids in the Human Aquaporin-1 Channel Involved in Activation of the Ionic Conductance and Inhibition by AqB011

*Mohamad Kourghi, Michael L. De Ieso, Saeed Nourmohammadi, Jinxin V. Pei and Andrea J. Yool**

Aquaporin Physiology and Drug Discovery Program, Adelaide Medical School, University of Adelaide, Adelaide, SA, Australia

***Correspondence:**
Andrea J. Yool
andrea.yool@adelaide.edu.au

Aquaporins are integral proteins that facilitate the transmembrane transport of water and small solutes. In addition to enabling water flux, mammalian Aquaporin-1 (AQP1) channels activated by cyclic GMP can carry non-selective monovalent cation currents, selectively blocked by arylsulfonamide compounds AqB007 (IC_{50} 170 μM) and AqB011 (IC_{50} 14 μM). *In silico* models suggested that ligand docking might involve the cytoplasmic loop D (between AQP1 transmembrane domains 4 and 5), but the predicted site of interaction remained to be tested. Work here shows that mutagenesis of two conserved arginine residues in loop D slowed the activation of the AQP1 ion conductance and impaired the sensitivity of the channel to block by AqB011. Substitution of residues in loop D with proline showed effects on ion conductance amplitude that varied with position, suggesting that the structural conformation of loop D is important for AQP1 channel gating. Human AQP1 wild type, AQP1 mutant channels with alanines substituted for two arginines (R159A+R160A), and mutants with proline substituted for single residues threonine (T157P), aspartate (D158P), arginine (R159P, R160P), or glycine (G165P) were expressed in *Xenopus laevis* oocytes. Conductance responses were analyzed by two-electrode voltage clamp. Optical osmotic swelling assays and confocal microscopy were used to confirm mutant and wild type AQP1-expressing oocytes were expressed in the plasma membrane. After application of membrane-permeable cGMP, R159A+R160A channels had a significantly slower rate of activation as compared with wild type, consistent with impaired gating. AQP1 R159A+R160A channels showed no significant block by AqB011 at 50 μM, in contrast to the wild type channel which was blocked effectively. T157P, D158P, and R160P mutations had impaired activation compared to wild type; R159P showed no significant effect; and G165P appeared to augment the conductance amplitude. These findings provide evidence for the role of the loop D as a gating domain for AQP1 ion channels, and identify the likely site of interaction of AqB011 in the proximal loop D sequence.

Keywords: major intrinsic protein, MIP, AQP1, water channel, non-selective cation channel, cyclic GMP, arylsulfonamide

INTRODUCTION

Aquaporins (AQPs) are a diverse family of channels for water and solutes, classified as major intrinsic proteins (MIPs) (Benga et al., 1986; Agre et al., 1993; Reizer et al., 1993). In mammals, classes of AQPs are differentially expressed in endothelial, epithelial and other cell types, and comprise key components of mechanisms for fluid homeostasis in single cells, barrier tissues, and organs (Nielsen et al., 1993; Boassa and Yool, 2005; Hachez and Chaumont, 2010). Some classes of aquaporin channels have been found shown to transport molecules other than water across the cell membrane, including glycerol, ammonia, urea, protons, as well as CO_2 and O_2 gases (Madeira et al., 2014; Kitchen et al., 2015), and ions (Yool, 2007; Yool and Campbell, 2012).

Aquaporin ion channel functions have been described for multiple members of the MIP family. Recent work has shown that a plant aquaporin channel (AtPIP2;1) serves as a non-selective cation channel that is sensitive to Ca^{2+} and pH (Byrt et al., 2016), addressing a mystery regarding the molecular basis of a Ca^{2+}-inhibited leak current known to be involved in environmental stress responses of roots (Demidchik and Tester, 2002). The insect aquaporin Big Brain (BIB) channel in *Drosophila* (Yanochko and Yool, 2002) and mammalian lens MIP (AQP0) have been characterized as ion channels (Zampighi et al., 1985; Ehring et al., 1990); their importance of these channels is evident from the consequences of genetic knockouts resulting in impaired nervous system development (Rao et al., 1992) and cataract formation (Berry et al., 2000), respectively. However the precise roles of their ion channel activities in cell signaling and development remain to be determined.

Controversy on the role of AQP1 as an ion channel, first proposed in 1996 (Yool et al., 1996), stemmed from a paradigm which stated AQP1 was nothing but a water channel (Tsunoda et al., 2004). An extensive body of work published since has shown: (i) AQP1 is a dual water and cation channel with a unitary conductance of 150 pS under physiological conditions, permeable to Na^+, K^+, and Cs^+, and gated by the binding of cGMP at the intracellular loop D domain (Anthony et al., 2000; Yu et al., 2006). (ii) AQP1 carries water through the individual intra-subunit pores, whereas cations pass through the central pore of the tetramer (Yu et al., 2006; Campbell et al., 2012). (iii) Single channel activity of natively expressed AQP1 is selectively lost after small interfering knockdown of AQP1 expression (Boassa et al., 2006). (iv) The availability of AQP1 to be activated as an ion channel is regulated by tyrosine kinase phosphorylation of the carboxyl terminal domain (Campbell et al., 2012). (v) AQP1 ion channel properties are altered by site-directed mutagenesis of the central pore domain, which changes the cationic selectivity of the current, and creates a gain-of-function blocking site by Hg^{2+} via introduction of a cysteine residue at the extracellular side (Campbell et al., 2012). (vi) Mutations of the carboxyl terminal domain of hAQP1 alter the efficacy of cGMP in activating the ionic conductance (Boassa and Yool, 2003). (vii) Molecular dynamic simulations confirmed it was theoretically feasible to move Na^+ ions through the AQP1 central pore and identified the cytoplasmic loop D domain as involved in gating of the ion channel; mutation of key loop D residues impaired ion channel activation without preventing water channel activity (Yu et al., 2006).

The ability to change specific ion channel properties of activation, ion selectivity, and block using site-directed mutations of the AQP1 amino acid sequence have provided convincing evidence that AQP1 directly mediates the observed ionic current (Anthony et al., 2000; Boassa and Yool, 2003; Yu et al., 2006; Campbell et al., 2012). The alternative suggestion that responses were due to unidentified native ion channels translocated into the membrane along with AQP1 was ruled out by these studies, which showed that the altered ion channel functions associated with mutations of AQP1 did not prevent normal assembly and plasma membrane expression of AQP1 channels as evidenced by immunolabeling, western blot, and measures of osmotic water permeability.

While the ion channel function of AQP1 was confirmed independently by other groups (Saparov et al., 2001; Zhang et al., 2007), the physiological relevance of AQP1 ion channel function remained uncertain, given the low proportion of ion conducting channels observed in reconstituted membrane assays. Mathematical modeling tested the premise, assuming only a tiny fraction of AQP1 acted as ion channels, and showed the predicted effects were sufficient for a meaningful impact on net transport in epithelial cells (Yool and Weinstein, 2002). Interestingly the relative amplitudes of ion currents and water fluxes for mammalian AQP6, also thought to be a dual water and ion channel (Yasui et al., 1999), were similar to those of AQP1, suggesting AQP6 similarly has a low proportion of functioning ion channels within the total population. Although high densities of water channels might be needed to move substantial fluid volumes, the apparently low ratios for aquaporins reinforce a basic concept in the ion channel field; relatively few charge-selective ion channels are needed to alter transmembrane voltage gradients (Hille, 2001).

With development of the first selective AQP1 ion channel inhibitor AqB011 (Kourghi et al., 2016), the question of the physiological function of the AQP1 ion channel could be directly addressed. Kourghi and colleagues showed AqB011 selectively inhibited migration in AQP1-expressing cancer cell lines, but not in those without AQP1, demonstrating that the AQP1 ion conductance can serve an essential role in cellular functions such as migration. Of the pharmacological inhibitors of AQP1 ion channel identified thus far, AqB011 is the most potent (IC_{50} 14 μM). Osmotic water fluxes in hAQP1-expressing oocytes were not altered by 200 μM AqB011, indicating the block is selective for AQP1 ion channel activity. Molecular docking models suggested loop D domain as a candidate binding site for the AqB011 (Kourghi et al., 2016), but the prediction remained to be tested.

The role of AQP1 loop D residues in ion conductance activation and in mediating block by AqB011 was tested here using site-directed mutations of amino acids. Conserved arginine residues at positions 159 and 160 in human AQP1 were mutated to alanines. As compared with wild type, the cGMP-mediated activation of the AQP1 ionic conductance response was significantly slower in R159A+R160A channels, the maximal amplitude of the activated current in the mutant construct was reduced as compared to wild type, and the mutant was insensitive to the inhibitor AqB011. Human AQP1 mutant constructs in which proline was substituted for conserved single residues threonine (T157P), aspartate (D158P), arginine (R159P, R160P), and glycine (G165P) showed differential effects on conductance activation depending on position, which suggested the conformation of loop D is important for AQP1 ion channel gating. Proline enables tight bends in peptide structures (Vanhoof et al., 1995). These results support the role of conserved loop D residues in AQP1 ion channel activation and inhibition

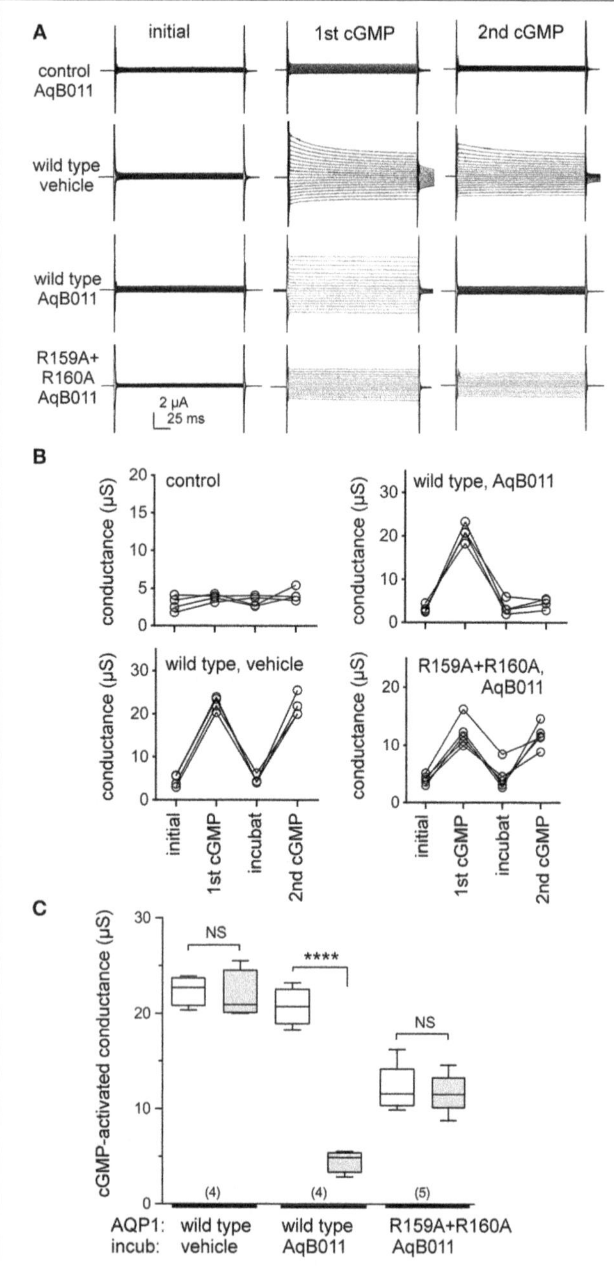

FIGURE 1 | Human AQP1 ionic conductances activated by cGMP differ in sensitivity to the inhibitor AqB011 in wild type and R159A+R160A expressing oocytes. **(A)** Electrophysiology traces showing currents recorded in control non-AQP oocytes, and in hAQP1 wild type and R159A+R160A expressing oocytes. The current traces are shown prior to stimulation (initial), after the first maximal response to CPT-cGMP (1st cGMP), and after the second maximal response (2nd cGMP) following a 2 h incubation with 50 μM AqB011 or vehicle (DMSO). **(B)** Trend plots show the ionic conductance amplitudes for individual oocytes through each series of treatments for AQP1 wild type, mutant, and non AQP-expressing control oocytes, measured before stimulation (initial), after the first CPT-cGMP (1st cGMP), after 2-h recovery in cGMP-free saline containing vehicle or 50 μM AqB011 ("incubat"), and after the second CPT-cGMP (2nd cGMP). **(C)** Compiled box plot data illustrate statistically significant block of AQP1 wild type but not R159A+R160 ion conductances following incubation in 50 μM AqB011. *n* values are above the x-axis. Boxes show 50% of data points; error bars show the full range; horizontal bars show median values. ****$p < 0.0001$.

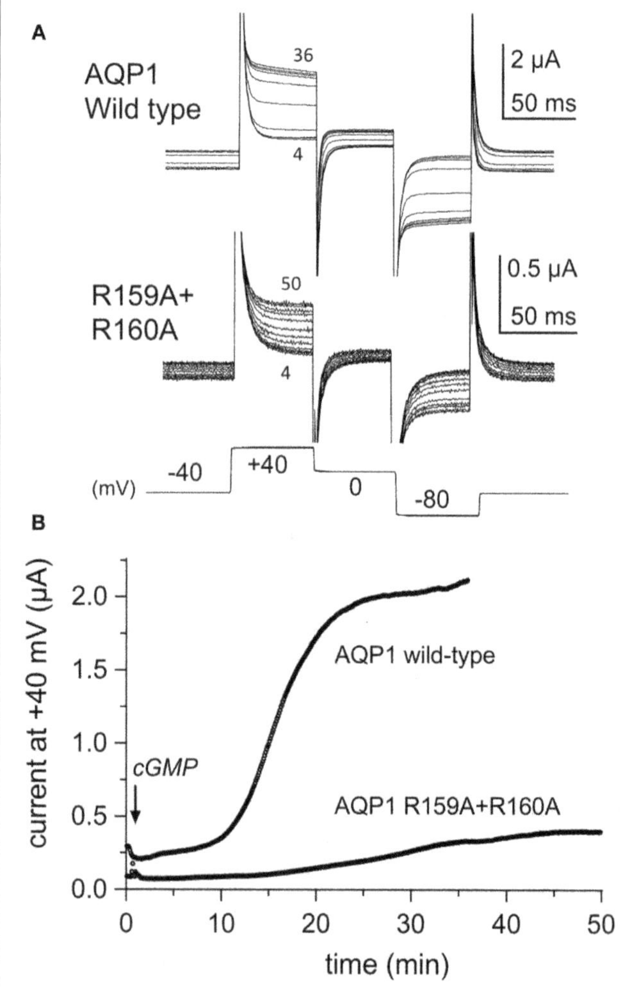

FIGURE 2 | Rates of activation of ion conductance responses to CPT-cGMP in oocytes expressing AQP1 wild type or R159A+R160A channels. **(A)** Ion current responses were monitored after application of CPT-cGMP using repeated series of brief steps to +40, 0, and −80 mV from a holding potential of −40 mV (10 per minute; 150 ms each). Traces are shown at 4 min intervals for clarity. Numbers indicate time in minutes post-application of CPT-cGMP. **(B)** The plot of steady state current amplitudes at +40 mV as a function of time after application of CPT-cGMP at time zero illustrates the difference in latency to activation in representative examples of AQP1 wild type and R159A+R160A expressing oocytes.

by AqB011, and provide further support for the concept that loop D is a gating domain for the AQP1 central ion pore.

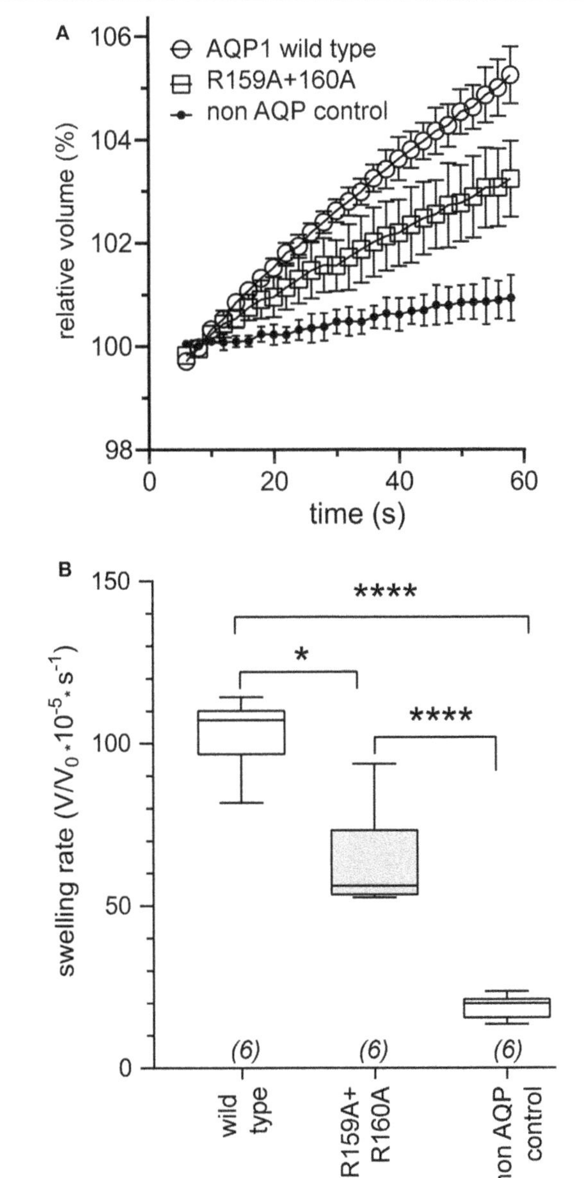

FIGURE 3 | Confirmation of expression of AQP1 wild type and AQP1 R159A+R160 mutant channels in oocyte plasma membranes by significantly increased osmotic water permeabilities as compared to non-AQP1 expressing controls. **(A)** Osmotic water permeabilities (mean ± SEM) assessed by quantitative swelling assays for AQP1 wild type (open circles) and AQP1 R159A+R160 mutant (squares) compared with non-AQP1 expressing control oocytes (filled circles). Relative volumes as a function of time after introduction into 50% hypotonic saline at time zero were measured from video-imaged cross-sectional areas. ($n = 6$ per group). **(B)** Box plot data showing osmotic swelling rates were higher in oocytes expressing AQP1 wild type and AQP1 R159A+R160 mutants than non-AQP1 expressing controls (one way ANOVA; *post-hoc* Bonferroni tests). $^{*}p < 0.05$; $^{****}p < 0.0001$; $n = 6$ per group. Boxes show 50% of data points; error bars show the full range; horizontal bars show median values.

MATERIALS AND METHODS

Oocyte Preparation and Injection

Unfertilized oocytes were harvested by partial ovariectomy from anesthetized *Xenopus laevis* frogs following national guidelines (Australian Code of Practice for the Care and Use of Animals for Scientific Purposes), and approved by the University of Adelaide Animal Ethics Committee (approval # M2013-167). Oocytes were defolliculated with collagenase (type 1A, 1 mg/ml; Sigma-Aldrich, St. Louis, MO) in the presence of trypsin inhibitor (0.05 mg/ml; Sigma-Aldrich, St. Louis, MO) for 1 to 1.5 h in OR-2 saline (96 mM NaCl, 2 mM KCl, 5 mM $MgCl_2$, penicillin 100 units/ml, streptomycin 0.1 mg/ml, and 5 mM HEPES; pH 7.6). Oocytes were then washed 4 times with OR-2 saline at ~10 min intervals, and kept at 16–18°C in isotonic Frog Ringers saline [96 mM NaCl, 2 mM KCl, 5 mM $MgCl_2$, 0.6 mM $CaCl_2$, 5 mM HEPES buffer, horse serum (5%; Sigma-Aldrich, St. Louis, MO), penicillin 100 units/ml streptomycin 0.1 mg/ml, and tetracycline 0.5 mg/ml, pH 7.6]. Oocytes were injected with 50 nl of water (control oocytes), or 50 nl of water containing 1 ng of AQP1 wild type cRNA, or 2 ng of AQP1 mutant cRNAs. Oocytes were then transferred to sterile dishes containing Frog Ringers saline and incubated at 16–18°C for 48 h or more to allow time for protein expression. Isotonic Na^+ saline used for electrophysiology and osmotic swelling assays contained (in mM): NaCl 96 mM, KCl 2 mM, $MgCl_2$ 5 mM, $CaCl_2$ 0.6 mM, and HEPES 5 mM, pH 7.3, without antibiotics or serum.

Site Directed Mutagenesis of AQP1

Site-directed mutations were generated in human AQP1 cDNA in the *Xenopus* expression vector (pxBGev), using the QuikChange site-directed mutagenesis kit (Agilent Technologies, Forest Hills, VIC, Australia) with custom-synthesized primers as described previously (Yu et al., 2006). The correct sequences of the constructs were confirmed by replicate DNA sequencing of the full-length cDNA constructs. Wild-type AQP1 and mutant cDNAs were linearized using BamHI and transcribed with T3 RNA polymerase using the mMessage mMachine kit (Ambion, Austin, TX).

Osmotic Swelling Assays and Confocal Microscopy

Swelling assays or confocal microscopy were used to confirm AQP1 wild type and mutant channels were expressed in oocyte plasma membranes. Swelling assays were performed in 50% hypotonic saline (isotonic Na^+ saline diluted with equal volume of water). Prior to swelling assays the control (non-AQP expressing), AQP1 wild type and AQP1 mutant expressing oocytes were rinsed in isotonic saline (without horse serum or antibiotics) for 10 min. Rates of swelling were imaged using a grayscale camera (Cohu, San Diego, CA) fixed on a dissecting microscope (Olympus SZ-PT; Olympus, Macquarie Park, Australia), and images were captured at 0.5 Hz using Image J software from National Institutes of Health (http://rsbweb.nih.gov/ij/). Swelling rates were determined from slope values of linear regression fits of relative volume as a function of time using Prism (GraphPad Software Inc., San

Diego, CA). For confocal microscopy, oocytes were fixed in 4% paraformaldehyde, permeabilized with 0.1% Triton X-100, and incubated with rabbit polyclonal anti-AQP1 antibody (provided by WD Stamer; Duke University, USA) diluted in buffered solution with 300 mM NaCl, 30 mM Na citrate, 1% bovine serum albumin, 0.05% TritonX-100, and 0.02% sodium azide. After secondary labeling with FITC-conjugated goat anti-rat antibody, preparations were imaged with a Leica (Nussloch, Germany) TCS-4D laser scanning confocal microscope.

Electrophysiological Recordings

Two-electrode voltage clamp recordings were performed at room temperature in standard isotonic Na^+ saline using a GeneClamp amplifier and Clampex 9.0 software (pClamp 9.0 Molecular Devices, Sunnyvale, CA, USA). Data were filtered at 2 kHz and stored to hard disk for analysis. Capillary glass pipettes ($\sim$1 MΩ) were filled with 1 M KCl. Initial conductance values were determined from current-voltage relationships measured prior to cGMP stimulation, by application of the nitric oxide donor sodium nitroprusside (SNP) at a final concentration of 7.5 mM, or by application of membrane permeable CPT-cGMP(8-(4-chlorophenylthio)-guanosine-3′,5′-cyclic monophosphate) at a final concentration of 10 μM, as per published methods (Boassa and Yool, 2003; Campbell et al., 2012). From a holding potential of −40, voltage steps from +60 to −110 mV were applied to measure conductance. Repeated steps to +40 mV at 6 s intervals were used to monitor changes in ion current responses as a function of time after application of an activator or inhibitor. For the studies of pharmacological inhibition by AqB011, after recording the conductance for the first response to CPT-cGMP, oocytes were transferred into isotonic Na^+ saline with either AqB011 or vehicle for 2 h. Incubation allowed recovery to initial conductance levels as well as time for AqB011 to cross the membrane to reach its intracellular site of action, as described previously (Kourghi et al., 2016). Recovery from block was very slow, taking hours after removal of the agent from the extracellular medium. Oocytes were then re-evaluated for responsiveness to a second application of CPT-cGMP to test for inhibition post-incubation without AqB011 present. AqB011 was synthesized by G Flynn (SpaceFill Enterprises LLC, Bozeman Montana USA) with preparation methods and chemical structure as previously published (Kourghi et al., 2016). AqB011 was prepared as a 1000x stock solution in the vehicle dimethylsulfoxide (DMSO) and diluted in recording saline to the final concentration; vehicle control saline was made with the equivalent amount of DMSO (0.1% V/V). Box plot histograms show 50% of data (boxes), the full range of data (error bars), and the median value (horizontal bar).

RESULTS

Reduced Sensitivity to Block by AqB011 in AQP1 R159A+R160A Channels

Voltage clamp recordings showed that application of extracellular CPT-cGMP activated ionic conductance responses in human AQP1 wild type and R159A+R160A mutant

GenBank ID		amino acid sequence		*Genus;* Common name
AAH22486.1	154	ATTDRRRRDLGGSAPLAIGLSVALGH	180	*Homo;* Human
AAH07125.1	154	ATTDRRRRDLGGSAPLAIGLSVALGH	180	*Mus;* Mouse
AAB46624.1	154	ATTDRRRRDLGGSAPLAIGLSVALGH	180	Rattus; Rat
XP_014989258.1	154	ATTDRRRRDLGGSAPLAIGLSVALGH	180	*Macaca;* Rhesus macaque
XP_012496173.1	154	ATTDRRRRDLGGSAPLAIGLSVALGH	180	*Propithecus;* Crowned sifaka
XP_012330551.1	154	ATTDRRRRDLGGSAPLAIGLSVALGH	180	*Aotus;* Night monkey
XP_008583141.1	154	ATTDRRRRDLGGSAPLAIGLSVALGH	180	*Galeopterus;* Malayan flying lemur
XP_005319226.1	154	ATTDRRRRDLGGSAPLAIGLSVALGH	180	*Ictidomys;* Thirteen lined ground squirrel
XP_022439712.1	156	ATTDRRRRDLGGSAPLAIGLSVALGH	182	*Delphinapteru;* Beluga whale
XP_010969922.1	156	ATTDRRRRDLSGSGPLAIGLSVALGH	182	*Camelus;* Bactrian camel
XP_005981267.1	156	ATTDRRRRDLGGSGPLAIGFSVALGH	182	*Pantholops;* Tibetan antelope
NP_777127.1	156	ATTDRRRRDLGGSGPLAIGFSVALGH	182	*Bos;* Cow
CAD92027.1	148	ATTDKRRRDVTGSAPLAIGLSVALGH	173	*Anguilla;* European eel
BAC82110.1	148	ATTDKRRRDVTGSAPLAIGLSVALGH	173	*Anguilla;* Japanese eel
ASW16810.1	144	ATTDKRRRDVAGSAPLAIGLSVALGH	169	*Coilia;* Grenadier anchovy
AIL02123.1	144	ATTDKRRRDVTGSAPLAIGLSVALGH	169	*Alosa;* Alewife (herring)
NP_996942.1	145	ATTDKRRRDVSGSAPLAIGLSVCLGH	171	*Danio;* Zebrafish
XP_020322871.1	147	AVTDKRRRDITGSAPLAIGLSVALGH	172	*Oncorhynchus;* Coho salmon
XP_013996040.1	147	AVTDKRRRDVTGSAPLAIGLSVALGH	172	*Salmo;* Atlantic salmon
XP_007242700.2	148	AATDKRRRDVMGSVPLAIGLSVALGH	174	*Astyanax;* Blind cavefish
XP_016109136.1	146	ATTDKRRRDVTGSAPLAIGLSVCLGH	171	*Sinocyclocheilus;* Golden line fish
XP_015474877.1	156	ATTDRRRNDVSGSAPLAIGLSVALGH	182	*Parus;* Great tit
KQK77783.1	156	ATTDRRRNDVSGSAPLAIGLSVALGH	182	*Amazona;* Blue-fronted parrot
XP_013808479.1	156	ATTDRRRNDVSGSAPLAIGLSVALGH	182	*Apteryx;* Brown kiwi
XP_009878414.1	156	ATTDRRRNDVSGSAPLAIGLSVALGH	182	*Charadrius;* Killdeer (plover)

FIGURE 4 | Amino acid sequence alignment for the loop D and flanking domains of AQP1 channels from diverse classes of vertebrates (mammals, fish, and birds). Amino acid sequences downloaded from the National Center for Biotechnology Information (NCBI) Protein database (www.ncbi.nlm.nih.gov/protein) were aligned using the NCBI BlastP online application (blast.ncbi.nlm.nih.gov) for multiple sequences. Residues in black are identical with the query sequence *Homo sapiens* AQP1. Variations in sequence are highlighted in red.

expressing oocytes (**Figure 1A**). Initial recordings measured before the application of CPT-cGMP showed uniformly low currents, comparable to those of non-AQP control oocytes. The ionic conductance increased after application of CPT-cGMP in AQP1 wild type and R159A+R160A expressing oocytes, but in not non-AQP control oocytes. After recording the first response, oocytes were transferred into isotonic Na^+ saline with 50 μM AqB011 or vehicle. **Figure 1B** shows trend plots of the conductance responses of individual oocytes through each series of treatments. After 2 h incubation, the ionic conductance responses recovered to initial levels, and a second application of CPT-cGMP was used to assess the level of reactivation of current (**Figures 1A,B**). CPT-cGMP activated currents were not observed in non-AQP expressing control oocytes. **Figure 1C** shows compiled box plot data for the ionic conductance values for human AQP1 wild type and R159A+R160A mutants. AQP1 wild type currents were strongly blocked after incubation in AqB011 but not after incubation with vehicle. The amplitude of maximal activation was lower in R159A+R160A mutant-expressing oocytes than wild type, and the R159A+R160A conductance was not sensitive to block by AqB011.

The recovery of the AQP1 wild type and mutant currents to baseline levels during the incubation period demonstrated that the responses were reversible, thus not due to oocyte damage or leak. Complete reactivation of wild type ionic conductance response to the second application of CPT-cGMP (after incubation in saline with vehicle) demonstrated that prior activation did not impair responsiveness of the AQP1-expressing oocytes to subsequent stimulation. AQP1 wild type-expressing oocytes incubated in saline with AqB011 were not re-activated by a second application of CPT-cGMP, confirming inhibition of the ion current as described previously

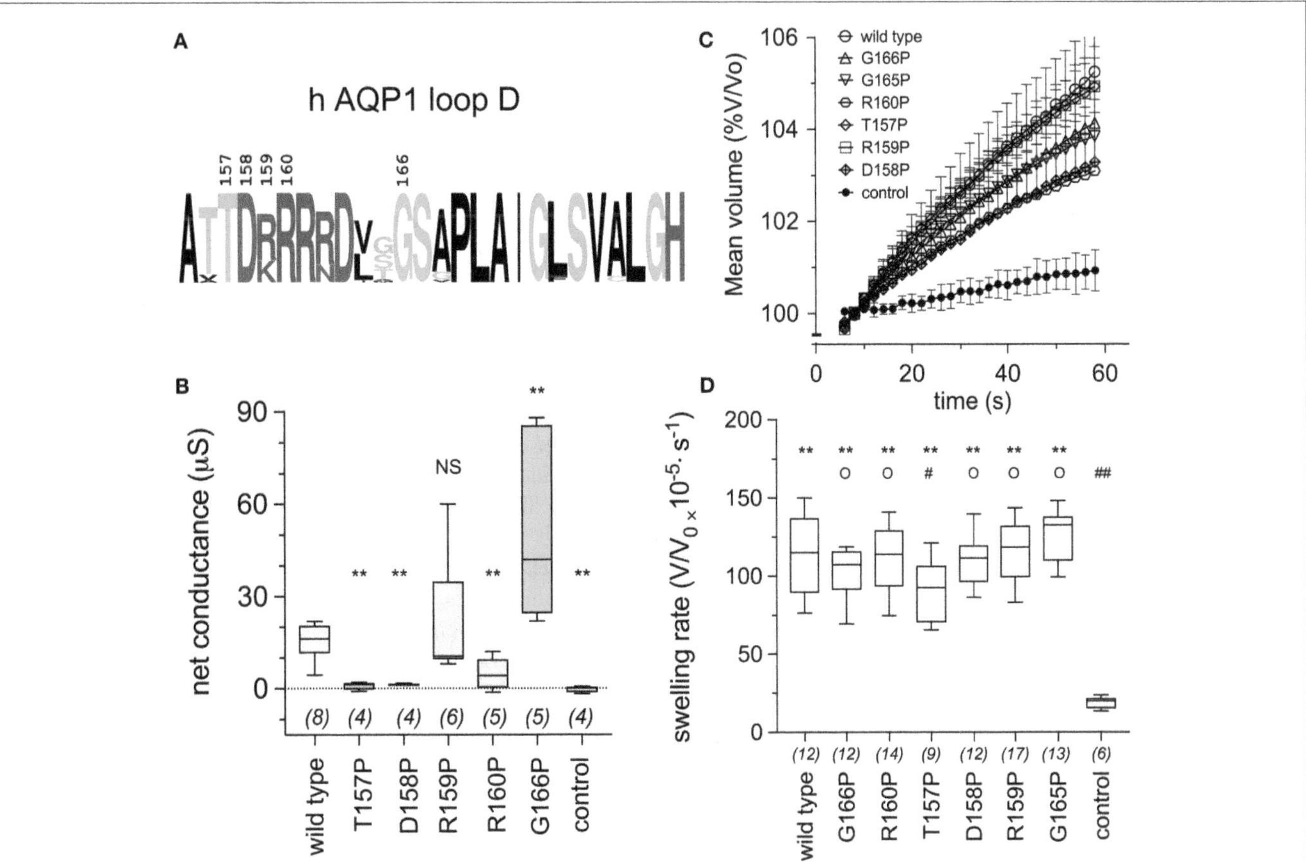

FIGURE 5 | Conserved amino acids in the AQP1 loop D domain influence the ion conductance response, as assessed by proline mutagenesis. **(A)** Schematic summary of the level of conservation of loop D amino acids in AQP1 sequences (data shown in **Figure 4**) created with the online WebLogo tool (http://weblogo.berkeley.edu/logo.cgi). Letter sizes represent corresponding relative frequencies of occurrence at that position in the sequence set. **(B)** Box plot data showing the net conductance values (maximal−initial) for hAQP1 wild type and proline substituted mutant channels. Position-specific effects of proline-scanning mutagenesis on ion conductance responses in human AQP1 suggested less conserved positions are more tolerant of proline substitution. Statistical significance was evaluated with ANOVA and *post-hoc* two-tailed Mann Whitney. $^{**}p < 0.01$; NS not significant, as compared with wild type; *n* values are above the x-axis. **(C)** Graph of mean volumes measured during optical swelling assays and standardized as a percentage of initial volume, for control oocytes and oocytes expressing wild type hAQP1 and proline-substituted mutants as a function of time after introduction of the oocyte into 50% hypotonic saline at time zero. (*n* values given in **D**). **(D)** Box plot histogram of swelling rates for hAQP1 wild type, proline mutant and control oocytes. Significant differences were determined by ANOVA ($p < 0.0001$) and *post-hoc* unpaired *T*-tests. ** indicates a significant difference from control, $p < 0.0001$. O indicates no significant difference from wild type, $p > 0.05$. A significant difference from wild type is indicated as # at $p < 0.05$, or ## for $p < 0.0001$.

(Kourghi et al., 2016). In contrast, the AQP1 R159A+R160A mutant channels showed no change in the second response to CPT-cGMP after incubation with or without AqB011, showing that sensitivity to the inhibitor was eliminated by the altered loop D sequence. The insensitivity of the R159A+R160A current furthermore demonstrated that the observed pharmacological block of wild type current by AqB011 cannot readily be ascribed to off-target effects on native oocyte channels or transporters, confirming the specificity of action of the antagonist compound.

Increased Latency to Activation for AQP1 R159A+R160A Channels

The conductance responses of wild type and R159A+R160A mutant channels differed in rates of activation after application of CPT-cGMP. Oocytes expressing AQP1 wild type activated more rapidly and reached a higher maximal current amplitude that did those expressing AQP1 R159A+R160A channels (**Figure 2A**). In wild type, the maximal response was reached by ~20–30 min after application of CPT-cGMP, whereas 50–60 min was needed for R159A+R160A expressing oocytes (**Figure 2B**). The latency to the onset of activation was considerably slower for the mutant construct. The long latency for R159A+R160A was consistent with prior work which reported no appreciable activation of the R159A+R160A mutant channels when assessed over a short time frame (within 8 min after application of the nitric oxide donor, sodium nitroprusside, which was used to stimulate endogenous oocyte cGMP production, and successfully activated AQP1 wild type ion currents) (Yu et al., 2006).

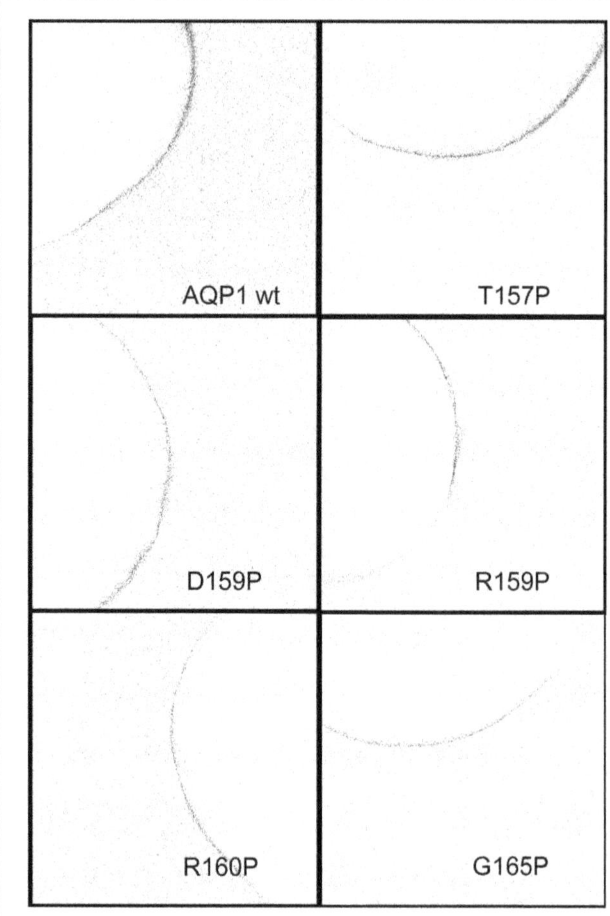

FIGURE 6 | Confocal images of anti-AQP1 immunolabeled oocytes expressing wild type and proline substituted mutant channels confirmed protein expression in the oocyte plasma membrane. See Methods for details.

Osmotic Water Permeability of AQP1 Wild Type and R159A+R160A Expressing Oocytes

Osmotic water permeability data (**Figure 3A**) confirmed successful expression of wild type and R159A+R160A mutant AQP1 channels in oocyte plasma membranes. The water channel activities of AQP1 wild type and R159A+R160A expressing oocytes were both were significantly greater than those of non-AQP1 expressing control oocytes (**Figure 3B**), confirming that both AQP1 channel types were expressed, assembled, and trafficked to the plasma membrane of oocytes. Expression levels for the R159A+R160A mutant channels estimated by osmotic water permeability were ~10% lower than wild type; however the mean conductance response in the arginine double mutant (**Figure 1C**) was half that of wild type, consistent with impairment of channel activation.

Effects of Proline Mutagenesis of the Loop D Amino Acid Sequence

Proline substituted mutant channels showed significant differences in response amplitudes that correlated with the degree of conservation of the amino acid residue in the loop D sequence. Sequence alignments for loop D and flanking domains illustrate the high level of identity for amino acids in AQP1 gene coding sequences from a diverse array of vertebrates, including mammals, fish, and birds (**Figure 4**). Net conductances, measured from amplitudes of the ionic conductance response, were calculated as the difference between the initial level and the final amplitude after SNP-mediated cGMP stimulation (**Figure 5**). Wild type AQP1 channels showed activation in response to SNP stimulation (**Figure 5B**) that was comparable in amplitude to that seen after application of CPT-cGMP (**Figure 1**). Control non-AQP-expressing oocytes showed no appreciable response. However, significantly impaired responses were seen for oocytes expressing AQP1 T157P, D158P, and R160P mutant channels (**Figure 5B**). T157, D158, and R160 residues exhibit complete identity across AQP1 sequences from diverse animals (**Figure 5A**). In contrast, AQP1 R159P expressing oocytes showed no significant difference from AQP1 wild type, which could fit with the observation that slightly more variation in amino acid sequence appears to be tolerated at that position. Interestingly, a significant difference also was observed for mutation to proline at the highly conserved G166, but the result was to promote rather than inhibit the activation of the conductance response as compared to wild type. The expression of functional channels in the oocyte membrane was confirmed

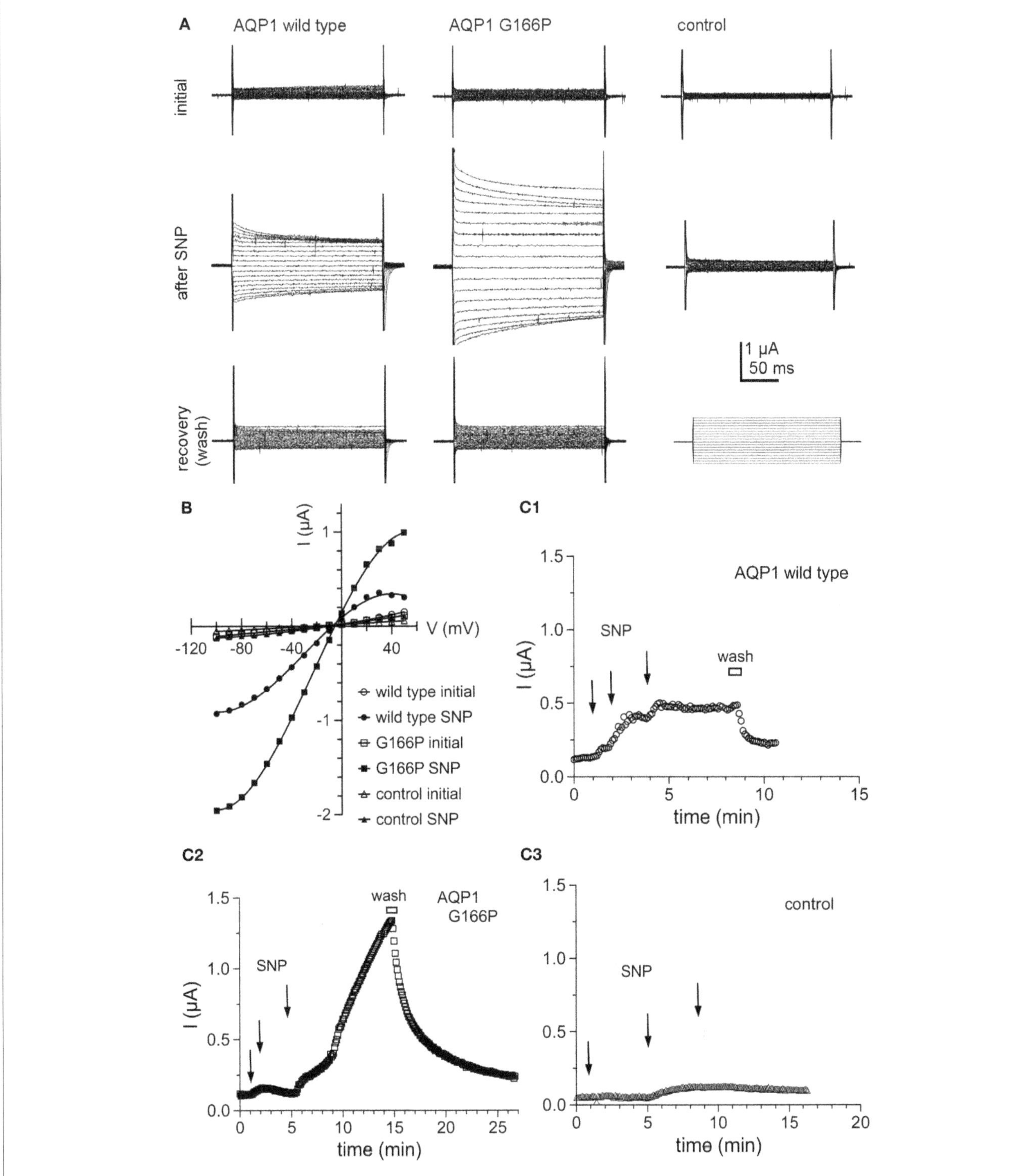

FIGURE 7 | Ion conductance responses of oocytes expressing human AQP1 wild type and G166P channels. **(A)** Currents recorded from wild type (left), G166P (middle), and non-AQP expressing control oocytes (right) by two-electrode voltage clamp before (initial) and after stimulation of intracellular cyclic GMP by application of the nitric oxide donor, sodium nitroprusside at a final concentration of 7.5 mM (after SNP). Perfusion of fresh bath saline without SNP (wash) promoted rapid recovery. **(B)** Current voltage relationships for the traces shown in **(A)**. **(C)** Steady state current amplitudes at +40 mV monitored as a function of time after three sequential applications of SNP (2.5 mM each) at times indicated by arrows, and after perfusion of bath saline without SNP (wash) shown by the horizontal bar, for wild type **(C1)**, G166P **(C2)**, and control **(C3)** oocytes. Data are from the same oocytes as shown in **(A)**.

by the demonstration of high osmotic water permeabilities for all the proline mutant constructs that were significantly greater that that of the non-AQP-expressing controls (**Figures 5C,D**). Confocal images of oocytes expressing AQP1 wild type and proline mutant channels confirmed that the constructs were expressed in the oocyte plasma membrane (**Figure 6**).

The conductance properties of AQP1 G166P-expressing oocytes, as compared with wild type and non-AQP control oocytes, are summarized in **Figure 7**. The ion conductance responses of AQP1 wild type and G166P-expressing oocytes showed an increase in amplitude but not in apparent kinetics (**Figure 7A**), reversal potential (**Figure 7B**), latency to activation, or reversibility of the responses after bath washout with fresh saline to remove SNP (**Figure 7C**). Control oocytes showed negligible responses to SNP (**Figures 7A,B**).

DISCUSSION

The aim of this study was to evaluate a candidate binding site for the AQP1 ion channel antagonist AqB011 suggested from prior *in silico* modeling, and to test the role of the intracellular loop D domain in AQP1 ion channel activation. Discovery of pharmacological tools for AQPs has been an area of keen interest for many years (Huber et al., 2012). As illustrated by the diagram in **Figure 8**, AQP1 ion channels are proposed to conduct solutes and water through pharmacologically distinct pathways (Saparov et al., 2001; Yool et al., 2002), with water transport mediated through the individual pores of the subunits (Jung et al., 1994), and ion transport proposed to be mediated by the central pore of the tetramer following activation by intracellular cGMP (Anthony et al., 2000; Yool and Weinstein, 2002; Campbell et al., 2012). The water channel function of hAQP1 is modulated by antagonists such as mercurial compounds (Preston et al., 1993); gold and silver compounds (Niemietz and Tyerman, 2002); the arylsulfonamide AqB013 (Migliati et al., 2009); medicinal herb compounds bacopasides I and II (Pei et al., 2016); aromatic carboxylic acid blockers referred to as CPD 1, 2, and 3 (Seeliger et al., 2013); and by agonist compounds such as AqF026 (Yool et al., 2013). Other inhibitors include TGN-020 for AQP4 (Igarashi et al., 2011), and gold-bipyridyl compounds for AQP3 (Martins et al., 2013; Graziani et al., 2017). The human AQP1 ion channel is pharmacologically distinct from the water pore, supporting the involvement of a separate pathway for ions through the central pore of the tetrameter (**Figure 8**). The AQP1 ion pore is blocked by Cd^{2+} (Boassa et al., 2006), other divalent cations (Kourghi et al., 2017b), and arylsulfonamide compounds AqB007 and AqB011 (Kourghi et al., 2016).

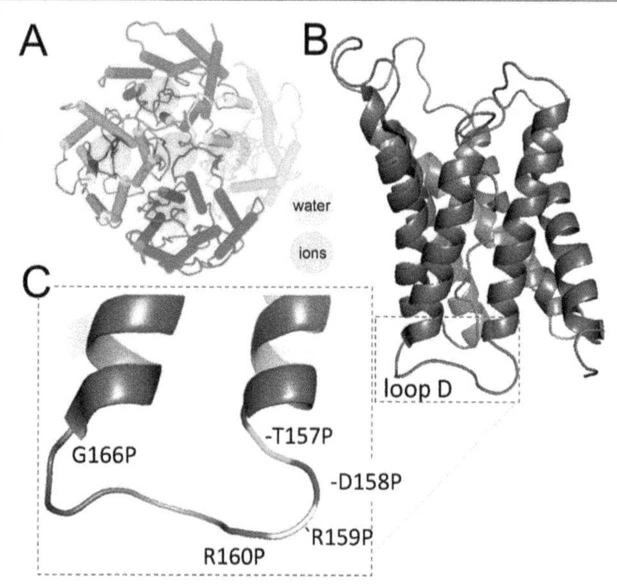

FIGURE 8 | Schematic diagrams illustrating the separate pathways proposed to mediate water and ion transport in the AQP1 tetrameric channel, and the position of the mutations tested in the loop D domain by proline mutagenesis. **(A)** AQP1 channels assemble as homomeric tetramers in the membrane bilayer. Water pores (blue) are located in each subunit; cations are thought to permeate via the central pore at the four-fold axis of symmetry in the channel (rose). **(B)** Loop D is a cytoplasmic loop between the 4 and 5th transmembrane domains in each subunit; loops D in the tetramer surround the central pore. **(C)** Amino acid residues in loop D tested by mutation to proline. Structural data used to create the diagrams were downloaded from the NCBI Structure database (www.ncbi.nlm.nih.gov/structure/), for PDB ID 1IH5 human AQP1 (Ren et al., 2001); and PDB 1JN4 bovine AQP1 (Sui et al., 2001).

AqB011 inhibits the human AQP1 ion current but not the water flux, and slows the migration of AQP1-expressing human colon cancer cells (Kourghi et al., 2016). Molecular docking studies suggested that AqB011 might interact with a conserved arginine residues located on loop D domain of AQP1, a region that has been suggested to be involved in gating of the central pore of the AQP1 channel (Yu et al., 2006). The role of the conserved loop D domain was tested using a mutant construct of the AQP1 channel in which the positively charged arginine residues in positions 159 and 160 of the human AQP1 amino acid sequence were replaced with alanine. The mutation R159A+R160A did not prevent the channel from being expressed on the membrane of oocytes, as demonstrated by measured osmotic water permeability. The hAQP1 R159A+R160A channel had previously been thought to be non-functional as an ion channel (Yu et al., 2006). However, work here showed the R159A+R160A ion conductance was activated by CPT-cGMP albeit at a significantly slower rate, to a lower maximal amplitude, and with a longer latency than for AQP wild type channels, which would have made it difficult to detect in protocols used previously. Nonetheless the residual ion channel function in the R159A+R160A mutant was significantly greater than in non-AQP controls and was sufficient to allow evaluation of a possible difference in sensitivity to block by AqB011.

The ion conductance in wild type AQP1 expressing oocytes was significantly inhibited by AqB011, confirming prior work (Kourghi et al., 2016). In contrast, AqB011 had no effect on the ion conductance response in R159A+R160A expressing oocytes. These results provide evidence that AqB011 is acting directly on the AQP1 channel, and not indirectly through hypothetical native oocyte channels or transporters associated with AQP1 proteins. The plant AQP AtPIP2;1 is a dual ion and water channel which also is insensitive to AqB011 (Kourghi et al., 2017b).

AtPIP2;1 has many amino acid sequence differences as compared to AQP1, but these include the absence of the poly-arginine series in loop D. Together these data suggest that selective pharmacological targeting of different classes of aquaporin ion channels will be possible, as structure-activity data for active agents continues to accrue, and discover of new agents expands the tools available for evaluating physiological roles of dual water and ion channels in the MIP family.

Proline scanning mutagenesis was used here to assess the role of the loop D domain in activation of the AQP1 ion conductance. Scanning mutagenesis is a method for analyzing the functional roles of amino acid residues in proteins by systematic replacement with another amino acid, such as alanine, cysteine, or proline (Cunningham and Wells, 1989; Kürz et al., 1995; Patel et al., 2013). Alanine is compact, lacking a bulky side group, and preserves 3D structure without influencing electrostatic characteristics (Cunningham and Wells, 1989). Alternatively, conformational structure can be deliberately altered by substituting residues with proline, which is distinctive in having the nitrogen atom covalently bound in a 5-membered ring, which impairs formation of intermolecular hydrogen bonds (Williams and Deber, 1991), and introduces "kinks" in secondary structure (Barlow and Thornton, 1988; Woolfson and Williams, 1990; Sankararamakrishnan and Vishveshwara, 1992). Proline scanning mutagenesis has been used to investigate gating mechanisms of ion channels such as the inward rectifier and transient receptor potential (TRP) channels (Sadja et al., 2001; Jin et al., 2002). Sadja et al. (2001) showed proline substitution in the second transmembrane domain of G-protein-coupled inwardly rectifying potassium channels shifted the channels into an active conformation, suggesting the site for Gβγ mediated gating. Dong et al. (2009) showed proline substitutions in the fifth transmembrane domain of TRPML1 ion channels locked the channels in an active state, which similarly allowed definition of the site of cation conductance gating. Proline scanning mutagenesis used here showed that the AQP1 cation channel is sensitive to mutations capable of altering the structure of the loop D domain, with both down- and upregulation of channel activity observed depending on the location of the mutation in the conserved amino acid sequence (**Figure 8**).

In sum, results here support the hypothesis that interaction of the inhibitor AqB011 depends on the structure of the loop D domain of the AQP1 channel, and that this domain is important for AQP1 ion channel gating. Aquaporin channels are more than simple pathways for the passive flux of water and glycerol. As a group they are increasingly being found to include highly specialized, regulated, multifunctional channels with diverse roles across the kingdoms of life (Gomes et al., 2009; Kourghi et al., 2017a). Results here contribute to understanding the structural basis for gating and pharmacological block of the human AQP1 ion channel, and add further evidence supporting the role of the central pore as the pathway for ion flux in human AQP1.

AUTHOR CONTRIBUTIONS

MK, JP, and AY: Participated in the research design. MK, SN, JP, and AY: Conducted experiments and performed data analysis. MK, MD, and AY: Wrote the manuscript. MK, MD, SN, JP, and AY: Reviewed and edited the manuscript.

FUNDING

Funding support for this research was provided by the Australian Research Council, grant DP160104641.

REFERENCES

Agre, P., Preston, G. M., Smith, B. L., Jung, J. S., Raina, S., Moon, C., et al. (1993). Aquaporin CHIP: the archetypal molecular water channel. *Am. J. Physiol.* 265, F463–F476. doi: 10.1152/ajprenal.1993.265.4.F463

Anthony, T. L., Brooks, H. L., Boassa, D., Leonov, S., Yanochko, G. M., Regan, J. W., et al. (2000). Cloned human aquaporin-1 is a cyclic GMP-gated ion channel. *Mol. Pharmacol.* 57, 576–588. doi: 10.1124/mol.57.3.576

Barlow, D. J., and Thornton, J. M.(1988). Helix geometry in proteins. *J. Mol. Biol.* 201, 601–619. doi: 10.1016/0022-2836(88)90641-9

Benga, G., Popescu, O., Pop, V. I., and Holmes, R. P. (1986). p-(Chloromercuri)benzenesulfonate binding by membrane proteins and the inhibition of water transport in human erythrocytes. *Biochemistry* 25, 1535–1538. doi: 10.1021/bi00355a011

Berry, V., Francis, P., Kaushal, S., Moore, A., and Bhattacharya, S. (2000). Missense mutations in MIP underlie autosomal dominant 'polymorphic' and lamellar cataracts linked to 12q. *Nat. Genet.* 25, 15–17. doi: 10.1038/75538

Boassa, D., Stamer, W. D., and Yool, A. J. (2006). Ion channel function of aquaporin-1 natively expressed in choroid plexus. *J. Neurosci.* 26, 7811–7819. doi: 10.1523/JNEUROSCI.0525-06.2006

Boassa, D., and Yool, A. J. (2003). Single amino acids in the carboxyl terminal domain of aquaporin-1 contribute to cGMP-dependent ion channel activation. *BMC Physiol.* 3:12. doi: 10.1186/1472-6793-3-12

Boassa, D., and Yool, A. J. (2005). Physiological roles of aquaporins in the choroid plexus. *Curr. Top. Dev. Biol.* 67, 181–206. doi: 10.1016/S0070-2153(05)67005-6

Byrt, C. S., Zhao, M., Kourghi, M., Bose, J., Henderson, S. W., Qiu, J., et al. (2016). Non-selective cation channel activity of aquaporin AtPIP2;1 regulated by Ca^{2+} and pH. *Plant Cell Environ.* 40, 802–815. doi: 10.1111/pce.12832

Campbell, E. M., Birdsell, D. N., and Yool, A. J. (2012). The activity of human aquaporin 1 as a cGMP-gated cation channel is regulated by tyrosine phosphorylation in the carboxyl-terminal domain. *Mol. Pharmacol.* 81, 97–105. doi: 10.1124/mol.111.073692

Cunningham, B. C., and Wells, J. A. (1989). High-resolution epitope mapping of hGH-receptor interactions by alanine-scanning mutagenesis. *Science* 244, 1081–1085. doi: 10.1126/science.2471267

Demidchik, V., and Tester, M. (2002). Sodium fluxes through nonselective cation channels in the plasma membrane of protoplasts from Arabidopsis roots. *Plant Physiol.* 128, 379–387. doi: 10.1104/pp.010524

Dong, X.-P., Wang, X., Shen, D., Chen, S., Liu, M., Wang, Y., et al. (2009). Activating mutations of the TRPML1 channel revealed by proline-scanning mutagenesis. *J. Biol. Chem.* 284, 32040–32052. doi: 10.1074/jbc.M109.037184

Ehring, G. R., Zampighi, G., Horwitz, J., Bok, D., and Hall, J. E. (1990). Properties of channels reconstituted from the major intrinsic protein of lens fiber membranes. *J. Gen. Physiol.* 96, 631–664. doi: 10.1085/jgp.96.3.631

Gomes, D., Agasse, A., Thiébaud, P., Delrot, S., Gerós, H., and Chaumont, F. (2009). Aquaporins are multifunctional water and solute transporters highly divergent in living organisms. *Biochim. Biophys. Acta* 1788, 1213–1228. doi: 10.1016/j.bbamem.2009.03.009

Graziani, V., Marrone, A., Re, N., Coletti, C., Platts, J. A., and Casini, A. (2017). A multi-level theoretical study to disclose the binding mechanisms of gold(III)-bipyridyl compounds as selective aquaglyceroporin inhibitors. *Chemistry* 23, 13802–13813. doi: 10.1002/chem.201703092

Hachez, C., and Chaumont, F. (2010). Aquaporins: a family of highly regulated multifunctional channels. *Adv. Exp. Med. Biol.* 679, 1–17. doi: 10.1007/978-1-4419-6315-4_1

Hille, B. (2001). *Ion Channels of Excitable Membranes, 3rd Edn.* Sunderland MA: Sinauer Associates Inc.

Huber, V. J., Tsujita, M., and Nakada, T. (2012). Aquaporins in drug discovery and pharmacotherapy. *Mol. Aspects Med.* 33, 691–703. doi: 10.1016/j.mam.2012.01.002

Igarashi, H., Huber, V. J., Tsujita, M., and Nakada, T. (2011). Pretreatment with a novel aquaporin 4 inhibitor, TGN-020, significantly reduces ischemic cerebral edema. *Neurol. Sci.* 32, 113–116. doi: 10.1007/s10072-010-0431-1

Jin, T., Peng, L., Mirshahi, T., Rohacs, T., Chan, K. W., Sanchez, R., et al. (2002). The βγ subunits of G proteins gate a K^+ channel by pivoted bending of a transmembrane segment. *Mol. Cell* 10, 469–481. doi: 10.1016/S1097-2765(02)00659-7

Jung, J. S., Preston, G. M., Smith, B. L., Guggino, W. B., and Agre, P. (1994). Molecular structure of the water channel through aquaporin CHIP. The hourglass model. *J. Biol. Chem.* 269, 14648–14654.

Kitchen, P., Day, R. E., Salman, M. M., Conner, M. T., Bill, R. M., and Conner, A. C. (2015). Beyond water homeostasis: diverse functional roles of mammalian aquaporins. *Biochim. Biophys. Acta* 1850, 2410–2421. doi: 10.1016/j.bbagen.2015.08.023

Kourghi, M., Pei, J. V., De Ieso, M. L., Flynn, G., and Yool, A. J. (2016). Bumetanide derivatives AqB007 and AqB011 selectively block the aquaporin-1 ion channel conductance and slow cancer cell migration. *Mol. Pharmacol.* 89, 133–140. doi: 10.1124/mol.115.101618

Kourghi, M., Pei, J. V., De Ieso, M. L., Nourmohammadi, S., Chow, P. H., and Yool, A. J. (2017a). Fundamental structural and functional properties of Aquaporin ion channels found across the kingdoms of life. *Clin. Exp. Pharmacol. Physiol.* 45, 401–409. doi: 10.1111/1440-1681

Kourghi, M., Pei, J. V., Qiu, J., Mcgaughey, S., Tyerman, S. D., Byrt, C. S., et al. (2017b). Divalent cations regulate the ion conductance properties of diverse classes of aquaporins. *Int. J. Mol. Sci.* 18:E2323. doi: 10.3390/ijms18112323

Kürz, L. L., Zühlke, R. D., Zhang, H.-J., and Joho, R. H. (1995). Side-chain accessibilities in the pore of a K^+ channel probed by sulfhydryl-specific reagents after cysteine-scanning mutagenesis. *Biophys. J.* 68, 900–905. doi: 10.1016/S0006-3495(95)80266-3

Madeira, A., Moura, T. F., and Soveral, G. (2014). Aquaglyceroporins: implications in adipose biology and obesity. *Cell Mol. Life Sci.* 72, 759–771. doi: 10.1007/s00018-014-1773-2

Martins, A. P., Ciancetta, A., De Almeida, A., Marrone, A., Re, N., Soveral, G., et al. (2013). Aquaporin inhibition by gold(III) compounds: new insights. *ChemMedChem* 8, 1086–1092. doi: 10.1002/cmdc.201300107

Migliati, E., Meurice, N., Dubois, P., Fang, J. S., Somasekharan, S., Beckett, E., et al. (2009). Inhibition of aquaporin-1 and aquaporin-4 water permeability by a derivative of the loop diuretic bumetanide acting at an internal pore-occluding binding site. *Mol. Pharmacol.* 76, 105–112. doi: 10.1124/mol.108.053744

Nielsen, S., Smith, B. L., Christensen, E. I., and Agre, P. (1993). Distribution of the aquaporin CHIP in secretory and resorptive epithelia and capillary endothelia. *Proc. Natl. Acad. Sci. U.S.A.* 90, 7275–7279. doi: 10.1073/pnas.90.15.7275

Niemietz, C. M., and Tyerman, S. D. (2002). New potent inhibitors of aquaporins: silver and gold compounds inhibit aquaporins of plant and human origin. *FEBS Lett.* 531, 443–447. doi: 10.1016/S0014-5793(02)03581-0

Patel, N., Exell, J. C., Jardine, E., Ombler, B., Finger, L. D., Ciani, B., et al. (2013). Proline scanning mutagenesis reveals a role for the flap endonuclease-1 helical cap in substrate unpairing. *J. Biol. Chem.* 288, 34239–34248. doi: 10.1074/jbc.M113.509489

Pei, J. V., Kourghi, M., De Ieso, M. L., Campbell, E. M., Dorward, H. S., Hardingham, J. E., et al. (2016). Differential inhibition of water and ion channel activities of mammalian aquaporin-1 by two structurally related bacopaside compounds derived from the medicinal plant *Bacopa monnieri*. *Mol. Pharmacol.* 90, 496–507. doi: 10.1124/mol.116.105882

Preston, G. M., Jung, J. S., Guggino, W. B., and Agre, P. (1993). The mercury-sensitive residue at cysteine 189 in the CHIP28 water channel. *J. Biol. Chem.* 268, 17–20.

Rao, Y., Bodmer, R., Jan, L. Y., and Jan, Y. N. (1992). The big brain gene of Drosophila functions to control the number of neuronal precursors in the peripheral nervous system. *Development* 116, 31–40.

Reizer, J., Reizer, A., and Saier, M. H. Jr. (1993). The MIP family of integral membrane channel proteins: sequence comparisons, evolutionary relationships, reconstructed pathway of evolution, and proposed functional differentiation of the two repeated halves of the proteins. *Crit. Rev. Biochem. Mol. Biol.* 28, 235–257. doi: 10.3109/10409239309086796

Ren, G., Reddy, V. S., Cheng, A., Melnyk, P., and Mitra, A. K. (2001). Visualization of a water-selective pore by electron crystallography in vitreous ice. *Proc. Natl. Acad. Sci. U.S.A.* 98, 1398–1403. doi: 10.1073/pnas.98.4.1398

Sadja, R., Smadja, K., Alagem, N., and Reuveny, E. (2001). Coupling Gβγ-dependent activation to channel opening via pore elements in inwardly rectifying potassium channels. *Neuron* 29, 669–680. doi: 10.1016/S0896-6273(01)00242-2

Sankararamakrishnan, R., and Vishveshwara, S. (1992). Geometry of proline-containing alpha-helices in proteins. *Chem. Biol. Drug Des.* 39, 356–363. doi: 10.1111/j.1399-3011.1992.tb01595.x

Saparov, S. M., Kozono, D., Rothe, U., Agre, P., and Pohl, P. (2001). Water and ion permeation of aquaporin-1 in planar lipid bilayers. Major differences in structural determinants and stoichiometry. *J. Biol. Chem.* 276, 31515–31520. doi: 10.1074/jbc.M104267200

Seeliger, D., Zapater, C., Krenc, D., Haddoub, R., Flitsch, S., Beitz, E., et al. (2013). Discovery of novel human aquaporin-1 blockers. *ACS Chem. Biol.* 8, 249–256. doi: 10.1021/cb300153z

Sui, H., Han, B.-G., Lee, J. K., Walian, P., and Jap, B. K. (2001). Structural basis of water-specific transport through the AQP1 water channel. *Nature* 414, 872–878. doi: 10.1038/414872a

Tsunoda, S. P., Wiesner, B., Lorenz, D., Rosenthal, W., and Pohl, P. (2004). Aquaporin-1, nothing but a water channel. *J. Biol. Chem.* 279, 11364–11367. doi: 10.1074/jbc.M310881200

Vanhoof, G., Goossens, F., Demeester, I., Hendriks, D., and Scharpé, S. (1995). Proline motifs in peptides and their biological processing. *FASEB J.* 9, 736–744. doi: 10.1096/fasebj.9.9.7601338

Williams, K. A., and Deber, C. M. (1991). Proline residues in transmembrane helixes: structural or dynamic role? *Biochemistry* 30, 8919–8923.

Woolfson, D. N., and Williams, D. H. (1990). The influence of proline residues on α-helical structure. *FEBS Lett.* 277, 185–188. doi: 10.1016/0014-5793(90)80839-B

Yanochko, G. M., and Yool, A. J. (2002). Regulated cationic channel function in *Xenopus* oocytes expressing Drosophila big brain. *J. Neurosci.* 22, 2530–2540. doi: 10.1523/JNEUROSCI.22-07-02530.2002

Yasui, M., Hazama, A., Kwon, T. H., Nielsen, S., Guggino, W. B., and Agre, P. (1999). Rapid gating and anion permeability of an intracellular aquaporin. *Nature* 402, 184–187. doi: 10.1038/46045

Yool, A. J. (2007). Aquaporins: multiple roles in the central nervous system. *Neuroscientist* 13, 470–485. doi: 10.1177/1073858407303081

Yool, A. J., Brokl, O. H., Pannabecker, T. L., Dantzler, W. H., and Stamer, W. D. (2002). Tetraethylammonium block of water flux in Aquaporin-1 channels expressed in kidney thin limbs of Henle's loop and a kidney-derived cell line. *BMC Physiol.* 2:4. doi: 10.1186/1472-6793-2-4

Yool, A. J., and Campbell, E. M. (2012). Structure, function and translational relevance of aquaporin dual water and ion channels. *Mol. Aspects Med.* 33, 443–561. doi: 10.1016/j.mam.2012.02.001

Yool, A. J., Morelle, J., Cnops, Y., Verbavatz, J. M., Campbell, E. M., Beckett, E. A., et al. (2013). AqF026 is a pharmacologic agonist of the water channel aquaporin-1. *J. Am. Soc. Nephrol.* 24, 1045–1052. doi: 10.1681/ASN.2012080869

Yool, A. J., Stamer, W. D., and Regan, J. W. (1996). Forskolin stimulation of water and cation permeability in aquaporin-1 water channels. *Science* 273, 1216–1218. doi: 10.1126/science.273.5279.1216

Yool, A. J., and Weinstein, A. M. (2002). New roles for old holes: ion channel function in aquaporin-1. *News Physiol. Sci.* 17, 68–72. doi: 10.1152/nips.01372.2001

Yu, J., Yool, A. J., Schulten, K., and Tajkhorshid, E. (2006). Mechanism of gating and ion conductivity of a possible tetrameric pore in aquaporin-1. *Structure* 14, 1411–1423. doi: 10.1016/j.str.2006.07.006

Zampighi, G. A., Hall, J. E., and Kreman, M. (1985). Purified lens junctional protein forms channels in planar lipid films. *Proc. Natl. Acad. Sci. U.S.A.* 82, 8468–8472. doi: 10.1073/pnas.82.24.8468

Zhang, W., Zitron, E., Hömme, M., Kihm, L., Morath, C., Scherer, D., et al. (2007). Aquaporin-1 channel function is positively regulated by protein kinase C. *J. Biol. Chem.* 282, 20933–20940. doi: 10.1074/jbc.M703858200

18

The Human SLC7A5 (LAT1): The Intriguing Histidine/Large Neutral Amino Acid Transporter and its Relevance to Human Health

Mariafrancesca Scalise[1], *Michele Galluccio*[1], *Lara Console*[1], *Lorena Pochini*[1] and *Cesare Indiveri*[1,2*]

[1] Unit of Biochemistry and Molecular Biotechnology, Department DiBEST (Biologia, Ecologia, Scienze della Terra), University of Calabria, Rende, Italy, [2] CNR Institute of Biomembranes, Bioenergetics and Molecular Biotechnology, Bari, Italy

***Correspondence:**
Cesare Indiveri
cesare.indiveri@unical.it

SLC7A5, known as LAT1, belongs to the APC superfamily and forms a heterodimeric amino acid transporter interacting with the glycoprotein CD98 (SLC3A2) through a conserved disulfide. The complex is responsible for uptake of essential amino acids in crucial body districts such as placenta and blood brain barrier. LAT1/CD98 heterodimer has been studied over the years to unravel the transport mechanism and the role of each subunit. Studies conducted in intact cells demonstrated that LAT1/CD98 mediates a Na^+ and pH independent antiport of amino acids. Some novel insights into the function of LAT1 derived from studies conducted in proteoliposomes reconstituted with the recombinant human LAT1. Using this experimental tool, it has been demonstrated that the preferred substrate is histidine and that CD98 is not required for transport being, plausibly, involved in routing LAT1 to the plasma membrane. Since a 3D structure of LAT1 is not available, homology models have been built on the basis of the AdiC transporter from *E.coli*. Crucial residues for substrate recognition and gating have been identified using a combined approach of bioinformatics and site-directed mutagenesis coupled to functional assays. Over the years, the interest around LAT1 increased because this transporter is involved in important human diseases such as neurological disorders and cancer. Therefore, LAT1 became an important pharmacological target together with other nutrient membrane transporters. Moving from knowledge on structure/function relationships, two cysteine residues, lying on the substrate binding site, have been exploited for designing thiol reacting covalent inhibitors. Some lead compounds have been characterized whose efficacy has been tested in a cancer cell line.

Keywords: LAT1, SLC7 family, histidine, drug design, pro-drugs, proteoliposomes, molecular docking

INTRODUCTION

SLC7A5 is a transporter dedicated to essential amino acids. In the pre-genomic era, it was known as LAT1, an acronym standing for Large Amino Acid Transporter 1, that has endured over the time (Christensen, 1990). LAT1 belongs to the SLC7 family included in the larger APC (Amino acid-Polyamine-organo Cation) superfamily. The SLC7 family consists of 15 members, two of which are pseudogenes. The 13 encoded proteins are classified in two subgroups: the cationic amino acid transporters and the light subunits (LATs) of the heterodimeric amino acid transporters. Molecular evolution studies show that the heterodimeric amino acid transporters and the cationic amino acid transporters have a common ancestor characterized by 12 trans-membrane domains. This structure is conserved in the heterodimeric amino acid transporters, while the cationic amino acid transporters evolved to 14 trans-membrane domain structures, resulting from duplication of the last two trans-membrane domains, plausibly after branching of eukaryotes and archea (Verrey et al., 2004; Palacin et al., 2005; Fotiadis et al., 2013). The cationic amino acid transporters are N-glycosylated membrane proteins and are responsible for transport of cationic amino acids in cells. The heterodimeric amino acid transporters are present only in eukaryotes and are characterized by a broader substrate specificity toward neutral amino acids (SLC7A5, A8, A10, A12), aromatic amino acids (SLC7A15), negatively charged amino acids (SLC7A11) and cationic amino acids plus neutral amino acids (SLC7A6, A7, A9) (Fotiadis et al., 2013) (and refs herein). The structural peculiarity of the heterodimeric amino acid transporters is that of being one of the few examples of transporters composed by two different subunits: the light subunit, LATs and the heavy subunit, i.e., a membrane glycoprotein belonging to the SLC3 family with a single transmembrane domain and a large extracellular domain. The mentioned interaction is well conserved through evolution occurring via a disulfide bridge between two cysteine residues of the proteins forming heterodimeric amino acid transporters (Bröer and Brookes, 2001; Wagner et al., 2001; Palacín and Kanai, 2004). It is interesting to note that the SLC3 family, which comprises only two members (SLC3A1 and SLC3A2), is included in the SLC classification even if the direct involvement of these proteins in transport is not proven. In the case of LAT1, the heavy subunit counterpart is the SLC3A2, also known as CD98 or 4F2hc. The 3D structure of the ectodomain of the human CD98 is solved (Fort et al., 2007). The mentioned interaction is described since the early LAT1 discovery in rat glioma (Kanai et al., 1998). Several studies describe the function/structure relationships of such intriguing molecular organization, including the human isoform isolated and cloned in 1999 (Prasad et al., 1999; Fotiadis et al., 2013 and refs herein). In this frame, the term "LAT1" is often used to indicate the heterodimer LAT1/CD98, as well. In the sake of clarity, in this review we will use the term "LAT1" or "CD98" to indicate each of the monomers; we will use the term "LAT1/CD98" to indicate the heterodimer. It is important to stress that LAT1 is a key protein in cell growth and development due to its involvement in distribution of eight out of the nine essential amino acids to specific body districts such as placenta and Blood Brain Barrier (BBB, see section Gene and Tissue Localization of LAT1 and CD98). On the contrary, due to its low expression level in intestine and to its relatively low transport capacity, LAT1 is not responsible for absorption of amino acids from diet. This function is mediated by other high capacity transport systems located in the microvilli brush-border (Bröer and Bröer, 2017). An important evidence of the crucial role of LAT1 in cell metabolism and growth derives from the lethal phenotype of knockout animal embryo, which cannot go beyond the mid-gestation stage (E11.5), i.e., when nervous cells start to differentiate (Ohgaki et al., 2017). Over the years, the interest around this transporter moved from biochemical to bio-medical issues due to its involvement in important diseases such as cancer and neurological disorders (Fuchs and Bode, 2005; del Amo et al., 2008). In fact, the number of clinical studies, reporting LAT1 alterations in human pathology, is continuously growing, even though the molecular bases of these phenomena are still far from being completely deciphered. During the last years, important metabolic and signaling clues are emerging, thanks to a better characterization of human LAT1 (see following sections). In particular, targeting of human LAT1 becomes a hot topic in drug discovery for advancing the treatment of diseases in which the protein is involved.

An overview of *status artis* on this transporter will be provided in the present review, shedding light on the "LATest" findings.

GENE AND TISSUE LOCALIZATION OF LAT1 AND CD98

The SLC7A5 gene, located at 16q24.2 (locus ID 8140), counts 39477 nucleotides with 10 exons (**Figure 1A**). Orthologs of this gene are present in 222 different organisms (https://www.ncbi.nlm.nih.gov/gene/8140). Two transcripts are reported in Ensemble (**Figure 1A**). One of these transcripts, NM_003486.6, codes for a protein of 507 amino acids, with a molecular mass of 55,010 Da. The other transcript derives from alternative splicing, but no evidence of a coded LAT1 protein is available, so far. Additional four transcripts are reported on NCBI databases, which, however, are only predicted. According to human protein Atlas project, RNA coding for SLC7A5 is ubiquitously expressed in all 27 tested tissues, even if at low levels (Fagerberg et al., 2014). Highest expression is measured in testis, bone marrow, brain and placenta (Prasad et al., 1999; Fotiadis et al., 2013). In polarized epithelia, LAT1 protein is mainly localized in basolateral membranes (Verrey et al., 2004; Fotiadis et al., 2013), with the exception of BBB where it is localized on both apical and basolateral membranes (Duelli et al., 2000). In placenta, LAT1 is on both maternal and fetal surfaces of syncytiotrophoblasts (Ohgaki et al., 2017). LAT1/CD98 heterodimer is also located in lysosomal membrane of HeLa cells (Milkereit et al., 2015).

The SLC3A2 gene, located at 11q12.3 (locus ID 6520), counts 32871 nucleotides with 13 exons (**Figure 1B**). Orthologous of this gene are present in 164 different organisms (https://www.ncbi.nlm.nih.gov/gene/6520). Four different transcripts are reported in Genbank database, coding for CD98 isoforms. The canonical isoform, NM_002394.5 (**Figure 1B**), results from 12 exons (exon 4 is not present) with total 2347 bp and encoding a protein of 630 amino acids, with a molecular mass of 67,994 Da. A three nucleotide longer isoform is also described, NM_001012662.2,

Abbreviations: LAT1, Large Amino Acid Transporter 1; BBB, Blood Brain Barrier; BCH, 2-aminobicyclo-(2,2,1)-heptane-2-carboxylic acid; IL-2, IL-17, interleukin-2, interleukin- 17; mTOR, mammalian Target of Rapamicyn; GCN2, general control nonderepressible 2; PET, Positron Emission Tomography; BNCT, Boron Neutron Capture Therapy.

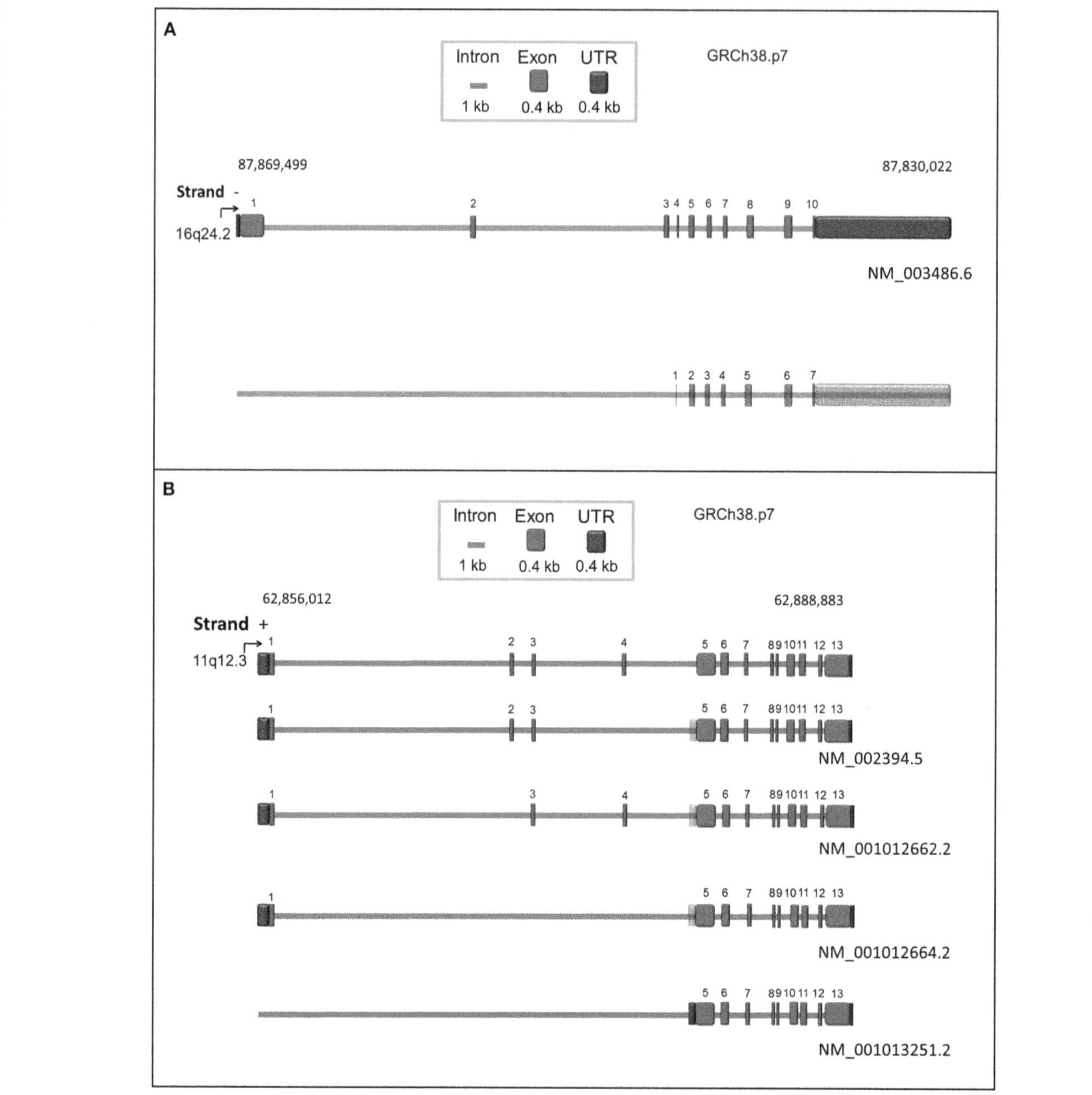

FIGURE 1 | Schematic representation of human SLC7A5 **(A)** and SLC3A2 **(B)** genes according to RCh38.p7 genome assembly. Intronic and exonic sequences are depicted in blue and red, respectively. UTR sequence is indicated in dark gray. Predicted UTR sequences or isoforms are in transparency. For each transcript, the relative Genbank accession number is indicated.

which derives from an alternative combination of 12 exons, i.e., the presence of exon 4 but not of exon 2 (**Figure 1B**). These little variations at transcriptional level generate proteins with 95% identity and 1 amino acid length difference, being the second isoform, 631 amino acids long. The third transcript, NM_001012664.2, results from transcription of 10 exons, lacking exons 2, 3 and 4, counts 2161 nucleotides and codes for a protein of 568 amino acids. The last transcript, NM_001013251.2 differs in the 5′ UTR and lacks the first four exons, counting 1938 nucleotides: the corresponding protein, composed by 529 amino acids, derives from translation starting at a downstream ATG (**Figure 1B**). According to human protein Atlas project (Fagerberg et al., 2014), RNA coding for CD98 is ubiquitously detected with the highest expression level in kidney, placenta, testis and bone marrow. Expression of CD98 correlates with that of LAT1 in terms of localization, as expected from the interaction between the two proteins. However, CD98 is also expressed in other tissues since it works as ancillary protein of other SLC7 members, as well (Fotiadis et al., 2013 and refs herein).

FUNCTION AND SUBSTRATE SPECIFICITY: THE DOUBLE FACE OF LAT1

The pioneer studies on LAT1/CD98 heterodimer are conducted in cell systems (such as *X. laevis* oocytes) measuring the uptake of essential amino acids using murine and human isoforms (Kanai et al., 1998; Mastroberardino et al., 1998; Prasad et al., 1999; Yanagida et al., 2001; Kim et al., 2002). These experiments establish that the transporter mediates an obligatory pH and Na^+ independent antiport of tryptophan, phenylalanine, leucine and histidine with high affinity (Km for human isoform ranging from 5 to 50 μM) (**Figure 2**). The Na^+ independence explains the relatively low transport capacity of this transporter and is in line with the low expression in the absorbent epithelia of intestine where, indeed, other transporters driven by Na^+ gradient, such as SNATs, $ATB^{0,+}$ and B^0AT1, guarantee a massive uptake of amino acids (Pochini et al., 2014; Bröer and Bröer, 2017) (**Figure 3**). The heterodimer is able to recognize much less efficiently also glutamine (Km in the mM range); while, alanine, proline and charged amino acids are not recognized as substrates (Kanai et al., 1998; Mastroberardino et al., 1998; Kim et al., 2002; Meier et al., 2002; del Amo et al., 2008). Several reports show that the non-metabolizable analog BCH is a substrate of LAT1/CD98 (**Figure 2**) (Mastroberardino et al., 1998; Prasad et al., 1999; Kim et al., 2002). LAT1/CD98 also catalyzes the transport of the thyroid hormones T3 and T4 (Friesema et al., 2001; del Amo et al., 2008), of the dopamine precursor L-DOPA as well as of amino acid-related exogenous compounds, such as the drugs melphalan, baclofen and gabapentin (Uchino et al., 2002; del Amo et al., 2008) (**Figure 2**). The Vmax of L-DOPA transport is reduced upon depletion of plasma membrane cholesterol by methyl-β-cyclodextrin (Dickens et al., 2017). The ability of the transporter to accept canonical amino acids and other substances with some basic features of amino acids (**Table 1**), awards LAT1 with a two-faced role in physiological and in pathological contexts (**Figure 2**). Several controversies, however, are unsolved concerning the specificity issue due to some technical restrictions in the studies performed with intact cell systems. Thus, a novel drive derived from the availability of the recombinant human LAT1 and CD98 over-expressed in *E.coli* (Galluccio et al., 2013). The two human proteins were purified in a large scale and functionally characterized in the *in vitro* model of proteoliposomes. This is a versatile experimental tool, constituted by phospholipid vesicles, which allows the operator to precisely control both the external and internal spaces (Scalise et al., 2013). This triggered clarification of a key point of human LAT1/CD98 physiology: LAT1 is the sole transport competent subunit of the heterodimer, able to mediate antiport of amino acids with the same properties of the heterodimer, while CD98 does not exhibit any intrinsic transport function (Napolitano et al., 2015). Moreover, the transport protein is inserted in the proteoliposomal membrane with the same orientation as in the cell membrane: this represents an important requisite for translating the results obtained *in vitro*, to a physiological context. In the same system, the preference of LAT1 for amino acids has been definitively assessed (**Figure 2**). Functional and kinetic asymmetry of the transporter has been demonstrated (Napolitano et al., 2015): histidine and tyrosine are the bidirectionally-transported substrates, while the others are preferentially inwardly transported and glutamine is a poor substrate. Proteoliposomes harboring hLAT1 revealed suitable for studying the effect of mercury compounds: both the inorganic ($HgCl_2$) and the organic (Methyl-Hg) forms of mercury strongly inhibit LAT1 mediated transport by binding to cysteine residue(s), in line with previous report on rabbit LAT1 (Boado et al., 2005; Napolitano et al., 2017a) (**Figure 2**). The results obtained with the purified protein substantiated the major role of LAT1 in histidine transport that, indeed, is already disclosed in the first important studies but then disregarded (Kanai et al., 1998; Mastroberardino et al., 1998; Prasad et al., 1999; Yanagida et al., 2001; Kim et al., 2002). The identification of histidine as LAT1 high affinity substrate *in vitro*, lays the groundwork for interpreting following important advances in human health (see section Regulation of LAT1 Expression). Histidine is, indeed, an essential amino acid eventually involved in aspartate and glutamate synthesis as well as in histamine production, thus being relevant for brain homeostasis and inflammatory response (Hasegawa et al., 2012; Sasahara et al., 2015). Interestingly, there is a concentration gradient for histidine across plasma membrane, being the plasma concentration of histidine one order of magnitude lower than the tissue concentration (Schmid et al., 1977). This gradient may constitute the driving force for extruding histidine in exchange with other essential amino

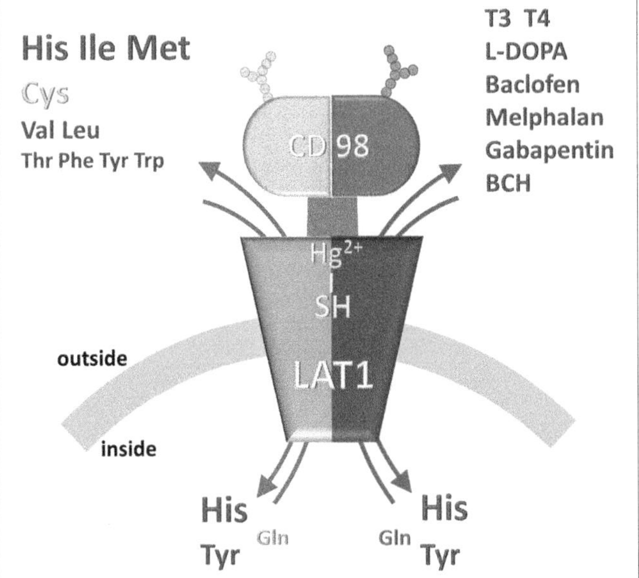

FIGURE 2 | Representation of LAT1/CD98 and its substrates. The protein heterodimer is asymmetrically inserted in the cell membrane. The double-face feature of LAT1 is indicated by two-color design of the model. The blue half represents the specificity toward amino acids which are colored in blue (Essential Amino Acids) and light blue (Non-Essential Amino Acids). The size is suggestive of the higher or the lower specificity toward the amino acids. The red half represents the known specificity toward non-amino acid substrates: hormones, drugs and inhibitors. The reactivity of –SH group(s) of the protein toward Hg^{2+} is also represented. Glycosylation of CD98 is depicted as "antennas".

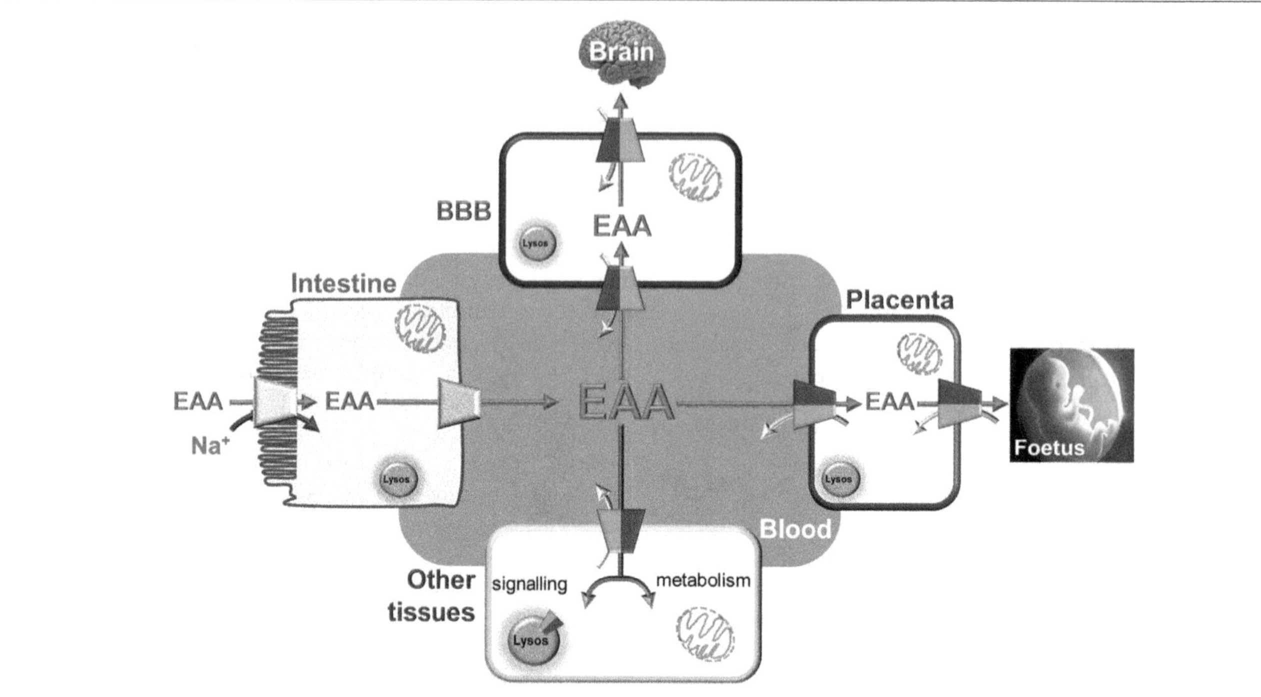

FIGURE 3 | The Essential Amino Acids distribution network through LAT1. Interplay among blood and epithelial polarized cells of intestine (apical membrane depicted as brush-border and basolateral membrane in contact with blood), placenta, BBB (Blood Brain Barrier) and other tissues. Essential Amino Acids are absorbed through intestine using Na^+ dependent transporters (indicated in gray) to allow their accumulation with high capacity. The same amino acids are conveyed to blood by other transporters present in the basolateral membrane of gut cells (indicated in light brown). From blood, Essential Amino Acids are accumulated in BBB and in placenta cells using LAT1 with an antiport reaction. In these cells, LAT1 is localized at both sides of cells allowing the flux of amino acids to Brain and Fetus, respectively. In other tissues, LAT1 is not highly expressed but plays the role of distributing Essential Amino Acids used both for signaling and metabolic purposes thanks also to alternative localization in lysosome membrane. These aspects became more important in tissues where LAT1 expression is strongly increased as in case of cancers. LAT1 is depicted as in **Figure 2** by two-colored half. Flux of Essential Amino Acids are indicated by blue arrows (from blood to tissues) and by gray arrows (from tissues to blood).

acid such as leucine that becomes an important metabolite in pathological conditions underlying LAT1 function (see section LAT1 and Diseases). Altogether, the studies on specificity of hLAT1 for substrates and their analogs, as well as the interaction with non-transported molecules, allow extrapolating the essential features for a molecule to plausibly be transported by hLAT1: vicinal carboxylic and amino groups are essential, as resumed in **Table 1**. Indeed, dopamine, serotonine and GABA, which lack of vicinal carboxylic or the amino groups are not transported (Tarlungeanu et al., 2016). Furthermore, a large side group is also important, validating the pioneering acronym Large Amino Acid Transporter 1 (LAT1). Moreover, hydrophobicity seems an additional requirement for the side group, since, besides small, also charged amino acids are not transported. These features are already hypothesized in preliminary studies conducted in intact cells using the rat isoform of LAT1 (Uchino et al., 2002). Importantly, the main properties described *in vitro* are also confirmed by studies in intact cells both in the presence and in the absence of the disulfide between C164 of hLAT1 and C109 of hCD98 (**Figure 2**), demonstrating that CD98 is not required for intrinsic transport activity of LAT1 neither for substrate specificity (Pfeiffer et al., 1998; Campbell and Thompson, 2001; Boado et al., 2005; Napolitano et al., 2015). Therefore, it can be argued that the most probable function of the ancillary subunit is that of trafficking LAT1 to its definitive location in plasma membrane as suggested for both murine and human isoforms (Nakamura et al., 1999; Wagner et al., 2001; Franca et al., 2005; Cormerais et al., 2016). The role of CD98 is described in the case of SLC7A8 (LAT2). Differently from LAT1, LAT2 needs CD98 for both purification and stabilization of the protein, for functional and structural studies (Rosell et al., 2014). However, additional studies are required to ascertain the regulation of LAT1 function and the molecular mechanism of trafficking.

KINETICS AND MOLECULAR MECHANISMS OF LAT1

Similarly to other human plasma membrane transporters, the 3D structure of LAT1 is not available. Homology models are built on the basis of the bacterial homolog AdiC from *E.coli* (Geier et al., 2013; Napolitano et al., 2017a). This is an arginine/agmatine transporter characterized by a LeuT-fold (Gao et al., 2010; Ilgü et al., 2016) and represents a paradigm structure for the APC superfamily. However, the sole model does not allow drawing conclusions on the kinetic mechanism of transport and the

TABLE 1 | The basic requirements for substrates of LAT1.

Substrate	Structure	References
HIS	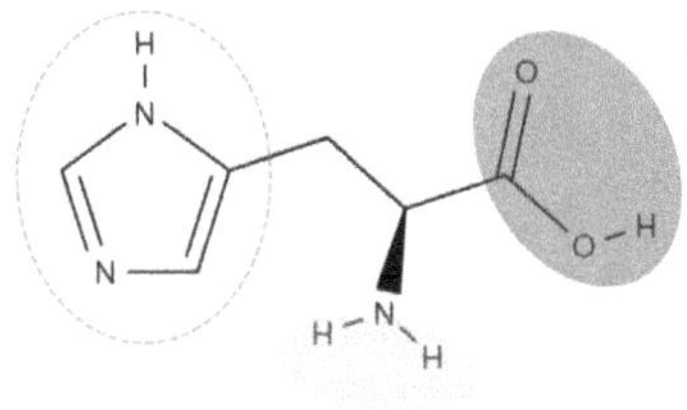	Mastroberardino et al., 1998; Napolitano et al., 2015
T3	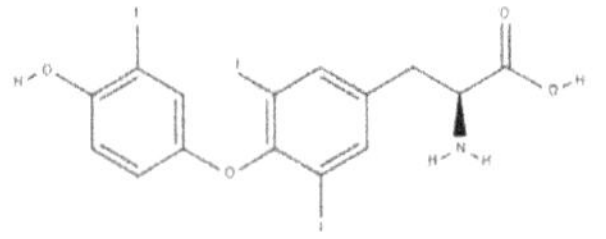	Friesema et al., 2001
T4	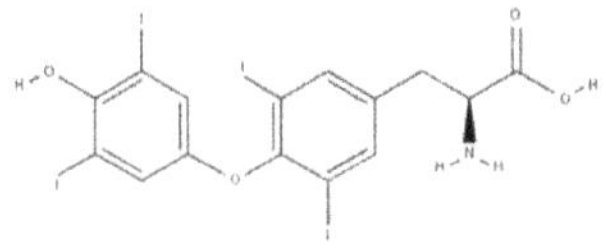	Friesema et al., 2001
L-DOPA	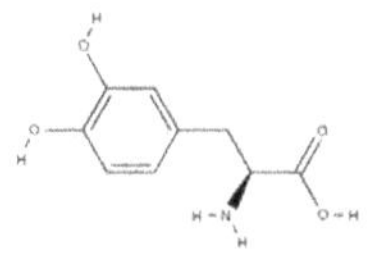	Kageyama et al., 2000
Baclofen	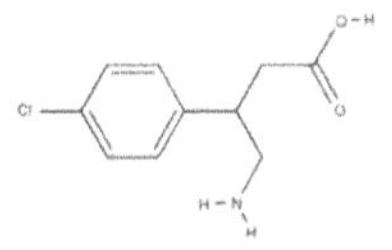	del Amo et al., 2008
Melphalan	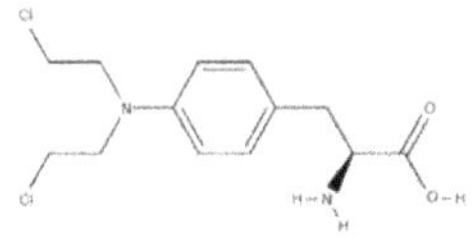	del Amo et al., 2008
Gabapentin	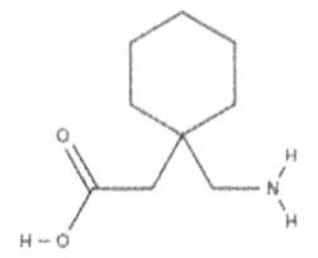	del Amo et al., 2008
BCH	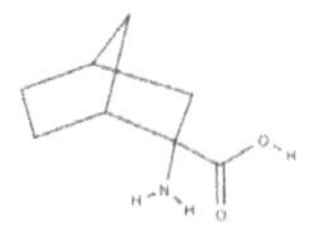	Mastroberardino et al., 1998

Table lists the structure of known LAT1 substrates; on the histidine structure, the carboxylic group is highlighted by red circle, the amino group by blue circle, the hydrophobic portion by dotted green line. The same groups are present in all the structures below.

molecular determinants of substrate recognition. To achieve this information, additional experimental approaches have been used in combination with bioinformatics. In this respect, the functionally active human recombinant protein has been employed in experiments conducted using proteoliposomes. Bi-substrate analysis, which could not be performed in intact cells, demonstrated that the amino acid antiport mediated by LAT1 occurs by a random simultaneous mechanism, i.e., with no preferential binding order of the substrates on the two opposed sides of the transporter. The collected data suggested that the internal and external substrates are translocated in a single transport cycle, implying the simultaneous exposure of binding sites for external and internal substrates (Napolitano et al., 2017a). This condition can be explained by the formation of functional homodimer whose existence has been proven by biochemical methodologies such as mild denaturing PAGE and cross-link approaches (Napolitano et al., 2017a). Noteworthy, this is in line with the oligomeric structure of the bacterial homologous AdiC (Gao et al., 2010) while it seems different from the data obtained with the LAT2/CD98 heterodimer that does not form homodimers (Rosell et al., 2014). Regarding the key determinants of the substrate binding site, some crucial residues that corresponded to those involved in gating of AdiC are predicted in previous study (Geier et al., 2013). These residues are F252, S342, and C407 in the human LAT1. More recently, using a combination of *in silico* methodologies, site directed mutagenesis and transport assay in proteoliposomes, we validated the predictions and identified the additional C335 residue as responsible for the interaction with the substrate (Napolitano et al., 2017a). Altogether, the combined approaches highlight that: (i) F252 plays the role of substrate gate opening and its aromaticity is essential to accomplish this function; (ii) S342 and C335 are crucial for histidine binding from the external side of the protein; (iii) C407 is, on the other hand, involved in substrate binding from the internal side (Napolitano et al., 2017a).

REGULATION OF LAT1 EXPRESSION

Notwithstanding the importance of LAT1 in mediating traffic of essential amino acids in both physiological and pathological conditions, little is known about regulation of its expression. In good agreement with the level of LAT1 protein in activated T lymphocytes, the cytokine IL-2 is able to up-regulate LAT1 expression (Sinclair et al., 2013). In rheumatoid arthritis, IL-17 is responsible for promoting LAT1-mediated migration of fibroblasts (Yu et al., 2018). Regulation by micro RNA (Miko et al., 2011) and long non-coding RNA is also reported (Yu et al., 2018). Moreover, DNA methylation occurring at promoter region seems to play a role in the regulation of LAT1 gene expression in human placenta across gestation (Simner et al., 2017). Glucose and insulin also modulate LAT1 expression: increase of glucose in diabetes induces a down-regulation of LAT1 expression with consequent sarcopenia in diabetes patients (Yamamoto et al., 2017). Conversely, glucose deprivation induces up-regulation of LAT1 in retina (Matsuyama et al., 2012). Interestingly, low insulin concentrations, upregulate LAT1 expression in muscle following mTORC1 activation (Walker et al., 2014). Vice versa, low expression of LAT1 in β-cells induces a strong reduction of insulin which is a protein constituted in large majority by the amino acids transported by LAT1 (Kobayashi et al., 2018).

The well documented over-expression of LAT1 in cancer is also explained by the presence, in the promoter region, of a canonical binding site for the proto-oncogene c-Myc (Hayashi et al., 2012) that, interestingly, regulates glucose metabolism (Kim et al., 2004). These evidences, even if fragmentary, suggest that a coordinate regulation of glucose and amino acid metabolism in cells may exist under both physiological and pathological conditions being in good agreement with the increased demand and transport of these nutrients in cancer (see section LAT1 and Diseases). Another pathway inducing expression of this transporter is mediated by YAP/TAZ, two transcriptional regulators which promote cell proliferation (Hansen et al., 2015). In renal carcinoma, LAT1 expression is increased by the hypoxia-inducible factor HIF2α that binds to LAT1 promoter (Elorza et al., 2012). In lung cancer, the activation of aryl hydrocarbon receptor pathway by diesel exhaust particles induces LAT1 up-regulation (Le Vee et al., 2016). It is also reported that in lung cancer LAT1 gives rise to a regulatory loop with the methyl transferase EZH2, involving the LAT1 negatively regulator RXRα, to control the methylation status of genes responsible for cell differentiation (Dann et al., 2015). In summary, from the mentioned works, a common denominator for regulation of LAT1 cannot be inferred at this stage. Anyway, the over-expression of this transporter in cancer cells refers to an increase of the protein amount and, hence, to an increased function as it occurs for glucose transporters (Ganapathy et al., 2009). Additional studies are needed to achieve a complete picture of the regulatory pathways involved in the control of LAT1 under physiological and pathological conditions.

LAT1 AND DISEASES

The link of LAT1 with cancer is nowadays well assessed. Indeed, over-expression of LAT1 is described in many human cancers and it certainly relates to metabolic changes occurring in cancer development and progression. In fact, transformed and malignant cells have specific metabolic requirements, which are collectively known as "Warburg effect" even if, over the years, this theory has been updated. A peculiar feature of cancer cells is the increased demand for nutrients such as glucose, essential amino acids and also glutamine, that becomes conditionally essential, for protein synthesis and/or energy supply (Ganapathy et al., 2009; Vander Heiden et al., 2009; Bhutia and Ganapathy, 2016; Scalise et al., 2017). Another hallmark of cancer cells is the requirement of leucine for mTOR activation in lysosome. Leucine is also a positive allosteric regulator of glutamate dehydrogenase in mitochondria, which, in turn, is responsible of glutamine fate (Scalise et al., 2017, and refs herein and see **Figure 3**). Thus, over-expression of LAT1 may respond to such specific needs together with other over-expressed amino acid transporters, such as ASCT2 and $ATB^{0,+}$ (Pochini et al., 2014). In the past, a functional cycle involving LAT1 and ASCT2 has been suggested. In this cycle, glutamine, entered through ASCT2, may furnish the driving force for leucine uptake through LAT1 (Nicklin et al., 2009); this picture needs to be updated since glutamine cannot be an actual driving force for LAT1 being a very low affinity substrate. (Scalise et al., 2017). The important role of LAT1 in cancer is substantiated by the finding that this transporter is expressed in cancers of most human tissues, according to GENT database (Shin et al., 2011). LAT1 over-expression is also a prognostic factor of metastasis (Hayashi and Anzai, 2017). It is important to note that in most of the corresponding non-cancer human tissues, LAT1 is poorly expressed or, in some cases, absent (see section Gene and Tissue Localization of LAT1 and CD98). The ancillary protein CD98 is greatly over-expressed in cancers as well, according to human genome U133A array used for the creation of the GENT database (Shin et al., 2011). However, the over-expression of the two proteins is not inevitably linked because LAT1 mediates amino acid transport independently from CD98 (Napolitano et al., 2015) and CD98 is a protein with pleiotropic roles ranging from immune system regulation, cell growth activation, cell adhesion to integrin signaling (Chillarón et al., 2001; Palacín and Kanai, 2004; Cantor and Ginsberg, 2012; Fotiadis et al., 2013). Thus, its over-expression in cancer may have molecular basis different from those of LAT1. In this respect, CD98 is used disjointedly from LAT1, as target of antibodies raised for counteracting cell proliferation and metastasis (Behrens et al., 2015; Hayes et al., 2015). Besides cancer, LAT1 is involved in other diseases related to its expression in placenta and BBB (**Figure 3**). As example, LAT1 expression is reduced in Intra-Uterine Growth Restriction (IUGR) (Pantham et al., 2016). This is a high risk condition for perinatal complications, characterized by reduced concentrations of leucine and phenylalanine. Moreover, intra-uterine growth restriction increases the risk of developing cardiovascular and metabolic diseases in childhood and adulthood. Conversely, maternal obesity is a possible cause of up-regulation of placental LAT1 in mouse model with consequent fetal overgrowth (Rosario et al., 2015). This represents a high risk condition for insulin resistance at birth and for developing type 2 diabetes in childhood and adulthood. Regarding the BBB, a decreased expression of LAT1 in this district is linked to onset and development of Parkinsons's disease (Ohtsuki et al., 2010). The molecular basis of the link is the reduced distribution of the dopamine precursor, L-DOPA, which is transported by LAT1, besides that of essential amino acids (Kageyama et al., 2000). The role of LAT1 in brain is also explained by transport of tryptophan, which is important for normal neurological development (Asor et al., 2015). More recently, alteration of LAT1 function in BBB caused by two natural mutations, has been described as the molecular determinant of Autism Spectrum Disorders (ASD); it is important to highlight that histidine, among the LAT1 substrates, exhibited in brain the greatest variation of concentration in the pathological phenotype (Tarlungeanu et al., 2016). This correlates well with the biochemical identification of histidine as the highest affinity LAT1 substrate confirming its relevance in underlying the pathophysiological role of LAT1 (Napolitano et al., 2015). On the basis of the experimental data, the molecular mechanism responsible for the pathological phenotype has been revealed: in particular, the defective mutants of LAT1 are not able to perform the exchange transport reaction resulting in a net accumulation of histidine in brain and a lack of other essential branched chain amino acids (Tarlungeanu et al.,

2016). Furthermore, LAT1 is involved in activation of T cells accompanied by metabolism enhancement (Hayashi et al., 2013). Finally, in inflammatory conditions, such as pancreatitis, LAT1 expression decreases (Rooman et al., 2013). This is linked to the function of LAT1 in acinar cells that allows accumulation of amino acids necessary to synthesize digestive enzymes (Rooman et al., 2013). Some previous works suggest that LAT1 can also mediate uptake of mercury compounds explaining their toxicity for fetal growth (Kajiwara et al., 1996; Bridges and Zalups, 2017); moreover, our inhibition studies by mercury compounds suggested that mercury-derivatives can impair essential amino acids transport in cells expressing LAT1 (Napolitano et al., 2017a). Also in BBB, the ability of LAT1 to mediate mercury compounds uptake may explain its toxicity in brain (Boado et al., 2005; Bridges and Zalups, 2017). Altogether, these findings highlight a crucial role of LAT1 in several human pathologies.

LINK OF LAT1 WITH AMINO ACID MOLECULAR SENSORS

Moving from the observations of tissue distribution and substrate specificity, it can be concluded that the physiological role of LAT1 consists in maintaining the concentration of essential amino acids, particularly in those body districts, such as brain and placenta (**Figure 3**), where these molecules are fundamental for normal growth and development (Fotiadis et al., 2013; Bröer and Bröer, 2017). Over the years, it became more and more clear that the same applies to cancers whose cells are addicted to amino acids (Ganapathy et al., 2009; Bhutia and Ganapathy, 2016).

All these features eventually merge into mTOR, a serine/threonine kinase belonging to the PI3K-related family (Milkereit et al., 2015; Cormerais et al., 2016; Saxton and Sabatini, 2017). In fact, genetic or chemical disruption of LAT1, but not CD98, triggers, on one hand, mTOR inhibition and, on the other, GCN2 activation enhancing amino acid stress response (Gallinetti et al., 2013; Cormerais et al., 2016). GCN2 is a serine/threonine kinase and together with mTOR are responsible for handling amino acids concentration in cells; their cooperation occurs with a different degree of cross talk depending on the stress conditions (Carroll et al., 2015).

The relationship between mTOR and LAT1 is a long lasting field of investigation also because mTOR hyper-activation is often described in cancers (Saxton and Sabatini, 2017; Wolfson and Sabatini, 2017). The network of proteins regulating and regulated by mTOR is very intricate and many efforts have been made over the years to dissect each player. The importance of amino acids in this scenario has been proposed very long ago, but only recently, the puzzle reached a quite complete form. Among the amino acids, glutamine, arginine and leucine are involved in activation of mTOR (Wang et al., 2015; Rebsamen and Superti-Furga, 2016). In this respect, the function of LAT1 is related to its ability in mediating uptake and accumulation of leucine in cells. The leucine taken up via LAT1, is sequestered by Sestrin2 causing an increase of free GATOR2 with consequent increase of mTOR signaling (Lee et al., 2010; Wolfson and Sabatini, 2017). Sestrin2, in fact, acts as a negative regulator of mTOR activity. Leucine sensed by Sestrin2 derives from plasma membrane uptake as well as by efflux from lysosomes. In this respect, it is worth of note that LAT1 mediates efflux of leucine from lysosomes as well (**Figure 3**) (Milkereit et al., 2015).

LAT1 DRUGGABILITY AND CLINICAL OUTCOMES

Given the above-described premises, it is not surprising that LAT1 is a relevant pharmacological target for several diseases. This protein is exploited for both drug delivery and chemical knocking-out, i.e., block of transport activity exerted by pharmacological compounds. The drug delivery issue is particularly relevant in the BBB due to the impermeability of this barrier to exogenous substances. This feature is responsible for inefficacy/low efficacy of several pharmacological treatments. Thus, the relatively wide substrate specificity of LAT1 is the pre-requisite for the "pro-drug" approach, searching for compounds fulfilling the requirement for transport competence (**Table 1**) and, hence, for crossing the BBB by a LAT1 mediated process (Peura et al., 2011; Zur et al., 2016). This strategy has the scope of improving pharmacodynamics of drugs targeting brain for neurological disorders (Puris et al., 2017). Several pro-drug compounds have been synthesized so far, whose chemical properties and, in some cases, delivery in specific tissues have been described. Among the compounds, LAT1 substrate derivatives of ketoprofene, valproate and perforin inhibitors seem to be efficiently delivered in model tissues (Gynther et al., 2008, 2010, 2016; Peura et al., 2011; Huttunen et al., 2016; Puris et al., 2017). Melphalan (**Table 1** and **Figure 2**), which is already used as a chemotherapy agent, can also be considered a LAT1 based prodrug (Kim et al., 2002; Ganapathy et al., 2009) even if some contradictory findings are reported (Uchino et al., 2002; Nakanishi and Tamai, 2011). The over-expression of LAT1 in several type of human cancers and its ability to transport modified substrates allow to exploit this protein in diagnostics and clinics, PET (Positron Emission Tomography) and BNCT (Boron Neutron Capture Therapy), respectively. PET allows the diagnosis of tumors by tracing accumulation of radiolabeled molecules specifically in cancer foci. The used molecules are tyrosine, phenylalanine and methionine derivatives, which are delivered to cells via LAT1 (Hayashi and Anzai, 2017) (and refs herein). BNCT is, on the contrary, an emerging anticancer therapy based on fission reactions that occur when boron is irradiated with neutron beams (Wongthai et al., 2015; Hayashi and Anzai, 2017). The essential condition for BNCT to work is the accumulation of boron that is guaranteed by the use of boronophenylalanine, another substrate derivative of LAT1, which is the most effective (Wongthai et al., 2015). Together with the efforts devoted to improve drug delivery and therapy, LAT1 is object of several studies aimed to identify potent and specific inhibitors able to chemically knockout the over-expressed protein. This important task, however, cannot be exhaustively performed using the virtual drug design approach, owing to the absence of a 3D crystallographic structure of LAT1 (see section Function and Substrate Specificity: The Double Face of LAT1). Indeed, all the works published so far dealing with bioinformatics, are based on homology models and require some validation by parallel approaches (Fang et al., 2009; Gao et al., 2010; Kowalczyk et al., 2011; Napolitano et al., 2017a). Two main strategies are followed searching for inhibitors: competitive inhibitors or non-competitive inhibitors design. In the first case, substrate-mimicking molecules are obtained, able to interact with the substrate binding site of the protein. It is worth to note that the tyrosine analog JPH203, previously known as KYT-0353, is a potent inhibitor (Oda et al., 2010) both *in vitro* and in mouse model of HT-29 tumors (colon cancer) (Oda et al., 2010; Wempe et al., 2012; Toyoshima et al., 2013). The molecular mechanism of action of JPH203, investigated using osteosarcoma cell line (Choi et al., 2017), consists in activating the mitochondrial pro-apoptotic pathway. This inhibitor is effective also in different type of cancers (Rosilio et al., 2015; Hayashi et al., 2016; Choi et al., 2017; Otsuki et al., 2017; Yothaisong et al., 2017). Moreover, a synergistic effect with metformin is observed in a cell line of HNC (Head and Neck Cancer) *in vitro* and in mouse-transplanted model (Ueno et al., 2016). Other ligands are proposed by using integrated approach of virtual screening of drug libraries and in *in vitro/ex vivo* models using cis-inhibition and trans-stimulation assays: phenylalanine and tyrosine analogs (Geier et al., 2013; Augustyn et al., 2016), triiodothyronine (T3) analogs (Kongpracha et al., 2017), tryptophan analogs (Ylikangas et al., 2014) and hydroxamic acids conjugated to LAT1 substrates (Zur et al., 2016); in the mentioned works, IC50 values are measured ranging from 1 μM to more than 300 μM. The effect of these ligands on cell proliferation is also evaluated to give information on potential pharmacological efficacy. Interestingly, the substrate analog strategy is also followed for other transporters such as ASCT2, that represents another key target for development of new anti-cancer drugs (Pochini et al., 2014; Bhutia and Ganapathy, 2016). In this case, glutamine and serine analogs have been designed and tested in cancer cell lines for their ability of blocking ASCT2 transport activity as recently reviewed (Pochini et al., 2014; Scalise et al., 2017). However, the described approaches can have some frailty if the concentration of natural amino acid substrates increases displacing the inhibitor and, thus, leading to less efficient effects (Augustyn et al., 2016). Then, after identification of two cysteine residues, i.e., C335 and C407, in the substrate binding site of LAT1 (Napolitano et al., 2017a) (see section Kinetics and Molecular Mechanisms of LAT1) we tried to apply an alternative strategy, i.e., design of inhibitors that could bind covalently to the cysteine residues leading to non-competitive inhibition. This study has been conducted *in vitro* in proteoliposomes carrying hLAT1 and validated in a cancer cell line (Napolitano et al., 2017b). The tested compounds belong to the dithiazole group, characterized by a favorable reactivity toward thiol functional groups of cysteine. Interestingly, some dithiazole derivatives are already known for their anti-fungal, anti-microbial and anti-tumor activities (Konstantinova et al., 2009). The inhibitors displaying the most potent effects react with C407, as demonstrated by the loss of efficacy on the C407A mutant. The action of these inhibitors on LAT1 may be related to the dithiazole moiety, which resembles the imidazole ring of histidine. Thus, inhibitor's recognition could be ascribed also to a "substrate-like" structure, but the molecular mechanism of stable inhibition is based on the disulfide bond with C407. In this case, in fact, the presence of substrate does not displace the inhibitor from the interaction with LAT1. The experimental data were corroborated by *in silico*-based analysis on the homology model of LAT1 (Napolitano et al., 2017b).

CONCLUSIONS

The relevance of LAT1 for human metabolism lies on the ability of this protein to recognize two classes of different substrates: essential amino acids and hormones as main physiological substrates and some drugs as non-physiological substrates. This two-faced feature elected LAT1 as a crossroad point in cell life. Indirect proof of such a statement is the occurrence of different kind of pathologies with wide degree of severity associated with alterations of function/expression of LAT1. The eminent position assumed by LAT1 is somewhat in contrast with the scarce depth of knowledge so far achieved. In fact, despite great efforts, which have been made to decipher the biology of LAT1, a complete scenario is not yet depicted. Combined approaches of bioinformatics, *in vitro* and *ex vivo* experimental approaches have been used to shed light on some dark sides of LAT1 transport mechanism, substrate specificity and regulation. These results gave a strong input to pharmacological studies, which led to identification of different classes of molecules able to interact with LAT1 either as non-transported inhibitors and as transported substrates with important outcome in human health. However, other biochemical aspects still need to be solved, such as the trafficking, the regulation of expression/function, and the effect of potential post-translational modifications on LAT1 stability/activity as well as the interaction with other transporters and enzymes. In fact, an integrated view of LAT1 activity in the cell context is necessary to completely understand the physiological role of this protein. An important issue regarding LAT1 and pharmacological outcomes is related to its peculiar expression in BBB, which is the physical barrier protecting the brain from xenobiotics but also the main route to provide this district with essential amino acids. In conclusion, the findings collectively derived from different works opened new perspectives also for translational medicine.

AUTHOR CONTRIBUTIONS

MS contributed in collecting bibliography, preparing figures and writing; MG, LC, and LP contributed in drawing structure figures and writing; CI contributed in writing and supervision of all the activities.

ACKNOWLEDGMENTS

This work was supported by funds from: Programma Operativo Nazionale [01_00937] - MIUR Modelli sperimentali biotecnologici integrati per lo sviluppo e la selezione di molecole di interesse per la salute dell'uomo to CI.

REFERENCES

Asor, E., Stempler, S., Avital, A., Klein, E., Ruppin, E., and Ben-Shachar, D. (2015). The role of branched chain amino acid and tryptophan metabolism in rat's behavioral diversity: Intertwined peripheral and brain effects. *Eur. Neuropsychopharmacol.* 25, 1695–1705. doi: 10.1016/j.euroneuro.2015.07.009

Augustyn, E., Finke, K., Zur, A. A., Hansen, L., Heeren, N., Chien, H. C., et al. (2016). LAT-1 activity of meta-substituted phenylalanine and tyrosine analogs. *Bioorg. Med. Chem. Lett.* 26, 2616–2621. doi: 10.1016/j.bmcl.2016.04.023

Behrens, C. R., Ha, E. H., Chinn, L. L., Bowers, S., Probst, G., Fitch-Bruhns, M., et al. (2015). Antibody-Drug Conjugates (ADCs) derived from interchain cysteine cross-linking demonstrate improved homogeneity and other pharmacological properties over conventional heterogeneous ADCs. *Mol. Pharm.* 12, 3986–3998. doi: 10.1021/acs.molpharmaceut.5b00432

Bhutia, Y. D., and Ganapathy, V. (2016). Glutamine transporters in mammalian cells and their functions in physiology and cancer. *Biochim. Biophys. Acta* 1863, 2531–2539. doi: 10.1016/j.bbamcr.2015.12.017

Boado, R. J., Li, J. Y., Chu, C., Ogoshi, F., Wise, P., and Pardridge, W. M. (2005). Site-directed mutagenesis of cysteine residues of large neutral amino acid transporter LAT1. *Biochim. Biophys. Acta* 1715, 104–110. doi: 10.1016/j.bbamem.2005.07.007

Bridges, C. C., and Zalups, R. K. (2017). Mechanisms involved in the transport of mercuric ions in target tissues. *Arch. Toxicol.* 91, 63–81. doi: 10.1007/s00204-016-1803-y

Bröer, S., and Bröer, A. (2017). Amino acid homeostasis and signalling in mammalian cells and organisms. *Biochem. J.* 474, 1935–1963. doi: 10.1042/BCJ20160822

Bröer, S., and Brookes, N. (2001). Transfer of glutamine between astrocytes and neurons. *J. Neurochem.* 77, 705–719. doi: 10.1046/j.1471-4159.2001.00322.x

Campbell, W. A., and Thompson, N. L. (2001). Overexpression of LAT1/CD98 light chain is sufficient to increase system L-amino acid transport activity in mouse hepatocytes but not fibroblasts. *J. Biol. Chem.* 276, 16877–16884. doi: 10.1074/jbc.M008248200

Cantor, J. M., and Ginsberg, M. H. (2012). CD98 at the crossroads of adaptive immunity and cancer. *J. Cell Sci.* 125, 1373–1382. doi: 10.1242/jcs.096040

Carroll, B., Korolchuk, V. I., and Sarkar, S. (2015). Amino acids and autophagy: cross-talk and co-operation to control cellular homeostasis. *Amino Acids* 47, 2065–2088. doi: 10.1007/s00726-014-1775-2

Chillarón, J., Roca, R., Valencia, A., Zorzano, A., and Palacin, M. (2001). Heteromeric amino acid transporters: biochemistry, genetics, and physiology. *Am. J. Physiol. Renal Physiol.* 281, F995–F1018. doi: 10.1152/ajprenal.2001.281.6.F995

Choi, D. W., Kim, D. K., Kanai, Y., Wempe, M. F., Endou, H., and Kim, J. K. (2017). JPH203, a selective L-type amino acid transporter 1 inhibitor, induces mitochondria-dependent apoptosis in Saos2 human osteosarcoma cells. *Korean J. Physiol. Pharmacol.* 21, 599–607. doi: 10.4196/kjpp.2017.21.6.599

Christensen, H. N. (1990). Role of amino acid transport and countertransport in nutrition and metabolism. *Physiol. Rev.* 70, 43–77. doi: 10.1152/physrev.1990.70.1.43

Cormerais, Y., Giuliano, S., Lefloch, R., Front, B., Durivault, J., Tambutte, E., et al. (2016). Genetic disruption of the multifunctional CD98/LAT1 complex demonstrates the key role of essential amino acid transport in the control of mTORC1 and tumor growth. *Cancer Res.* 76, 4481–4492. doi: 10.1158/0008-5472.CAN-15-3376

Dann, S. G., Ryskin, M., Barsotti, A. M., Golas, J., Shi, C., Miranda, M., et al. (2015). Reciprocal regulation of amino acid import and epigenetic state through lat1 and ezh2. *EMBO J.* 34, 1773–1785. doi: 10.15252/embj.201488166

del Amo, E. M., Urtti, A., and Yliperttula, M. (2008). Pharmacokinetic role of L-type amino acid transporters LAT1 and LAT2. *Eur. J. Pharm. Sci.* 35, 161–174. doi: 10.1016/j.ejps.2008.06.015

Dickens, D., Chiduza, G. N., Wright, G. S., Pirmohamed, M., Antonyuk, S. V., and Hasnain, S. S. (2017). Modulation of LAT1 (SLC7A5) transporter activity and stability by membrane cholesterol. *Sci. Rep.* 7:43580. doi: 10.1038/srep43580

Duelli, R., Enerson, B. E., Gerhart, D. Z., and Drewes, L. R. (2000). Expression of large amino acid transporter LAT1 in rat brain endothelium. *J. Cereb. Blood Flow Metab.* 20, 1557–1562. doi: 10.1097/00004647-200011000-00005

Elorza, A., Soro-Arnaiz, I., Melendez-Rodriguez, F., Rodriguez-Vaello, V., Marsboom, G., De Carcer, G., et al. (2012). HIF2alpha acts as an mTORC1 activator through the amino acid carrier SLC7A5. *Mol. Cell* 48, 681–691. doi: 10.1016/j.molcel.2012.09.017

Fagerberg, L., Hallstrom, B. M., Oksvold, P., Kampf, C., Djureinovic, D., Odeberg, J., et al. (2014). Analysis of the human tissue-specific expression by genome-wide integration of transcriptomics and antibody-based proteomics. *Mol. Cell. Proteomics* 13, 397–406. doi: 10.1074/mcp.M113.035600

Fang, Y., Jayaram, H., Shane, T., Kolmakova-Partensky, L., Wu, F., Williams, C., et al. (2009). Structure of a prokaryotic virtual proton pump at 3.2 A resolution. *Nature* 460, 1040–1043. doi: 10.1038/nature08201

Fort, J., De La Ballina, L. R., Burghardt, H. E., Ferrer-Costa, C., Turnay, J., Ferrer-Orta, C., et al. (2007). The structure of human 4F2hc ectodomain provides a model for homodimerization and electrostatic interaction with plasma membrane. *J. Biol. Chem.* 282, 31444–31452. doi: 10.1074/jbc.M704524200

Fotiadis, D., Kanai, Y., and Palacin, M. (2013). The SLC3 and SLC7 families of amino acid transporters. *Mol. Aspects Med.* 34, 139–158. doi: 10.1016/j.mam.2012.10.007

Franca, R., Veljkovic, E., Walter, S., Wagner, C. A., and Verrey, F. (2005). Heterodimeric amino acid transporter glycoprotein domains determining functional subunit association. *Biochem. J.* 388, 435–443. doi: 10.1042/BJ20050021

Friesema, E. C., Docter, R., Moerings, E. P., Verrey, F., Krenning, E. P., Hennemann, G., et al. (2001). Thyroid hormone transport by the heterodimeric human system L amino acid transporter. *Endocrinology* 142, 4339–4348. doi: 10.1210/endo.142.10.8418

Fuchs, B. C., and Bode, B. P. (2005). Amino acid transporters ASCT2 and LAT1 in cancer: partners in crime? *Semin. Cancer Biol.* 15, 254–266. doi: 10.1016/j.semcancer.2005.04.005

Gallinetti, J., Harputlugil, E., and Mitchell, J. R. (2013). Amino acid sensing in dietary-restriction-mediated longevity: roles of signal-transducing kinases GCN2 and TOR. *Biochem. J.* 449, 1–10. doi: 10.1042/BJ20121098

Galluccio, M., Pingitore, P., Scalise, M., and Indiveri, C. (2013). Cloning, large scale over-expression in *E. coli* and purification of the components of the human LAT 1 (SLC7A5) amino acid transporter. *Protein J.* 32, 442–448. doi: 10.1007/s10930-013-9503-4

Ganapathy, V., Thangaraju, M., and Prasad, P. D. (2009). Nutrient transporters in cancer: relevance to Warburg hypothesis and beyond. *Pharmacol. Ther.* 121, 29–40. doi: 10.1016/j.pharmthera.2008.09.005

Gao, X., Zhou, L., Jiao, X., Lu, F., Yan, C., Zeng, X., et al. (2010). Mechanism of substrate recognition and transport by an amino acid antiporter. *Nature* 463, 828–832. doi: 10.1038/nature08741

Geier, E. G., Schlessinger, A., Fan, H., Gable, J. E., Irwin, J. J., Sali, A., et al. (2013). Structure-based ligand discovery for the Large-neutral Amino Acid Transporter 1, LAT-1. *Proc. Natl. Acad. Sci. U.S.A.* 110, 5480–5485. doi: 10.1073/pnas.1218165110

Gynther, M., Jalkanen, A., Lehtonen, M., Forsberg, M., Laine, K., Ropponen, J., et al. (2010). Brain uptake of ketoprofen-lysine prodrug in rats. *Int. J. Pharm.* 399, 121–128. doi: 10.1016/j.ijpharm.2010.08.019

Gynther, M., Laine, K., Ropponen, J., Leppanen, J., Mannila, A., Nevalainen, T., et al. (2008). Large neutral amino acid transporter enables brain drug delivery via prodrugs. *J. Med. Chem.* 51, 932–936. doi: 10.1021/jm701175d

Gynther, M., Pickering, D. S., Spicer, J. A., Denny, W. A., and Huttunen, K. M. (2016). Systemic and Brain Pharmacokinetics of Perforin Inhibitor Prodrugs. *Mol. Pharm.* 13, 2484–2491. doi: 10.1021/acs.molpharmaceut.6b00217

Hansen, C. G., Ng, Y. L., Lam, W. L., Plouffe, S. W., and Guan, K. L. (2015). The Hippo pathway effectors YAP and TAZ promote cell growth by modulating amino acid signaling to mTORC1. *Cell Res.* 25, 1299–1313. doi: 10.1038/cr.2015.140

Hasegawa, S., Ichiyama, T., Sonaka, I., Ohsaki, A., Okada, S., Wakiguchi, H., et al. (2012). Cysteine, histidine and glycine exhibit anti-inflammatory effects in human coronary arterial endothelial cells. *Clin. Exp. Immunol.* 167, 269–274. doi: 10.1111/j.1365-2249.2011.04519.x

Hayashi, K., and Anzai, N. (2017). Novel therapeutic approaches targeting L-type amino acid transporters for cancer treatment. *World J. Gastrointest. Oncol.* 9, 21–29. doi: 10.4251/wjgo.v9.i1.21

Hayashi, K., Jutabha, P., Endou, H., and Anzai, N. (2012). c-Myc is crucial for the expression of LAT1 in MIA Paca-2 human pancreatic cancer cells. *Oncol. Rep.* 28, 862–866. doi: 10.3892/or.2012.1878

Hayashi, K., Jutabha, P., Endou, H., Sagara, H., and Anzai, N. (2013). LAT1 is a critical transporter of essential amino acids for immune reactions in activated human T cells. *J. Immunol.* 191, 4080–4085. doi: 10.4049/jimmunol.1300923

Hayashi, K., Jutabha, P., Maeda, S., Supak, Y., Ouchi, M., Endou, H., et al. (2016). LAT1 acts as a crucial transporter of amino acids in human thymic carcinoma cells. *J. Pharmacol. Sci.* 132, 201–204. doi: 10.1016/j.jphs.2016.07.006

Hayes, G. M., Chinn, L., Cantor, J. M., Cairns, B., Levashova, Z., Tran, H., et al. (2015). Antitumor activity of an anti-CD98 antibody. *Int. J. Cancer* 137, 710–720. doi: 10.1002/ijc.29415

Huttunen, K. M., Huttunen, J., Aufderhaar, I., Gynther, M., Denny, W. A., and Spicer, J. A. (2016). L-Type amino acid transporter 1 (lat1)-mediated targeted delivery of perforin inhibitors. *Int. J. Pharm.* 498, 205–216. doi: 10.1016/j.ijpharm.2015.12.034

Ilgü, H., Jeckelmann, J. M., Gapsys, V., Ucurum, Z., De Groot, B. L., and Fotiadis, D. (2016). Insights into the molecular basis for substrate binding and specificity of the wild-type L-arginine/agmatine antiporter AdiC. *Proc. Natl. Acad. Sci. U.S.A.* 113, 10358–10363. doi: 10.1073/pnas.1605442113

Kageyama, T., Nakamura, M., Matsuo, A., Yamasaki, Y., Takakura, Y., Hashida, M., et al. (2000). The 4F2hc/LAT1 complex transports L-DOPA across the blood-brain barrier. *Brain Res.* 879, 115–121. doi: 10.1016/S0006-8993(00)0 2758-X

Kajiwara, Y., Yasutake, A., Adachi, T., and Hirayama, K. (1996). Methylmercury transport across the placenta via neutral amino acid carrier. *Arch. Toxicol.* 70, 310–314. doi: 10.1007/s002040050279

Kanai, Y., Segawa, H., Miyamoto, K., Uchino, H., Takeda, E., and Endou, H. (1998). Expression cloning and characterization of a transporter for large neutral amino acids activated by the heavy chain of 4F2 antigen (CD98). *J. Biol. Chem.* 273, 23629–23632. doi: 10.1074/jbc.273.37.23629

Kim, D. K., Kanai, Y., Choi, H. W., Tangtrongsup, S., Chairoungdua, A., Babu, E., et al. (2002). Characterization of the system L amino acid transporter in T24 human bladder carcinoma cells. *Biochim. Biophys. Acta* 1565, 112–121. doi: 10.1016/S0005-2736(02)00516-3

Kim, J. W., Zeller, K. I., Wang, Y., Jegga, A. G., Aronow, B. J., O'donnell, K. A., et al. (2004). Evaluation of myc E-box phylogenetic footprints in glycolytic genes by chromatin immunoprecipitation assays. *Mol. Cell. Biol.* 24, 5923–5936. doi: 10.1128/MCB.24.13.5923-5936.2004

Kobayashi, N., Okazaki, S., Sampetrean, O., Irie, J., Itoh, H., and Saya, H. (2018). CD44 variant inhibits insulin secretion in pancreatic beta cells by attenuating LAT1-mediated amino acid uptake. *Sci. Rep.* 8:2785. doi: 10.1038/s41598-018-20973-2

Kongpracha, P., Nagamori, S., Wiriyasermkul, P., Tanaka, Y., Kaneda, K., Okuda, S., et al. (2017). Structure-activity relationship of a novel series of inhibitors for cancer type transporter L-type amino acid transporter 1 (LAT1). *J. Pharmacol. Sci.* 133, 96–102. doi: 10.1016/j.jphs.2017.01.006

Konstantinova, L. S., Bol'shakov, O. I., Obruchnikova, N. V., Laborie, H., Tanga, A., Sopena, V., et al. (2009). One-pot synthesis of 5-phenylimino, 5-thieno or 5-oxo-1,2,3-dithiazoles and evaluation of their antimicrobial and antitumor activity. *Bioorg. Med. Chem. Lett.* 19, 136–141. doi: 10.1016/j.bmcl.2008.11.010

Kowalczyk, L., Ratera, M., Paladino, A., Bartoccioni, P., Errasti-Murugarren, E., Valencia, E., et al. (2011). Molecular basis of substrate-induced permeation by an amino acid antiporter. *Proc. Natl. Acad. Sci. U.S.A.* 108, 3935–3940. doi: 10.1073/pnas.1018081108

Lee, J. H., Budanov, A. V., Park, E. J., Birse, R., Kim, T. E., Perkins, G. A., et al. (2010). Sestrin as a feedback inhibitor of TOR that prevents age-related pathologies. *Science* 327, 1223–1228. doi: 10.1126/science.1182228

Le Vee, M., Jouan, E., Lecureur, V., and Fardel, O. (2016). Aryl hydrocarbon receptor-dependent up-regulation of the heterodimeric amino acid transporter LAT1 (SLC7A5)/CD98hc (SLC3A2) by diesel exhaust particle extract in human bronchial epithelial cells. *Toxicol. Appl. Pharmacol.* 290, 74–85. doi: 10.1016/j.taap.2015.11.014

Mastroberardino, L., Spindler, B., Pfeiffer, R., Skelly, P. J., Loffing, J., Shoemaker, C. B., et al. (1998). Amino-acid transport by heterodimers of 4F2hc/CD98 and members of a permease family. *Nature* 395, 288–291. doi: 10.1038/26246

Matsuyama, R., Tomi, M., Akanuma, S., Tabuchi, A., Kubo, Y., Tachikawa, M., et al. (2012). Up-regulation of L-type amino acid transporter 1 (LAT1) in cultured rat retinal capillary endothelial cells in response to glucose deprivation. *Drug Metab. Pharmacokinet.* 27, 317–324. doi: 10.2133/dmpk.DMPK-11-RG-122

Meier, C., Ristic, Z., Klauser, S., and Verrey, F. (2002). Activation of system L heterodimeric amino acid exchangers by intracellular substrates. *EMBO J.* 21, 580–589. doi: 10.1093/emboj/21.4.580

Miko, E., Margitai, Z., Czimmerer, Z., Varkonyi, I., Dezso, B., Lanyi, A., et al. (2011). miR-126 inhibits proliferation of small cell lung cancer cells by targeting SLC7A5. *FEBS Lett.* 585, 1191–1196. doi: 10.1016/j.febslet.2011.03.039

Milkereit, R., Persaud, A., Vanoaica, L., Guetg, A., Verrey, F., and Rotin, D. (2015). LAPTM4b recruits the LAT1-4F2hc Leu transporter to lysosomes and promotes mTORC1 activation. *Nat. Commun.* 6:7250. doi: 10.1038/ncomms8250

Nakamura, E., Sato, M., Yang, H., Miyagawa, F., Harasaki, M., Tomita, K., et al. (1999). 4F2 (CD98) heavy chain is associated covalently with an amino acid transporter and controls intracellular trafficking and membrane topology of 4F2 heterodimer. *J. Biol. Chem.* 274, 3009–3016. doi: 10.1074/jbc.274.5.3009

Nakanishi, T., and Tamai, I. (2011). Solute carrier transporters as targets for drug delivery and pharmacological intervention for chemotherapy. *J. Pharm. Sci.* 100, 3731–3750. doi: 10.1002/jps.22576

Napolitano, L., Galluccio, M., Scalise, M., Parravicini, C., Palazzolo, L., Eberini, I., et al. (2017a). Novel insights into the transport mechanism of the human amino acid transporter LAT1 (SLC7A5). Probing critical residues for substrate translocation. *Biochim. Biophys. Acta* 1861, 727–736. doi: 10.1016/j.bbagen.2017.01.013

Napolitano, L., Scalise, M., Galluccio, M., Pochini, L., Albanese, L. M., and Indiveri, C. (2015). LAT1 is the transport competent unit of the LAT1/CD98 heterodimeric amino acid transporter. *Int. J. Biochem. Cell Biol.* 67, 25–33. doi: 10.1016/j.biocel.2015.08.004

Napolitano, L., Scalise, M., Koyioni, M., Koutentis, P., Catto, M., Eberini, I., et al. (2017b). Potent inhibitors of human LAT1 (SLC7A5) transporter based on dithiazole and dithiazine compounds for development of anticancer drugs. *Biochem. Pharmacol.* 143, 39–52. doi: 10.1016/j.bcp.2017.07.006

Nicklin, P., Bergman, P., Zhang, B., Triantafellow, E., Wang, H., Nyfeler, B., et al. (2009). Bidirectional transport of amino acids regulates mTOR and autophagy. *Cell* 136, 521–534. doi: 10.1016/j.cell.2008.11.044

Oda, K., Hosoda, N., Endo, H., Saito, K., Tsujihara, K., Yamamura, M., et al. (2010). L-type amino acid transporter 1 inhibitors inhibit tumor cell growth. *Cancer Sci.* 101, 173–179. doi: 10.1111/j.1349-7006.2009.01386.x

Ohgaki, R., Ohmori, T., Hara, S., Nakagomi, S., Kanai-Azuma, M., Kaneda-Nakashima, K., et al. (2017). Essential roles of L-type amino acid transporter 1 in syncytiotrophoblast development by presenting fusogenic 4F2hc. *Mol. Cell. Biol.* 37:e00427-16. doi: 10.1128/MCB.00427-16

Ohtsuki, S., Yamaguchi, H., Kang, Y. S., Hori, S., and Terasaki, T. (2010). Reduction of L-type amino acid transporter 1 mRNA expression in brain capillaries in a mouse model of Parkinson's disease. *Biol. Pharm. Bull.* 33, 1250–1252. doi: 10.1248/bpb.33.1250

Otsuki, H., Kimura, T., Yamaga, T., Kosaka, T., Suehiro, J. I., and Sakurai, H. (2017). Prostate cancer cells in different androgen receptor status employ different leucine transporters. *Prostate* 77, 222–233. doi: 10.1002/pros.23263

Palacín, M., and Kanai, Y. (2004). The ancillary proteins of HATs: SLC3 family of amino acid transporters. *Pflugers Arch.* 447, 490–494. doi: 10.1007/s00424-003-1062-7

Palacin, M., Nunes, V., Font-Llitjos, M., Jimenez-Vidal, M., Fort, J., Gasol, E., et al. (2005). The genetics of heteromeric amino acid transporters. *Physiology* 20, 112–124. doi: 10.1152/physiol.00051.2004

Pantham, P., Rosario, F. J., Weintraub, S. T., Nathanielsz, P. W., Powell, T. L., Li, C., et al. (2016). Down-regulation of placental transport of amino acids precedes the development of intrauterine growth restriction in maternal nutrient restricted baboons. *Biol. Reprod.* 95:98. doi: 10.1095/biolreprod.116.141085

Peura, L., Malmioja, K., Laine, K., Leppanen, J., Gynther, M., Isotalo, A., et al. (2011). Large amino acid transporter 1 (LAT1) prodrugs of valproic acid: new prodrug design ideas for central nervous system delivery. *Mol. Pharm.* 8, 1857–1866. doi: 10.1021/mp2001878

Pfeiffer, R., Spindler, B., Loffing, J., Skelly, P. J., Shoemaker, C. B., and Verrey, F. (1998). Functional heterodimeric amino acid transporters lacking cysteine residues involved in disulfide bond. *FEBS Lett.* 439, 157–162. doi: 10.1016/S0014-5793(98)01359-3

Pochini, L., Scalise, M., Galluccio, M., and Indiveri, C. (2014). Membrane transporters for the special amino acid glutamine: structure/function relationships and relevance to human health. *Front. Chem.* 2:61. doi: 10.3389/fchem.2014.00061

Prasad, P. D., Wang, H., Huang, W., Kekuda, R., Rajan, D. P., Leibach, F. H., et al. (1999). Human LAT1, a subunit of system L amino acid transporter: molecular cloning and transport function. *Biochem. Biophys. Res. Commun.* 255, 283–288. doi: 10.1006/bbrc.1999.0206

Puris, E., Gynther, M., Huttunen, J., Petsalo, A., and Huttunen, K. M. (2017). L-type amino acid transporter 1 utilizing prodrugs: how to achieve effective brain delivery and low systemic exposure of drugs. *J. Control. Release* 261, 93–104. doi: 10.1016/j.jconrel.2017.06.023

Rebsamen, M., and Superti-Furga, G. (2016). SLC38A9: A lysosomal amino acid transporter at the core of the amino acid-sensing machinery that controls MTORC1. *Autophagy* 12, 1061–1062. doi: 10.1080/15548627.2015.1091143

Rooman, I., Lutz, C., Pinho, A. V., Huggel, K., Reding, T., Lahoutte, T., et al. (2013). Amino acid transporters expression in acinar cells is changed during acute pancreatitis. *Pancreatology* 13, 475–485. doi: 10.1016/j.pan.2013.06.006

Rosario, F. J., Kanai, Y., Powell, T. L., and Jansson, T. (2015). Increased placental nutrient transport in a novel mouse model of maternal obesity with fetal overgrowth. *Obesity* 23, 1663–1670. doi: 10.1002/oby.21165

Rosell, A., Meury, M., Alvarez-Marimon, E., Costa, M., Perez-Cano, L., Zorzano, A., et al. (2014). Structural bases for the interaction and stabilization of the human amino acid transporter LAT2 with its ancillary protein 4F2hc. *Proc. Natl. Acad. Sci. U.S.A.* 111, 2966–2971. doi: 10.1073/pnas.1323779111

Rosilio, C., Nebout, M., Imbert, V., Griessinger, E., Neffati, Z., Benadiba, J., et al. (2015). L-type amino-acid transporter 1 (LAT1): a therapeutic target supporting growth and survival of T-cell lymphoblastic lymphoma/T-cell acute lymphoblastic leukemia. *Leukemia* 29, 1253–1266. doi: 10.1038/leu.2014.338

Sasahara, I., Fujimura, N., Nozawa, Y., Furuhata, Y., and Sato, H. (2015). The effect of histidine on mental fatigue and cognitive performance in subjects with high fatigue and sleep disruption scores. *Physiol. Behav.* 147, 238–244. doi: 10.1016/j.physbeh.2015.04.042

Saxton, R. A., and Sabatini, D. M. (2017). mTOR signaling in growth, metabolism, and disease. *Cell* 169, 361–371. doi: 10.1016/j.cell.2017.03.035

Scalise, M., Pochini, L., Galluccio, M., Console, L., and Indiveri, C. (2017). Glutamine transport and mitochondrial metabolism in cancer cell growth. *Front. Oncol.* 7:306. doi: 10.3389/fonc.2017.00306

Scalise, M., Pochini, L., Giangregorio, N., Tonazzi, A., and Indiveri, C. (2013). Proteoliposomes as tool for assaying membrane transporter functions and interactions with xenobiotics. *Pharmaceutics* 5, 472–497. doi: 10.3390/pharmaceutics5030472

Schmid, G., Fricke, L., Lange, H. W., and Heidland, A. (1977). Intracellular histidine content of various tissues (brain, striated muscle and liver) in experimental chronic renal failure. *Klin. Wochenschr.* 55, 583–585. doi: 10.1007/BF01490512

Shin, G., Kang, T. W., Yang, S., Baek, S. J., Jeong, Y. S., and Kim, S. Y. (2011). GENT: gene expression database of normal and tumor tissues. *Cancer Inform.* 10, 149–157. doi: 10.4137/CIN.S7226

Simner, C., Novakovic, B., Lillycrop, K. A., Bell, C. G., Harvey, N. C., Cooper, C., et al. (2017). DNA methylation of amino acid transporter genes in the human placenta. *Placenta* 60, 64–73. doi: 10.1016/j.placenta.2017.10.010

Sinclair, L. V., Rolf, J., Emslie, E., Shi, Y. B., Taylor, P. M., and Cantrell, D. A. (2013). Control of amino-acid transport by antigen receptors coordinates the metabolic reprogramming essential for T cell differentiation. *Nat. Immunol.* 14, 500–508. doi: 10.1038/ni.2556

Tarlungeanu, D. C., Deliu, E., Dotter, C. P., Kara, M., Janiesch, P. C., Scalise, M., et al. (2016). Impaired amino acid transport at the blood brain barrier is a cause of autism spectrum disorder. *Cell* 167, 1481–1494 e1418. doi: 10.1016/j.cell.2016.11.013

Toyoshima, J., Kusuhara, H., Wempe, M. F., Endou, H., and Sugiyama, Y. (2013). Investigation of the role of transporters on the hepatic elimination of an LAT1 selective inhibitor JPH203. *J. Pharm. Sci.* 102, 3228–3238. doi: 10.1002/jps.23601

Uchino, H., Kanai, Y., Kim, D. K., Wempe, M. F., Chairoungdua, A., Morimoto, E., et al. (2002). Transport of amino acid-related compounds mediated by L-type amino acid transporter 1 (LAT1): insights into the mechanisms of substrate recognition. *Mol. Pharmacol.* 61, 729–737. doi: 10.1124/mol.61.4.729

Ueno, S., Kimura, T., Yamaga, T., Kawada, A., Ochiai, T., Endou, H., et al. (2016). Metformin enhances anti-tumor effect of L-type amino acid transporter 1 (LAT1) inhibitor. *J. Pharmacol. Sci.* 131, 110–117. doi: 10.1016/j.jphs.2016.04.021

Vander Heiden, M. G., Cantley, L. C., and Thompson, C. B. (2009). Understanding the Warburg effect: the metabolic requirements of cell proliferation. *Science* 324, 1029–1033. doi: 10.1126/science.1160809

Verrey, F., Closs, E. I., Wagner, C. A., Palacin, M., Endou, H., and Kanai, Y. (2004). CATs and HATs: the SLC7 family of amino acid transporters. *Pflugers Arch.* 447, 532–542. doi: 10.1007/s00424-003-1086-z

Wagner, C. A., Lang, F., and Broer, S. (2001). Function and structure of heterodimeric amino acid transporters. *Am. J. Physiol. Cell Physiol.* 281, C1077–C1093. doi: 10.1152/ajpcell.2001.281.4.C1077

Walker, D. K., Drummond, M. J., Dickinson, J. M., Borack, M. S., Jennings, K., Volpi, E., et al. (2014). Insulin increases mRNA abundance of the amino acid transporter SLC7A5/LAT1 via an mTORC1-dependent mechanism in skeletal muscle cells. *Physiol. Rep.* 2:e00238. doi: 10.1002/phy2.238

Wang, S., Tsun, Z. Y., Wolfson, R. L., Shen, K., Wyant, G. A., Plovanich, M. E., et al. (2015). Metabolism. Lysosomal amino acid transporter SLC38A9 signals arginine sufficiency to mTORC1. *Science* 347, 188–194. doi: 10.1126/science.1257132

Wempe, M. F., Rice, P. J., Lightner, J. W., Jutabha, P., Hayashi, M., Anzai, N., et al. (2012). Metabolism and pharmacokinetic studies of JPH203, an L-amino acid transporter 1 (LAT1) selective compound. *Drug Metab. Pharmacokinet.* 27, 155–161. doi: 10.2133/dmpk.DMPK-11-RG-091

Wolfson, R. L., and Sabatini, D. M. (2017). The Dawn of the Age of Amino Acid Sensors for the mTORC1 Pathway. *Cell Metab.* 26, 301–309. doi: 10.1016/j.cmet.2017.07.001

Wongthai, P., Hagiwara, K., Miyoshi, Y., Wiriyasermkul, P., Wei, L., Ohgaki, R., et al. (2015). Boronophenylalanine, a boron delivery agent for boron neutron capture therapy, is transported by ATB0,+, LAT1 and LAT2. *Cancer Sci.* 106, 279–286. doi: 10.1111/cas.12602

Yamamoto, Y., Sawa, R., Wake, I., Morimoto, A., and Okimura, Y. (2017). Glucose-mediated inactivation of AMP-activated protein kinase reduces the levels of L-type amino acid transporter 1 mRNA in C2C12 cells. *Nutr. Res.* 47, 13–20. doi: 10.1016/j.nutres.2017.08.003

Yanagida, O., Kanai, Y., Chairoungdua, A., Kim, D. K., Segawa, H., Nii, T., et al. (2001). Human L-type amino acid transporter 1 (LAT1): characterization of function and expression in tumor cell lines. *Biochim. Biophys. Acta* 1514, 291–302. doi: 10.1016/S0005-2736(01)00384-4

Ylikangas, H., Malmioja, K., Peura, L., Gynther, M., Nwachukwu, E. O., Leppanen, J., et al. (2014). Quantitative insight into the design of compounds recognized by the L-type amino acid transporter 1 (LAT1). *ChemMedChem* 9, 2699–2707. doi: 10.1002/cmdc.201402281

Yothaisong, S., Dokduang, H., Anzai, N., Hayashi, K., Namwat, N., Yongvanit, P., et al. (2017). Inhibition of l-type amino acid transporter 1 activity as a new therapeutic target for cholangiocarcinoma treatment. *Tumour Biol.* 39:1010428317694545. doi: 10.1177/1010428317694545

Yu, Z., Lin, W., Rui, Z., and Jihong, P. (2018). Fibroblast-like synoviocyte migration is enhanced by IL-17-mediated overexpression of L-type amino acid transporter 1 (LAT1) via the mTOR/4E BP1 pathway. *Amino Acids* 50, 331–340. doi: 10.1007/s00726-017-2520-4

Zur, A. A., Chien, H. C., Augustyn, E., Flint, A., Heeren, N., Finke, K., et al. (2016). LAT1 activity of carboxylic acid bioisosteres: Evaluation of hydroxamic acids as substrates. *Bioorg. Med. Chem. Lett.* 26, 5000–5006. doi: 10.1016/j.bmcl.2016.09.001

Permissions

All chapters in this book were first published by Frontiers; hereby published with permission under the Creative Commons Attribution License or equivalent. Every chapter published in this book has been scrutinized by our experts. Their significance has been extensively debated. The topics covered herein carry significant findings which will fuel the growth of the discipline. They may even be implemented as practical applications or may be referred to as a beginning point for another development.

The contributors of this book come from diverse backgrounds, making this book a truly international effort. This book will bring forth new frontiers with its revolutionizing research information and detailed analysis of the nascent developments around the world.

We would like to thank all the contributing authors for lending their expertise to make the book truly unique. They have played a crucial role in the development of this book. Without their invaluable contributions this book wouldn't have been possible. They have made vital efforts to compile up to date information on the varied aspects of this subject to make this book a valuable addition to the collection of many professionals and students.

This book was conceptualized with the vision of imparting up-to-date information and advanced data in this field. To ensure the same, a matchless editorial board was set up. Every individual on the board went through rigorous rounds of assessment to prove their worth. After which they invested a large part of their time researching and compiling the most relevant data for our readers.

The editorial board has been involved in producing this book since its inception. They have spent rigorous hours researching and exploring the diverse topics which have resulted in the successful publishing of this book. They have passed on their knowledge of decades through this book. To expedite this challenging task, the publisher supported the team at every step. A small team of assistant editors was also appointed to further simplify the editing procedure and attain best results for the readers.

Apart from the editorial board, the designing team has also invested a significant amount of their time in understanding the subject and creating the most relevant covers. They scrutinized every image to scout for the most suitable representation of the subject and create an appropriate cover for the book.

The publishing team has been an ardent support to the editorial, designing and production team. Their endless efforts to recruit the best for this project, has resulted in the accomplishment of this book. They are a veteran in the field of academics and their pool of knowledge is as vast as their experience in printing. Their expertise and guidance has proved useful at every step. Their uncompromising quality standards have made this book an exceptional effort. Their encouragement from time to time has been an inspiration for everyone.

The publisher and the editorial board hope that this book will prove to be a valuable piece of knowledge for researchers, students, practitioners and scholars across the globe.

List of Contributors

Chris N. J. Young
Molecular Medicine Laboratory, Institute of Biomedical and Biomolecular Sciences, School of Pharmacy and Biomedical Sciences, University of Portsmouth, Portsmouth, United Kingdom
Faculty of Health and Life Sciences, The School of Allied Health Sciences, De Montfort University, Leicester, United Kingdom

Dariusz C. Górecki
Molecular Medicine Laboratory, Institute of Biomedical and Biomolecular Sciences, School of Pharmacy and Biomedical Sciences, University of Portsmouth, Portsmouth, United Kingdom
The General Karol Kaczkowski Military Institute of Hygiene and Epidemiology, Warsaw, Poland

Andrea Magrì and Simona Reina
Section of Molecular Biology, Department of Biological, Geological and Environmental Sciences, University of Catania, Catania, Italy
Section of Biology and Genetics, Department of Biomedicine and Biotechnology, National Institute for Biomembranes and Biosystems, Section of Catania, Catania, Italy

Vito De Pinto
Section of Biology and Genetics, Department of Biomedicine and Biotechnology, National Institute for Biomembranes and Biosystems, Section of Catania, Catania, Italy

Francesco Tadini-Buoninsegni, Serena Smeazzetto and Maria Rosa Moncelli
Department of Chemistry "Ugo Schiff," University of Florence, Florence, Italy

Roberta Gualdani
Laboratory of Cell Physiology, Institute of Neuroscience, Université Catholique de Louvain, Louvain-la-Neuve, Belgium

Rachel A. North
School of Biological Sciences, University of Canterbury, Christchurch, New Zealand
Biomolecular Interaction Centre, University of Canterbury, Christchurch, New Zealand
Department of Chemistry and Molecular Biology, University of Gothenburg, Gothenburg, Sweden

S. Ramaswamy
The Institute for Stem Cell Biology and Regenerative Medicine, Bangalore, India

Weixiao Y. Wahlgren and Rosmarie Friemann
Department of Chemistry and Molecular Biology, University of Gothenburg, Gothenburg, Sweden
Centre for Antibiotic Resistance Research, University of Gothenburg, Gothenburg, Sweden

Daniela M. Remus and Sarah A. Kessans
School of Biological Sciences, University of Canterbury, Christchurch, New Zealand
Biomolecular Interaction Centre, University of Canterbury, Christchurch, New Zealand

Mariafrancesca Scalise and Cesare Indiveri
Unit of Biochemistry and Molecular Biotechnology, Department DiBEST (Biologia, Ecologia, Scienze della Terra), University of Calabria, Arcavacata di Rende, Italy

Elin Dunevall and Elin Claesson
Department of Chemistry and Molecular Biology, University of Gothenburg, Gothenburg, Sweden

Tatiana P. Soares da Costa and Matthew A. Perugini
Department of Biochemistry and Genetics, La Trobe Institute for Molecular Science, La Trobe University, Melbourne, VIC, Australia

Jane R. Allison
Biomolecular Interaction Centre, University of Canterbury, Christchurch, New Zealand
Centre for Theoretical Chemistry and Physics, Institute of Natural and Mathematical Sciences, Massey University, Auckland, New Zealand
Maurice Wilkins Centre for Molecular Biodiscovery, University of Auckland, Auckland, New Zealand

Renwick C. J. Dobson
School of Biological Sciences, University of Canterbury, Christchurch, New Zealand
Department of Biochemistry and Molecular Biology, Bio21 Molecular Science and Biotechnology Institute,University of Melbourne, Parkville, VIC, Australia

Anna Rita Cappello, Rosita Curcio, Rosamaria Lappano, Marcello Maggiolini and Vincenza Dolce
Department of Pharmacy, Health and Nutritional Sciences, University of Calabria, Rende, Italy

Angela Tesse
Centre National de La Recherche Scientifique, Institut National de la Santé et de la Recherche Médicale, l'Institut du Thorax, Universitè de Nantes, Nantes, France

Elena Grossini
Laboratory of Physiology, Department of Translational Medicine, University East Piedmont, Novara, Italy

Grazia Tamma and Giuseppe Calamita
Department of Biosciences, Biotecnhologies and Biopharmaceutics, University of Bari "Aldo Moro", Bari, Italy

Catherine Brenner
Institut National de la Santé et de la Recherche Médicale UMR-S 1180-LabEx LERMIT, Université Paris-Sud, Université Paris-Saclay, Châtenay Malabry, France

Piero Portincasa
Clinica Medica "A. Murri", Department of Biomedical Sciences and Human Oncology, Medical School, University of Bari "Aldo Moro", Bari, Italy

Raul A. Marinelli
Instituto de Fisiología Experimental, CONICET, Facultad de Ciencias Bioquímicas y Farmacéuticas, Universidad Nacional de Rosario, Rosario, Argentina

Sina Schmidl and Mislav Oreb
Institute of Molecular Biosciences, Goethe University Frankfurt, Frankfurt am Main, Germany

Cristina V. Iancu and Jun-yong Choe
Department of Biochemistry and Molecular Biology, Rosalind Franklin University of Medicine and Science, North Chicago, IL, United States

Mohamad Kourghi, Michael L. De Ieso, Saeed Nourmohammadi, Jinxin V. Pei and Andrea J. Yool
Aquaporin Physiology and Drug Discovery Program, Adelaide Medical School, University of Adelaide, Adelaide, SA, Australia

Rupert Abele
Institute of Biochemistry, Biocenter, Goethe University Frankfurt, Frankfurt, Germany

Robert Tampé
Institute of Biochemistry, Biocenter, Goethe University Frankfurt, Frankfurt, Germany
Cluster of Excellence -Macromolecular Complexes, Goethe University Frankfurt, Frankfurt, Germany

Rosella Scrima, Claudia Piccoli and Nazzareno Capitanio
Department of Clinical and Experimental Medicine, University of Foggia, Foggia, Italy

Darius Moradpour
Service of Gastroenterology and Hepatology, Centre Hospitalier Universitaire Vaudois, University of Lausanne, Lausanne, Switzerland

Anna Meier, Holger Erler and Eric Beitz
Department of Pharmaceutical and Medicinal Chemistry, Christian-Albrechts-University of Kiel, Kiel, Germany

Anna Hucke, Georg Beyer, Dorothea Zeeh, Rita Schröter, Marta Kantauskaitè and Giuliano Ciarimboli
Experimental Nephrology, Medical Clinic D, University Hospital, University of Münster, Münster, Germany

Ga Young Park and Stephen J. Lippard
Department of Chemistry, Massachusetts Institute of Technology, Cambridge, MA, United States

Oliver B. Bauer, Christina Köppen, Christoph A. Wehe and Uwe Karst
Institute of Inorganic and Analytical Chemistry, University of Münster, Münster, Germany

Michael Sperling
Institute of Inorganic and Analytical Chemistry, University of Münster, Münster, Germany
European Virtual Institute for Speciation Analysis, Münster, Germany

Yohannes Hagos
PortaCellTec Biosciences GmbH, Göttingen, Germany

Michael L. De Ieso and Andrea J. Yool
Department of Physiology, Adelaide Medical School, University of Adelaide, Adelaide, SA, Australia

Ana Galán-Cobo, Elena Arellano-Orden, Rocío Sánchez Silva, Nela Suárez-Luna and Miriam Echevarría
Departamento de Fisiología Médica y Biofísica, Instituto de Biomedicina de Sevilla, Hospital Universitario Virgen del Rocío, CSIC, Universidad de Sevilla, Sevilla, Spain

José Luis López-Campos
Unidad Médico-Quirúrgica de Enfermedades Respiratorias, Hospital Universitario Virgen del Rocio, Sevilla, Spain
Centro de Investigación Biomédica en Red sobre Enfermedades Respiratorias (CIBERES), Madrid, Spain

César Gutiérrez Rivera and José A. Rodríguez Portal
Unidad Médico-Quirúrgica de Enfermedades Respiratorias, Hospital Universitario Virgen del Rocio, Sevilla, Spain

María Molina-Molina
Centro de Investigación Biomédica en Red sobre Enfermedades Respiratorias (CIBERES), Madrid, Spain
Laboratorio de Neumologia Experimental, Servicio de Neumologia, Institut d'Investigació Biomédica de Bellvitge, Hospital Universitario de Bellvitge, Barcelona, Spain

Lourdes Gómez Izquierdo
Servicio Anatomía Patológica, HU Virgen del Rocío Sevilla, Seville, Spain

André Gomes, Inês V. da Silva, Cecília M. P. Rodrigues, Rui E. Castro and Graça Soveral
Research Institute for Medicines (iMed.ULisboa), Faculty of Pharmacy, Universidade de Lisboa, Lisbon, Portugal
Department Bioquimica e Biologia Humana, Faculty of Pharmacy, Universidade de Lisboa, Lisbon, Portugal

Leire Méndez-Giménez, Silvia Ezquerro and Amaia Rodríguez
Metabolic Research Laboratory, University of Navarra, Pamplona, Spain
CIBER Fisiopatología de la Obesidad y Nutrición, Instituto de Salud Carlos III, Madrid, Spain

Sofie V. Hellsten, Rekha Tripathi, Mikaela M. Ceder and Robert Fredriksson
Molecular Neuropharmacology, Department of Pharmaceutical Biosciences, Uppsala University, Uppsala, Sweden

Gema Frühbeck
Metabolic Research Laboratory, University of Navarra, Pamplona, Spain
CIBER Fisiopatología de la Obesidad y Nutrición, Instituto de Salud Carlos III, Madrid, Spain
Department of Endocrinology and Nutrition, Clínica Universidad de Navarra, Pamplona, Spain

Mariafrancesca Scalise, Michele Galluccio, Lara Console and Lorena Pochini
Unit of Biochemistry and Molecular Biotechnology, Department DiBEST (Biologia, Ecologia, Scienze della Terra), University of Calabria, Rende, Italy

Cesare Indiveri
Unit of Biochemistry and Molecular Biotechnology, Department DiBEST (Biologia, Ecologia, Scienze della Terra), University of Calabria, Rende, Italy
CNR Institute of Biomembranes, Bioenergetics and Molecular Biotechnology, Bari, Italy

Index

A

Actin Polymerization, 180-182, 188

Acute Lung Injury, 68-69, 72, 147, 196

Aerobic Glycolysis, 11, 133, 138, 169

Alpinetin, 147, 149, 155, 157

Alzheimer's Disease, 69-70, 73, 163, 165, 169-174

Amoebiasis, 43-44, 64

Aquaglyceroporins, 63-65, 70-72, 75, 79, 82-83, 146, 150, 156, 176, 189-190, 192, 214

Aquaporins, 59, 66, 71-77, 81-83, 145-146, 154-155, 175-176, 179, 181-183, 186-193, 195-196, 203-205, 213-214

B

Bariatric Surgery, 74, 79, 82

C

Calcium Channels, 51, 65, 133, 135-136, 141

Cancer Invasion, 175-179, 184, 186, 193

Cardiovascular Disease, 67, 145, 151, 176, 193

Cell Membranes, 23, 66, 74-75, 115, 122, 138, 142, 155, 173, 189

Cell Migration, 68-69, 72, 147-148, 152-153, 155-156, 175, 177-194, 202-203, 214

Cell Proliferation, 28, 66, 68, 70-71, 77-78, 80, 148-149, 151, 157, 164, 168, 171-172, 176, 178, 181, 188-189, 192, 196, 202, 222, 224, 227

Cell-matrix Adhesion, 180, 182

Cellular Dissociation, 175, 179, 186

Cerebrospinal Fluid, 148, 156, 177, 191

Chagas Disease, 43-44

Chemotaxis, 103, 105, 111, 187-188, 192

Clotrimazole, 164-165, 168, 170, 172-174

Curcuminoids, 146-147

Cytoplasm, 15-16, 24, 67-68, 77, 96, 100, 102, 110, 139-140, 180

E

Entamoeba Histolytica, 43-44

Epidermal Growth Factor, 98, 110, 179, 189-190

Epithelial-mesenchymal Transition, 179, 186-187, 189-190, 193, 195-196, 203

Extracellular Matrix, 7, 176, 178, 182, 188, 200, 202

G

Gene Therapy, 107-110, 112

Glycerol Permeability, 46, 60, 72, 79-81, 83, 156, 193

Glycolysis, 11, 77-78, 102, 104-106, 109, 111,126, 133, 137-138, 140, 161, 165, 169-170, 172, 174

H

Hepatocellular Carcinoma, 69-71, 133, 140, 170, 172, 174, 177, 179, 190-191, 193

Hesperetin, 147, 149, 155-156

Hesperidin, 154, 156, 166, 170, 174

Homeostasis, 7, 15, 17, 19-20, 66, 70, 75, 82, 93, 97-103, 107, 109-110, 133, 136, 141, 145, 148, 151, 155, 158, 183, 205, 214, 219, 225

Hypoxia, 97, 101, 104, 108, 111, 137-138, 141-144, 148, 151, 157, 160, 176-179, 187, 189, 192, 196, 202-203, 222

I

Indirect Targeting, 45-46

Insulin Resistance, 19, 72, 74-75, 77, 79-83, 108, 156

Ischemic Stroke, 68, 73, 151, 190

K

Kinetoplastids, 43-44, 50-51

L

Leishmaniasis, 12, 43-44, 63-65

Lipogenesis, 75, 81, 108, 133, 137, 140, 144

Lipopolysaccharide, 11, 68, 72-73, 122-123, 149

Liquiritigenin, 147, 150, 155

Liver Cirrhosis, 69, 133

M

Major Facilitator Superfamily, 29, 32, 111, 114

Metastasis, 9-10, 98, 110, 165, 168, 174-184, 186-194, 222

Microscale Thermophoresis, 115, 118-119, 123, 164

Mitochondria Associated Membranes, 133

Mitochondrial Dysfunctions, 133, 136

Mitophagy, 137, 140-144

N

Naringenin, 147-150, 156-157

Neurodegeneration, 158, 162-163, 168

O

Oligonucleotides, 67, 70, 114, 167, 173

Osteoporosis, 102, 151

Oxidative Phosphorylation, 77, 133, 135-138

Oxidative Stress, 43, 45, 50, 59, 62, 66, 72, 106, 133, 136, 143, 145, 149-150, 153, 155-156, 160, 166, 170, 191

P

Pancreatic Ductal Adenocarcinoma, 69-70, 77, 179

Pancreatic Steatosis, 74, 76-77, 79, 82-83

Paromomycin, 44

Peripheral Targeting, 45-46
Pharmacology, 9, 11, 14, 64, 175, 183-184, 188
Phytochemicals, 28, 145-146, 151, 153-156
Plasmodium Berghei, 45, 59, 63
Plasmodium Falciparum, 20, 43, 59-65
Plasmodium Knowlesi, 44
Plasmodium Vivax, 43, 60, 63
Polarization, 36, 180, 188
Polyphenols, 145-146, 148-150, 154-156
Proteoliposomes, 16, 25-27, 38, 41, 100-101, 116, 119, 121, 183, 193, 216, 219, 221, 224, 227
Protozoa, 43
Protrusion, 177, 180-182
Pulmonary Edema, 70, 149
Pyruvate Dehydrogenase, 138-139, 142-143

Q
Quercetin, 147-150, 155-156

R
Redox Signaling, 133, 140
Ruthenium Red, 134-135, 139, 141, 164, 168, 170

S
Sleeping Sickness, 43-44, 65
Sodium Solute Symporter, 113-114
Stilbenes, 146-147, 150

T
Toxoplasmosis, 43-44, 52, 61, 63
Triglyceride, 70, 75, 83, 139
Trypanosomiasis, 44, 58, 60, 65
Tumor Angiogenesis, 170, 175, 178, 186-188

U
Ultracentrifugation, 115, 117, 121-122

V
Verapamil, 51, 56, 58, 62-64
Viroporin, 133, 135-136, 142
Voltage-dependent Anion Channel, 135, 141, 143, 158, 168-174

Printed in the USA
CPSIA information can be obtained
at www.ICGtesting.com
JSHW050846251023
50683JS00018B/94